118.75
10€

D1684375

PROGRESS IN BRAIN RESEARCH

VOLUME 64

THE OCULOMOTOR AND SKELETALMOTOR SYSTEMS:
DIFFERENCES AND SIMILARITIES

Recent volumes in PROGRESS IN BRAIN RESEARCH

Volume 46:	Membrane Morphology of the Vertebrate Nervous System. A Study with Freeze-etch Technique, by C. Sandri, J. M. Van Buren and K. Akert — *revised edition* — 1982
Volume 53:	Adaptive Capabilities of the Nervous System, by P. S. McConnell, G. J. Boer, H. J. Romijn, N. E. Van de Poll and M. A. Corner (Eds.) — 1980
Volume 54:	Motivation, Motor and Sensory Processes of the Brain: Electrical Potentials, Behaviour and Clinical Use, by H. H. Kornhuber and L. Deecke (Eds.) — 1980
Volume 55:	Chemical Transmission in the Brain. The Role of Amines, Amino Acids and Peptides, by R. M. Buijs, P. Pévet and D. F. Swaab (Eds.) — 1982
Volume 56:	Brain Phosphoproteins, Characterization and Function, by W. H. Gispen and A. Routtenberg (Eds.) — 1982
Volume 57:	Descending Pathways to the Spinal Cord, by H. G. J. M. Kuypers and G. F. Martin (Eds.) — 1982
Volume 58:	Molecular and Cellular Interactions Underlying Higher Brain Functions, by J.-P. Changeux, J. Glowinksi, M. Imbert and F. E. Bloom (Eds.) — 1983
Volume 59:	Immunology of Nervous System Infections, by P. O. Behan, V. Ter Meulen and F. Clifford Rose (Eds.) — 1983
Volume 60:	The Neurohypophysis: Structure, Function and Control, by B. A. Cross and G. Leng (Eds.) — 1983
Volume 61:	Sex Differences in the Brain: The Relation Between Structure and Function, by G. J. De Vries, J. P. C. De Bruin, H. B. M. Uylings and M. A. Corner (Eds.) — 1984
Volume 62:	Brain Ischemia: Quantitative EEG and Imaging Techniques, by G. Pfurtscheller, E. J. Jonkman and F. H. Lopes da Silva — 1984
Volume 63:	Molecular Mechanisms of Ischemic Brain Damage, by K. Kogure, K.-A. Hossmann, B. K. Siesjö and F. A. Welsh (Eds.) — 1985
Volume 64:	The Oculomotor and Skeletalmotor Systems: Differences and Similarities, by H.-J. Freund, U. Büttner, B. Cohen and J. Noth (Eds.) — 1986
Volume 65:	Psychiatric Disorders: Neurotransmitters and Neuropeptides, by J. M. Van Ree and S. Matthysse (Eds.) — 1986
Volume 66:	Peptides and Neurological Disease, by P. C. Emson, M. N. Rossor and M. Tohyama (Eds.) — 1986
Volume 67:	Visceral Sensation, by F. Cervero and J. F. B. Morrison (Eds.) — 1986
Volume 68:	Coexistence of Neuronal Messengers — A New Principle in Chemical Transmission, by T. G. M. Hökfelt, K. Fuxe and B. Pernow (Eds.) — 1986

PROGRESS IN BRAIN RESEARCH

VOLUME 64

THE OCULOMOTOR AND SKELETAL-MOTOR SYSTEMS: DIFFERENCES AND SIMILARITIES

Edited by

H.-J. Freund

Department of Neurology, University of Düsseldorf, Moorenstrasse 5, D-4000 Düsseldorf 1, F.R.G.

U. Büttner

Department of Neurology, Ludwig-Maximilians University, Marchioninstrasse 15, D-8000 Munich 70, F.R.G.

B. Cohen

Department of Neurology, Mount Sinai School of Medicine of the City University of New York, Annenberg 21-74, 1 Gustave Levy Place, New York, NY 10029, U.S.A.

and

J. Noth

Department of Neurology and Clinical Neurophysiology, Alfried Krupp Krankenhaus, D-4300 Essen, F.R.G.

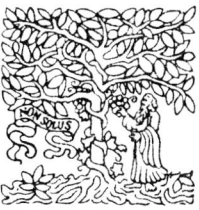

ELSEVIER
AMSTERDAM – NEW YORK – OXFORD
1986

© 1986, Elsevier Science Publishers B.V. (Biomedical Division)

All rights reserved. No part of this publication may be reproduced, stored in a retrieval system or transmitted in any form or by any means, electronic, mechanical, photocopying, recording or otherwise without the prior written permission of the publisher, Elsevier Science Publishers B.V./Biomedical Division, P.O. Box 1527, 1000 BM Amsterdam, The Netherlands.

Special regulations for readers in the USA:
This publication has been registered with the Copyright Clearance Center Inc. (CCC), Salem, Massachusetts. Information can be obtained from the CCC about conditions under which photocopying of parts of this publication may be made in the USA. All other copyright questions, including photocopying outside of the USA, should be referred to the copyright owner, Elsevier Science Publishers B.V. (Biomedical Division) unless otherwise specified.
ISBN 0-444-80655-5 (volume)
ISBN 0-444-80104-9 (series)

Published by:
Elsevier Science Publishers B.V. (Biomedical Division)
P.O. Box 211
1000 AE Amsterdam
The Netherlands

Sole distributors for the USA and Canada:
Elsevier Science Publishing Company, Inc.
52 Vanderbilt Avenue
New York, NY 10017
USA

Library of Congress Cataloging in Publication Data
Main entry under title:

The Oculomotor and skeletalmotor systems.

(Progress in brain research; v. 64)
Based on symposium held at Schloss Hugenpoet on Oct. 15-18, 1984.
Includes bibliographies and index.
1. Motor neurons — Congresses. 2. Efferent pathways — Congresses. 3. Eye — Movements — Regulation — Congresses. 4. Muscles — Innervation — Congresses. I. Freund, H. J. II. Series. [DNLM: 1. Muscles — physiology — congresses. 3. Oculomotor Muscles — physiology — congresses.
W1 PR667J v. 64 / WW 400 019 1984]
QP376.P7 vol. 64 612'.82 s [612'.846] 85-25384 [QP369.5]

ISBN 0-444-80655-5 (U.S.)

Printed in The Netherlands

List of Contributors

G. E. Alexander, Departments of Neurology and Neuroscience, The Johns Hopkins University School of Medicine, Baltimore, MD 21205, U.S.A.

R. Baker, Department of Physiology, New York University Medical Center, 550 First Avenue, New York, NY 10016, U.S.A.

E. Bauswein, Division of Biocybernetics, Department of Biophysics, University of Düsseldorf, D-4000 Düsseldorf, F.R.G.

A. Berthoz, Laboratoire de Physiologie Neurosensorielle, CNRS, 15 Rue de l'Ecole de Médecine, 75270 Paris cedex 06, France

E. Bizzi, Massachusetts Institute of Technology, Department of Psychology and Whitaker College, Cambridge, MA 02139, U.S.A.

R. Boyle, Department of ORL, Washington University School of Medicine, St. Louis, MO 63110, U.S.A.

C. J. Bruce, Department of Neurology, Georgetown University School of Medicine, Washington, DC 20057, and Section of Neuroanatomy, Yale University School of Medicine, New Haven, CT 06520, U.S.A.

U. Büttner, Department of Neurology, Ludwig-Maximilians University, Marchioninstrasse 15, D-8000 Munich 70, F.R.G.

J. Büttner-Ennever, Institute of Neuropathology, University of Munich, Thalkirchnerstrasse 36, 8000 Munich, F.R.G.

P. D. Cheney, Department of Physiology and Biophysics, and Regional Primate Research Center SJ-50, University of Washington, Seattle, WA 98195, U.S.A.

B. Cohen, Department of Neurology, Mount Sinai School of Medicine of the City University of New York, Annenberg 21-74, 1 Gustave Levy Place, New York, NY 10029, U.S.A.

M. R. DeLong, Departments of Neurology and Neuroscience, The Johns Hopkins University School of Medicine, Baltimore, MD 21205, U.S.A.

J. Dichgans, University Neurological Clinic, Liebermeisterstrasse 18–20, D-7400 Tübingen, F.R.G.

J. C. Eccles, Max-Planck-Institut für Biophysikalische Chemie, Göttingen, F.R.G.

R. Eckmiller, Division of Biocybernetics, Department of Biophysics, University of Düsseldorf, D-4000 Düsseldorf, F.R.G.

E. E. Fetz, Department of Physiology and Biophysics, and Regional Primate Research Center SJ-50, University of Washington, Seattle, WA 98195, U.S.A.

B. Fischer, Department of Clinical Neurology and Neurophysiology, University of Freiburg, Hansastrasse 9, 7800 Freiburg, F.R.G.

H.-H. Friedemann, Department of Neurology and Clinical Neurophysiology, Alfried Krupp Krankenhaus, D-4300 Essen, F.R.G.

H.-J. Freund, Neurologische Klinik der Universität Düsseldorf, Moorenstrasse 5, D-4000 Düsseldorf, F.R.G.

M. E. Goldberg, Laboratory of Sensimotor Research, National Eye Institute, National Institutes of Health, Bethesda, MD 20205, U.S.A.

A. Grantyn, Laboratoire de Physiologie Neurosensorielle, CNRS, 15 Rue de l'Ecole de Médecine, 75270 Paris cedex 06, France

O.-J. Grüsser, Department of Physiology, Freie Universität, Arnimallee 22, 1000 Berlin 33, Germany

V. Henn, Neurology Department, University Hospital, CH-8091 Zürich, Switzerland

K. Hepp, Physics Department, Swiss Federal Institute of Technology, CH-8093 Zürich, Switzerland

O. Hikosaka, Department of Physiology, Toho University, School of Medicine, Tokyo, Japan

K.-P. Hoffmann, Abteilung für Vergleichende Neurobiologie, Biologie IV, Universität Ulm, Oberer Eselsberg, 7900 Ulm, F.R.G.

N. Hogan, Department of Mechanical Engineering, Massachusetts Institute of Technology, Cambridge, MA 02139, U.S.A.

G. Holstege, Department of Neuroanatomy, Medical Faculty, Erasmus University, Rotterdam, The Netherlands

J. Hore, Departments of Physiology and Ophthalmology, University of Western Ontario, London, Ontario, Canada N6A 5C1

M. Horne, Departments of Anatomy and Neurobiology, Neurology and Neurosurgery, and The McDonnell

Center for Study of Higher Brain Function, Washington University School of Medicine, St. Louis, MO 63110, U.S.A.

J. Hounsgaard, Department of Neurophysiology, The Panum Institute, Blegdamsvej 3, DK-2200 Copenhagen, Denmark

H. Hultborn, Department of Physiology, The Panum Institute, Blegdamsvej 3, DK-2200 Copenhagen, Denmark

M. F. Jay, Department of Physiology and The Neurosciences Program, University of Alabama in Birmingham, University Station, Birmingham, AL 35294, U.S.A.

M. Jeannerod, Laboratoire de Neuropsychologie Expérimentale, INSERM, Unité 94, 16 Avenue du Doyen Lépine, Bron, France

D. Kane, Departments of Anatomy and Neurobiology, Neurology and Neurosurgery, and The McDonnell Center for Study of Higher Brain Function, Washington University School of Medicine, St. Louis, MO 63110, U.S.A.

D. Kernell, Department of Neurophysiology, University of Amsterdam, 1054 BW Amsterdam, The Netherlands

O. Kiehn, Department of Physiology, The Panum Institute, Blegdamsvej 3, DK-2200 Copenhagen, Denmark

G. E. Loeb, Laboratory of Neural Control, IRP, National Institute of Neurological and Communicative Disorders and Stroke, National Institutes of Health, 9000 Rockville Pike, Bethesda, MD 20205, U.S.A.

G. Markert, Department of Neurology, University of Düsseldorf, Moorenstrasse 5, D-4000 Düsseldorf, F.R.G.

V. Matsuo, National Eye Institute, Clinical Branch, National Institutes of Health, Bethesda, MD 20205, U.S.A.

P. B. C. Matthews, Laboratory of Physiology, Oxford University, Parks Road, Oxford OX1 3PT, U.K.

K.-H. Mauritz, Neurologischeklinik, Universität Düsseldorf, D-4000 Düsseldorf, F.R.G.

F. A. Miles, Laboratory of Sensorimotor Research, National Eye Institute, Building 10, Room 6C420, National Institutes of Health, Bethesda, MD 20205, U.S.A.

J. Mink, Departments of Anatomy and Neurobiology, Neurology and Neurosurgery, and The McDonnell Center for Study of Higher Brain Function, Washington University School of Medicine, St. Louis, MO 63110, U.S.A.

S. J. Mitchell, Departments of Neurology and Neuroscience, The Johns Hopkins University School of Medicine, Baltimore, MD 21205, U.S.A.

F. A. Mussa-Ivaldi, Massachusetts Institute of Technology, Department of Psychology and Whitaker Institute, Cambridge, MA 02139, U.S.A.

J. Noth, Department of Neurology and Clinical Neurophysiology, Alfried Krupp Krankenhaus, D-4300 Essen, F.R.G.

S. S. Palmer, Department of Physiology and Biophysics, and Regional Primate Research Center SJ-50, University of Washington, Seattle, WA 98195, U.S.A.

W. Precht[†], Institute für Hirnforschung der Universität Zürich, August-Forelstrasse 1, 8029 Zürich, Switzerland

R. T. Richardson, Departments of Neurology and Neuroscience, The Johns Hopkins University School of Medicine, Baltimore, MD 21205, U.S.A.

D. A. Robinson, Departments of Ophthalmology and Biomedical Engineering, The Johns Hopkins University, 601 North Broadway, Baltimore, MD 21205, U.S.A.

J. Schlag, Department of Anatomy, and Brain Research Institute, University of California, Los Angeles, CA 90024, U.S.A.

M. Schlag-Rey, Department of Anatomy, and Brain Research Institute, University of California, Los Angeles, CA 90024, U.S.A.

M. H. Schreiber, Departments of Anatomy and Neurobiology, Neurology and Neurosurgery, and The McDonnell Center for Study of Higher Brain Function, Washington University School of Medicine, St. Louis, MO 63110, U.S.A.

D. L. Sparks, Department of Physiology and Biophysics, University of Alabama in Birmingham, University Station, Birmingham, AL 35294, U.S.A.

P. L. Strick, Research Service, V. A. Medical Centre, Departments of Neurosurgery and Physiology, SUNY-Upstate Medical Center, Syracuse, NY 13210, U.S.A.

W. T. Thach, Departments of Anatomy and Neurobiology, Neurology and Neurosurgery, and The McDonnell Center for Study of Higher Brain Function, Washington University School of Medicine, St. Louis, MO 63110, U.S.A.

T. Vilis, Departments of Physiology and Ophthalmology, University of Western Ontario, London, Ontario, Canada N6A 5C1

D. M. Waitzman, University of California at San Francisco, San Francisco, CA 94143, U.S.A.

Michael Weinrich, Department of Neurology, Stanford University Medical School, Stanford, CA 94305, U.S.A.

M. Wiesendanger, Institut de Physiologie, Université de Fribourg, Pérolles, CH-1700 Fribourg, Switzerland

S. P. Wise, Laboratory of Neurophysiology, National Institute of Mental Health, Building 36, Room 2D-10, Bethesda, MD 20205, U.S.A.

R. H. Wurtz, Laboratory of Sensimotor Research, National Eye Institute, National Institutes of Health, Bethesda, MD 20205, U.S.A.

Preface

Although eye and body movements are both motor acts, their investigation is conducted along different lines. This is the consequence of the different research strategies required for the analysis of distinctly different sensory control modes and mechanical demands. In addition, control system theory has played an important role in formulating the theoretical basis for understanding the oculomotor and vestibular systems. In spite of the differences, the two motor subsystems share common organizational principles. A comparative evaluation of what is different and what is similar in the skeletalmotor and oculomotor systems offers the opportunity to recognize how the various functional demands are hardwired in the neuronal circuitries.

This book is the outcome of a symposium held at Schloss Hugenpoet near Düsseldorf from October 15th to 18th, 1984. It was conceived to provide a platform for an intense communication between scientists specialized in oculomotor or skeletalmotor research. A step by step comparison was made of the functional and structural organization of the two systems at different levels of complexity. The more general aspects of motor control strategies were discussed on the background of the demands imposed by the sensory inputs and the biomechanical requirements. The cooperative aspects of eye-head and eye-hand coordination, adaptive control mechanisms and psychophysical phenomena were issues that were also evaluated.

A comparison of this kind was meant to stimulate new approaches based on comparative aspects rather than to provide an update about the state of the art in either field.

Contents

List of Contributors	V
Preface	IX

Special Introduction

Learning in the motor system
    J. C. Eccles 3

Section I — Final Common Pathway

Organization and properties of spinal motoneurones and motor units
    D. Kernell 21

Extraocular motoneuron behavior in synergistic action
    K. Hepp and V. Henn 31

Transmitter-controlled properties of α-motoneurones causing long-lasting motor discharge to brief excitory inputs
    J. Hounsgaard, H. Hultborn and O. Kiehn 39

Discussion
    P. B. C. Matthews 51

Section II — Sensory Information Used by the Motor System

What are the afferents of origin of the human stretch reflex, and is it a purely spinal reaction?
    P. B. C. Matthews 55

Experimental evidence for the existence of a proprioceptive transcortical loop
    M. Wiesendanger 67

Visual inputs relevant for the optokinetic nystagmus in mammals
    K.-P. Hoffmann 75

Discussion
    O.-J. Grüsser 85

Section III — Neuroanatomical Substrates of Premotor Centres

Anatomy of premotor centers in the reticular formation controlling oculomotor, skeletomotor and autonomic motor systems
    J. Büttner-Ennever and G. Holstege 89

The organization of thalamic inputs to the "premotor" areas
P. L. Strick 99

Discussion
S. P. Wise.. 111

Section IV-A — Specialized Areas in Motor Control: Supratentorial

Movement-related activity in the premotor cortex of rhesus macaques
S. P. Wise, M. Weinrich and K.-H. Mauritz 117

Activity of forelimb motor units and corticomotoneuronal cells during ramp-and-hold torque responses: comparisons with oculomotor cells
E. E. Fetz, P. D. Cheney and S. S. Palmer... 133

The role of the arcuate frontal eye fields in the generation of saccadic eye movements
M. E. Goldberg and C. J. Bruce 143

Express saccades in man and monkey
B. Fischer... 155

The contribution of basal ganglia to limb control
M. R. DeLong, G. E. Alexander, S. J. Mitchell and R. T. Richardson...... 161

Role of the basal ganglia in the initiation of saccadic eye movements
R. H. Wurtz and O. Hikosaka 175

Role of the central thalamus in gaze control
J. Schlag and M. Schlag-Rey... 191

Discussion
P. L. Strick 203

Section IV-B — Specialized Areas in Motor Control: Infratentorial

A comparison of disorders in saccades and in fast and accurate elbow flexions during cerebellar dysfunction
T. Vilis and J. Hore.. 207

Cerebellar relation to muscle spindles in hand tracking
W. T. Thach, M. H. Schreiber, J. Mink, S. Kane and M. Horne............... 217

Cerebellar control of eye movements
U. Büttner, R. Boyle and G. Markert 225

The functional organization of the primate superior colliculus: A motor perspective
   D. L. Sparks and M. F. Jay 235

Horizontal saccades and the central mesencephalic reticular formation
   B. Cohen, D. M. Waitzman, J. A. Büttner-Ennever and V. Matsuo 243

Brainstem neurons are peculiar for oculomotor organization
   R. Baker 257

Spinal programs for locomotion
   G. E. Loeb 273

Discussion
   J. Dichgans 281

Section V — Functional Organisation of Movements

Time control of hand movements
   H.-J. Freund 287

Reflex control of hand muscles
   J. Noth and H.-H. Friedemann 295

Pathophysiology of rapid eye movement generation in the primate
   V. Henn and K. Hepp 303

Smooth pursuit eye movements
   R. Eckmiller and E. Bauswein 313

Neuronal mechanisms underlying eye-head coordination
   A. Berthoz and A. Grantyn 325

Regulation of multi-joint arm posture and movement
   E. Bizzi, F. A. Mussi-Ivaldi and N. Hogan 345

Are corrections in accurate arm movements corrective?
   M. Jeannerod 353

Discussion
   D. A. Robinson 361

Section VI — Adaptive Control and Psychophysical Aspects

Parametric adjustments in the oculomotor system
   F. A. Miles 367

Recovery of some vestibuloocular and vestibulospinal functions following unilateral labyrinthectomy
W. Precht 381

The effect of gaze motor signals and spatially directed attention on eye movements and visual perception
O.-J. Grüsser 391

Discussion
A. Berthoz 405

Section VII — General Concepts

Is the oculomotor system a cartoon of motor control?
D. A. Robinson 411

Some concluding remarks about general concepts in studies of the skeletomotor system
M. Wiesendanger 419

Final discussion
B. Cohen 425

Subject Index 427

SPECIAL INTRODUCTION

Learning in the motor system

John C. Eccles

Max-Planck-Institut für Biophysikalische Chemie, Göttingen 2841, F.R.G.

Introduction

It is proposed that three distinct classes of phenomena are included in the general theme of motor learning. Examples of each will be considered in turn.

Firstly, there is the learning of automatic movements, in which the whole process is subconscious from the beginning. A much investigated learnt movement of this type is the learning of a corrective vestibulo-ocular reflex. Similarly, the movements of a conditioned reflex are automatic from the start.

Secondly, there is the learning of motor skills by animals. There is an enormous literature on the training of animals in motor skills by operant conditioning techniques. However, attention is focussed on animal studies of the neuronal responses of the cerebrum and cerebellum. From mere behavioural descriptions we shall never come to understand how the brain is effective in the learning of a motor skill.

Thirdly, there is the learning of human skills. In this learning it is essential to have mental concentration with a planned strategy of action and a subsequent evaluation and correction of errors in successive attempts. When well learned, the skills can be accomplished without voluntary attention, as in walking, swimming, cycling, skiing. The performance of the skilled action has become automatic. Today, the list of learned motor skills is enormous. There is much more interest in motor skills as exhibited in all the sports than in intellectual and artistic performances, with the exception of ballet. No doubt television is responsible in part for this bias.

It would be generally agreed that the cerebral cortex is primarily involved in human motor learning, but the cerebellum is most importantly involved, and also the basal ganglia and presumably brain stem nuclei.

Learning of automatic movements

There is a very ancient part of the cerebellum, the flocculus, that controls the eye movements when the head is turned. One can think that the function of this part of the cerebellum is to maintain, as far as possible, a fixed position of the visual image on the retina. The movements of the head are sensed by the semicircular canals of the vestibular system. For our present purpose we have only to consider the horizontal canal because in the experiments of Ito et al. (1974), to which we here refer, the head of the rabbit was rotated about a vertical axis. The pathway diagram of Fig. 1 shows the direct projection of the vestibular nerve to the vestibular nucleus (VN) that in turn projects directly to the oculomotor nucleus (OM) for the eye muscles. By itself, this pathway can achieve some stabilization of the retinal image, but the control is much more regular in operation when it is aided by the pathway through the cerebellar flocculus. In Fig. 1 there are two mossy fibre (MF) inputs, one directly from the vestibular nerve, and the other a feedback from the visual system, which probably acts as a controlling device on the vestibulo-ocular reflex, improving the stability of the visual field during head movements. So far we have neglected the role of the climbing

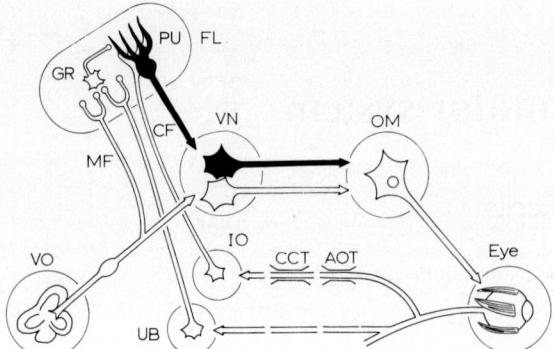

Fig. 1. Construction of the flocculo-vestibulo-ocular system. OM, oculomotor neuron; IO, inferior olive; CCT, central tegmental tract; AOT, accessory optic tract; VO vestibular organ; FL, flocculus; VN, second-order vestibular neurons; PU, Purkinje cells; GR, granule cell; UB, pontine nucleus. Modified from Ito (1975).

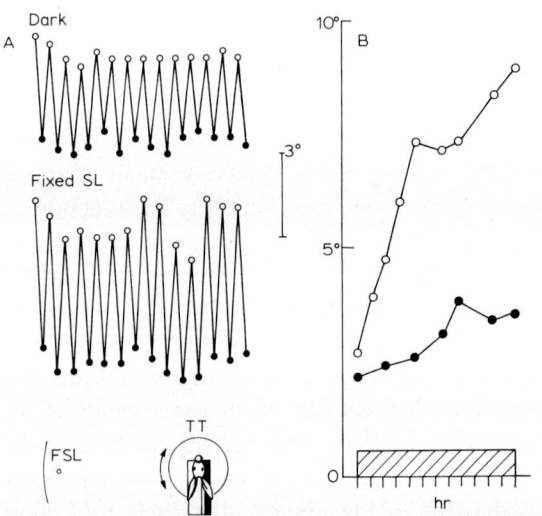

Fig. 2. Horizontal eye movement induced by sinusoidal head rotation and its modification during presentation of slit lights in the visual field. A. Open circles indicate the most nasal, and closed circles the most temporal, positions of the cornea mark on the left eye during each cycle of 14 head rotations. Plottings on the top indicate the eye movement in darkness and provide the control for the immediately succeeding measurement with slit light (SL) to the left eye, as plotted below. Diagrams at the bottom indicate dorsal views of the turntable (TT) mounting the rabbit, fixed-slit light (FSL) (Ito et al., 1974a). B. Changes of rabbit's horizontal vestibulo-ocular reflex during sustained head rotation with the fixed-slit light presented. Normal rabbit. Ordinate, mean angular amplitudes of the horizontal eye movement during 10° head rotation; abscissa, time; ○, eye movements measured with the fixed-slit light shown; ●, that measured in temporary darkness (Ito et al., 1974).

fibre (CF) input, which is predominantly activated by the visual input, via the pathway indicated to the inferior olive via the accessory optic tract (Fig. 1, AOT) (Maekawa and Simpson, 1973).

In Fig. 2 the head of the rabbit is subjected to a sine wave horizontal rotation with a standard amplitude of 10° and a frequency of 0.15 Hz. The plotted left eye movements (Fig. 2A) show that the compensation for the head rotation was much better when there was a fixed vertical strip of light than in darkness, but it was well below the 10° requirement for complete compensation. It was of great interest that when the head rotation was continued for many hours (Fig. 2B) there was a progressive increase in the compensation when tested with an illuminated slit (open circles). After several hours it became almost perfect for eliminating the retinal image slip. Evidently, there had been learning of the adaptive change, and this was very much less with the continual rotation when the measurements were carried out in darkness (filled circles).

These observations provide clear evidence of the automatic learning process that over some hours tends to improve the stability of the retinal image. Two experiments define the neural pathways concerned in this learning. In the first experiment, after ablation of the flocculus there was no learning. The second experiment showed that learning did not occur, or only rarely, in a minor later form, when the inferior olive was destroyed. Thus, we have good evidence that the CF input to the cerebellar Purkinje cells of the flocculus (Fig. 1) is effective in causing a learned cerebellar modification that gives improvement in the stabilization of the retinal image over and above that achieved by the vestibulo-ocular reflex. A remarkable feature is that in Fig. 2 about 1300 trials were required for the good adaptive response.

Gonshor and Melvill Jones (1976a, b) performed similar experiments on human vestibulo-ocular reflexes that were disturbed by a horizontal visual inversion by dove prisms. Again, there was learning that minimized retinal image slip and that presumably is similarly explained by the responses of the flocculus (cf. Robinson, 1976).

Marr (1969) developed a most challenging theory of the neuronal events involved in cerebellar learning. He proposed that the single climbing fibre input into a Purkinje cell played the role of a teacher for the enormous number of parallel fibre synapses (about 100,000) on the dendrites of that same cell. This enormous excitatory synaptic input is dominant in evoking the discharges of that Purkinje cell,

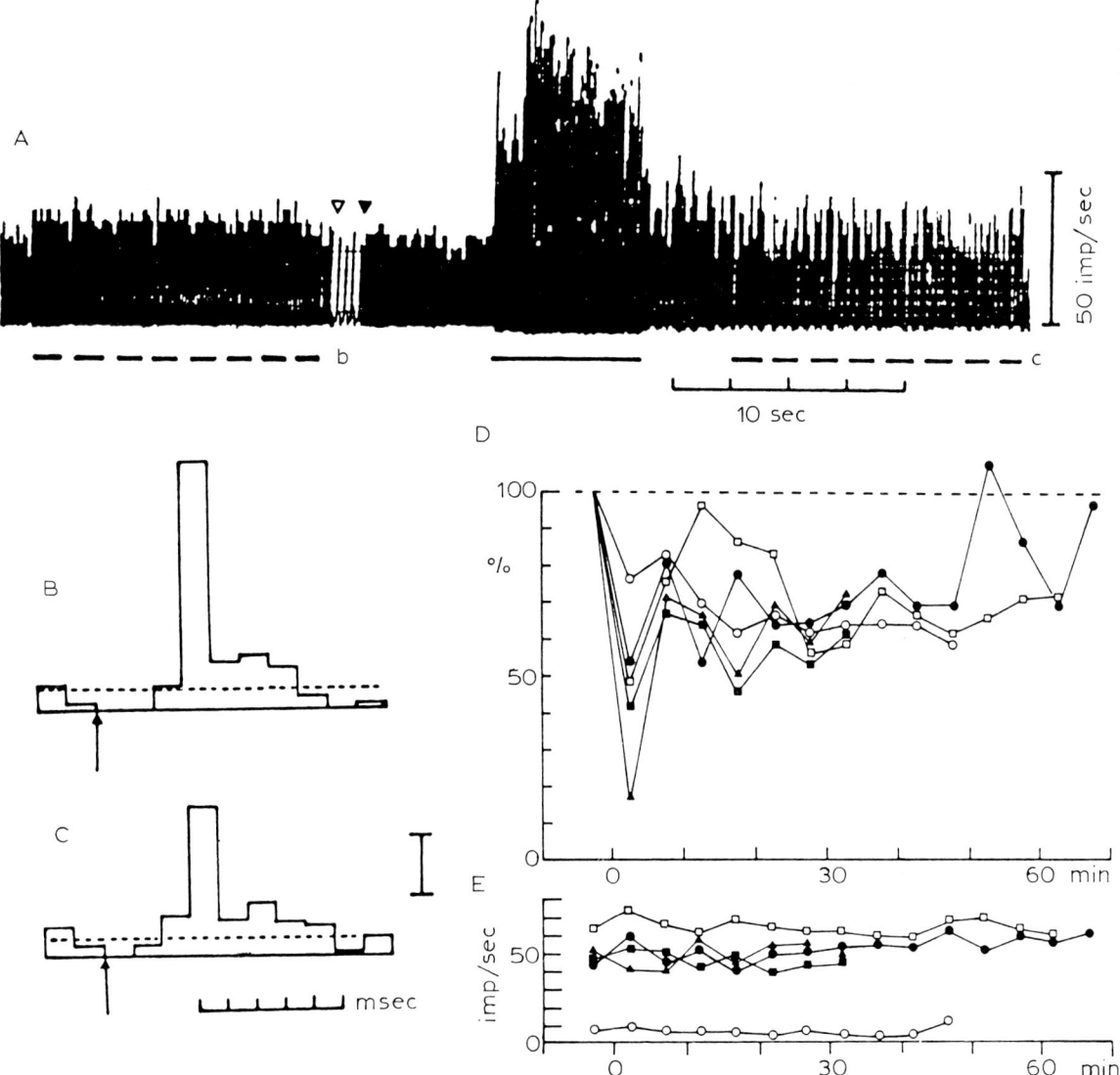

Fig. 3. Effect of conjunctive stimulation of a vestibular nerve and the inferior olive. A. Strip chart record of simple spike discharge from a Purkinje cell. Bin width, 0.5 second. Between ▽ and ▼ was a gap for 3 minutes. Horizontal dashed lines, period of 2/sec stimulation of the ipsilateral vestibular nerve. Horizontal continuous line, period of 4/sec conjunctive stimulation of the inferior olive and 20/sec stimulation of the ipsilateral vestibular nerve. B, C. Peristimulus histograms constructed during the periods b and c, respectively, in A. Calibration for B, C: 10 impulses/bin/100 sweeps. D. Ordinate, values of the firing index measured from peaks of the peristimulus histograms shown in B and C. The average values of two to three trials performed during each 5-minute period are plotted. Note that plotted values of the firing index were normalized by control values before conjunctive stimulation. The dashed line is drawn at 100%. E. Spontaneous discharge rate, averaged for each 5-minute period. Measurements from five different Purkinje cells (Ito et al., 1982).

which give simple spike discharges (SS), usually at a frequency of about 50/sec. In contrast, the single CF impulse exerts a powerful excitation generating a brief burst of impulses, which is called a complex spike (CS). In the Marr hypothesis, learning was effected because the CS response (the teacher) increased the potency of those parallel fibre synapses that were activated at about the same time, which ensured a very sharp selective effect for the learned potentiation. A little later, Albus (1971), on the basis of perceptron theory, proposed a diametrically opposite plastic influence, namely that there was a prolonged depression of those parallel fibre synapses activated at about the same time as the CS response. CS responses are infrequent, usually at 1–2 Hz.

With recording from the individual Purkinje cells of the flocculus during the head rotation, Ghelarducci et al. (1975) studied the phase relationship of simple spikes (SS) to complex spikes (CS). Their evidence suggested a depressant influence of CS on SS, which is in accord with the Albus hypothesis. However, we now turn to a more direct testing procedure devised by Ito et al. (1982).

The plastic influence of a CF impulse on the excitatory synapses made by parallel fibres on the dendrites of that same Purkinje cell was first demonstrated (Ito et al., 1982) by utilizing a vestibular nerve stimulus to set up a mossy fibre input into the flocculus that activated the Purkinje cells via granule cells and parallel fibres (cf. Fig. 1). The interacting CF impulse was set up by stimulation of the inferior olive. Conjunction was effected by simultaneous stimulation for 25 seconds of the inferior olive at 4 Hz and the vestibular nerve at 25 Hz, which are in the normal physiological ranges. Any change in the effectiveness of parallel fibre synapses on the Purkinje cells was evaluated by observing the impulses generated by a test vestibular nerve stimulus at 2/sec in comparison with the number before the conjunction (Fig. 3A). The firing index, as it is called, sharply diminished for some minutes (Fig. 3B,C), then partly recovered, to be followed by a depression for over 1 hour (Fig. 3D). This was a clear demonstration of the Albus version of the conjunction phenomenon, namely, a prolonged synaptic depression of the parallel fibre synapses on the Purkinje cell dendrites. It is of interest that a similar conjunctive stimulation did not depress the synapses on basket cells.

The defect of this pioneering investigation was that the vestibular nerve stimulation was remote from the actual site of the presumed interaction on the Purkinje cell dendrites (Fig. 1). Therefore, Ito and Kano (1982) set up the parallel fibre volley by direct stimulation and recorded the field potentials that the parallel fibre volley generated synaptically in the Purkinje cells at the presumed site of interaction. Again, conjunction often resulted in a significant synaptic depression that lasted more than an hour.

Fig. 4A illustrates a still further refinement by Ekerot and Kano (1983). Both climbing fibres and parallel fibres were directly activated, the parallel fibres by two microelectrodes setting up beams projecting to the Purkinje cell whose impulse discharges were being selectively recorded. Conjunction was effected by stimulation both of the climbing fibre and of parallel fibres by one of the electrodes at 4 Hz for 1 minute. The responses by the other PF electrode served as a control. The peristimulus time histograms in Fig. 4B were constructed from the responses of the Purkinje cell to the PF stimulation, 60 stimuli at 2 Hz. The post-conjunctional response was less than half the control shown above, whereas to the right there was no depression of the response evoked from the parallel fibre beam not activated in the conjunction. The importance of this restriction of the CF depressant action on PF synapses cannot be overestimated. It is the key to the selectivity that is an essential requisite for an effective learning mechanism. It is also observed in the long-term potentiation in the hippocampus (Eccles, 1983).

The time course of depression is shown in Fig. 4C for two conjunctions with the inactive control and then with 4 Hz stimulation for 1 minute of the control parallel fibre beam alone. In Fig. 4D a more prolonged depression was exhibited after conjunction in another two Purkinje cells. Depressions of

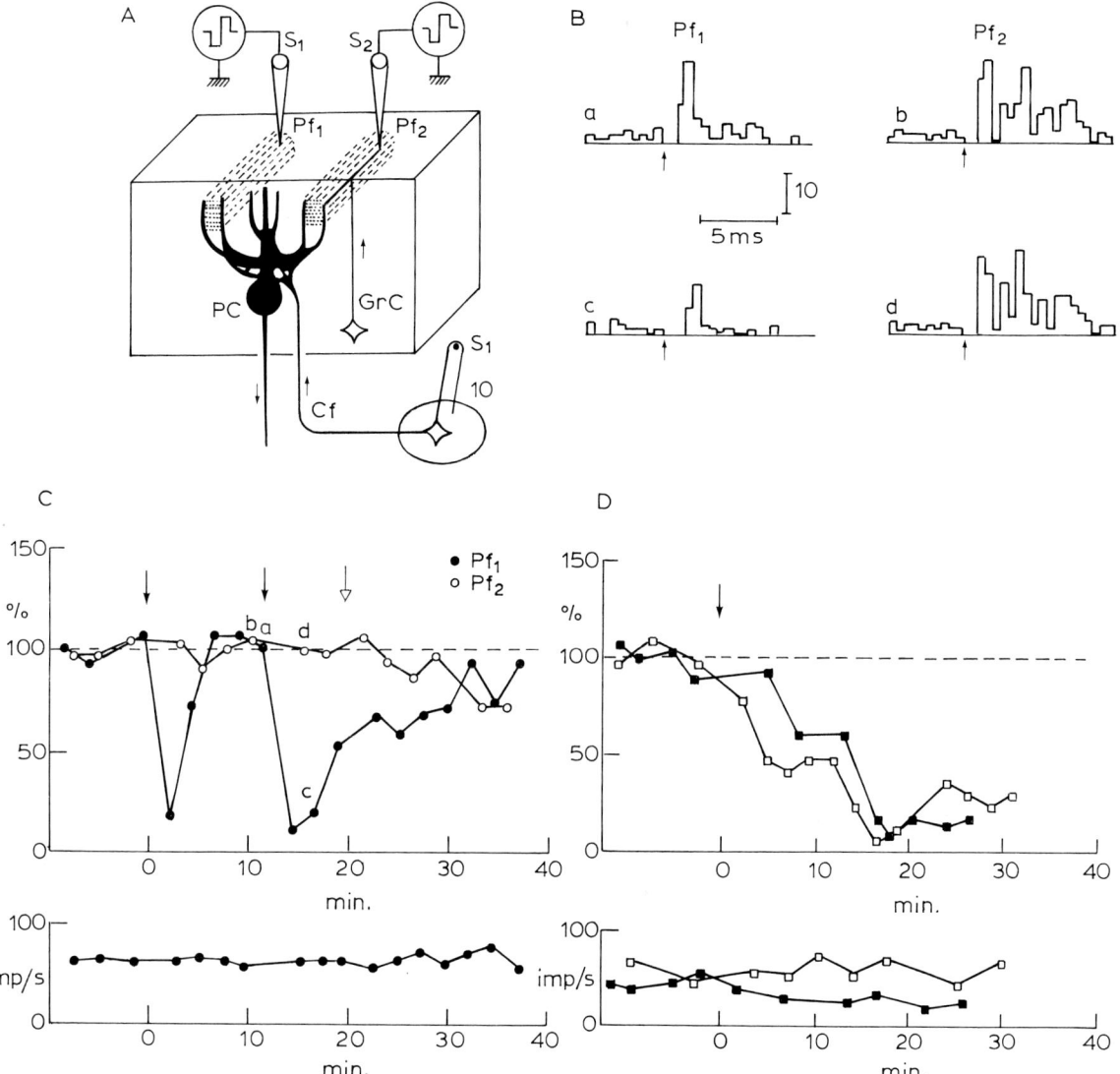

Fig. 4. Effect of conjunctive activation of parallel fibres and climbing fibres on the parallel fibre-Purkinje cell transmission. A. Experimental arrangement for stimulating two beams of parallel fibres in the molecular layer and climbing fibres in the inferior olive and for extracellularly recording from a Purkinje cell (PC). S_1 and S_2 microelectrodes for stimulation. GrC, granule cell. B. Peristimulus histogram for discharge from the Purkinje cell. Upper diagrams, control. Lower diagrams, after conjunctive activation of the beam (Pf_1) with climbing fibres. C plots the firing index at the peaks of the peristimulus histograms. Closed arrows indicate the moments of conjunctive stimulation of IO with Pf_1 at 4 Hz for 1 minute, and the open arrow indicates the moment of activation of Pf_2 alone with the same stimulus parameters. Lower histogram in C, spontaneous firing level. D. Similar to C but for another two Purkinje cells separately tested with only one beam of parallel fibres (Ekerot and Kano, 1983).

parallel fibre synapses have been recorded for up to 2 hours. An interesting additional observation is that the amount of depression progressively declined, with conjunction intervals of CF leading PF by 20 mseconds up to 375 mseconds, the conjunction stimulation being then at 2 Hz. Thus, the CF opens for a limited time (no more than 0.5 seconds) a window (Ito et al., 1982), for its depressant influ-

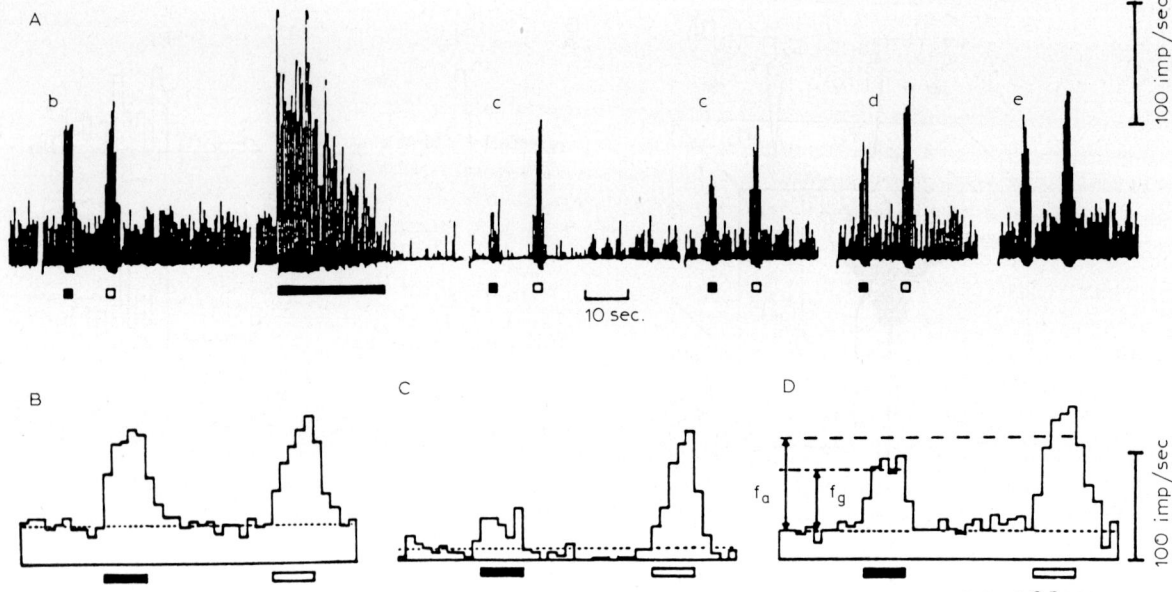

Fig. 5. Responses of a Purkinje cell to amino acids and changes due to conjunctive application of glutamate and stimulation of the inferior olive. A. Strip chart record showing simple spike discharges of a Purkinje cell. Bin widths, 0.5 second. Filled squares underneath the records indicate application of glutamate with a 9 nA current. Open squares indicate application of aspartate with 69 nA of current. Filled band: 9 nA glutamate ionophoresis plus stimulation of the inferior olive at 4/sec. Record is interrupted between c' and d, and between d and e. d, 5 minutes after onset of conjunctive stimulation; e, 30 minutes. B, C, D. Spike density histograms expanding records b, c and d in A, respectively. The methods of measuring f_g and f_a are indicated in D. Dotted lines in B and C show spontaneous discharge rates calculated from the intitial 10 bins. Two dashed lines in D indicate average discharge rates during application of glutamate and aspartate, respectively.

ence on a presently activated parallel fibre synapse.

It has been demonstrated by Ito et al. (1982) and Ito (1984) that the synaptic depression is due to a lowered sensitivity of the postsynaptic membrane to the synaptic transmitter, glutamate. Moreover, an hour-long desensitization to applied glutamate followed a conjunction of climbing fibre stimulation at 4 Hz with a prolonged (25–50 seconds) glutamate iontophoresis (Fig. 5A,B,C). It is of special interest that there was no depression of the much lower aspartate sensitivity. These iontophoretic experiments are thus closely analogous to the conjunction tests of Figs. 3 and 4.

We now confront the intriguing question of how the climbing fibre impulse is instrumental in producing a depression of those parallel fibre synapses with which it is in conjunction. There is a spatial problem in the interaction because the synapses of the CF fibre are restricted to the proximal two-thirds of the Purkinje dendrites, while the PF synapses are at all levels (Eccles et al., 1967). Ekerot and Oscarsson (1980, 1981) discovered a solution to this problem. Intracellular recording from a proximal dendrite of the Purkinje cell revealed that the response to a climbing fibre impulse is composed of an initial complex spike response followed by a plateau depolarization for about 100 mseconds (Fig. 6A). Prolonged depolarization of more distal

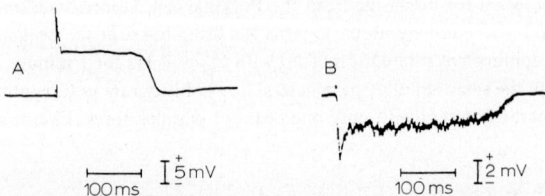

Fig. 6. Plateau potentials evoked in Purkinje cell dendrites by impulses in climbing fibres. A. Intracellular recording from proximal dendrite. B. Extracellular recording from distal dendrites (Ekerot, 1985).

dendrites was also produced by the climbing fibre impulse, as indicated by the negative potential recorded extracellularly (Fig. 6B), but it was more variable in duration, from a few mseconds to several hundreds of mseconds. They suggested that a prolonged increase in Ca^{2+} conductance could be responsible for the depolarization, citing the finding of Stöckle and Ten Bruggencate (1978) that climbing fibre activation decreased the extracellular calcium.

Llinás and Sugimori (1982) also investigated the Purkinje cell responses produced by CF inputs, but in in vitro slice preparations. They observed a prolonged depolarization both in intrasomatic and in intradendritic recording. It was shown to be due to Ca^{2+} input since it was reduced and abolished by progressive $CdCl_2$ addition to the bath. The more complex bursts of spike responses are not seen in vivo, which raises the question of the effects of possible dendritic injury by the slicing technique. Ekerot and Oscarsson (1980, 1981) suggested that the increased intracellular Ca^{2+} could depress the receptor sensitivity in the manner described by Miledi (1980) for the ACh receptors at motor endplates.

Ito (1984) illustrated this calcium hypothesis (Fig. 7). Depolarization by the climbing fibre impulse opens calcium channels across the postsynaptic membrane, with the consequence that there is a partial self-regenerative depolarization that keeps the Ca^{2+} channels open for 100 or more mseconds. The increased intradendritic Ca^{2+} sets in train various metabolic reactions, including generating a second messenger system which then acts on the postsynaptic receptor sites of the parallel fibre synapses, reducing their sensitivity to the transmitter (glutamate) and so depressing the synaptic effectiveness of the parallel fibres in the manner described by Ito et al. (1982) and Ekerot (1985). However, there is the crucial problem of accounting for the selectivity of the depression, namely that only the activated parallel fibre synapses are depressed by the conjunction, yet all the dendritic synapses would be subjected to increased Ca^{2+}.

The hypothetic diagram (Fig. 7) can account for the finding that although the CF synapses are only on the proximal two-thirds of the dendrites, all of the activated parallel fibre synapses are depressed. By electrotonic transmission the Purkinje dendrites would be depolarized through their whole length, and hence there is an increased Ca^{2+} input that would depress the sensitivity of even the most distal synapses. It also accounts for the finding of Campbell et al. (1983a) that if, by stimulation of parallel fibres, an intense depolarization is produced, there is opening of the calcium channels, with the consequent plateau after-depolarization. Furthermore, if the parallel fibre volley activated inhibitory cells (basket or stellate), and so diminished the initial excitatory depolarization by the climbing fibre impulse or by the massed parallel fibres, then there was depression or inhibition of the prolonged plateau, presumably because there was inadequate depolarization to open the calcium channels (Campbell et al., 1983b).

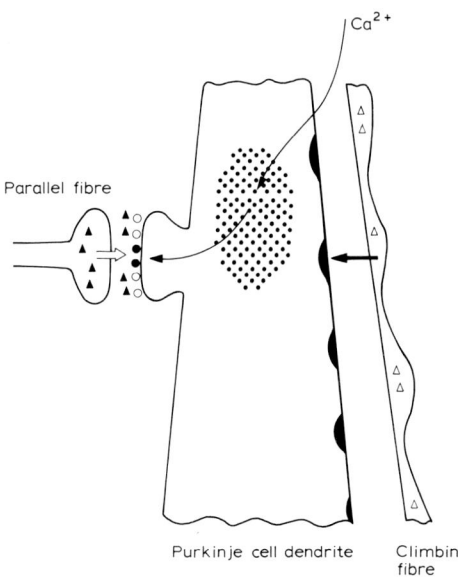

Fig. 7. Diagram showing proposed action of CF impulse in depolarizing Purkinje cell dendrites and so opening channels for Ca^{2+} entry. This Ca^{2+} activates a second messenger system that depresses sensitivity of the spine synapse to the transmitter released by the parallel fibre impulse (Ito, 1984).

The responses of the vestibulo-ocular reflex exhibit an adaptive learning response over many hours, and there is good evidence that the role of the climbing fibre input into the flocculus is to depress the parallel fibre synapses with which it is in conjunction, which is the Albus hypothesis. In the sine wave head rotation the input by CF into Purkinje cells tends to be out of phase with the mossy fibre input (Ghelarducci et al., 1975), and possibly the adaptation results from the conjunction depression. This depression is caused by a reduction of the glutamate sensitivity of the parallel fibre synapses. Furthermore, there is evidence that this depression is brought about by the increase in dendritic Ca^{2+} consequent on the opening of the Ca^{2+} channels by strong depolarization. This complex hypothetical explanation of the automatic learning involved in the adaptive vestibulo-ocular reflex needs much more experimental testing. Yet it will be helpful in attempting to understand motor learning in the two higher classes. Since by all evidence, anatomical, physiological and pharmacological, all parts of the cerebellar cortex are similar, it can be assumed that the vermis, pars intermedia and the hemispheres have plastic properties similar to that demonstrated in Figs. 3–6 for the flocculus and paraflocculus. This conclusion will be most significant in the subsequent two sections.

The learning of motor skills by animals

Most significant experimental observations on the learning of a motor skill have been described by Sasaki and Gemba (1981, 1982, 1983). The learning procedure is a very simple operant conditioning. A monkey is presented with a visual stimulus by a small green electric bulb which is turned on for 900 mseconds at random time intervals of 2.5–6 seconds. The monkey has to learn that if it lifts a lever by wrist extension during the light stimulus, there is a small juice reward. Initially, the monkey lifts the lever at random, with an occasional reward, but, gradually, after some weeks of training with about a thousand trials a week, there is motor learning and, eventually, the monkey lifts the lever on every light stimulus and at a progressively diminishing latency, which reaches a uniform short time. There is still full success when the light stimulus is shortened to 500 mseconds.

Before the onset of the operant conditioning, and under anaesthesia, several bipolar recording electrodes had been implanted in the cerebral cortex of the monkey, one on the pial surface, the other 2.5–3 mm deeper (Fig. 8). Each bipolar electrode thus led from a localized area of the cortex an electrical potential with recording of surface to depth, which is derived by subtraction, as indicated in Fig. 8 (S–D).

Figs. 9A–E are bipolar recordings from the sites indicated on the cerebral cortex in Fig. 8. In columns I–IV there are the responses at various stages

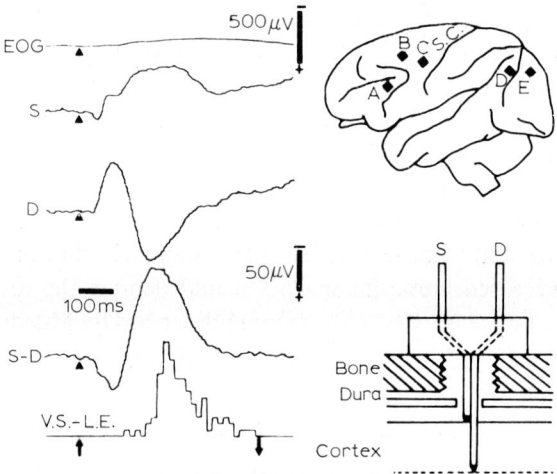

Fig. 8. Specimen potentials recorded on the surface (S) and in the depth (D) (2.5–3.0 mm below the surface) of the forelimb motor cortex contralateral to the moving hand. S–D gives surface potential minus depth potential and is the same as the record of IV, C in Fig. 9. Simultaneously recorded electrooculogram (EOG) (at the rostrolateral edge of the frontal bone above the orbita on the left side) is presented. Cortical potentials and EOG were led against the indifferent electrode in the bone just behind the ear, amplified by AC amplifiers of 2.0 seconds time constant and averaged 100 times with the time pulse of the onset of the light stimulus. Reaction times measured from the stimulus onset to the movement of lever elevation (V.S.–L.E.) are plotted for the same 100 samples in the histogram at every 16 mseconds. Calibrations are 500 μV for EOG and 50 μV for cortical potentials; and 100 mseconds for all traces. Triangles and upward arrow indicate the stimulus onset, and downward arrow the end of the stimulus. Five sites for recording in the left hemisphere are illustrated in the upper right diagram (A–E) and correspond to those in Fig. 9. The lower right scheme illustrates a chronic recording electrode implanted on the surface (S) and in the depth (D) of the cortex (Sasaki and Gemba, 1981).

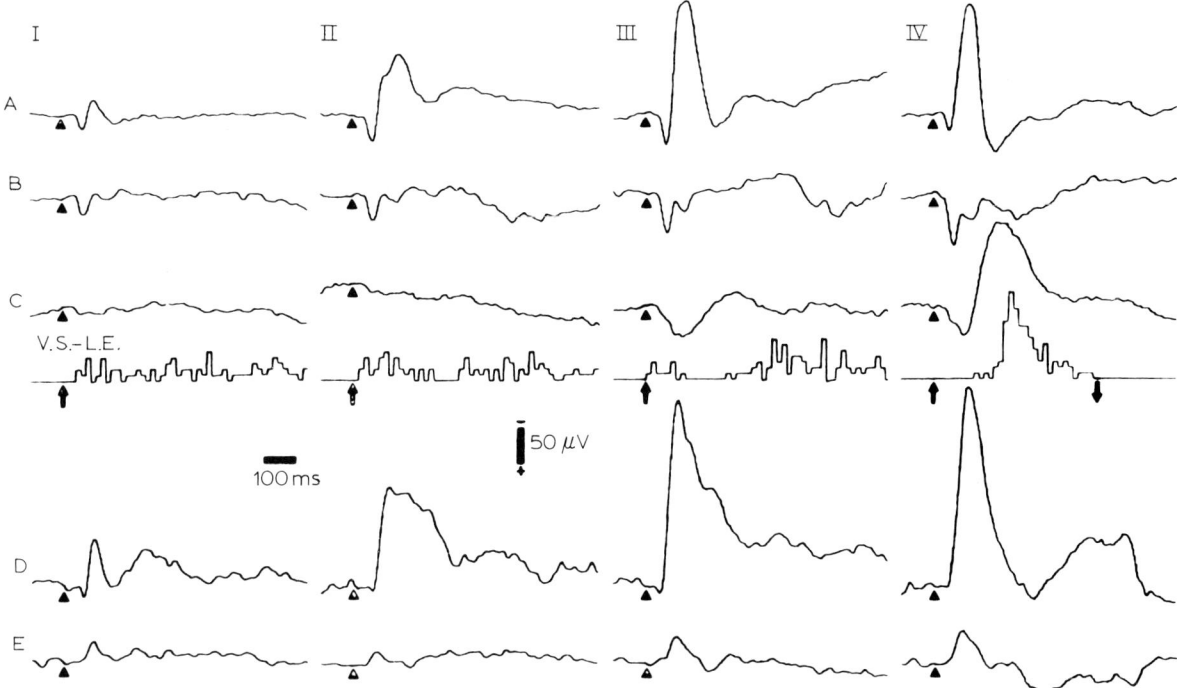

Fig. 9. Specimen records from five sites (A–E, see Fig. 8) in the cortex contralateral to the moving hand in one and the same monkey. Columns I–IV present four different stages in the learning process of visually initiated hand movements, respectively, 3, 21, 24 and 59 days after the commencement of training. Only S–D records are presented with the average of 100 times. The histogram under C gives reaction times of the same 100 samples, but some parts were curtailed in I–III, as the light stimulus was 900 mseconds in I–III and the end was out of the trace presented. Calibrations are 50 μV for all potentials and 100 mseconds for all traces (Sasaki and Gemba, 1981).

of the learning procedure, after approximately 500, 3000, 4000 and 9000 trials. The row V.S.–L.E. gives the reaction times measured from the light stimulus onset to the movement of the lever. In stages I and II the lever movement is random relative to the light stimulus, but by stage III there is a clear bunching of the motor responses, with a latency of 250–600 mseconds, and in stage IV the monkey was performing well, with a latency as brief as 200 mseconds and a mean latency of about 250 mseconds. It is surprising that many thousands of trials were necessary for this effective learning of a simple motor act, but eventually the monkey performs the lifting of the lever in a skilled manner.

The responses of the cerebral cortex develop with the learning. It was surprising to find that the prefrontal cortex (A in Fig. 9) exhibited an increased response early in the learning procedure, and that very large responses developed in area 18 (Fig. 9D), whereas in area 17 (Fig. 9E) there was a much smaller response. However, this could depend on the unfavourable location of electrode E (cf. Fig. 8, upper right). Attention should be focussed on the responses of the forelimb motor area, row C in Fig. 9. Only at the stage of an effective motor reaction (III) does a delayed negative wave appear, and it becomes large in IV, preceding by about 50 msec the averaged reaction times (V.S.–L.E.). In contrast to the bilateral responses at the recording sites from the association cortex, the forelimb motor cortex was strictly contralateral to the activated forelimb, which was also observed for the somatosensory cortex. Evidently, there was much cerebral activity in various cortical regions (rows A and D of Fig. 9) before this learned response developed, the forelimb motor cortex only responding when the conditioned activity developed to a high level.

Sasaki, Gemba and coworkers recognized that the late surface negative wave of the motor cortex resembled the response to projection from the neocerebellum via the ventrolateral (VL) thalamic nucleus (Sasaki et al., 1976, 1979). This identification was tested by excising the opposite cerebellar hemisphere (Sasaki et al., 1982). As shown in Fig. 10A, the large negative potential of the motor cortex (Preop.) was completely eliminated (Postop.), and at the same time the conditioned response was greatly delayed. Instead of a quick skilled lifting of the lever, there was a late disordered response, which is also seen in Fig. 10B for three other hemispherectomies. In Fig. 10A the interpositus nucleus was not excised, so a recovery of cerebello-thalamo-cerebral circuity was possible with further training, as is seen in the responses at 11, 21 and 49 postoperative days. The negative potential was restored to about half of the preoperative size and there was a full recovery of the response latency. After complete operative removal of the cerebellar hemisphere and intermediate lobe, there was no recovery.

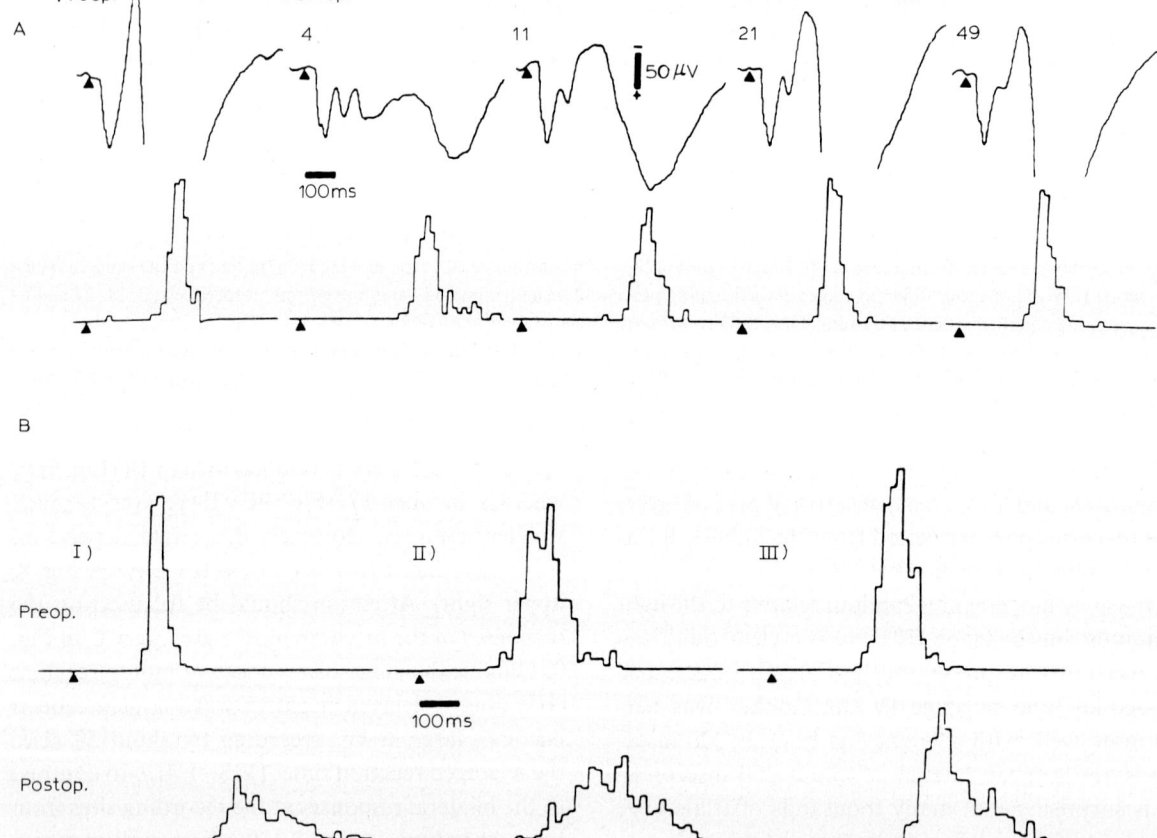

Fig. 10. A. Visually initiated premovement potentials (S–D) in the forelimb motor cortex (upper row) and histograms of reaction times (lower row) as influenced by cerebellar hemispherectomy when the interpositus was spared: Preop. before and Postop. at indicated days later. 50 μV calibration for potentials and 100 msec scale for potentials and histograms. 100 samples for all potentials and histograms. B. Influence of cerebellar hemispherectomy on reaction times of visually initiated movements. Control data before operation (upper row, Preop.) and those after (lower row, Postop.) are presented for three monkeys (I, II, III). Histograms of 300 movements (lever elevation) after onset of the visual stimulus (triangle) were calculated for 16 mseconds time bins, 100 mseconds scale for all records (Sasaki et al., 1982).

It can be concluded that in the fast skilled lever lifting of the trained monkey the contralateral neocerebellum plays a key role in instructing the motor cortex. In support of this conclusion is the finding (Sasaki and Gemba, 1982) that in two monkeys hemispherectomized before the training procedure, there was failure to develop the negative wave over the contralateral motor cortex. The visually initiated hand movement required a much longer training procedure and the learned movement was irregular, with a long latency and often failure.

In learning this simple skill of a visually initiated hand movement the visual input to the cerebral cortex resulted in responses in several areas of the association cortex (Fig. 9, rows A and D) that appear eventually to bring the contralateral neocerebellum into the response. It is postulated that, in Fig. 9, with continued training the cerebro-cerebello-thalamic pathway grows in effectiveness so that the hand movement becomes more skilful and at a progressively shorter latency (Fig. 9, row V.S.–L.E.).

It is an attractive hypothesis that this increased cerebellar influence arises because of learning in the cerebellum, which has already been established in the flocculus by direct experimental investigation (Figs. 3 and 4). There it was seen that, by conjunction of the climbing fibre and parallel fibre inputs into a Purkinje cell, there was initiated a prolonged depression (>1 hour) of the activated parallel fibre synapses on that Purkinje cell (Figs. 3 and 4). Since the sole output by Purkinje cells is to inhibit the nuclear cells, depression of the mossy fibre excitation of Purkinje cells results in a disinhibition of the nuclear cells, which is an excitation. Thus, there would be an increase in the excitatory dentatus-interpositus input into the VL thalamus. This would result in a thalamo-cortical input into the motor cortex that is postulated to produce the negative wave in Fig. 9, row C, IV, and in Fig. 10A (Preop.).

In accord with this dentate → motor cortex proposal, Thach (1975) had already found that in fast wrist movements in trained monkeys the activity of the dentate neurones tended to be earlier than the motor cortex activity, the mean values being respectively 70 and 54 mseconds before the muscle contraction. When the dentate nucleus was cooled (Meyer-Lohmann et al., 1977) there was a delay of 0.05 to 0.15 second in the movement, which was in accord with a proposed chain of command: cerebellum → dentatus nucleus → thalamus → motor cortex. However, in this experiment an earlier stage must be added. The GO signal must initially activate the cerebral cortex, the association areas projecting the command to the cerebellum, as proposed by Sasaki and Gemba (1981) on the basis of Fig. 9.

A very different motor learning task from that of Sasaki and Gemba was investigated by Gilbert and Thach (1977). The right hand of the monkey grasped a handle that alternately gave a flexor and extensor force to the wrist of a variable duration of 1.5–4.0 seconds and the task of the monkey was to return the handle to the midposition, success being indicated by a signal light. After training, this return was accomplished skilfully in about 0.5 second. Then the paradigm was altered by an increase or decrease in either the flexor or extensor force, the other being unaltered. The smooth learnt response was disturbed by the changed force, but a good compensation was learnt in 12 to 100 trials, whereas at the same time there was little disturbance in the response to the unchanged force in the opposite direction. Recording of single P-cell responses was simultaneously performed through an electrode assembly which had been implanted previously in the ipsilateral cerebellar cortex, usually in the pars intermedia of the anterior lobe. With adjustment of the recording electrode the complex spikes (CS) due to climbing fibre input could be clearly distinguished from the simple spikes (SS) due to the mossy fibre-parallel fibre inputs to that same Purkinje cell. Because of the changed force some Purkinje cells were subjected to a CF input of short latency, often with a later prolonged increase. In some cells it was this increased extensor load that triggered the increased CF input, in other cells a decreased extensor load was effective; similarly, other Purkinje cells were responsive to changes in flexor loads. The brief increase in CF responses corresponded to the learning time for the changed force and there was an associated decrease in SS spikes, which continued indefinitely during the increased or decreased forces, the CF input meanwhile having ceased.

Gilbert and Thach (1977) concluded that the increase in CS in conjunction with parallel fibre inputs probably was responsible for the depression of the Purkinje cell responses (SS) to parallel fibre inputs, as proposed in the Albus (1971) version of cerebellar learning. Subsequently (cf. the previous section), this hypothesis has been tested by the Ito and Ekerot groups, with results in accord with the prediction. Moreover, the experiments of Gilbert and Thach on the cerebellar responses have been complemented by the studies of Sasaki and Gemba on the responses of the cerebral cortex.

The learning of motor reactions to a changed force was quite fast (Gilbert and Thach, 1977), in great contrast to the learning of the visually initiated response (Fig. 9). Changed forces in rhythmic animal movements would be a common experience, as for example in walking on a terrain with changing slopes; hence, a rapid learning is essential. The learning of lever movement to irregularly presented light flashes is a much more esoteric experience for the animal, hence presumably the extreme slowness of that learning. This slowness was advantageous to Sasaki and Gemba in their study of the stages of learning. In further investigations they are recording the cerebral potentials from many more areas, including the supplementary motor area. Brinkman and Porter (1983) suggest that the premotor area may be specially involved in motor learning, but the premotor responses were not large and augmented but little in the Sasaki and Gemba experiments (Fig. 9, row B).

Fig. 11 represents diagrammatically the cerebral-cerebellar contributions to the responses described in this section when an animal is learning a motor task in an operant conditioning. It is the basis of an hypothesis of motor learning. All training of animals by operant conditioning involves some sensory input — visual, auditory, somatosensory — so there will be, as shown, an initial involvement of primary sensory cortex, and secondarily of various association areas. With a visual input Sasaki and Gemba found the peristriate cortex strongly excited

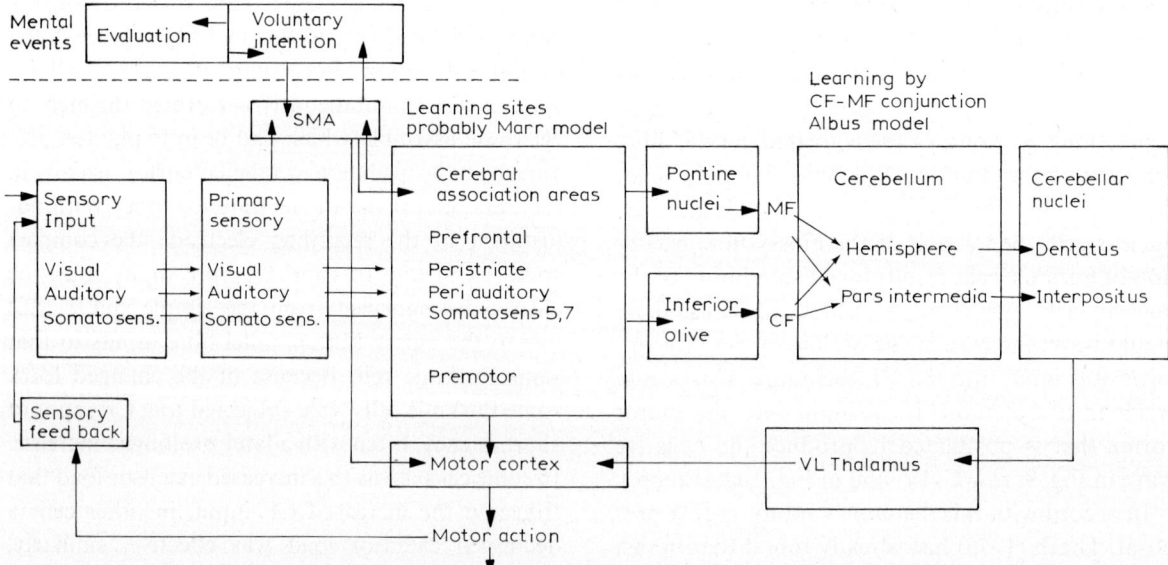

Fig. 11. Diagrammatic representation of the proposed mental and neural events in learning a skilled movement. Mental events for human motor learning are shown above the broken line separating them from the neural events. The role of mental events in animal motor learning is left undefined. The arrows indicate directions of main pathways of action. Full description in text. All pathways are excitatory except for the inhibitory action of the cerebellum on the cerebellar nuclei.

(Fig. 9, row D), but for other sensory inputs there presumably would be other association areas. However, a prefrontal involvement (Fig. 9A) could be common to all. There is progressive augmentation through learning stages I to IV (Fig. 9A and D). It is proposed that this learning response of the association cortices could be an example of the Marr (1970) model for conjunction potentiation in cerebral cortex (cf. Eccles, 1981, 1983). At the next stage there is projection from these association cortices to the motor cortex, giving a rather crude learnt response, as is seen after cerebellectomy (Fig. 10). For a skilled learnt response the cerebellum seems to be necessary. As shown in Fig. 11, there would be projection to the contralateral hemisphere and pars intermedia by both mossy fibres and climbing fibres (Sasaki et al., 1977). It is proposed that there is a learnt response (Gilbert and Thach, 1977) from their interaction in the Albus manner of conjunction, so producing a prolonged depression of the mossy fibre response. At a further stage of the cerebro-cerebellar-cerebrum circuit (Fig. 11) there is activation by disinhibition of the neurones of the dentate and interpositus nuclei (Allen et al., 1977, 1978), which in turn project to the VL thalamus and so to the motor cortex for a skilled response (Figs. 8, 9, 10).

It is thus proposed in Fig. 11 that motor learning is accomplished in two stages, the cerebral, possibly on the Marr (1970) conjunction model, and the cerebellar, on the Albus (1971) model. This hypothesis is presented as a challenge for rigorous testing. For example, it is essential to have much more investigation, in the manner of Sasaki and Gemba, of the responses of the association cortices and particularly of the premotor area and the supplementary motor cortex. Again, the cerebellar cortex and nuclei must be studied in various learning procedures in the manner of Gilbert and Thach. Further outstanding problems relate to the responses of the thalamic nuclei. However, the most significant deficiency derives from the as yet largely unknown learning responses of the basal ganglia (cf. De Long and Georgopoulos, 1983).

The learning of human motor skills

The two preceding sections on motor learning, culminating in the diagram of Fig. 11, provide a basis for our enquiry into the learning of the much more complex human motor skills, involving as they must a predominantly neocortical location. This enquiry will provide some important insight, but, because of inadequate knowledge, the emerging story will be more fragmentary than in the two preceding sections.

In learning a motor skill it is essential to concentrate on the planned action, so it can be postulated that the supplementary motor area (SMA) is initially activated by the intention (Eccles, 1982a, b), with subsequent excitation of other neocortical areas, particularly the premotor, with their stored motor programs. There is then excitation of the motor cortex to generate a discharge down the pyramidal tract that evokes the first "naïve" movement. Feedback by vision and somatosensory systems would be the basis of further intentions initiated by the SMA.

Meanwhile, on the basis of the discoveries of Sasaki and Gemba, it is postulated that the various cortical association areas are activated in a progressively enhanced manner (Fig. 9A, D) and in turn project to the neocerebellum and pars intermedia as in Fig. 11, with an interaction of CF and MF inputs in the Albus model. Just as with the animal studies in the previous section, it can be expected that there is initiated from the Purkinje cell/nuclear cell interaction a discharge up to the VL thalamus and so by relay to the motor cortex (Fig. 11). Thus, as learning proceeds, the motor cortex will be provided with a patterned input incorporating more and more of the learned information, which results in a pyramidal tract discharge giving the desired movement. The responses shown in Fig. 9C display the animal equivalent for this proposed cerebellar projection via the VL thalamus to the motor cortex.

The learning of an animal skill was postulated to be due to two distinct learning phenomena, in the cerebrum and in the cerebellum, as illustrated in

Fig. 11. Unfortunately, there is little evidence on the neuronal machinery involved in human motor learning. It is not possible to carrry out precise electrical recording in the manner of Gilbert and Thach (1977) or of Sasaki and Gemba (1981) (Figs. 8, 9, 10). However, there are studies on clinical lesions, especially of the cerebellum, which result in clumsy and inefficient movements, as originally described by Holmes (1939). Brooks (1979) has given a comprehensive review of Holmes's descriptions of the motor disabilities resulting from cerebellar lesions, and of clinical investigations since that time. Of necessity the clinical material cannot be investigated by precise neuronal studies so one has to rely on monkey experiments, as partly described in the previous section.

It can be suggested that the readiness potential of Deecke and Kornhuber (1977, 1978) gives evidence of a cerebellar input to the motor cortex resembling that of Fig. 9C, stage IV. After being symmetrical over the ipsi- and contralateral motor cortices in the early stages, asymmetry develops in the later stages. The readiness potential over the motor cortex that is involved in the movements becomes considerably increased, and this leads on to the motor potential. This developing asymmetry may be due at least in part to the cerebello-thalamo-cortical input which is seen in Fig. 9C, stages III and IV, and in the Preop. response of Fig. 10A.

Studies by radio-emission tomography have disclosed areas of the cerebrum and deeper nuclei that are involved in voluntary movement as distinct from automatic movement (Roland et al., 1980, 1982; Roland 1984). All these movements had to be learnt, but the neuronal processes involved in that learning are unknown. However, all voluntary movements seemed to be initiated in the supplementary motor area (SMA), with perhaps some help from the premotor cortex (Eccles, 1982a, b). Brinkman and Porter (1983) concluded from their studies on conscious monkeys that the premotor cortex may be specially involved in learning new motor programs. The visual input would seem to be of special importance for the premotor area.

It can therefore be assumed that in the learning of some movement, the SMA is primarily involved by the mental intention (Fig. 11), with perhaps some premotor assistance, and that there is a continuous conscious judgement or appraisal (evaluation box in Fig. 11) of the successive trials. This appraisal is based on the sensory feedback (Fig. 11) and results in intentions to carry out the movement more and more skilfully by action through the SMA. So, in the learning of a human skill, mind-brain interaction is a key factor. Mental activities such as critical evaluation, redesigning of the intended movement, a further critical evaluation of the new movement and so on are experienced by all who try to learn a new skill or to improve an existing one. This conscious activity is diagrammed in the upper box of Fig. 11, together with its proposed action on the SMA. The SMA is shown also to be influenced by the primary sensory areas, in accord with the findings of Tanji and Kurata (1982).

In contrast to the poverty of the data on cerebral and cerebellar involvement in human motor learning, there is a large literature on behavioural studies with mechanical and EMG recordings. However, there has been no coherent attempt to understand the learning at the neuronal and synaptic level. For human motor learning the diagram of Fig. 11 derived from studies on monkeys can be accepted provisionally. It is evident that the learning of motor skills provides an immense challenge for investigation of both monkeys and humans.

It is probable that the learned responses of the association cortex with their progressive augmentation (Fig. 9A, D) are dependent on the same neuronal factors, as with cognitive memories (Eccles, 1981, 1983), namely, the Marr (1970) type of conjunction potentiation, as indicated in Fig. 11. However, in contrast to cognitive learning, motor learning is not dependent on the hippocampus. The well-known subject of bilateral hippocampectomy (H.M.) was able to learn a complex motor skill despite an extreme disability in cognitive learning. For example, he learned in normal time (3 days) to draw a line between the parallel lines of a double lined star, the whole process being learned through vision in a mirror. In subsequent days he had no recollection of learning the task; nevertheless, he had retained the motor skill (Milner, 1966). The hippocampus does not appear in Fig. 11.

The hypothesis illustrated in Fig. 11, with the addition of mental events for humans, is offered not as some final story, but provisionally. It is in need of testing at every level, but at least it is a coherent story of motor learning, where previously there were unrelated conjectures. It is of interest that an increase of intradendritic calcium is proposed as a key factor for both cerebellar learning (Fig. 7) and for hippocampal and cerebral learning (Eccles, 1983). The difference is that Ca^{2+} is responsible for conjunction depression in the cerebellum, the Albus model, and for conjunction potentiation, in the long-term potentiation of the hippocampus and for the Marr model (1970) in the neocerebrum. This difference in synaptic design presumably relates to the inhibitory action of the cerebellar Purkinje cells and to the excitatory action of all cerebral pyramidal cells.

References

Albus, J. S. (1971) A theory of cerebellar function. Math. Biosci., 10: 25–61.
Allen G. I., Gilbert, P. F. C., Marini, R., Schultz, W. and Yin, T. C. T. (1977) Integration of cerebral and peripheral inputs by interpositus neurons in monkey. Exp. Res., 27: 81–99.
Allen, G. I., Gilbert, P. F. C., Marini, R. and Yin, T. C. T. (1978) Convergence of cerebral inputs onto dentate neurons in monkey. Exp. Brain Res., 32: 151–170.
Brinkman, C. and Porter, R. (1983) Supplementary motor area and premotor area of the monkey cerebral cortex: functional organisation and activities of single neurons during performance of a learned movement. In J. E. Desmedt (Ed.), Motor Control Mechanisms in Health and Disease, Raven Press, New York, pp. 393–420.
Brooks, V. B. (1979) Control of intended limb movements by the lateral and intermediate cerebellum. In H. Asanuma and V. J. Wilson (Eds.), Integration in the Nervous System, Igaku-Shoin, Tokyo, pp. 321–356.
Campbell, N. C., Ekerot, C.-F., Hesslow, G. and Oscarsson, O. (1983a) Dendritic plateau potentials evoked in Purkinje cells by parallel fibre volleys in the cat. J. Physiol., 340: 209–223.
Campbell, N. C., Ekerot, C.-F. and Hesslow, G. (1983b) Interaction between responses in Purkinje cells evoked by climbing fibre impulses and parallel fibre volleys in the cat. J. Physiol., 340: 225–238.
Deecke, L. and Kornhuber, H. H. (1977) Cerebral potentials and the initiation of voluntary movement. In J. E. Desmedt (Ed.), Attention, Voluntary Contraction and Event-related Cerebral Potentials, Progress in Clinical Neurophysiology, Vol. 1, Karger, Basel, pp. 132–150.
Deecke, L. and Kornhuber, H. H. (1978) An electrical sign of participation of the mesial "supplementary" motor cortex in human voluntary finger movement. Brain Res., 159: 473–496.
De Long, M. R. and Georgopoulos, A. P. (1983) Motor functions of the basal ganglia. Am. Soc. Handb., 21: 1017–1061.
Eccles, J. C. (1981) The modular operation of the cerebral neocortex considered as the material basis of mental events. Neuroscience, 6: 1839–1856.
Eccles, J. C. (1982a) The initiation of voluntary movements by the supplementary motor area. Arch. Psychiatr., 231: 423–441.
Eccles, J. C. (1982b) How the Self acts on the brain. Psychoneuroendocrinology, 7: 271–283.
Eccles, J. C. (1983) Calcium in long-term potentiation as a model for memory. Neuroscience, 10: 1071–1081.
Eccles, J. C., Ito, M. and Szentágothai, J. (1967) The Cerebellum as a Neuronal Machine, Springer Verlag, Heidelberg.
Ekerot, C. F. (1985) Climbing fibre actions on Purkinje cells — plateau potentials and long-lasting depression of parallel fibre responses. In J. Dichgans, J. Bloedel and W. Precht (Eds.), Cerebellar Functions, Springer Verlag, Berlin, in press.
Ekerot, C. F. and Kano, M. (1983) Climbing fibre induced depression of Purkinje cell responses to parallel fibre stimulation. Proc. Int. Union Physiol. Sci., 15: 393.
Ekerot, C. F. and Oscarsson, O. (1980) Prolonged dendritic depolarizations evoked in Purkinje cells by climbing fibre impulses. Brain Res., 192: 272–275.
Ekerot, C. F. and Oscarsson, O. (1981) Prolonged depolarization elicited in Purkinje cell dendrites by climbing fibre impulses in the cat. J. Physiol., 318: 207–221.
Ghelarducci, B., Ito, M. and Yagi, N. (1975) Impulse discharges from flocculus Purkinje cells of alert rabbits during visual stimulation combined with horizontal head rotation. Brain Res. 87: 66–72.
Gilbert, P. F. C. and Thach, W. T. (1977) Purkinje cell activity during motor learning. Brain Res., 128: 309–328.
Gonshor, A. and Melvill-Jones, G. (1976a) Short-term adaptive changes in the human vestibulo-ocular reflex arc. J. Physiol., 256: 361–379.
Gonshor, A. and Melvill-Jones, G. (1976b) Extreme vestibulo-ocular adaptation induced to prolonged optical reversal of vision. J. Physiol., 256: 381–414.
Holmes, G. (1939) The cerebellum of man. Brain, 62: 1–30.
Ito, M. (1984) The Cerebellum and Neural Control, Raven Press, New York, p. 580.

Ito, M. and Kano, M. (1982) Long-lasting depression of parallel fiber-Purkinje cell transmission induced by conjunctive-stimulation of parallel fibers and climbing fibers in the cerebellar cortex. Neurosci. Lett., 33: 253–258.

Ito, M., Sakurai, M. and Tongroach, P. (1982) Climbing fibre-induced depression of both mossy fibre responsiveness and glutamate sensitivity of cerebellar Purkinje cell. J. Physiol., 324: 113–134.

Ito, M., Shiida, T., Yagi, N. and Yamamoto, M. (1974) The cerebellar modification of rabbits horizontal vestibulo-ocular reflex induced by sustained head rotation combined with visual stimulation. Proc. Jpn. Acad. Sci., 50: 85–89.

Llinás, R. and Sugimori, M. (1982) Functional significance of the climbing fibre input to Purkinje cells: An in vitro study in mammalian cerebellar slice. In S. L. Palay and V. Chan-Palay (Eds.) The Cerebellum, New Vistas. Springer Verlag, Berlin, pp. 402–410.

Maekawa, K. and Simpson, J. I. (1973) Climbing fibre responses evoked in the vestibulocerebellum of rabbit from visual system. J. Neurophysiol., 36: 649–666.

Marr, D. (1969) A theory of the cerebellar cortex. J. Physiol. Lond. 202: 437–470.

Marr, D. (1970) A theory for cerebral neocortex. Proc. Roy, Soc. Lond. B, 176: 161–234.

Meyer-Lohmann, J., Hore, J. and Brooks, V.B. (1977) Cerebellar participation in generation of prompt arm movement. J. Neurophysiol., 38: 871–908.

Miledi, R. (1980) Intracellular calcium and desensitization of acetylcholine receptors. Proc. Roy. Soc. Lond. B, 209: 447–452.

Milner, B. (1966) Amnesia following operation on the temporal lobes. In C. W. M. Whitty and O. L. Zangwill (Eds), Amnesia, Butterworths, London, pp. 109–133.

Robinson, D. A. (1976) Adaptive gain control of vestibuloocular reflex by the cerebellum. J. Neurophysiol., 39: 954–969.

Roland, P. E. (1984) Organization of motor control by normal human brain. Human Neurobiol., 2: 205–216.

Roland, P. E., Larsen, B., Lassen, N. A. and Skinhøj, E. (1980) Supplementary motor area and other cortical areas in organization of voluntary movements in man. J. Neurophysiol., 43: 118–136.

Roland, P. E., Meyer, E., Shibasaki, T., Yamamoto, Y. L. and Thompson, C. J. (1982) Regional cerebral blood flow changes in cortex and basal ganglia during voluntary movements in normal human volunteers. J. Neurophysiol., 48: 467–480.

Sasaki, K. and Gemba, H. (1981) Changes of premovement field potentials in the cerebral cortex during learning processes of visually initiated hand movements in the monkey. Neurosci. Lett., 27: 125–130.

Sasaki, K. and Gemba, H. (1982) Development and change of cortical field potentials during learning processes of visually initiated hand movement in the monkey. Exp. Brain Res., 48: 429–437.

Sasaki, K. and Gemba, H. (1983) Learning of fast and stable hand movement and cerebro-cerebellar interactions in the monkey. Brain Res., 277: 41–46.

Sasaki, K., Kawaguchi, S., Oka, H., Sakai, M. and Mizuno, N. (1976) Electrophysiological studies on the cerebellocerebral projections in monkeys. Exp. Brain Res., 24: 495–507.

Sasaki, K., Oka, H., Kawaguchi, S., Jinnai, K. and Yasuda, T. (1977) Mossy fibre and climbing fibre responses produced in the cerebellar cortex by stimulation of the cerebral cortex in monkeys. Exp. Brain Res. 29: 419–428.

Sasaki, K., Jinnai, K., Gemba, H., Hashimoto, S. and Mizuno, N. (1979) Projection of the cerebellar dentate nucleus onto the frontal association cortex in monkeys. Exp. Brain Res., 37: 193–198.

Sasaki, K., Gemba, H. and Mizuno, N. (1982) Cortical field potentials preceding visually initiated hand movements and cerebellar actions in the monkey. Exp. Brain Res., 46: 29–36.

Stöckle, H. and Ten Bruggencate, G. (1978) Climbing fibre mediated rhythmic modulations of potassium and calcium in cat cerebellar cortex. Exp. Neurol., 61: 226–230.

Tanji, J. and Kurata, K. (1982) Comparison of movement-related activity in two cortical motor areas of primates. J. Neurophysiol., 48: 633–653.

Thach, W. T. (1975) Timing of activity in cerebellar dentate nucleus and cerebral motor cortex during prompt volitional movement. Brain Res., 88: 233–241.

SECTION I

Final Common Pathway

Organization and properties of spinal motoneurones and motor units

D. Kernell

Department of Neurophysiology, University of Amsterdam, AMC, Meibergdreef 15, 1105 AZ Amsterdam, The Netherlands

Introduction

In the present contribution I will give a brief survey of some known facts and current problems concerning motoneurones and motor units of the cat's hindlimb. Particular attention will be devoted to properties which are of importance for the rate- and recruitment-gradation of muscle force.

Contractile properties of motor units

The main task of muscle fibres and motor units is to produce controllable amounts of force. In reflex and voluntary movements, motor unit force may be graded by varying the rate of repetitive activation. Fig. 1 illustrates this well-known way of modulating force for two motor units from the hindlimb muscle m. peroneus longus (Kernell et al., 1983c). For each unit, a number of superimposed contractions are shown, as produced by different stimulus rates up to and including the frequencies needed for maximum tetanic tension. The two units were markedly different from each other. Firstly, unit A had a smaller maximum force than unit B. Secondly, a lower range of rates was needed for modulating the force of unit A than for that of unit B. Thirdly, when stimulated by repeated bursts during a couple of minutes, force was maintained much better in A than in B (not illustrated). Thus, the units of a muscle may differ from each other with respect to at least three major contractile properties: force, speed and endurance. These three properties are largely dependent on different mechanisms but, statistically, they do not vary independently of each other. In practically all limb muscles studied so far (see Burke, 1981), the force, speed and endurance show a co-variation similar to that schematically indicated in Fig. 2 (diameter of symbols proportional to maximum force): at one end of the distribution the units are slow, fatigue-resistant and weak, and at the other extreme they are fast, fatigue-sensitive and strong. In between, the units tend to be fast, intermediate in force and variously resistant to fatigue. This characteristic distribution of contractile properties was first described clearly by Burke and his group (1971, 1973), and

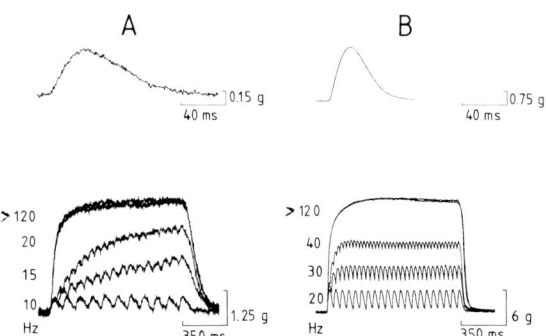

Fig. 1. Isometric contractions from a slow-twitch (A) and a fast-twitch (B) unit from the same peroneus longus muscle. Upper recordings show the single twitch (average of 21 and 14 sweeps, respectively). Lower recordings show superimposed responses to repetitive stimuli at rates indicated to the left of each record. In both units, about the same force-response was produced by stimulation at 120.5 and 151.5 Hz, respectively (both responses included in each record). From Kernell et al. (1983c).

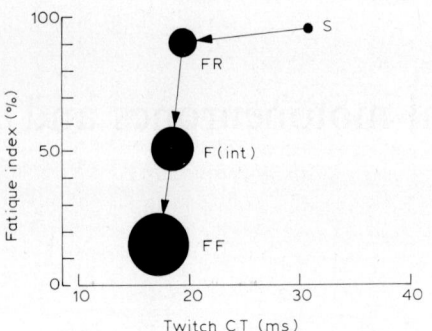

Fig. 2. Plot of fatigue resistance (fatigue index, %) versus twitch contraction time (msec) for 80 motor units of cat m. peroneus longus. Mean values are shown for motor units of the categories S, FR, F(int) and FF, respectively, as classified according to the criteria of Burke et al. (1973). Plotted symbols have diameters in direct proportion to the maximum tetanic tension of the respective group of units (mean maximum tension for FF units: 27.9 g). Arrows indicate presumed order of recruitment in most kinds of contractions (cf. Burke, 1981). Data from results of Kernell et al. (1983b).

they assigned the well-known terms of S units for the slow ones, FR units for the fast-twitch, fatigue-resistant ones and FF units for the fast-twitch, fatigue-sensitive ones. Commonly a fourth category of fast-twitch, intermediate-fatigue units, F(int), is included as well (Burke, 1981). For all the three contractile parameters of Fig. 2, physiological measurements give values that may vary continuously over the whole encountered range (cf. fatigue indices of Fig. 5). It is still a matter of discussion, however, whether the S, FR and FF unit categories should be regarded as distinct "types" (cf. Fleshman et al., 1981) or as descriptive categories from a continuous distribution.

Data such as those of Figs. 1 and 2 illustrate that even a single skeletal muscle is quite a complex machine to handle for the nervous system. An optimum use of a muscle requires that the nervous system takes into account how the various muscle units differ in their properties. This is done in two major ways: (i) there is a "speed-match" between the rhythmic properties of a motoneurone and the contractile speed of its muscle fibres, (ii) there is a "recruitment-match" between the apparent excitability of a motoneurone and the contractile properties of its muscle fibres. These two aspects of motoneurone-muscle-matching will be separately discussed below.

The matching between motoneuronal discharge properties and contractile speed

Quite a long time ago, it was noted by Denny-Brown (1929) that the motoneurones of a slow muscle (soleus) were capable of discharging steadily at what we now know to be comparatively slow rates (5–10 Hz). In gradually increasing reflex contractions of mixed muscles, motoneurones of fast-twitch units tend to start discharging at higher rates than neurones innervating units with a slower twitch (Kernell and Sjöholm, 1975; Grimby et al., 1979). This difference between fast- and slow-twitch units does not primarily depend on synaptic circuitry, because corresponding differences in minimum firing rate are found if individual motoneurones are steadily activated by intracellularly injected current (Kernell, 1979; injected currents used as substitute for steady post-synaptic currents, see Kernell, 1984). In each case, a motoneurone typically starts discharging at a minimum rate which is close to the lowest rate producing some summation of consecutive twitches. This type of speed-match tends to maximize the capability of motoneurones to grade force by a modulation of discharge rate: the relation between contractile tension and activation frequency is particularly steep over a range of rates just above that needed for a commencing twitch summation (cf. Fig. 1; Cooper and Eccles, 1930; Kernell et al., 1983c).

In spinal motoneurones which are subjected to steady excitation, the minimum rate of steady firing depends primarily on an intrinsic membrane property: the duration of after-hyperpolarization (AHP) (Kernell, 1965b). Some time ago, it had already been noted by Eccles et al. (1958) that the AHP tends to be particularly long-lasting in motoneurones with slow-twitch muscle fibres and slowly conducting (i.e., small-diameter) axons. It should be stressed that the AHP is of particular importance for the minimum rate and not for the maximum one; the maximum steady rate at which a continuously excited motoneurone may be made to discharge depends mainly on its spike generating mechanisms. Also, the maximum rate tends to be greater for fast-twitch motoneurones than for slow-twitch ones (Kernell, 1979; cf. also Kernell, 1965b).

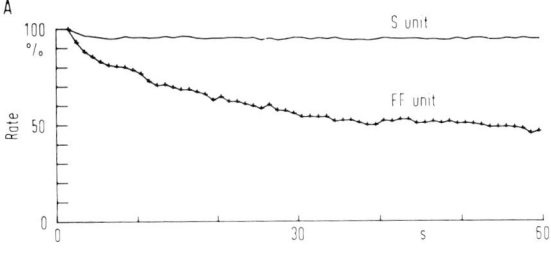

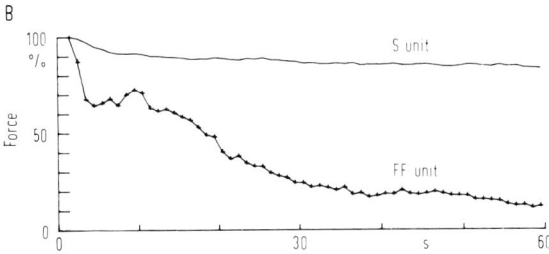

Fig. 3. Late adaptation in two individual motoneurones from m. gastrocnemius medialis. The cells were activated by currents injected through the intracellular microelectrode. Force production of their units simultaneously monitored from the muscle (tendon connected to sensitive force transducer, muscle kept at optimum length for a twitch). The muscle unit of the S motoneurone had a twitch contraction time of 53 mseconds and a fatigue index of 97%. The muscle unit of the FF motoneurone had a twitch contraction time of 25 mseconds and a fatigue index of 7%. Values plotted in the illustration were derived from repetitive discharges elicited by constant injected currents lasting >1 minute. A. Plot of firing rate (%) versus time (seconds) for first minute of discharges produced by current of 5 nA above threshold for rhythmic firing. For consecutive seconds of discharge, mean firing rates have been connected by straight lines. Firing rates given as percentage of rate during second second of discharge (= first value plotted = 16.1 Hz for the S unit and 28.9 Hz for the FF unit). B. Contractile force produced by the discharges in A. Force given as percentage of value for second second of discharge. For non-fused contractions, plotted values refer to mean force, as calculated over time periods of 1 second. Control measurements showed that most of the force-decline of the FF unit was indeed caused by the decreased firing rate and not by muscle fatigue. From Kernell and Monster (1982b).

We have recently been re-investigating another aspect of the rhythmic properties of motoneurones: how they discharge in response to a constant intracellular stimulation lasting for several tens of seconds (cf. Granit et al., 1963; Kernell, 1965a). In most previous studies, the analysis of rhythmic properties was limited to durations of 1 or a few seconds and, when studied over such brief times, discharge rate seemed to have become rather steady already after a few hundred mseconds ("initial adaptation"). Studies at a longer time base revealed, however, that most motoneurones show a marked and slowly progressive drop in discharge rate during, in particular, the first 0.5–1 minute of constant stimulation ("late adaptation") (Kernell and Monster, 1982a). For cells activated by the same amount of supra-threshold current, the late adaptation was much more prominent among fast-twitch motoneurones than among slow-twitch ones (Kernell and Monster, 1982b). Typical examples are shown in Fig. 3. In Fig. 3A, the changes in discharge rate during the course of 1 minute of constant stimulation are shown for an S motoneurone and an FF motoneurone of gastrocnemius. In the FF-cell there was a marked drop in discharge rate (A) and motor unit tension (B). In the S-cell, rate as well as tension remained almost constant. Thus, also in this respect, the S motoneurones are well equipped for one of their major tasks: the maintenance of prolonged postural contractions (see the following section). Among the fast-twitch motoneurones, we found no differences in late adaptation between FF and FR cells.

The observed differences in late adaptation between fast and slow motoneurones (Fig. 3) probably were mainly a direct consequence of the differences in impulse rate at the beginning of the respective discharges (Kernell and Monster, 1982b). The late adaptation seems to depend on cumulative aftereffects of the discharging spikes (activation of electrogenic sodium pump as a result of sodium entry?; cf. Sokolove and Cooke, 1971). The higher the discharge rate, the more cumulative aftereffects per unit time and the greater becomes the late adaptation.

relationships for m. peroneus longus by aid of the technique of glycogen depletion (Donselaar et al., 1985).

Motoneuronal excitability and recruitment order

When stimulated directly via an intracellular microelectrode, the threshold current for a single spike discharge (Fleshman et al., 1981) or for repetitive firing (Kernell and Monster, 1981) is small for S neurones, larger for FR cells and still larger for the FF motoneurones. How do these differences in electrical excitability arise?

When stimulated with steady current, the stimulus intensity needed to reach threshold will at least depend on (i) the amount of depolarization needed for eliciting (repetitive) action potentials (V_{thr}) and (ii) the input resistance of the cell (cf. Ohm's law).

Among motoneurones that were readily discharged by dorsal root stimulation (synaptic excitation), the same average V_{thr} was found for slow-twitch and fast-twitch (mainly FR?) motoneurones (Pinter et al., 1983; cf. discussion of Gustafsson and Pinter, 1984b). However, the V_{thr} of S motoneurones might possibly tend to be somewhat lower than that of the opposite extreme, the FF motoneurones. Such a view is supported by comparisons between electrophysiologically characterized motoneurones (Gustafsson and Pinter, 1984b) as well as by the relationships between input resistance and current threshold among muscle-unit-identified motoneurones (Fleshman et al., 1981). Especially when stimulated by relatively long-lasting currents, "active" membrane properties might be of considerable importance for differences in current threshold (cf. Schwindt and Crill, 1980; Gustafsson and Pinter, 1984b). When stimulated by slowly rising currents, an accommodative increase of V_{thr} seems to take place in many fast-twitch motoneurones (Burke and Nelson, 1971).

It has been known for a long time that the input resistance is higher for motoneurones with a slow axonal conduction velocity and a long-lasting AHP than for those with faster axons and briefer AHPs (Kernell, 1966). This difference as well as the resulting difference in threshold current for slow and fast cells might be caused partly by the fact that the soma-dendrite size of slow cells generally tends to be smaller than that of the fast ones (cf. Fig. 4). However, when we made a direct comparison between neuronal size and input resistance in the same cells we discovered that the difference in input resistance between large and small cells was much greater than one would expect from the differences in size alone (Kernell and Zwaagstra, 1981). Hence, these findings indicated that the mean specific membrane resistance tends to be lower in large (fast) cells than in smaller (often slower) ones. In essence, these results have been confirmed by others (Burke et al., 1982; Gustafsson and Pinter, 1984a), and the findings indicate that even if all cells had the same V_{thr} and were excited by the same density of equivalent synapses, small and slow cells generally would tend to be more easily activated than larger and faster ones in response to an asynchronous steady synaptic input (for further discussion, see Kernell and Zwaagstra, 1981).

The above-mentioned considerations suggest that differences in intrinsic membrane properties are of considerable importance for the way in which the recruitment occurs within a motoneurone pool. There is no direct causal relationship between these membrane properties (e.g., specific membrane resistance) and motoneuronal size. Still, for reasons which we do not yet understand, some of these membrane properties show a more or less evident tendency to co-vary with aspects of neuronal size (cf. Kernell and Zwaagstra, 1981; Burke et al., 1982; Gustafsson and Pinter, 1984a). Such a covariation, and not size itself, might constitute the main basis for the correlation between axonal size and recruitment order in reflexes (Henneman et al., 1965; Henneman and Mendell, 1981). It should be stressed that an ascending-size-order of recruitment does not only exist with respect to comparisons between different type-categories of units (e.g., fast vs. slow), but it may also be very strikingly present within a single category (e.g., slow-twitch units, Bawa et al., 1984). It remains to be proven whether there is a correspondingly close correlation, within such a subpopulation, between axonal conduction velocity and intrinsic excitability. However, it is also of importance to realize that marked differences in intrinsic excitability may occur independently of differences in axonal or soma-dendritic size. The most evident example concerns the FR and FF motoneurones of cat triceps surae. There is experimental evidence indicating that, in triceps surae as well as in other muscles, FR motoneurones are more easily reflex-activated than are the FF cells (see Burke, 1981). In triceps surae, the two classes of cell have, on average, nearly the same axonal conduction velocity (Burke et al., 1973) as well as soma-dendrite size (no statistically significant differences found, Burke et al., 1982; Ulfhake and Kellerth, 1982). However, the average input resistance is greater for FR than for FF motoneurones (Fleshman et al., 1981). Thus, the two classes of cell apparently differ in mean specific membrane resistance, and such differences are likely to be partly responsible for the fact that, on average, the threshold current is lower for FR than for FF motoneurones (Fleshman et al., 1981; Kernell and Monster, 1981).

Effects of chronic stimulation

In an effort to understand more about the mechanisms by which the mutual matching arises between motoneuronal and muscle properties, we have recently embarked upon studies of the long-term effects of impulse activity (Kernell et al., 1983a; Eerbeek et al., 1984). We then used a portable ministimulator for producing chronic electrical activation of the deafferented common peroneal nerve. In each cat, stimulation lasted 4–8 weeks. In a final acute experiment we investigated the contractile properties of m. peroneus longus.

Our experiments with chronic stimulation have confirmed that the more a fast (mixed) muscle is activated via its nerve, the further its properties change toward those of slow units (Salmons and Vrbová, 1969; Salmons and Henriksson, 1981). These changes do not only concern contractile speed and endurance, but also the maximum tetanic force becomes markedly smaller after a prolonged period of substantially enhanced activity (cf. Salmons and Vrbová, 1969; Salmons and Henriksson, 1981). The weakening is partly caused by a decrease in diameter of the musle fibres (Salmons and Henriksson, 1981; Donselaar, Eerbeek, Kernell and Verhey, unpublished data). Furthermore, our results have shown that when given during the same amount of total time per day, fast and slow pulse rates of chronic stimulation had practically the same effect on isometric aspects of muscle speed. Even pulse rates as fast as 100 Hz were capable of producing an evident slowing of muscle contraction (Fig. 6) as well as marked histochemical changes (staining for myofibrillar ATPase). In innervated mixed muscles of the cat we found no evidence for the interesting kinds of frequency-specificity that have been observed in rat denervated soleus muscle (Lømo et al., 1980).

Findings from experiments with chronic stimulation are consistent with the idea that the matching between usage and contractile properties of motor units arise, to a great extent, via long-term effects of motor unit activity on motor unit properties. Thus, the ascending-force-order of recruitment might exist (partly) because the most easily recruited motoneurones tend, as a result of great amounts of activation, to become equipped with weak muscle fibres. Similarly, the difference in force and endurance between FF and FR units (cf. Fig. 2) might be a secondary result of differences in the daily amount of activation of these two kinds of motoneurones. Our results should not be taken to mean, however, that differences in muscle fibre properties are determined only by differences in activation patterns: long-term changes in activity can probably only alter the various contractile properties of muscle fibres within a limited "adaptive range", and this range is likely to have been set, different for different muscles, at an early stage of development. The importance of such a presetting is, for instance, suggested as one compares the properties of limb and eye muscles.

The extraocular muscles tend to be used throughout the waking hours. Most of the fast units of

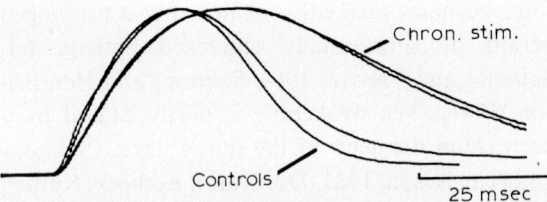

Fig. 6. Effects of high-frequency chronic stimulation on time course of isometric twitch. Twitches recorded from four different peroneus longus muscles of two cats. The two twitches labelled "Chron. stim." were from muscles that had been chronically activated via the nerve during 8 weeks prior to the illustrated recordings. The two twitches labelled "Controls" were from the contra-lateral (non-stimulated) side of the same animals. Chronic stimulation was given as 100 Hz bursts of 0.1 second duration repeated every 2 seconds (activation during 5% of total time). The illustrated recordings were obtained in a final acute experiment. In each case, the tendon of the muscle was connected to a force transducer and kept at the optimum length for a twitch. Each record represents the average of ten sweeps. In order to facilitate comparisons of time course, the force records are shown at a common time scale, but with normalized amplitudes. Prior to the period of chronic stimulation, the cats had been subjected to a dorsal rhizotomy and a hemispinalization on the experimental side. In the absence of subsequent chronic stimulation, these operations did not affect the time course of the twitch (Eerbeek et al., 1984). From data of Kernell et al. (1983a).

mixed limb muscles are probably used much more incidentally (cf. Walmsley et al., 1978). Still, in spite of their great amount of usage per day, the twitch of eye muscles remains faster than that of the fastest hindlimb muscles (Cooper and Eccles, 1930). Hindlimb muscles become considerably slowed down by treatment with even moderate amounts (5% of total time) of pulse rates as fast as those commonly used by eye motoneurones (100 Hz; cf. Robinson, 1970; Fig. 6). Hence, it is unlikely that the twitch of the eye muscles remains brief, thanks to the high impulse rates of the extraocular motoneurones. Such comparisons strongly indicate that the effects of increased usage on twitch speed occur within a completely different "adaptive range" for eye and for limb muscles.

Summary

A survey is given of experimental results concerning the organization and properties of motoneurones and motor units of cat hindlimb. Particular attention is devoted to properties of importance for the rate- and recruitment-gradation of muscle force. Two kinds of motoneurone-muscle matching are described and analyzed: (i) the "speed-match" between the isometric speed of muscle fibres and intrinsic rhythmic properties (frequency range, late adaptation) of their motoneurones, (ii) the "recruitment-match" between contractile properties of muscle units (force, speed, endurance) and excitability-related intrinsic properties of their motoneurones. The most easily recruited motoneurones of a pool are generally known to be equipped with relatively weak, slow and fatigue-resistant muscle units. Experiments with long-term muscle activation suggest that this recruitment-match is (partly) produced by the fact that great amounts of daily activity tend to make muscle fibres weaker, slower and more fatigue resistant.

Acknowledgement

The investigations were supported in part by the Foundation for Medical Research (FUNGO), which is subsidized by the Netherlands Organization for the Advancement of Pure Research (ZWO).

References

Bawa, P., Binder, M. D., Ruenzel, P. and Henneman, E. (1984) Recruitment order of motoneurons in stretch reflexes is highly correlated with their axonal conduction velocity. J. Neurophysiol., 52: 410–420.

Brown, M. C. and Booth, C. M. (1983) Postnatal development of the adult pattern of motor axon distribution in rat muscle. Nature, 304: 741–742.

Burke, R. E. (1981) Motor units: anatomy, physiology and functional organization. In V. B. Brooks (Ed.), Handbook of Physiology — The Nervous System II, Part 1, American Physiological Society, Bethesda, MD, pp. 345–422.

Burke, R. E. and Nelson, P.G. (1971) Accommodation to current ramps in motoneurons of fast and slow twitch motor units. Int. J. Neurosci., 1, 347–356.

Burke, R. E., Levine, D. N., Zajac, F. E., Tsairis, P. and Engel, W. K. (1971) Mammalian motor units: physiological-histochemical correlation in three types in cat gastrocnemius. Science, 174: 709–712.

Burke, R. E., Levine, D. N., Tsairis, P. and Zajac, F. E. (1973) Physiological types and histochemical profiles in motor units of the cat gastrocnemius. J. Physiol. (Lond.), 234: 723–748.

Burke, R. E., Strick, P. L., Kanda, K., Kim, C. C. and Walmsley, B. (1977) Anatomy of medial gastrocnemius and soleus motor nuclei in cat spinal cord. J. Neurophysiol., 40: 667–680.

Burke, R. E., Dum, R. P., Fleshman, J. W., Glen, L. L., Lev-Tov, A., O'Donovan, M. J. and Pinter, M. J. (1982) An HRP study of the relation between cell size and motor unit type in cat ankle extensor motoneurons. J. Comp. Neurol., 209: 17–28.

Clamann, H. P. and Kukulka, C. G. (1977) The relation between size of motoneurons and their position in the cat spinal cord. J. Morphol., 153: 461–466.

Cooper, S. and Eccles, J. C. (1930) The isometric responses of mammalian muscles. J. Physiol. (Lond.), 69: 377–385.

Cullheim, S. (1978) Relations between cell body size, axon diameter and axon conduction velocity of cat sciatic alpha-motoneurons stained with horseradish peroxidase. Neurosci. Lett., 8: 17–20.

Denny-Brown, D. (1929) On the nature of postural reflexes. Proc. Roy. Soc. B, 104: 252–301.

Donselaar, Y., Kernell, D., Eerbeek, O. and Verhey, B. A. (1985) Somatotopic relations between spinal motoneurones and muscle fibres of the cat's m. peroneus longus. Brain Res., 335: 81–88.

Eccles, J. C., Eccles, R. M. and Lundberg, A. (1958) The action potentials of the alpha motoneurones supplying fast and slow muscles. J. Physiol. (Lond.), 142: 275–291.

Eerbeek, O., Kernell, D. and Verhey, B. A. (1984) Effects of fast and slow patterns of tonic long-term stimulation on contractile properties of fast muscle in the cat. J. Physiol. (Lond.), 352: 73–90.

Fleshman, J. W., Munson, J. B., Sypert, G. W. and Friedman, W. A. (1981) Rheobase, input resistance and motor-unit type in medial gastrocnemius motoneurons in the cat. J. Neurophysiol., 46: 1326–1338.

Granit, R., Kernell, D. and Shortess, G. K. (1963) The behaviour of mammalian motoneurones during long-lasting orthodromic, antidromic and trans-membrane stimulation. J. Physiol. (Lond.), 169: 743–754.

Grimby, L., Hannerz, J. and Hedman, B. (1979) Contraction time and voluntary discharge properties of individual short toe extensor motor units in man. J. Physiol. (Lond.), 289: 191–201.

Gustafsson, B. and Pinter, M. J. (1984a) Relations among passive electrical properties of lumbar alpha-motoneurones of the cat. J. Physiol. (Lond.), 356: 401–431.

Gustafsson, B. and Pinter, M. J. (1984b) An investigation of threshold properties among cat spinal alpha-motoneurones. J. Physiol. (Lond.), 357: 453–483.

Henneman, E. and Mendell, L. M. (1981) Functional organization of motoneuron pool and its inputs. In V. B. Brooks (Ed.), Handbook of Physiology — The Nervous System II, Part 1, American Physiological Society, Bethesda, MD, pp. 423–507.

Henneman, E. and Olson, C. B. (1965) Relations between structure and function in the design of skeletal muscle. J. Neurophysiol., 28: 581–598.

Henneman, E., Somjen, G. and Carpenter, D. O. (1965) Functional significance of cell size in spinal motoneurons. J. Neurophysiol., 28: 560–580.

Jami, L. and Petit, J. (1975) Correlation between axonal conduction velocity and tetanic tension of motor units in four muscles of the cat hind limb. Brain Res., 96: 114–118.

Kernell, D. (1965a) The adaptation and the relation between discharge frequency and current strength of cat lumbosacral motoneurones stimulated by long-lasting injected currents. Acta Physiol. Scand., 65: 65–73.

Kernell, D. (1965b) The limits of firing frequency in cat lumbosacral motoneurones possessing different time course of afterhyperpolarization. Acta Physiol. Scand., 65: 87–100.

Kernell, D. (1966) Input resistance, electrical excitability, and size of ventral horn cells in cat spinal cord. Science, 152: 1637–1640.

Kernell, D. (1979) Rhythmic properties of motoneurones innervating muscle fibres of different speed in m. gastrocnemius medialis of the cat. Brain Res., 160: 159–162.

Kernell, D. (1984) The meaning of discharge rate: excitation-to-frequency transduction as studied in spinal motoneurones. Arch. Ital. Biol., 122: 5–15.

Kernell, D. and Monster, A. W. (1981) Threshold current for repetitive impulse firing in motoneurones innervating muscle fibres of different fatigue sensitivity in the cat. Brain Res., 229: 193–196.

Kernell, D. and Monster, A. W. (1982a) Time course and properties of late adaptation in spinal motoneurones in the cat. Exp. Brain Res., 46: 191–196.

Kernell, D. and Monster, A. W. (1982b) Motoneurone properties and motor fatigue. An intracellular study of gastrocnemius motoneurones of the cat. Exp. Brain Res., 46: 197–204.

Kernell, D. and Sjöholm, H. (1975) Recruitment and firing rate modulation of motor unit tension in a small muscle of the cat's foot. Brain Res., 98: 57–72.

Kernell, D. and Zwaagstra, B. (1981) Input conductance, axonal conduction velocity and cell size among hindlimb motoneurones of the cat. Brain Res., 204: 311–326.

Kernell, D., Eerbeek, O., Donselaar, Y. and Verhey, B. A. (1983a) Effects of moderate amounts of fast and slow rates of chronic stimulation on the contractile properties of a fast hindlimb muscle in the cat. Proc. Int. Union Physiol. Sci., 15: 189.

Kernell, D., Eerbeek, O. and Verhey, B. A. (1983b) Motor unit categorization on basis of contractile properties: an experimental analysis of the composition of the cat's m. peroneus longus. Exp. Brain Res., 50: 211–219.

Kernell, D., Eerbeek, O. and Verhey, B. A. (1983c) Relation between isometric force and stimulus rate in cat's hindlimb motor units of different twitch contraction time. Exp. Brain Res., 50: 220–227.

Kernell, D., Verhey, B. A. and Eerbeek, O. (1985) Neuronal and muscle unit properties at different rostro-caudal levels of cat's motoneurone pool. Brain Res., 335: 71–79.

Lømo, T., Westgaard, R. H. and Engebretsen, L. (1980) Different stimulation patterns affect contractile properties of denervated rat soleus muscles. In D. Pette (Ed.), Plasticity of Muscle, Walter de Gruyter and Co., Berlin, pp. 297–309.

Lüscher, H.-R., Ruenzel, P. and Henneman, E. (1979) How the size of motoneurones determines their susceptibility to discharge. Nature, 282: 859–861.

Lüscher, H.-R., Ruenzel, P. and Henneman, E. (1980) Topographic distribution of terminals of IA and group II fibers in spinal cord, as revealed by postsynaptic population potentials. J. Neurophysiol., 43: 968–985.

Pinter, M. J., Curtis, R. L. and Hosko, M. J. (1983) Voltage threshold and excitability among variously sized cat hindlimb motoneurons. J. Neurophysiol., 50: 644–657.

Robinson, D. A. (1970) Oculomotor unit behavior in the monkey. J. Neurophysiol., 33: 393–404.

Salmons, S. and Henriksson. J. (1981) The adaptive response of skeletal muscle to increased use. Muscle Nerve, 4: 94–105.

Salmons, S. and Vrbová, G. (1969) The influence of activity on some contractile characteristics of mammalian fast and slow muscles. J. Physiol. (Lond.), 201: 535–549.

Schwindt, P. C. and Crill, W. E. (1980) Properties of a persistent inward current in normal and TEA-injected motoneurons. J. Neurophysiol., 43: 1700–1724.

Sokolove, P. G. and Cooke, I. M. (1971) Inhibition of impulse activity in a sensory neuron by an electrogenic pump. J. Gen. Physiol., 57: 125–163.

Swett, J. E., Eldred, E. and Buchwald, J. S. (1970) Somatotopic cord-to-muscle relations in efferent innervation of cat gastrocnemius. Am. J. Physiol., 219: 762–766.

Ulfhake, B. and Kellerth, J.-O. (1982) Does alpha-motoneurone size correlate with motor unit type in cat triceps surae? Brain Res., 251: 201–209.

Walmsley, B., Hodgson, J. A. and Burke, R. E. (1978) Forces produced by medial gastrocnemius and soleus muscles during locomotion in freely moving cats. J. Neurophysiol., 41: 1203–1216.

Zwaagstra, B. and Kernell, D. (1980) The duration of after-hyperpolarization in hindlimb alpha motoneurones of different sizes in the cat. Neurosci. Lett., 19: 303–307.

Extraocular motoneuron behavior in synergistic action

K. Hepp and V. Henn

Physics Department, Swiss Federal Institute of Technology, and Neurology Department, University of Zürich, CH-8093 Zürich, Switzerland

Introduction

The oculomotor system is unique and different from all skeletomotor systems in several aspects. It is a two-ball-joint system equipped with a set of 12 muscles which over a limited range operate in six rotatory degrees of freedom in the configuration space of two rotators. Although there is no mechanical coupling between the two eyes, the central innervation reduces the number of degrees of freedom. For example, conjugate eye movements obeying Listing's law (cyclotorsion uniquely determined by horizontal and vertical eye position) have only two degrees of freedom. Due to the small inertia of the almost spherical eye in its well protected enclosure, eye movements can be very rapid and very precise. The force needed to execute the same eye movements at different times remains constant, within small limits. This led to the creation of models which can be checked against actual measurements.

Dynamics of eye movements in one dimension

Robinson was the first to describe the basic innervation pattern which extraocular muscles need in order to execute different eye movement programs (Robinson, 1964, 1975a). Single cell recordings in alert monkeys (Fuchs and Luschei, 1970; Schiller, 1970; Keller and Robinson, 1972; Henn and Cohen, 1972) and electromyographic recordings in humans (Collins et al., 1975) confirmed the basic concept of a tonic discharge as a function of eye position and a phasic component related to velocity during slow or rapid movements. Several reviews of eye movement organization have been published recently (Carpenter, 1977; Robinson, 1982; Henn et al., 1982; Leigh and Zee, 1983); the cellular organization of extraocular motoneurons has been reviewed by Keller (1981), and the anatomy and role of extraocular sensory afferents has been surveyed by Porter et al. (1983).

The basic equation to describe motoneuron behavior (Robinson, 1975a) has the form

$$f(t - \tau) = a(p(t) - p_0) + b\dot{p}(t) + c\ddot{p}(t) \quad (1)$$

where f is the firing rate of the motoneuron, p the component of eye position (e.g., one direction angle of the visual axis) in the pulling direction of the respective muscle, $\dot{p}$ the velocity, $\ddot{p}$ the acceleration at time t with a time delay τ of approximately 5 mseconds. Average values are: position sensitivity, $a = 4$ Hz/deg; velocity sensitivity, $b = 1$ Hz/deg/sec; and acceleration sensitivity, $c = 0.01$ Hz/deg/sec^2. The above equation is typical for a temporal code which relates the firing rate of a motoneuron to the trajectory of the eye. The equation is a very useful first approximation to explain many neuro-ophthalmological observations. Below we shall discuss aspects of behavior which cannot be reduced to this equation. In order to generalize this equation to include different programs of eye movements into arbitrary directions, a more complex description

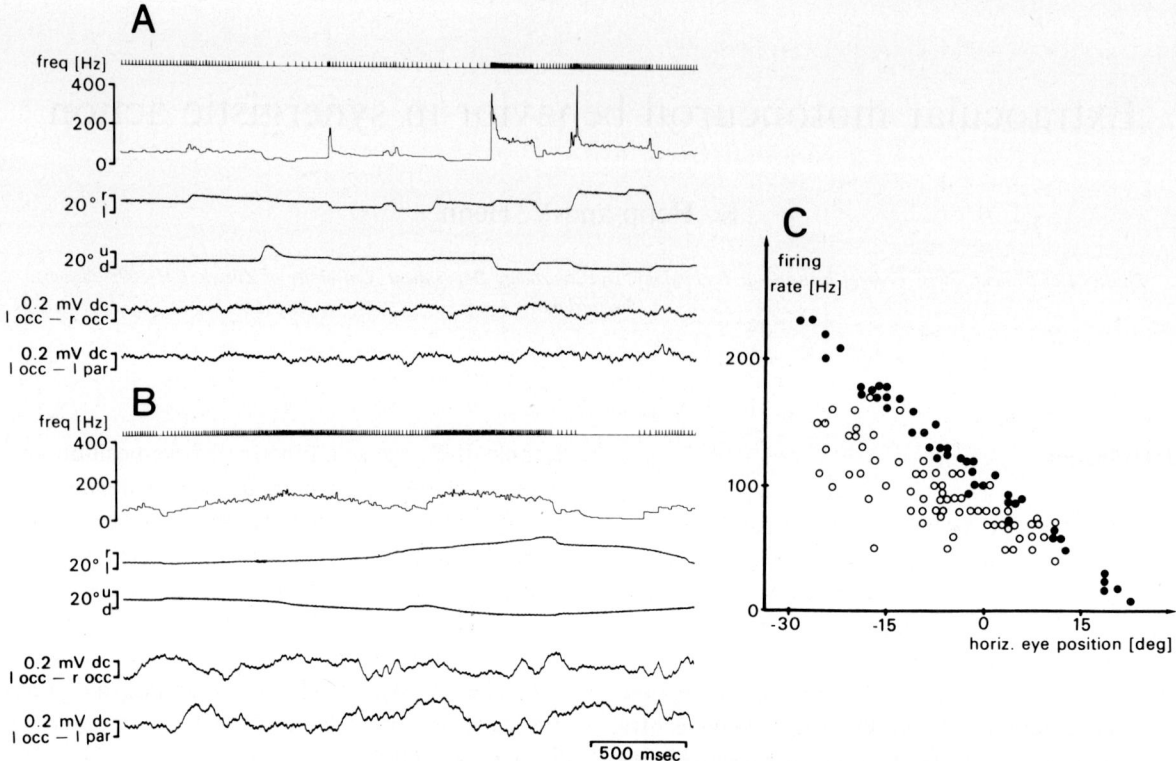

Fig. 1. A and B are recordings from the same trochlear motoneuron during wakefulness (A) and light sleep (B). From above, blips indicating the occurrence of a spike, instantaneous firing rate of the neuron, horizontal and vertical eye position, and electroencephalographic traces. C. Rate-position relation for a medial rectus motoneuron during alertness (filled circles) and light sleep (open circles). From Henn et al. (1984).

is necessary, as well as more precise neurophysiological measurements, including all freedoms of rotations of the eyes. For example, f is not only dependent on the direction of the visual axis, but will vary with cyclotorsion.

State of alertness

Just as a drifting pattern of slow eye movements indicates decreased vigilance before falling asleep, the firing rate of motoneurons is strongly dependent on the state of alertness (Henn et al., 1984). In the state of light sleep, input to the motoneurons is reduced and the co-contraction of eye muscles is relaxed. From this state of light sleep the animal can immediately switch back to alertness, usually accompanied by a saccade. Firing rates in motoneurons then immediately return to their normal alert state values described in equation 1. The difference between alertness and light sleep is shown in Figs. 1A and B for a trochlear motoneuron. In Fig. 1C the rate position relation for a medial rectus motoneuron is shown during fixation. Filled circles were measurements in the alert state and open circles in states of light sleep. The fact that for a certain eye position the firing rate cannot exceed the value as determined by equation 1 has to be explained by the neural control of the "integrator" which provides the tonic input to the motoneurons.

Hysteresis

There is an ongoing discussion about hysteresis phenomena leading to higher frequencies when a given position has been reached from the off-direction. Eckmiller (1974) originally reported an effect on the firing rate in the order of 10%. From Fig. 1 it becomes clear that for such experiments the state of alertness has to be carefully monitored and eye position has to be measured with a higher precision than is possible with skin electrodes. Results from recent experiments incorporating such controls by Goldstein and Robinson (1982) arrive at much smaller — and at times negligible — values.

Absence of breaking pulse

For rapid limb movements Wachholder and Altenburg (1926; reviewed in Hallett and Marsden, 1979) found an acceleration burst of innervation in the agonist muscle, then a deceleration burst in the antagonist and finally another agonist burst. We have rarely found a significant breaking activity in the antagonist at the end of a saccade without a corresponding overshoot. Such a breaking activity can be found in burst and burst-tonic premotor neurons of the oculomotor system (see, e.g., Figs. 1B and 2 of Van Gisbergen et al., 1981), but the damping and the innervation of the eye is extremely well balanced so that such a signal is not needed for the extraocular muscles.

Frequency saturation in motoneurons

An important non-linear correction to equation 1 is the saturation of the firing rate in motoneurons during saccades. During large rapid movements maximum velocities of 800 deg/sec over about 20 mseconds can be reached. Eye acceleration is then negligible due to the small value of c. The maximal burst rate of a typical motoneuron is about 500 Hz, while equation 1 would predict a typical rate of 800 Hz. On the right side of Fig. 2 we have analyzed the stationary velocity-firing rate of a motoneuron during large saccades with different velocities (ranging from 300 to 800 deg/sec) at fixed eye position and with negligible acceleration or deceleration corrections. In this range, the firing rate only varied from 300 to 500 Hz.

Saccade interaction with vestibulo-ocular reflex

The discussion above has been restricted to eye movements when the monkey's head was fixed.

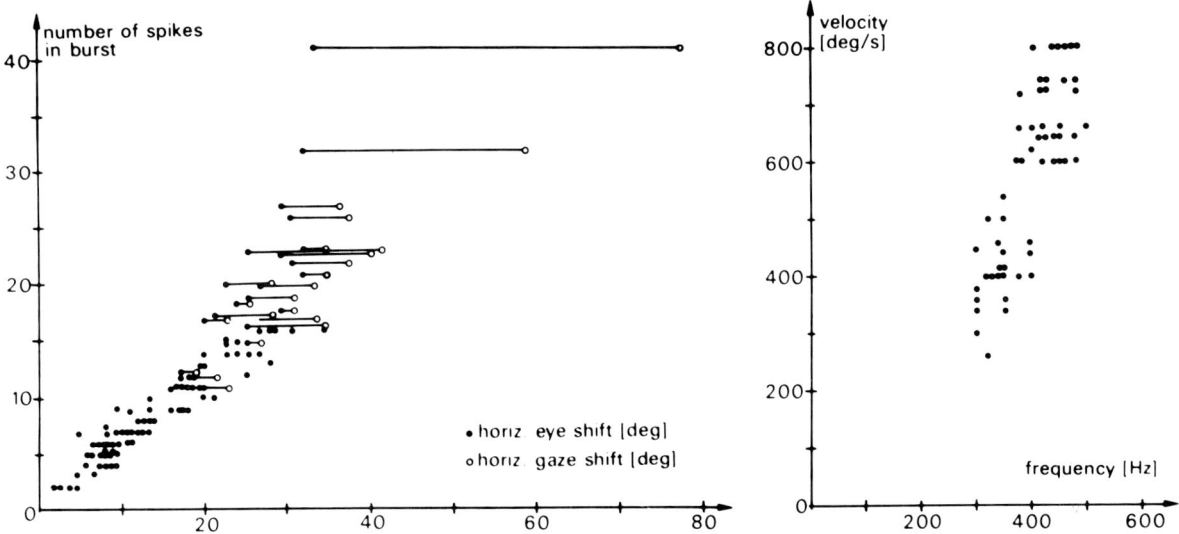

Fig. 2. Left. Horizontal eye or gaze shift (connected by a line) versus number of spikes in the burst of a motoneuron. Right. Average frequency in the burst of a motoneuron versus average velocity, taken over an interval of 10 mseconds, which is separated by at least 10 mseconds from the saccade on- and off-set. In this interval the frequency and velocity were approximately constant.

When the head is free to move in the horizontal plane, there is dynamic interaction between saccade motor programs and the vestibulo-ocular reflex (VOR). There is still controversy to what extent during combined eye-head movements the VOR superimposes on the saccade and thus slows it when both go into the same direction during voluntary movements, or whether, particularly during large movements, the VOR is shut off. There are certainly many examples when saccades are slowed during synergistic head movements (Morasso et al., 1973). The left side of Fig. 2 shows recordings from a motoneuron related either to eye shift (filled circles) or gaze shift (i.e., head plus eye shift, open circles) in an alert monkey.

Whereas for saccades up to about 20 degrees amplitude the relation between number of spikes in a burst and movement component in the pulling direction of the respective muscle can be approximated by a straight line (Fig. 2, left side), for larger movements the frequency saturation of motoneurons around 500 Hz introduces a systematic deviation from this relationship. If, instead of the eye movement component, the gaze shift (eye plus head movement) is plotted against number of spikes (open circles), the points obtained can be approximated by a straight line. This, of course, makes no sense as extraocular motoneurons cannot move the head. It teaches us one thing in the search for neurons which might code eye, head or gaze movements: If a relation between neuronal activity and one movement parameter yields a more linear relation than with another movement parameter, such a relation does not necessarily imply causality. Therefore, any such investigations have to be coupled with anatomical and lesion studies. For motoneurons, such information is available, and for central structures we have always stressed the need for such comparative studies to arrive at valid interpretations. Therefore, we are very reluctant to accept the hypothesis of a class of medium-lead burst neurons representing "gaze-shift" as proposed by Whittington et al. (1984).

Two-dimensional representation of eye movements

Points in a two-dimensional plane can be represented in a Cartesian or in a polar coordinate system. We chose a Cartesian coordinate system with the anterior axis in the primary direction of the eye orthogonal to a horizontal and vertical orbital direction. Then, the horizontal eye deviation h is the angle by which the anterior-vertical plane has to be rotated around the vertical axis to pass through a given visual direction, and similarly the vertical eye deviation v is the angle for the rotation of the anterior-horizontal plane around the horizontal axis. Up to small corrections, (h,v) are the polar coordinates of Robinson (1975b).

As pointed out above, the degrees of freedom of eye movements are clearly reduced relative to the movements which are possible mechanically. It has been suggested that this is due primarily to restrictions in the innervation pattern. To obtain more quantitative information, we recorded from motoneurons while the animals were trained to shift their fixation systematically through all secondary and tertiary eye positions (Hepp and Henn, 1985). As a first result we will describe the relationship between static firing rate, f, and eye position. Recordings were obtained from axons of the IIIrd, IVth, and VIth nerves. Fig. 3 gives a typical result from a trochlear motoneuron. The horizontal plane rep-

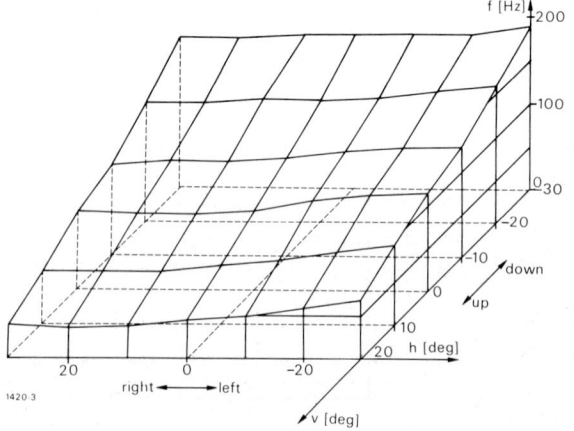

Fig. 3. Innervation surface of a trochlear motoneuron. The horizontal plane represents eye position and the elevation above the firing rate at the respective eye positions.

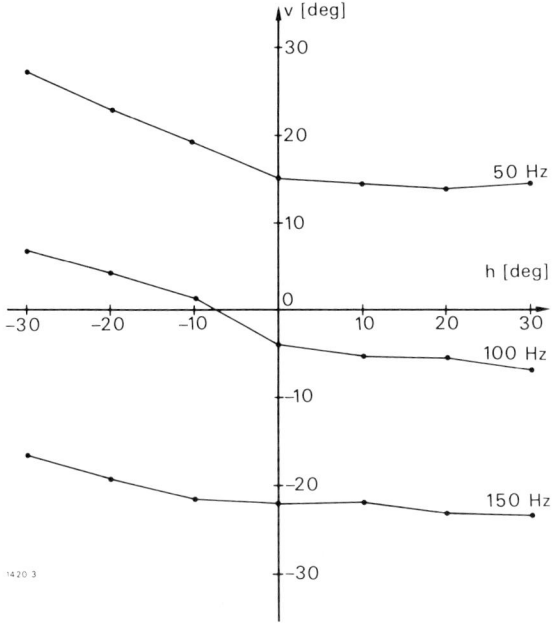

Fig. 4. Iso-frequency curves of the same trochlear motoneuron as shown in Fig. 3.

resents eye position and the elevation of the surface above the respective firing rate. A more transparent representation of the same data is given by iso-frequency curves which are the intersections of the *f-h-v* surface (the innervation surface) at fixed values of *f* as shown in Fig. 4. The innervation gradient of this neuron is directed orthogonally to this family of iso-frequency curves and points downward in the

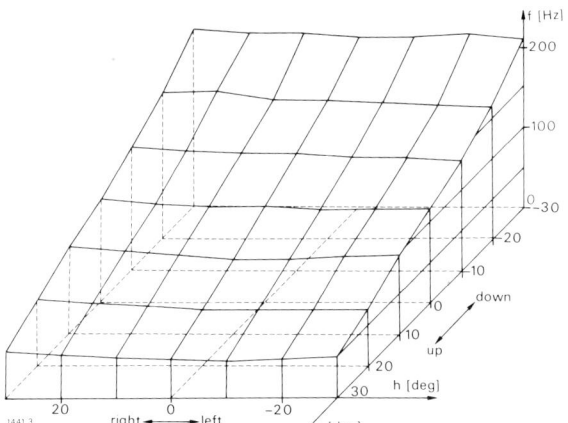

Fig. 5. Innervation surface of an inferior rectus motoneuron.

medial and downward and 20 degrees outwards in the lateral hemifield. Notice that the curves are convex from the low frequency side and are remarkably parallel. Figs. 5 and 6 give a similar sample for a typical inferior rectus motoneuron. Note that the curves are almost parallel to the horizontal in the lateral hemifield and only slightly curved in the medial hemifield. We were not able to separate motoneurons for upward pulling muscles, as fibers for superior rectus and inferior oblique lie intermingled in the oculomotor nerve. In our sample of motoneurons with upward on-directions it is remarkable that curves at low frequencies tend to be concave, and at higher frequencies form straight lines (Figs. 7 and 8). Curves do not fall into two families of mirror images to inferior rectus and trochlear neurons. This poses the question to what extent vertical neurons can be paired to form antagonistic yoke muscles and whether they obey Sherington's law of antagonistic innervation. Medial and lateral rectus motoneurons display iso-frequency curves which in mid-position are essentially straight lines running almost parallel to the vertical meridian.

The question of how muscles should be yoked in antagonistic pairs cannot be judged directly from

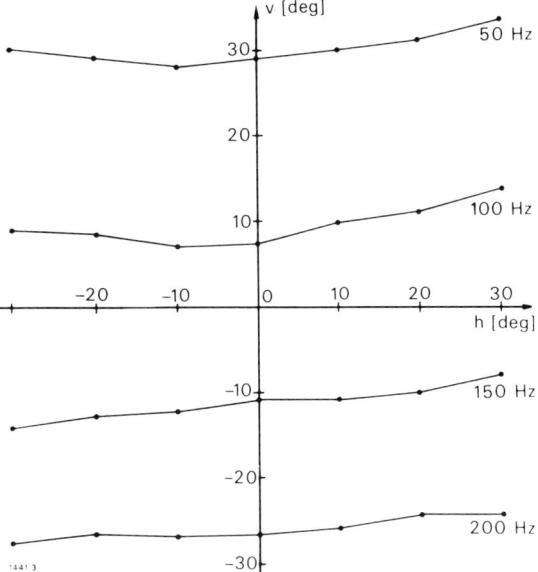

Fig. 6. Iso-frequency curves of the inferior rectus motoneuron as shown in Fig. 5.

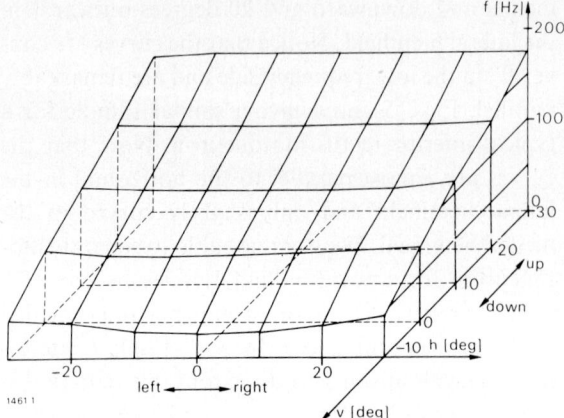

Fig. 7. Innervation surface of a motoneuron with an upward on-direction.

our curves in the h-v plane. This would have to be computed from the innervation as a function of muscle length which we have not made, since for the monkey the length-position data are not available. For humans, Robinson (1975b) has computed the iso-innervation curves of all six eye muscles, with pairing of the horizontal recti, the vertical recti and the vertical obliques. Our curves are qualitatively similar, but show some systematic deviations. The question has not been solved of how rigid the antagonistic pairing is far away from primary position. Also, vestibular projections prove to be more complex than the original idea of connecting one canal with one yoked muscle pair for each eye. For instance, in the cat, and probably also in monkey and man, the anterior canal excites disynaptically both superior recti and the contralateral inferior oblique, and inhibits both inferior recti and the contralateral superior oblique (Uchino et al., 1980, reviewed in Ito, 1984). Clearly, one sees from the very different iso-frequency curves of inferior rectus and superior oblique that there is no rigid yoking of the left inferior rectus muscle with the right trochlear muscle. We think that during conjugate eye movements which obey Listing's law, namely during fixation and saccades, the visual system generates an eye displacement signal which is transformed into sustained activity in motoneurons by the integrators for the different muscles, where position-dependent corrections are added by adaptive circuits through the cerebellum (see Vilis and Hore, Section IVB).

Which central signal is required by a motoneuron?

For generation of rapid eye movements, the medium-lead burst neurons seem to be the essential link to transmit their information via an integrator to motoneurons. Medium-lead burst neurons carry an eye displacement signal in the respective pulling directions of motoneurons. As an aid to compare further the behavior of motoneurons and medium-lead burster, we present the analysis of a trochlear motoneuron (Fig. 9). The change of firing rate $\Delta f = f_2 - f_1$, between two fixations (f_1, h_1, v_1) and (f_2, h_2, v_2) is plotted as a function of the gaze shift $(\Delta h, \Delta v) = (h_2 - h_1, v_2 - v_1)$. Such measurements might be useful in deciding whether fixed populations of pre-motor neurons are coupled to fixed populations of motoneurons. This leads to the more general question of how angular acceleration in three-dimensional space as detected by the vestibular system is tranformed via a minimum of only

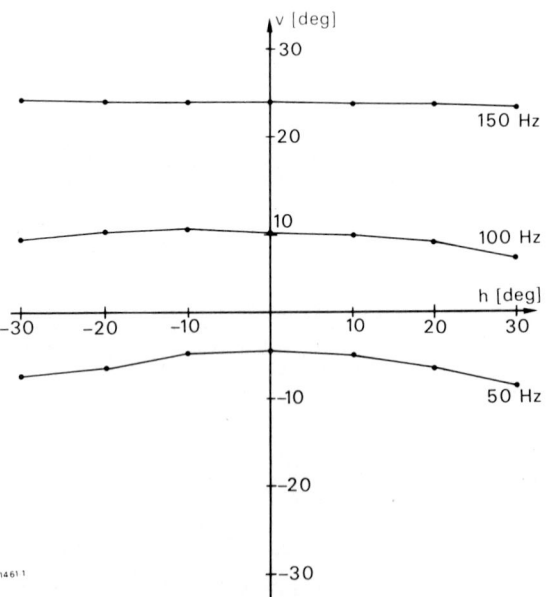

Fig. 8. Iso-frequency curves of the motoneuron shown in Fig. 7 with an upward on-direction.

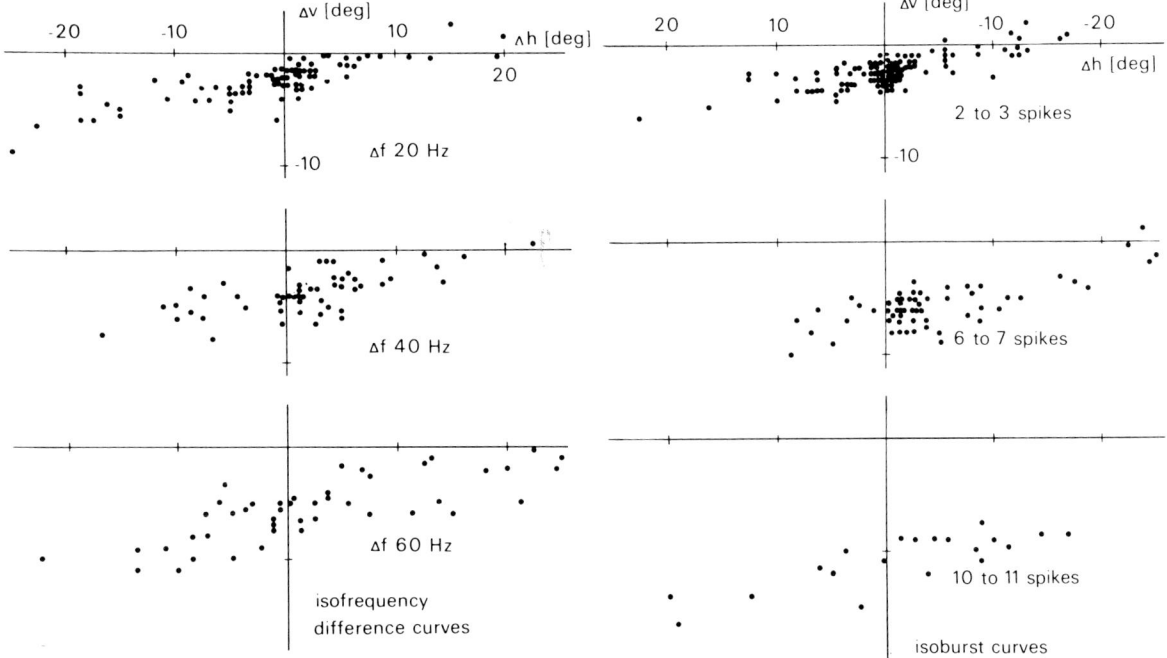

Fig. 9. Iso-frequency difference curves (left) and iso-burst curves (right) for a trochlear motoneuron. Instead of absolute values, differences in motoneuron activity are plotted. Therefore, these values correspond to the distance between iso-frequency curves. One obtains almost straight lines, indicating that iso-frequncy lines are shifted almost in parallel for different levels of activation. From Henn et al. (1982).

two synapses to a compensatory eye movement, and whether the vestibular coordinate system defined by the orientation of the three semi-circular canals constitutes the general reference system for the nervous system to code angular movement in space. To decide this we would need precise measurements of the geometry of the labyrinths and eye muscle insertions. It seems that there are enough deviations from a strictly orthogonal Cartesian coordinate system that we have to check the alternative solution that on the sensory input side the vestibular and visual systems use their own specialized systems to represent space as compared to motor output systems. We would propose that in this direction much can still be learnt from peripheral systems about central organization.

Summary and conclusions

As a first approximation firing rate in extraocular motoneurons is linearly related to eye position, velocity, and acceleration if movement in the respective on-direction of a motoneuron is considered. However, there are systematic deviations: the firing frequency often saturates in single neurons; during interaction with the vestibulo-ocular reflex saccades are frequently slowed down, if the head is free to move; and in states of reduced alertness neuronal activity changes in specific ways. Empirically, Listing's law has been found to describe well cyclotorsion as a function of eye position. This reduces the theoretical six degrees of freedom for the eyes during conjugate gaze down to two. To investigate how eye muscles interact to move and hold the eyes in tertiary position, we recorded motoneuron activity and presented results as iso-frequency curves indicating all possible eye positions for a given frequency in a motoneuron. This gives a picture of how motoneurons interact in a synergistic fashion to hold the eyes in tertiary positions.

References

Carpenter, R. H. S. (1977) Movements of the Eyes, Pion, London.

Collins, C. C., O'Meara, D. and Scott, A. B. (1975) Muscle tension during unrestrained human eye movements. J. Physiol. (Lond.), 245: 351–369.

Eckmiller, R. (1974) Hysteresis in the static characteristics of eye position coded neurons in the alert monkey. Pflügers Arch., 350: 249–258.

Fuchs, A. F. and Luschei, E. S. (1970) Firing patterns of abducens neurons of alert monkeys in relationship to horizontal eye movement. J. Neurophysiol., 33: 382–392.

Goldstein, H. P. and Robinson, D. A. (1982) The fine structure of oculomotor motoneuron activity during saccades. Soc. Neurosci., 8: 156.

Hallett, M. and Marsden, C. D. (1979) Ballistic flexion movements of the human thumb. J. Physiol. (Lond.), 294: 33–50.

Henn, V. and Cohen, B. (1972) Eye muscle motor neurons with different functional characteristics. Brain Res., 45: 561–568.

Henn, V., Büttner-Ennever, J. A. and Hepp, K. (1982) The primate oculomotor system. I. Motoneurons. A synthesis of anatomical, physiological, and clinical data. Human Neurobiol., 1: 77–85.

Henn, V., Baloh, R. W. and Hepp, K. (1984) The sleep-wake transition in the oculomotor system. Exp. Brain Res., 54: 166–176.

Hepp, K. and Henn, V. (1985) Iso-frequency curves of oculomotor neurons in the Rhesus monkey. Vision Res., 25: 493–499.

Ito, M. (1984) The Cerebellum and Neural Control, Raven Press, New York.

Keller, E. L. (1981) Oculomotor neuron behavior. In B. L. Zuber (Ed.), Models of Oculomotor Behavior and Control, CRC Press, Boca Raton, FL, pp. 1–19.

Keller, E. L. and Robinson, D. A. (1972) Abducens unit behavior in the monkey during vergence movements. Vision Res., 12: 369–382.

Leigh, R. J. and Zee, D. S. (1983) The Neurology of Eye Movements, Davis, Philadelphia.

Morasso, P. Bizzi, E. and Dichgans, J. (1973) Adjustment of saccade characteristics during head movements. Exp. Brain Res., 16: 492–500.

Porter, J. D., Guthrie, B. L. and Sparks, D. L. (1983) Innervation of monkey extraocular muscles: localization of sensory and motor neurons by retrograde transport of horseradish peroxidase. J. Comp. Neurol., 218: 208–219.

Robinson, D. A. (1964) The mechanics of human saccadic eye movement. J. Physiol. (Lond.), 174: 245–264.

Robinson, D. A. (1975a) Oculomotor control signals. In G. Lennerstrand and P. Bach-y-Rita (Eds.), Basic Mechanisms of Ocular Motility and Their Clinical Implications, Pergamon Press, Oxford, pp. 337–374.

Robinson, D. A. (1975b) A quantitative analysis of extraocular muscle cooperation and squint. Inv. Ophthal., 14: 801–825.

Robinson, D. A. (1982) Control of eye movements. In Handbook of Physiology, The Nervous System, Vol. II/2, American Physiological Society, Bethesda, MD, pp. 1275–1320.

Schiller, P. H. (1970) The discharge characteristics of single units in the oculomotor and abducens nuclei of the unanesthetized monkey. Exp. Brain Res., 10: 347–362.

Uchino, Y., Suzuki, S. and Watanabe, S. (1980) Vertical semicircular canal inputs to cat extraocular motoneurons. Exp. Brain Res., 41: 45–53.

Van Gisbergen, J. A. M., Robinson, D. A. and Gielen, S. (1981) A quantitative analysis of saccadic eye movements by burst neurons. J. Neurophysiol., 45: 417–442.

Wacholder, K. and Altenburg, H. (1926) Beiträge zur Physiologie der willkürlichen Bewegung. XI. Mitteilung. Ueber die Genese der Antagonistentätigkeit. Pflügers Arch., 215: 622–626.

Whittington, D. A., Lestienne, F. and Bizzi, E. (1984) Behavior of preoculomotor burst neurons during eye-head coordination. Exp. Brain Res., 55: 215–222.

Transmitter-controlled properties of α-motoneurones causing long-lasting motor discharge to brief excitatory inputs

J. Hounsgaard, H. Hultborn and O. Kiehn

Department of Neurophysiology, The Panum Institute, Blegdamsvej 3, DK-2200 Copenhagen, Denmark

Introduction

Brief sensory inputs to intact conscious subjects commonly trigger complex long-lasting motor responses in which higher cerebral mechanisms — or even voluntary action — may be integrative parts. However, long-lasting motor discharge following brief afferent stimulation is also observed in reduced preparations, such as decerebrate or spinal animals. In his book "Integrative action of the nervous system" Sherrington (1906) described the after-discharge in the flexion reflex and the crossed extension reflex. He wrote that a "characteristic difference between conduction in nerve-trunks and in reflex-arcs is the less close correspondence in the latter between moment of cessation of stimulus and moment of cessation of end effect. The reflex-arc shows marked "after-discharge", the nerve-trunk does not". He gave examples of reflex contractions that persisted for 5 seconds or more after the cessation of the stimulus (see further, in Creed et al., 1932). Forbes (1922) suggested that the persisting motor discharge was due to "delay paths" in the spinal cord, by which the motoneurones could receive a long-lasting bombardment of excitatory impulses in response to a single afferent volley. If these delay paths were organized with recurrent excitatory connections reverberating activity in closed loops could provide a maintained excitatory drive of motoneurones (cf. Forbes, 1929).

Reverberating activity in closed neuronal loops has been postulated to be an important integral mechanism underlying various phenomena, ranging from temporal integration in the vestibulo-ocular reflex (Robinson, 1968, 1971) to maintenance of "initial" memory (Hebb, 1949). Such far-reaching notions stand in sharp contrast to the virtual absence of experimental evidence for sustained reverberating activity in well-defined neuronal circuits (however, cf. Tsukahara, 1972).

In 1975 Hultborn et al. described that selective stimulation of muscle spindle Ia afferents could trigger a motor discharge of maintained duration to the same (homonymous) and synergic muscles. Because of the well-defined input and output, it seemed within reach to identify and analyse the network supposed to maintain reverberating activity. However, in our recent analysis of this phenomenon (Hounsgaard and Kiehn, 1985; Hounsgaard et al., 1984) we found that the sustained motor discharge was caused by intrinsic membrane properties of the motoneurones themselves, rather than reverberating activity in interneuronal loops.

Results

Motor discharge of maintained duration evoked by impulses in muscle spindle Ia afferents

Many years ago Granit and his collaborators (1957)

discovered that repeated brief pulls of the triceps muscles potentiated the tonic stretch reflex during a subsequent ramp-and-hold stretch. Since this potentiation by brief pulls was shared for several different reflexes to triceps (the tonic stretch-reflex, the crossed extensor reflex and the pinna reflex) they interpreted their finding as being due to a (post-tetanic) potentiation at a common pre-motoneuronal level. Almost 20 years later, Hultborn et al. (1975) observed a phenomenon which almost certainly was an expression of the same basic mechanism. They found that a short train of brief stretches (vibration; typically 100 μm at 200 Hz for 100–1000 mseconds) to the appropriately prestretched soleus muscle, in the decerebrated cat, triggered a sustained increase in the EMG activity in addition to the ordinary short latency (monosynaptic) response (Hultborn et al., 1975; Hultborn and Wigström, 1980). Since an amplitude of vibration as small as 10 μm was sufficient, the effect was attributed to activation of muscle spindle Ia afferents (Lundberg and Winsbury, 1960; Fetz et al., 1979). From these results it was still uncertain whether the maintained activity was due to mechanisms in the CNS. It could also be explained by a positive feedback through a peripheral loop including Ia afferents, fusimotor neurones (γ- or β-motoneurones) and muscle spindles. However, direct recording from the Ia afferents refuted this notion (Hultborn and Wigström, 1980); actually, their firing frequency decreased (by unloading) rather than increased as required if the long-lasting motor activity was maintained through the peripheral loop.

The necessity and importance of central mechanisms for the maintenance of prolonged excitation was established in experiments in which the fusimotor-loop was opened either by curarization or by sectioning the soleus nerve (Hultborn and Wigström, 1980). In these experiments the prolonged excitability increase was monitored by recording the efferent activity from the peripheral motor nerves (electroneurogram, ENG). Fig. 1 illustrates the rectified ENG from the nerve to the soleus muscle (SOL) following a train of group I volleys in the nerve from the medial gastrocnemius (MG). As expected from the pattern of monosynaptic Ia excitation (Eccles et al., 1957), a strong activity in the SOL nerve was evoked during the MG train. The surprising finding was the maintained activity after the stimulus period. On many occasions the prolonged activity slowly fell off, but under "optimal" conditions — seen in most animals for at least some time — the activity outlasting the excitatory stimulus stayed at a constant level even for several minutes. In such cases the motor discharge could be terminated, at any time, by a short train of stimuli to group II muscle afferents or cutaneous afferents. Fig. 1 illustrates that a brief train of stimuli to the nerves from peroneus brevis and tertius muscle (Per) reset the activity to the level seen before the MG group I train. In the following we will refer to trains of stimuli to Ia afferents and to high threshold muscle afferents/cutaneous afferents as the "on" stimulus and "off" stimulus, respectively (cf. Fig. 1).

The experiments described above demonstrated the existence of a central mechanism that maintained a lasting excitability increase when activated

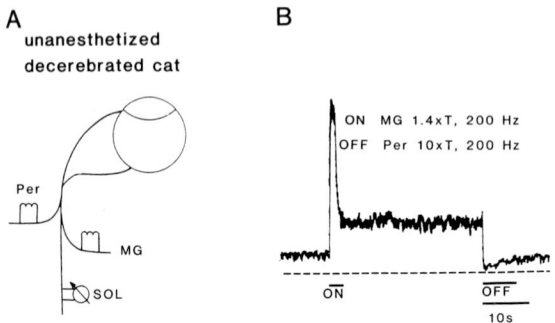

Fig. 1. Long-lasting excitability increase in SOL motoneurones following a stimulus train to the MG nerve. A. Experimental arrangement. Unanesthetized, anaemically decerebrate preparation. the nerves to medial gastrocnemius (MG) and peroneus brevis/tertius (Per) were mounted for stimulation and the soleus nerve (SOL) for recording. B. Rectified and filtered SOL electroneurogram (ENG). The interrupted time below the record shows the baseline with no ENG activity. The timing of the "on" stimulus (MG, 1.4 × cf2 T, 200 Hz) and "off" stimulus (Per, 10 × T, 200 Hz) are shown by thick lines below the record. The strength of stimulation is expressed in multiples of threshold ($\times T$) for the lowest threshold afferent fibres. (Crone, Hultborn and Mazieres, unpublished data.)

by a train in Ia afferents. Since all the experiments discussed above were performed on decerebrate cats (either intercollicular decerebration or anaemic decerebration ad modum, Pollock and Davis, 1930) it was an open question in which part of the remaining CNS this mechanism was located. Since an acute spinal transection at lower thoracic level immediately abolished the long-lasting excitability increase by an "on" stimulus (Hultborn and Wigström, 1980), the brainstem seemed to be involved either by mediating the effect or by maintaining a supraspinal facilitation of primarily intrinsic spinal mechanisms. Several years ago it was demonstrated (Engberg et al., 1968b) that an active serotonergic raphe-spinal projection is of importance for maintaining the control of spinal mechanisms in the decerebrate state. Therefore, we tested whether the serotonin blocker methysergide (3 mg/kg, intravenously) interfered with the long-lasting excitability increase following an "on" stimulus. Indeed, sustained firing was abolished, thus implying that the serotonergic system was normally involved. In addition to these "negative signs", following interruption of serotonergic transmission there is also positive support for the involvement of the serotonergic system. Intravenous administration of the serotonin precursor 5-hydroxytryptophan (5-HTP) is supposed to cause transmitter liberation from serotonergic nerve terminals (cf. Andén et al., 1964). When 5-HTP (50–100 mg/kg) is given to acute spinal preparations several aspects of the decerebrate control of spinal mechanisms are restored (Engberg et al., 1968a; Ahlman et al., 1971). Following this treatment it was also possible to elicit the long-last-

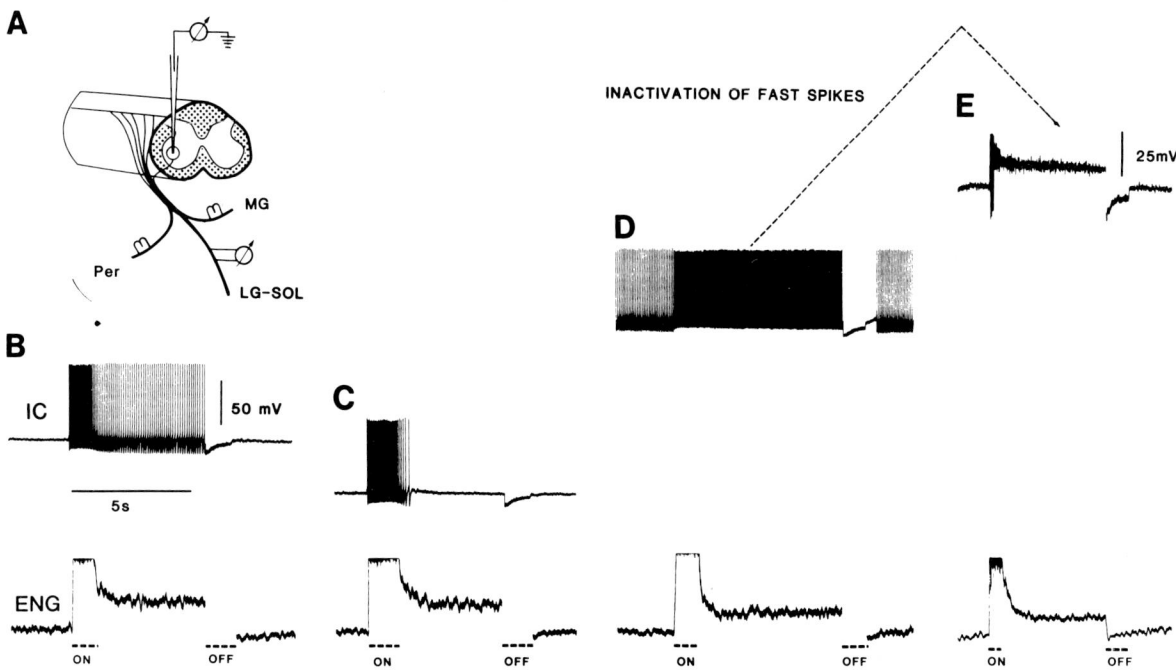

Fig. 2. Sustained shifts in excitability of cat α-motoneurones triggered by postsynaptic excitation and inhibition. A. Experimental arrangement. Same preparation as in Fig. 1. B–E show simultaneous recording from a sampled motoneurone (intracellular, IC, upper traces) and from the nerve (ENG, lower traces) innervating the lateral gastrocnemius and soleus (LG-SOL) muscles. The excitability increase is induced and terminated by short trains of stimuli to the MG nerve and Per nerve, respectively. The timing of the "on" stimulus (MG, $1.7 \times T$, 300 Hz) and the "off" stimulus (Per, $10 \times T$, 200 Hz) are marked by interrupted lines below the ENG. The upper traces in B–E show the intracellular responses to "on" and "off" stimuli at different holding potentials. Voltage calibrations refer to intracellular recordings. Time calibration in B applies for all records. Records in B, C and D are from the same cell. Adapted from Hounsgaard et al. (1984).

ing excitability increase (Fig. 6), suggesting that the serotonergic system was indeed of pivotal importance (Hultborn and Wigström, 1980). The experiments also demonstrated that the basic mechanism responsible for the maintenance of the excitability increase was located at segmental level.

Plateau potentials in cat α-motoneurones

As the next step in the analysis of the assumed interneuronal network we decided to investigate the prolonged excitability increase by intracellular recording from the α-motoneurones (unanesthetized decerebrate cats, Hounsgaard et al., 1984). In these experiments intracellular recording from a sampled motoneurone (innervating LG-SOL, upper records in Fig. 2B–E) and the ENG recording from the whole LG-SOL nerve (lower records in B–E) were always performed in parallel.

As expected, the sustained ENG activity following the "on" stimulus was paralleled by a corresponding sustained firing in the motoneurone (Fig. 2B). In both cases the maintained activity was terminated by an "off" stimulation to the Per nerve. In order to visualize the presumed EPSP underlying the repetitive firing we then hyperpolarized the motoneurone by a continuous bias current through the recording microelectrode to keep the membrane potential below firing level (Fig. 2C). The "on" stimulus again increased the ENG activity (cf. lower records in B and C). However, in the motoneurone spikes were only triggered during the "on" stimulus and the membrane potential then rapidly returned to the level before the "on" stimulus. A possible explanation for this paradoxical finding was that motoneurones near their threshold of activation were reactivated by the small depolarizing overswing following the afterhyperpolarization (Eccles et al., 1958), so that once activated, spike activity would continue at a fixed slow frequency. To test this notion we depolarized the motoneurone with a continuous bias current (Fig. 2D) to achieve a low-frequency background firing before testing the effects of the "on" and "off" stimuli: the "on" stimulus now caused a step increase in the firing rate, while the "off" stimulus returned the motoneurone to the slow discharge rate. We suggested that the "on" stimulus triggered a drive not seen in the hyperpolarized state. This conclusion was strengthened further by the following experiment. The generation of normal fast action potentials was first inactivated by long-lasting depolarizing current (40–100 nA through the recording microelectrode); this current was then decreased rapidly and the membrane potential returned to a value somewhat above the original threshold level. With this regime the generation of spikes often remained inactivated for a long period. In this state the "on" stimulus triggered a long-lasting depolarization which was terminated by the "off" stimulus (Fig. 2E). The plateau depolarization, which was on the order of 5–15 mV, could not be graded. Whether the strength or the train duration of the MG "on" stimulus was graded, the plateau depolarization always appeared as an all-or-none response. This behaviour, together with the absence of any subthreshold depolarization in the hyperpolarized state, shows that the sustained excitability increase of α-motoneurones following an "on" stimulus was not due to continuous synaptic excitation. The experiments illustrated in Fig. 3, using intracellular current pulses to stimulate the motoneurones, showed that intrinsic properties of the motoneurones were indeed responsible.

Fig. 3A shows self-sustained discharge following a short depolarizing pulse through the microelectrode; the firing was then terminated by a short hyperpolarizing pulse. When the spike mechanism was inactivated, brief intracellular current pulses generated maintained potential shifts (Fig. 3B) similar to those evoked synaptically.

In addition to the above described "on" and "off" responses to short-lasting current pulses we also observed a peculiar firing behaviour in response to long-lasting triangular current pulses. The firing frequency for any given current was much larger during the descending phase than during the initial ascending phase (Fig. 3C). When the instantaneous frequency was plotted against injected current the frequency/current relation showed

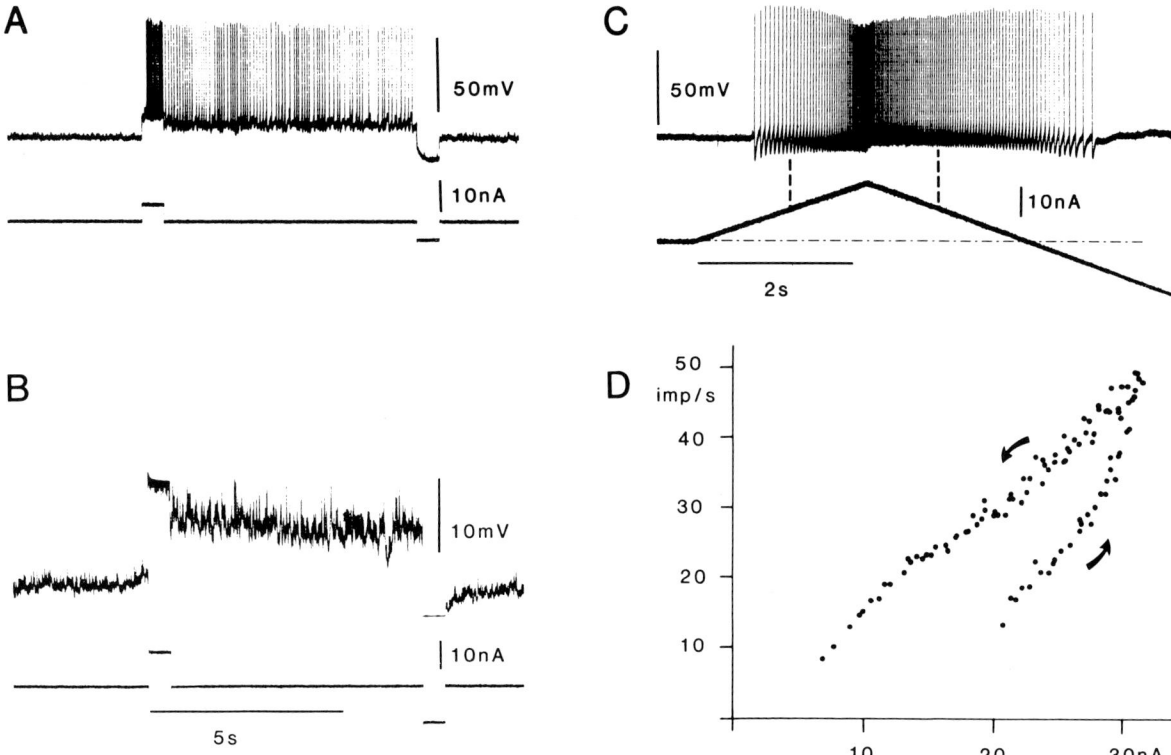

Fig. 3. Sustained shifts in excitability triggered by depolarizing and hyperpolarizing currents injected intracellularly. In A–C, intracellular recordings from motoneurones are displayed in upper traces and injected current in lower traces. A. Sustained firing initiated by a short depolarizing current pulse and terminated by a short hyperpolarizing current pulse. B. In the same cell this sequence of current pulses evoked and terminated a depolarizing shift after prior inactivation of the spike-generating mechanism by excessive depolarization. C. Hysteretic firing during a triangular current pulse. The intracellular signal was passed through a 5 Hz AC filter for reproduction. D. The instantaneous frequency as a function of current during triangular current injection. Data taken from the records in C; arrows indicate the time sequence. From Hounsgaard et al. (1984).

an obvious hysteresis (Fig. 3D) in the direction opposite to that expected from the late adaptation described by Kernell and Monster (1982). It seemed likely that the two phenomena illustrated in Fig. 3 (the sustained excitability increase to short-lasting current pulses and the hysteresis during triangular pulses) were due to the same basic mechanism.

It may be asked why the bistable properties of cat α-motoneurones have been overlooked by intense research over the last 30 years? Actually, self-sustained firing (as in Fig. 3A) has been well documented by Schwindt and Crill (1980a) during experimental epilepsy by topical application of penicillin. In voltage clamp experiments on normal motoneurones the same authors (1980a,b) have described a region of "negative resistance" which may correspond to bistable properties (see further, in the next subsection). The reason why the bistability has not attracted more attention seems related to the fact that it is not seen in the most commonly used preparations, i.e., spinalized and/or nembutalized animals. Thus, the bistability (Fig. 2, Fig. 3A,B) and the hysteretic firing during triangular pulses (Fig. 3C,D) disappeared after an acute spinal transection, but returned after injection of 5-HTP. The suppression of the bistability by small doses of barbiturates to decerebrate cats most probably is an indirect effect secondary to a depression of the activity in the raphe-spinal projection (cf. below).

Serotonin-dependent plateau potentials in turtle motoneurones in vitro

The experiments in the cat, summarized above, identified the motoneuronal membrane as the determining locus for the long-lasting motor discharge following a brief excitatory input and suggested that the response was serotonin dependent. While the possible functional significance of the findings is currently being investigated using the cat preparation, technical limitations inherent in in vivo experiments preclude direct answers to certain questions concerning the underlying membrane mechanisms. In consequence, attention was focused on the possibility of reproducing the basic phenomenology under study in an in vitro preparation of the spinal cord. These aims were met in experiments on motoneurones in sections of turtle spinal cord (Hounsgaard and Kiehn, 1985). This preparation was chosen because recent experiments indicated that substantial pieces of isolated brain tissue from the turtle remain viable in vitro (Mori and Shepherd, 1979).

Fig. 4 documents the validity of the preparation for the present purpose. In intracellular recordings from motoneurons in normal medium a depolarizing current pulse evoked a train of action potentials adapting from a high initial firing rate to a lower steady-state level (Fig. 4A). After addition of serotonin to the medium the firing frequency instead accelerated during a train of action potentials evoked by a similar stimulus. This acceleration was invariably associated with a depolarizing afterpotential (plateau potential) following termination of the depolarizing current pulse. The afterpotential increased in duration and exceeded threshold at holding membrane potentials depolarized from rest (Fig. 4B). Finally, in the 10 mV range, just below threshold, the plateau persisted until terminated by a brief hyperpolarization (Fig. 4C). In the presence of serotonin turtle motoneurones responded to triangular current pulses with the same hysteretic firing pattern as described in the cat (Fig. 3C,D). The changes induced by serotonin were not affected markedly by addition of barbiturate. This supports

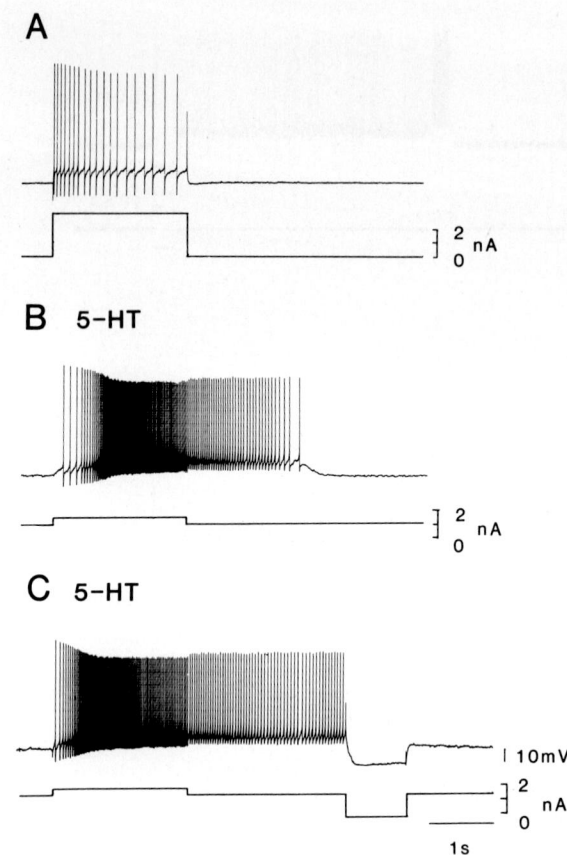

Fig. 4. Serotonin-induced changes in response properties of turtle motoneurones. Intracellular recordings from motoneurones (identified by antidromic invasion following ventral root stimulation) in an in vitro preparation of the isolated turtle spinal cord. In A–C, intracellular recordings are displayed in upper traces and injected current in lower traces. A. Adaptation of rhythmic firing in normal medium. B. Acceleration of firing during the depolarizing current pulse and afterdischarge following the termination of the pulse, when serotonin (10^{-4} M) was added to the medium. C. More prominent acceleration and shift of motoneuronal activity between two stable states (bistability) induced by depolarizing and hyperpolarizing current pulses. The holding membrane potential slightly depolarized from the level in B. Voltage and time calibrations apply to all records. All records from the same cell. Adapted from Hounsgaard and Kiehn (1985).

the earlier suggestion that barbiturates suppress bistability in the cat by reducing raphe-spinal activity, rather than by a direct action on motoneurones.

These experiments strengthened the idea that serotonin was directly responsible for the sustained

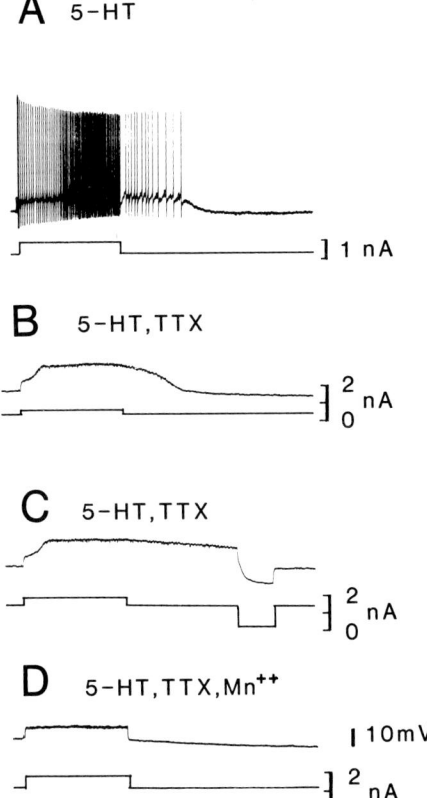

Fig. 5. Ionic mechanism of serotonin-induced plateau potential and bistability in turtle motoneurones. Same experimental arrangement and preparation as in Fig. 4. Serotonin and tetrodotoxin administered to the reservoir in concentration of 10^{-4} and 10^{-6} M, respectively. In D, $CaCl_2$ was replaced by $MnCl_2$. Upper traces: intracellular recordings from motoneurones. Lower traces: injected current. A. Control sweep in serotonin (5-HT) containing medium. B. Tetrodotoxin (TTX) -resistant plateau potential corresponding to the phase of acceleration during the pulse and to the afterdischarge following the pulse (see Figs. 4B and 5A). C. Bistable behaviour of motoneurone initiated and terminated by brief depolarizing and hyperpolarizing current pulses in 5-HT and TTX. The cell was more depolarized than in B. D. Plateau potential disappeared in Mn^{2+}, TTX and 5-HT medium. Voltage and time calibration applies to all records. All records from the same cell. Adapted from Hounsgaard and Kiehn (1985).

motor activity after a short-lasting excitation. In addition, the remarkable similarity between the behaviour of motoneurones in the cat and the turtle suggested that transmitter modulation of the intrinsic membrane properties was a common feature for vertebrate motoneurones.

In a fairly straightforward manner the ionic mechanisms underlying the depolarizing plateau potential were now open for study (Fig. 5A–D). The plateau potential, present in serotonin-containing medium, was clearly independent of spike generation and sodium conductance, since it persisted after addition of tetrodotoxin (Fig. 5B) and after substitution of Na^+ with choline (unpublished observations). The duration of the plateau after the initiating depolarizing pulse depended on the background membrane potential as in normal serotonin-containing medium (Fig. 5B,C). Finally, Fig. 5D shows that the depolarizing plateau potential was blocked by Mn^{2+}, and therefore attributed to a Ca^{2+} conductance.

It is of interest to notice that a Ca^{2+} conductance is normally operative in motoneurones even in the absence of sustained afterdischarges (Barrett and Barrett, 1976; Schwindt and Crill, 1980c). The "negative resistance" region in the steady-state current voltage curve described in voltage clamped cat motoneurones is supposedly explained by this Ca^{2+} conductance (Schwindt and Crill, 1980b,c). We predict that the negative resistance region is enhanced by serotonin. The bistable behaviour of motoneurones is explained if the "negative resistance" region crosses the zero current level (i.e., becomes a second stable membrane potential). This prediction is currently under study in the turtle preparation using voltage clamp. These experiments are also aimed at clarifying whether serotonin enhances a Ca^{2+} conductance or reduces a K^+ conductance (see Hounsgaard and Kiehn, 1985, for discussion).

Discussion

At this moment we are obviously far from understanding the functional role of the transmitter-controlled bistability of vertebrate motoneurones. Actually we do not know whether self-sustained firing without concommittant synaptic excitation represents a normal functional state or whether it is an extreme situation seen with unphysiologically strong serotonergic action onto the motoneuronal membrane. However, it can hardly be doubted that the voltage-dependent non-inactivating Ca^{2+} conductance will serve to "amplify" ongoing excitatory synaptic input. The neurotransmitter serotonin seems to control the gain, be it by acting directly on this particular Ca^{2+} conductance or indirectly by reduction of a K^+ conductance. It is interesting that several authors already have attributed "gain-setting" functions to the descending monoaminergic innervation of the spinal cord (McCall and Aghajanian, 1979; VanderMaelen and Aghajanian, 1982; Kuypers, 1982; Kuypers and Huisman, 1982). Actually, Kuypers refers to the monoaminergic descending systems as a special "gain-setting" component of the motor system "instrumental in providing motivational drive in the execution of movements".

The early mapping of the monoaminergic pathways with the histofluorescence techniques (Dahlström and Fuxe, 1964, 1965) already demonstrated a strong serotonergic projection from the raphe nuclei to the spinal cord; this pathway was also seen to terminate profusely among spinal somatic motoneurones. Studies using techniques of retrograde and anterograde transport (see Björklund and Skagerberg, 1982; Bowker et al., 1982; Holstege and Kuypers, 1982; Huisman et al., 1982; Kuypers and Huisman, 1982; Skagerberg and Björklund, 1985) have greatly increased the present knowledge of the raphe-spinal system. Thus, it is now established that the innervation of the ventral horn originates mainly from neurones in the caudal medulla (nc. raphe obscurus and pallidus and nc. reticularis ventralis) which descend through the ventrolateral funiculus. In addition, the recent immuno-histochemical studies by Kojima and collaborators (Kojima et al., 1982, 1983a,b; Kojima and Sano, 1983) have given a detailed picture of the termination of serotonergic fibres in the mammalian spinal cord. There is a dense termination in the ventral horn and a fine reticular plexus of varicose serotonin fibres is evident around the motoneurones of each investigated species.

The prominent plateau-potentials in α-motoneurones in the decerebrate preparation may be of pivotal importance for the classical tonic stretch reflex. During the ramp-and-hold stretch the dynamic sensitivity of muscle spindle Ia afferents causes an efficient synaptic excitation during the ramp phase. When motoneurones are recruited during this phase they maintain a remarkably constant firing rate despite the continuing extension of the muscle (Grillner and Udo, 1971). This behaviour would be expected if the Ia excitation triggered the plateau-potential, which is much larger than the Ia excitation per se (Crone, Hultborn, Kiehn, Mazieres and Wigström, unpublished data). Also, the sustained low-frequency firing during the holding phase may be caused by the maintained plateau potential, supported by a much weaker synaptic excitation (the lower static sensitivity of muscle spindle Ia afferents). If so, the plateau should be rather unstable, and terminated by even short-lasting synaptic inhibition, permanently derecruiting the motor unit. Actually, it seems likely that this mechanism contributes to the lasting derecruitment of motor units in the clasp knife phenomenon, since the afferent input triggering that reaction should be of rather short duration (however, cf. Rymer et al., 1979).

Present quantitative knowledge of the sensory input and efferent output in the vestibulo-ocular reflex has prompted several investigators to postulate a neuronal integrator in the intervening CNS (Robinson, 1968, 1971; Skavenski and Robinson, 1973). There have been several attempts to model this neuronal integrator (Rosen, 1972; Kamath and Keller, 1976; Cannon et al., 1983). The assumption common for all these models is a network of neurones with positive feedback loops. Some of our observations point to a very different possibility. The bistable properties of motoneurones allow them to act as very simple integrators, like flip-flops, which are set at one of two levels by short excitatory or inhibitory inputs. However, when the whole motoneuronal pool is considered, many different levels can be maintained by recruitment of new units. Fig. 6 illustrates an experiment in which the activity in the soleus motoneuronal pool was monitored by recording the rectified soleus EMG

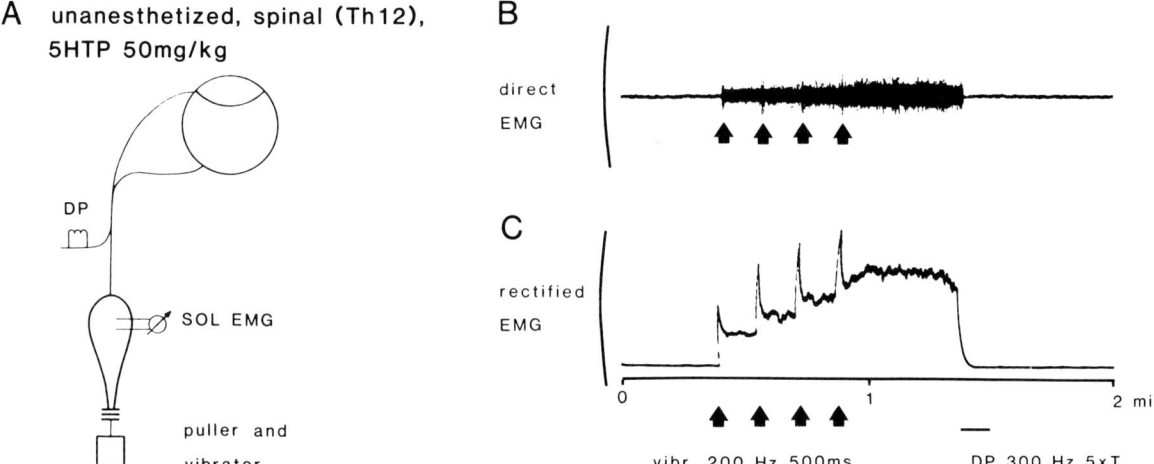

Fig. 6. "Staircase" phenomena following repeated vibrations of soleus muscle. A. Experimental arrangement. Unanesthetized decerebrate cat, with an acute spinal transection and 5-HTP (50 mg/kg, intravenously). The soleus muscle was freed and its tendon fixed to a puller. The SOL-EMG was recorded from copper wires inserted into the muscle. The soleus muscle was vibrated (100 μm at 200 Hz for 500 mseconds; arrows in B and C). Stimulation of the deep peroneal nerve (DP; 300 Hz, 5 × T) was used as an "off" stimulus. B. Direct SOL-EMG showing the stepwise increase in EMG activity induced by repeated vibrations and the reset of activity by stimulation of DP nerve. C. The same SOL-EMG response as in B but rectified and filtered. From Hultborn and Wigström, unpublished data.

activity. In response to repeated "on" stimuli (stimulus parameters remained constant) a stepwise increase of the lasting maintained activity was recorded. Each step implied activation of plateau-potentials in an additional fraction of the motoneuronal pool. Although the integration in the vestibulo-ocular reflex seems to take place at premotoneuronal level, the experimental finding of Fig. 6 emphasizes that intrinsic membrane properties may be crucial parts in a neuronal integrator.

Acknowledgements

This work was supported by the Danish Medical Research Council and the Danish Multiple Sclerosis Society.

References

Ahlman, H., Grillner, S. and Udo, M. (1971) The effect of 5-HTP on the static fusimotor activity and the tonic stretch reflex of an extensor muscle. Brain Res., 27: 393–396.

Andén, N.-E., Jukes, M. G. M. and Lundberg, A. (1964) Spinal reflexes and monoamine liberation. Nature, 202: 1222–1223.

Barrett, E. F. and Barrett, J. N. (1976) Separation of two voltage-sensitive potassium currents, and demonstration of a tetrodotoxin-resistant calcium current in frog motoneurons. J. Physiol. (Lond.), 255: 737–774.

Björklund, A. and Skagerberg, G. (1982) Descending monoaminergic projections to the spinal cord. In B. Sjölund and A. Björklund (Eds.), Brain Stem Control of Spinal Mechanisms, Elsevier Biomedical Press, Amsterdam, pp. 55–88.

Bowker, R. M., Westlund, K. N., Sullivan, M. C. and Coulter, J. D. (1982) Organization of descending serotonergic projections to the spinal cord. In H. G. J. M. Kuypers and G. F. Martins (Eds.), Descending Pathways to the Spinal Cord, Progress in Brain Research, Vol. 57, Elsevier Biomedical Press, Amsterdam, pp. 239–265.

Cannon, S. C., Robinson, D. A. and Shamma, S. (1983) A proposed neural network for the integrator of the oculomotor system. Biol. Cyper., 49: 127–136.

Creed, R. S., Denny-Brazon, D., Eccles, J. C., Liddell, E. G. and Sherrington, C. S. (1932) Reflex Activity of the Spinal Cord. Oxford University Press, Oxford.

Dahlström, A. and Fuxe, K. (1964) Evidence for the existence of monoamine-containing neurons in the central nervous system. I. Demonstration of monoamines in the cell bodies of brain stem neurons. Acta Physiol. Scand., Suppl. 232: 5–55.

Dahlström, A. and Fuxe, K. (1965) Evidence for the existence of monoamine neurons in the central nervous system. II. Experimentally induced changes in the intraneuronal amine levels of bulbospinal neuron systems. Acta Physiol. Scand., Suppl. 247: 6–37.

Eccles, J. C., Eccles, R. M. and Lundberg, A. (1957) The convergence of monosynaptic excitatory afferents on to many different species of alpha motoneurones. J. Physiol. (Lond.), 137: 22–50.

Eccles, J. C., Eccles, R. M. and Lundberg, A. (1958) The action potentials of motoneurones supplying fast and slow muscles. J. Physiol. (Lond.), 142: 275–291.

Engberg, I., Lundberg, A. and Ryall, R. W. (1968a) The effect of reserpine on transmission in the spinal cord. Acta Physiol. Scand., 72: 115–122.

Engberg, I., Lundberg, A. and Ryall, R. W. (1968b) Is the tonic decerebrate inhibition of reflex paths mediated by monoaminergic pathways? Acta Physiol. Scand., 72: 123–133.

Fetz, E. E., Jankowska, E., Johannisson, T. and Lipski, J. (1979) Autogenetic inhibition of motoneurones by impulses in group Ia muscle spindle afferents. J. Physiol. (Lond.), 293: 173–195.

Forbes, A. (1922) The interpretation of spinal reflexes in terms of present knowledge of nerve conduction. Physiol. Rev., 2: 361.

Forbes, A. (1929) The Foundations of Experimental Psychology. Clark University Press, Worcester.

Granit, R., Phillips, C. G., Skoglund, S. and Steg, G. (1957) Differentiation of tonic from phasic alpha ventral horn cells by stretch, pinna and crossed extensor reflexes. J. Neurophysiol., 20: 470–481.

Grillner, S. and Udo, M. (1971) Motor unit activity and stiffness of the contracting muscle fibres in the tonic stretch reflex. Acta Physiol. Scand., 81: 422–424.

Holstege, G. and Kuypers, H. G. J. M. (1982) The anatomy of brain stem pathways to the spinal cord in cat. A labeled amino acid tracing study. In H. G. J. M. Kuypers and G. F. Martin (Eds.), Descending Pathways to the Spinal Cord, Progress in Brain Research, Vol. 57, Elsevier Biomedical Press, Amsterdam, pp. 145–175.

Hebb, D. O. (1949) The Organization of Behavior. A Neuropsychological Theory. John Wiley and Sons, New York/Chapman and Hall, London.

Hounsgaard, J. and Kiehn, O. (1985) Ca^{++} dependent bistability induced by serotonin in spinal motoneurons. Exp. Brain Res., 57: 422–425.

Hounsgaard, J., Hultborn, H., Jespersen, B. and Kiehn, O. (1984) Intrinsic membrane properties causing a bistable behaviour of α-motoneurones. Exp. Brain Res., 55: 391–394.

Huisman, A. M., Kuypers, H. G. J. M. and Verburgh, C. A. (1982) Differences in collateralization of the descending spinal pathways from red nucleus and other brain stem cell groups in cat and monkey. In H. G. J. M. Kuypers and G. F. Martin (Eds.), Descending Pathways to the Spinal Cord, Progress in Brain Research, Vol. 57, Elsevier Biomedical Press, Amsterdam, pp. 185–217.

Hultborn, H. and Wigström, H. (1980) Motor response with long latency and maintained duration evoked by activity in Ia afferents. In J. E. Desmedt (Ed.), Progress in Clinical Neurophysiology, Spinal and Supraspinal Mechanisms of Voluntary Motor Control and Locomotion, Vol. 8, Karger, Basel, pp. 99–115.

Hultborn, H., Wigstrom, H. and Wangberg, B. (1975) Prolonged activation of soleus motoneurones following a conditioning train in soleus Ia afferents — a case for a reverberating loop? Neurosci. Lett., 1: 147–152.

Kamath, B. Y. and Keller, E. L. (1976) A neurological integrator for the oculomotor control system. Math. Biosci., 30: 341–352.

Kernell, D. and Monster, A. W. (1982) Time course and properties of late adaptation in spinal motoneurones of the cat. Exp. Brain Res., 46: 191–196.

Kojima, M. and Sano, Y. (1983) The organization of serotonin fibers in the anterior column of the mammalian spinal cord. Anat. Embryol., 167: 1–11.

Kojima, M., Takeuchi, Y., Goto, M. and Sano, Y. (1982) Immunohistochemical study on the distribution of serotonin fibers in the spinal cord of the dog. Cell Tissue Res., 226: 477–491.

Kojima, M., Takeuchi, Y., Goto, M. and Sano, Y. (1983a) Immunohistochemical study on the localization of serotonin fibers and terminals in the spinal cord of the monkey (*Macaca fuscata*). Cell Tissue Res., 229: 23–36.

Kojima, M., Takeuchi, Y., Kawata, M. and Sano, Y. (1983b) Motoneurons innervating the cremaster muscle of the rat are characteristically densely innervated by serotonergic fibers as revealed by combined immunohistochemistry and retrograde fluorescence DAPI-labelling. Anat. Embryol., 168: 41–49.

Kuypers, H. G. J. M. (1982) A new look at the organization of the motor system. In H. G. J. M. Kuypers and G. F. Martins (Eds.), Descending Pathways to the Spinal Cord, Progress in Brain Research, Vol. 57, Elsevier Biomedical Press, Amsterdam, pp. 381–403.

Kuypers, H. G. J. M. and Huisman, A. M. (1982) The new anatomy of the descending brain pathways. In B. Sjölund and A. Björklund (Eds.), Brain Stem Control of Spinal Mechanisms, Fernstrom Foundation Series, Elsevier Biomedical Press, Amsterdam, pp. 29–54.

Lundberg, A. and Winsbury, G. (1960) Selective adequate activation of large afferents from muscle spindles and Golgi tendon organs. Acta Physiol. Scand., 49: 155–164.

McCall, R. B. and Aghajanian, G. K. (1979) Serotonergic facilitation of facial motoneuron excitation. Brain Res., 169: 11–27.

Mori, K. and Shepherd, G. M. (1979) Synaptic excitation and long-lasting inhibition of mitral cells in the in vitro turtle olfactory bulb. Brain Res., 172: 155–159.

Pollock, I. J. and Davis, L. (1930) The reflex activities of a decerebrate animal. J. Comp. Neurol., 50: 377–411.

Robinson, D. A. (1968) Eye movement control in primates. Science, 161: 1219–1224.

Robinson, D. A. (1971) Models of oculomotor neural organization. In P. Bach-y-Rita, C. C. Colins and J. E. Hyde (Eds.), The Control of Eye Movements, Academic Press, New York, pp. 519–538.

Rosen, M. J. (1972) A theoretical neural integrator. IEEE Trans. Biomed. Eng., 19: 362–367.

Rymer, W. Z., Houk, J. C. and Crago, P. E. (1979) Mechanisms of the clasp-knife reflex studied in an animal model. Exp. Brain Res., 37: 93–113.

Schwindt, P. C. and Crill, W. E. (1980a) Role of a persistent inward current in motoneuron bursting during spinal seizures. J. Neurophysiol., 43: 1296–1318.

Schwindt, P. C. and Crill, W. E. (1980b) Properties of a persistent inward current in normal and TEA-injected motoneurons. J. Neurophysiol., 43: 1700–1724.

Schwindt, P. C. and Crill, W. E. (1980c) Effects of barium on cat spinal motoneurons studied by voltage clamp. J. Neurophysiol., 44: 827–846.

Sherrington, C. (1906) The Integrative Action of the Nervous System. Yale University Press, New Haven, CT.

Skagerberg, G. and Björklund, A. (1985) Topographic principles in the spinal projections of serotonergic and non-serotonergic brainstem neurons in the rat. Neuroscience, 15: 445–480.

Skavenski, A. A. and Robinson, D. A. (1973) Role of abducens neurons in vestibulocular reflex. J. Neurophysiol., 36: 724–738.

Tsukahara, N. (1972) The properties of the cerebello-pontine reverberating circuit. Brain Res., 40: 67–71.

VanderMaelen, C. P. and Aghajanian, G. K. (1982) Serotonin-induced depolarization of rat facial motoneurons in vivo: comparison with amino acid transmitters. Brain Res., 239: 139–152.

Discussion

P. B. C. Matthews

Laboratory of Physiology, Oxford University, Parks Road, Oxford OX1 3PT, U.K.

Kernell was asked whether his description of somatic motoneurones applied equally to oculomotor neurones, and in his reply he stressed various differences. Baker emphasized that in many properties the two sets of neurones were very similar and Kernell concurred. Hepp stressed that to understand non-linearities of behaviour one must analyse them quantitatively and not just describe them qualitatively. Robinson commented on the particular non-linearity of the hysteresis in firing rates. As it is only about 5% it can often be ignored.

The vigorous discussion of Hultborn's paper centred on the question of the normal physiological role of the bistable motoneuronal behaviour that he had observed under high degrees of serotonergic drive. Under more normal conditions, he reiterated that he saw its role as likely to be to act as a gain control of motoneurones, but one with little spatial specificity. He had emphasized its possible role as an "integrator" partly because the means by which the second integration is achieved in the vestibulo-ocular reflex remains to be established and rather little attention seems to have been paid to the possible role of peculiar membrane properties of individual neurones in achieving it. However, he did not see the oculomotor neurones as performing this operation, and it remained to be established whether interneurones could behave in the way he had described for motoneurones. Those present who had recorded from oculomotor neurones in the awake animal agreed that there was no possibility of these neurones performing the required integration.

SECTION II

Sensory Information Used by the Motor System

What are the afferents of origin of the human stretch reflex, and is it a purely spinal reaction?

Peter B. C. Matthews

Laboratory of Physiology, Oxford University, Parks Road, Oxford OX1 3PT, U.K.

Introduction

The stretch reflex is such a ubiquitous response of skeletal muscle that its apparent complete absence from the oculomotor system is a matter of some interest. From the mechanical point of view such a difference in design between the two systems seems natural since the eyes have no need of any such load compensation reaction. However, from the neurological point of view the difference is tremendously challenging since human extraocular muscles are richly endowed with muscle spindles. Thus, the muscle spindle cannot exist simply to mediate the stretch reflex, and the information it provides about what is happening in the muscle must also have other important uses; this is suggested equally by the wealth of projections to higher centres of the spindle afferent signals from limb muscles. The hope is that the study of the oculomotor system will disclose something about these functions, not only for this system itself but also to open the way for a better understanding of the skeletomotor system. However, the functions of the extraocular spindles still seem to be a matter for speculation. A complementary approach to the same goal is to try to understand the stretch reflex sufficiently well to be able to strip away its contribution from a complex somatic response in the whole animal so as to identify the genuinely higher level reactions and subject them to analysis. This has proved surprisingly difficult, but only after we have understood the relatively dull low-level response of the stretch reflex can we hope to be able to move on to more interesting things.

My present thesis is that in man the spinal stretch reflex is more complex than hitherto supposed and receives its excitatory drive from the slow spindle afferents as well as the fast spindle afferents. This has the inevitable consequence, in a species of such considerable size, that simple spinal components of response will occur with an initial latency far above that of the tendon jerk, by virtue of the delay produced by the slower conduction along the smaller afferents. It also complicates analysis of higher activity, since measurement of latency is blunted as a tool for separating supraspinal from spinal responses. A general principle that emerges, which is likely to be applicable equally to the oculomotor system, is that different sized spindle afferents (with different types of sensory termination within the spindle) may co-operate to produce an integrated central response, rather than producing quite different sorts of effect as supposed in so much of the classical analysis of reflexes. The evidence for my case is indirect and I accept entirely that it is not yet proven, and that some of the new findings may be open to alternative interpretation. But that is quite different from disproving the hypothesis which provides the simplest unitary explanation for a range of experimental findings, and is contradicted by none. Most of the detailed evidence has already been published (Matthews, 1984a,b,c) so the present account can concentrate on the essentials of the argument and skip over various controls. A minimum of reference is provided to the voluminous related literature since so many excellent reviews already exist (Matthews, 1972, 1985; Desmedt, 1978; Marsden et al., 1978, 1983; Baldissera et al, 1981; Evarts, 1981; Wiesendanger and Miles, 1982). I apologise to all those who recognise a reference to their work or views without the text being cited; this has been done simply to help the reader get to the heart of the matter without continual interruption.

Background

Muscle spindles contain two morphologically distinct types of sensory ending, namely the primary endings supplied by the group Ia afferents and the secondary endings supplied by the smaller and thus slower group II afferents. Both are excited by stretch but the classical description of the stretch reflex over at least the period 1945–1970 attributes it entirely to the activity of the Ia afferents, on the basis of work on the cat. Latterly, there has been some loosening of this view following the suggestion that in the decerebrate cat the group II afferents contribute significantly (Matthews, 1969), but the matter has remained sub judice. In other preparations, group II afferents have been found to excite the motoneurones of their own muscle monosynaptically, but the effects have been weak in comparison with those of the Ia afferents and their significance remains debatable. What cannot be doubted is that if the group II afferents were to produce excitation then it would inevitably occur with a latency greater than that produced by the Ia afferents excited by the same stimulus, because of the difference in afferent conduction time. In the cat, the group II afferents conduct at about half to a third of the speed of the Ia afferents; but with the shortness of the neural pathways involved this would introduce only a few mseconds delay between their reflex responses, and this might not be readily detectable when mechanical stimuli are being used. In man, however, the much greater conduction distances involved mean that the postulated two separate components of response to stretch should be separated by 10–20 mseconds when distal muscles are studied. Thus, the present hypothesis predicts that there will be a long-latency stretch reflex in addition to a short-latency stretch reflex.

Whether there is such a long-latency stretch reflex in man is already a matter of intense controversy. On the one hand, there are those who believe fervently that there is one. They then almost invariably interpret it as due to a "long-loop" reflex, with the initial Ia volley producing a delayed action on the motoneurones by virtue of being routed via the motor cortex. The same initial Ia input is thus suggested to produce a double excitation of the motoneurones, first by monosynaptic short-latency action and then by long-loop action. Animal work shows that the requisite fast pathways certainly exist to the motor cortex and back, and the question is whether they are organised merely to produce a simple "stretch reflex", and if they do do this whether they have sufficient potency to produce the observed responses. On the other hand, sceptics emphasize that a continued Ia monosynaptic bombardment of the motoneurone pool, elicited by continuing stretch, might be expected to produce a continued motor discharge and for various adventitious reasons this could be "segmented" so as to give the appearance of a series of separate reflex responses; such segmentation might reflect partly a bursting of Ia firing dependent upon muscle resonances and so on, and partly the operation of refractory and inhibitory mechanisms within the spinal cord. Investigation restricted to studying just the response to the onset of a gross stretch seems unlikely to resolve the matter.

Results

The present approach has been to use high-frequency vibration (100–150 Hz) as the stimulus in addition to muscle stretch produced by joint displacement. The rationale for this is that, in both animals and man, vibration has a powerful excitatory action on the Ia afferents, much more than it does upon the group II afferents, whereas stretch excites both types of afferent; the selectivity of vi-

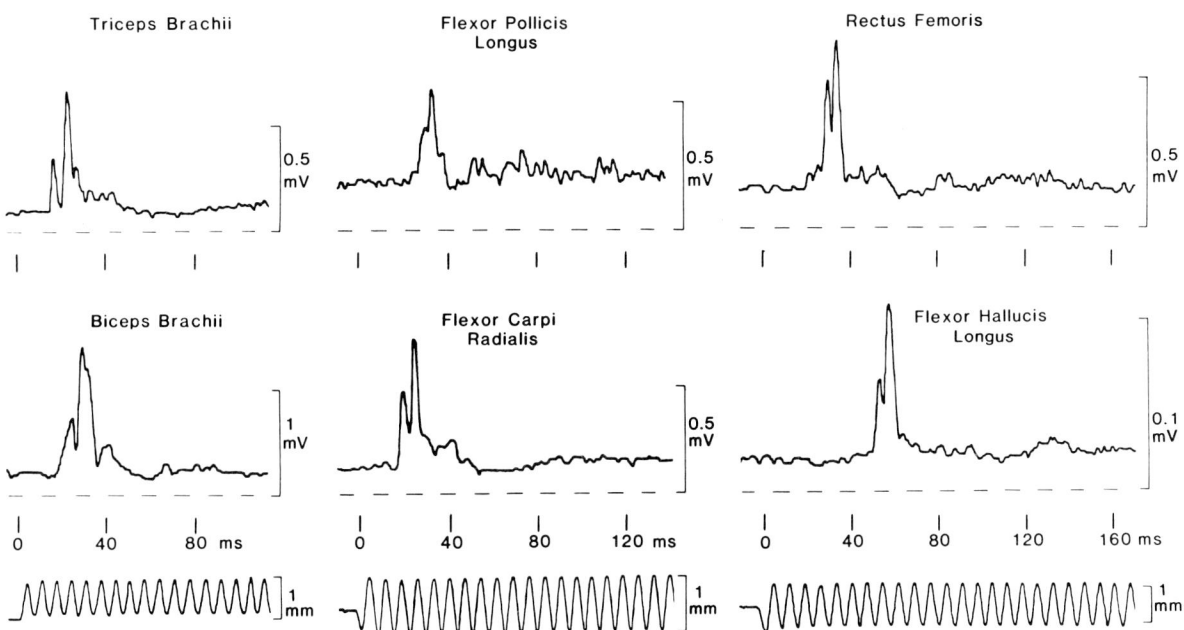

Fig. 1. The phasic reflex response occurring at the onset of vibration seen in the averaged rectified surface electromyogram of various muscles. For the large limb muscles the vibration was applied by pressing a vibrator percutaneously upon their tendons. For the flexors of the thumb and toes the whole digit was moved. In each case the subject was initially voluntarily contracting the muscle isometrically so as to develop about 20% of its maximal force. The subjects made no voluntary response to the stimulus and simply "let it happen". Short periods of vibration were repeated at regular intervals (typically 300 mseconds every 800 mseconds) and 64 to 128 individual responses averaged. The vibration recording was obtained from a length transducer incorporated in the vibrator. From Matthews (1984c).

bration is not absolute, but that does not matter for the present argument. If the stretch reflex, including any long-latency components, depends solely upon Ia action then it should be produced equally by vibration and by stretch. But if it possesses long-latency components that depend upon group II action then they should be largely in abeyance with vibration. Fig. 1 shows that for a number of human muscles, vibration produces a brief phasic response in the electromyogram with little significant sign of a long-latency response, and certainly nothing which would draw attention to itself if there were no expectation of such a response. Various later waves may be seen on occasion with vibration, as in Fig. 2; but when the matter has been tested they were abolished by shortening the duration of the period of vibration, suggesting that they depended upon continued short-latency Ia action rather than upon long-loop activity. It bears emphasis that such phasic responses do not imply that the vibration failed to produce a continued Ia excitation. Simple theoretical considerations show that a pool of motoneurones that are already discharging tonically, as in the present case, would be expected to behave in just this way on the sudden arrival of a maintained increase in excitation (Matthews, 1984c). This is because the initial step of excitation will immediately trigger the discharge of all those motoneurones which were already nearing their threshold and they will then be refractory; Renshaw inhibition can also be expected to contribute.

Direct comparison of stretch and vibration for the long thumb flexor

To gain force, such observation of the effect of vibration needs to be combined with observations on the genuine stretch reflex elicited from the same

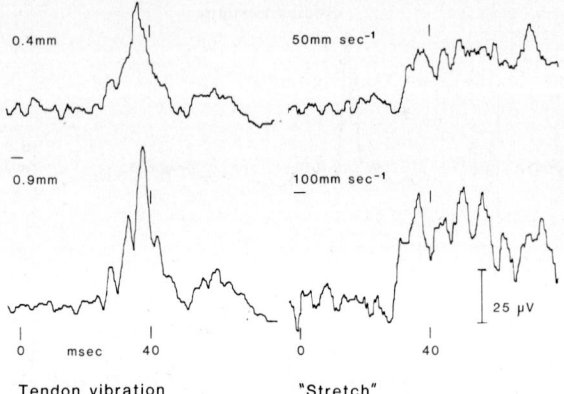

Fig. 2. The contrasting reflex responses of flexor pollicis longus (FPL) to vibration (applied in this case percutaneously to its tendon), and to a ramp-and-hold stretch (applied by forcibly extending the terminal phalanx while the proximal phalanx was clamped), Time zero corresponds to the beginning of the stimulus (cf. Fig. 1). The stretch response is much more prolonged and continues while the initial vibration response is decaying. The velocity of "stretch" refers to the movement of the thumb, measured at the base of the nail, and should be multiplied by 3 to convert to degrees angular movement at the interphalangeal joint; the total such movement was 9°. The zero of the upper EMG records is given by the short horizontal lines below; those for the lower records were similar. Other details as in Fig. 1. From Matthews (1984a).

muscle of the same subject by a frank stretch. There is considerable variation in the prominence and behaviour of the late stretch-evoked waves from muscle to muscle and subject to subject, and considerable doubt has been raised as to whether a genuine delayed "long-latency" reflex is always present even with stretch. Fig. 2 shows such a comparison for the human flexor pollicis longus which very regularly showed late waves with stretch. The records on the left show the usual phasic response to vibration, with activity falling back to the base line at 40 mseconds, which is when the long-latency response is suggested to begin (Marsden et al., 1976). The records on the right show that stretch elicits the same sort of short-latency excitation at about 30 mseconds, but activity now continues over the period 40–50–60 mseconds, when the response to vibration has dropped right down. This is readily interpreted as due to the motoneurone pool being progressively excited by the arrival of new inputs via the long-latency pathway. These act in conjunction with the continued excitation delivered by the short-latency pathway and so prevent the reduction of the response from its initial peak, which would have occurred if the short-latency pathway had acted alone to provide a steady level of excitatory drive. The stretch responses in Fig. 2 show a series of minor segments which might perhaps be due to the arrival of successive separate excitatory volleys at the pool, but other possibilities seem equally likely; thus, in this case, as often, it is quite impossible to decide upon the precise latency of the long-latency excitation which is suggested to underlie the continued motor discharge. In other subjects the initial short-latency response may be less prominent and an apparently fresh response is seen starting at about 40 mseconds, as in Fig. 3 (middle), allowing a tentative estimate to be made of the la-

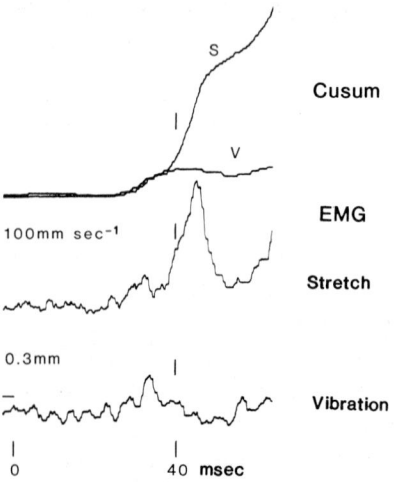

Fig. 3. Comparison of the "long-latency" responses of FPL to stretch and to vibration when the initial short-latency responses were the same. The matching of the short-latency responses was achieved by choosing appropriate parameters of stimulation (velocity of stretch, amplitude of vibration). The middle record shows the response to a ramp stretch in the same way as in Fig. 2, but from a different subject with a prominent long-latency response with a latency of just under 40 mseconds. The bottom record shows his response to the weak vibration that elicited the same initial motor discharge; as in Fig. 1, the vibration was applied to the thumb. At the top, the "cusums" of these two responses are superimposed; the "cusum" is the integral of the rectified EMG after subtracting the initial level throughout. From Matthews (1984a).

tency of the delayed route. This was especially so for slower velocities of stretch, as extensively described by Marsden et al. (1976); in this situation, however, interpretation is complicated by the uncertainty whether, due to mechanical lags, the Ia discharge picks up slowly and whether any appreciable central facilitation is required to produce an appreciable response, as could occur if the Ia short-latency pathway was mediated by one or two interneurones as well as monosynaptically.

The essential present point is that the temporal profile of the reflex response to stretch is quite different from that to vibration; the latter is markedly more phasic, with activity falling away over the period 40–50 mseconds from the beginning of stimulation, whereas stretch-evoked activity continues throughout this period or even appears de novo. Fig. 3 shows that this difference does not depend upon any differences in the strength of the initial Ia excitation in the two cases; for example, the vibration might have been so much the more powerful stimulus that many more motoneurones were made refractory in the short-latency response and thus unable to respond to long-latency activation. The responses in Fig. 3 have been selected so that the initial short-latency discharges (in the period 30–40 mseconds) are closely similar for the two modes of stimulation, while the later responses can be seen to differ in the usual way. The selection was done from among a number of responses obtained at the same session using different velocities of stretching and amplitudes of vibration. Such observations seem incompatible with the long-loop hypothesis of the genesis of the response at 40 mseconds. On the evidence of the similarity of the short-latency responses, the initial Ia volleys were similar for stretch and vibration. Thus, any delayed long-loop action of these same volleys should also have been closely similar. Since the observed responses are not, the hypothesis would seem contradicted, or at least to require rescue by the introduction of ad hoc assumptions to explain this particular result. However, the findings are precisely those to be expected upon the group II hypothesis with the delayed excitation attributable to the delayed arrival at the spinal cord of the group II activity set up at the beginning of stretch, but which was not elicited by vibration. All these responses can still be seen after locally anaesthetising the thumb, and so seem likely to be attributable to intramuscular receptors. Of these, the spindle group II afferents provide the only plausible candidates for the delayed response. However, in view of the uncertainties both about their conduction velocity in man and about the precise latency of the later response, it is impossible to decide upon the central reflex latency, and thus the extent to which interneurones are involved. But there seems no possibility of the central delay being sufficient for the response at 40–50 mseconds to be attributable to the postulated group II action being mediated supraspinally.

Responses to termination of stimulus

On the assumption that a genuine and distinct long-latency stretch reflex does exist then the above findings provide reasonably cogent evidence that it should be attributed to spindle group II afferents acting spinally, rather than to Ia afferents acting supraspinally. However, on the evidence adduced so far, the initial proposition might reasonably be denied and all the responses attributed to continued short-latency Ia action and the group II hypothesis dismissed. This is because in the absence of microneuronographic recordings it cannot be guaranteed that the level of Ia activity elicited by the two modes of stimulation continues to remain the same after the initial discharge at the beginning of stimulation. In other words, the response in the period 40–50 mseconds could be suggested to be due to the afferent Ia discharge in the period 10–20 mseconds from the beginning of the stimulus acting spinally, rather than to that in the period 0–10 mseconds acting supraspinally. Inhibitory pathways might also be suggested to be differentially activated by the two modes of stimulation. In the absence of direct evidence there is no point in further debating such possibilities.

However, the problem can be largely sidestepped by switching attention to the effect of terminating

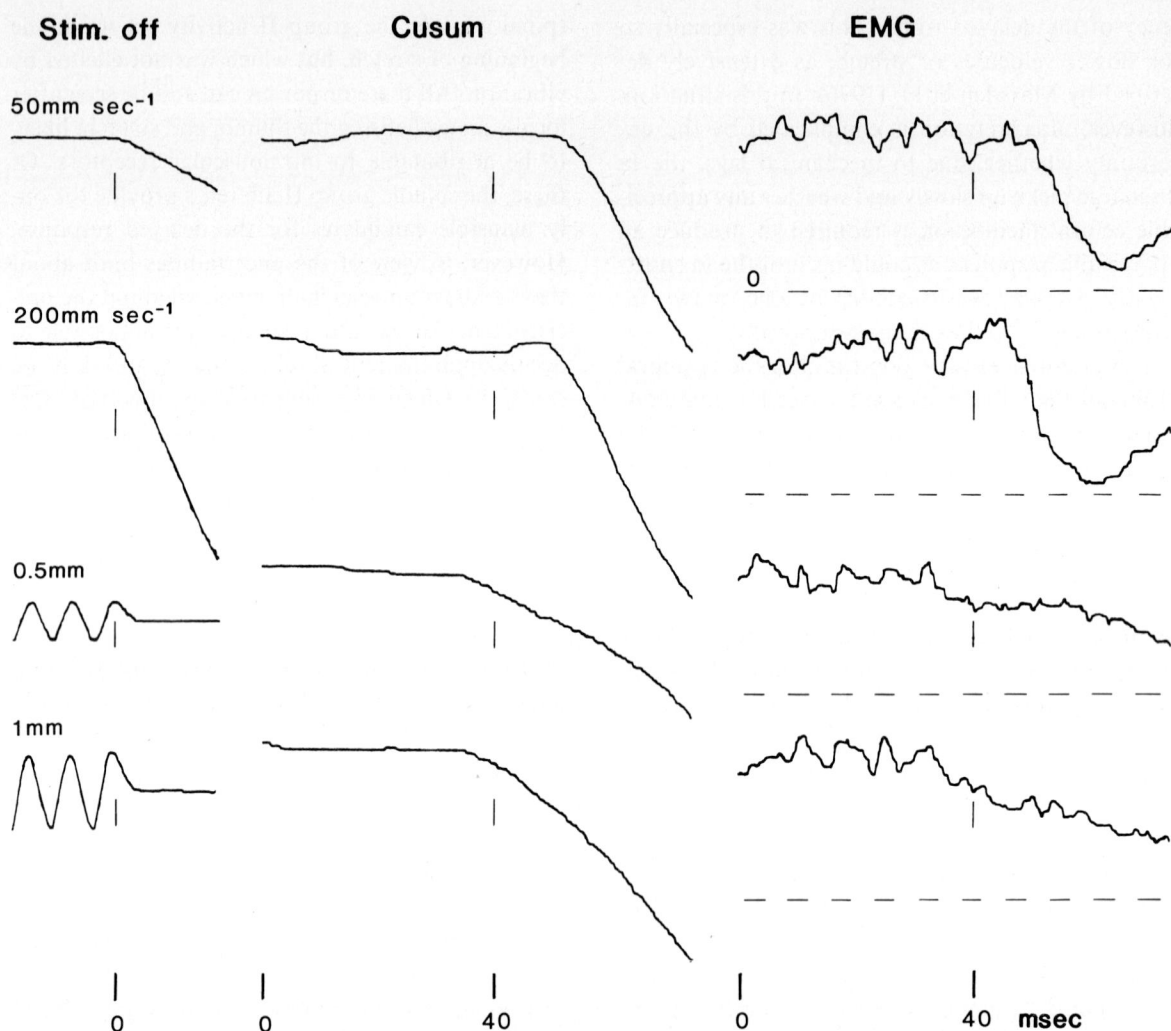

Fig. 4. "Off" responses on cessation of pre-existing stretch or vibration of FPL. The consequent reduction of activity is attributed to a disfacilitation resulting from the withdrawal of reflex excitation. The major effect with stretch occurs at much longer latency than that for vibration. Left, stimuli; middle, cusums; right, rectified EMGs. The gain for the bottom two records is half that of those above. From Matthews (1984a).

the stimulus, rather than of initially applying it. With both types of stimuli there should then be a reduction of Ia firing, with consequent disfacilitation of the motoneurones but with fewer possibilities for spurious late responses. As illustrated in Fig. 4, the findings again support the group II hypothesis. On terminating vibration (lower records) there is a short latency "off" effect attributable to withdrawal of the vibration-evoked Ia bombardment of the motoneurones by short-latency pathways. There is no appreciable separate long-latency "off" response at beyond 40 mseconds. The smallness of the effect is notable, and may well be partly due to the central action of the Ia afferents having been scaled down by autogenetically elicited presynaptic inhibition. In contrast, release of stretch shows a well-marked long-latency "off" response at above 40 mseconds while the short-latency effect cannot be detected with any certainty against the prevailing level of the background noise. On other occasions it has been observed for flexor pollicus longus, along with the delayed response, but it is always small. The large size of the delayed response is remarkable and fits with the suggestion that, unlike the Ia afferents, the group II afferents were producing a considerable maintained excitation of the motoneurone pool. The delayed "off" response on release of stretch did not depend upon delays in the reduction of afferent firing due to mechanical factors since, as illustrated, it occurred with much the same latency on releasing the pre-existing stretch at different velocities. Various further control experiments make it very unlikely that the "off" effect of stretch is attributable to a delayed inhibition of the motoneurones, rather than to the suggested disfacilitation. Ia inhibition, elicited by the concomitant stretch of the antagonist, would be expected to occur with a short latency, close to that for monosynaptic action.

These findings argue yet more cogently than before, firstly, that there is a genuine delayed component of the stretch reflex which cannot be explained by continued Ia spinal action and, secondly, that neither can it be attributed to supraspinal Ia action, as otherwise it should also have been elicited by vibration. It is the fortunate fact that flexor pollicis longus typically has such a small short-latency response at "off" that makes it so certain that the delayed response is a distinct entity requiring special explanation, since the latter is then seen virtually on its own. This makes its interpretation much more definite than on the application of stretch; not all other muscles behave so simply.

Behaviour of other muscles, especially semitendinosus

On the transcortical hypothesis the long-latency response might be expected to be particularly well developed for muscles under a high degree of cortical control, such as those operating upon the primate hand, and whose motoneurones may be presumed to be richly innervated by the pyramidal tract. In this respect, however, the short flexor of the human thumb is anomalous. When acting in conjunction with the long flexor to resist movement its stretch reflex response may be dominated by the short-latency component mediated spinally, even

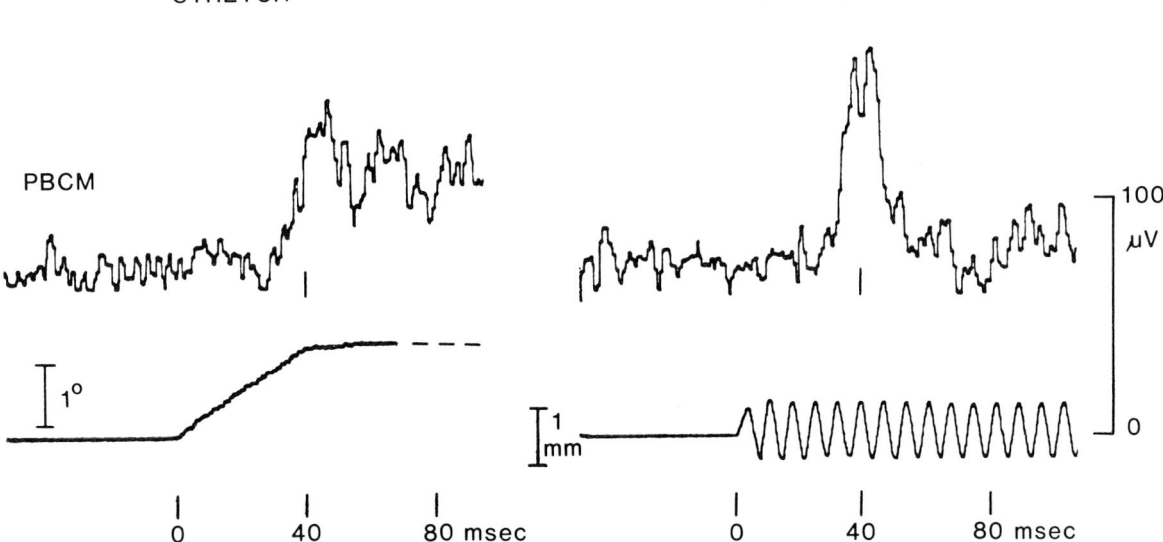

Fig. 5. Comparison of the responses of the hamstring muscle, semitendinosus, to stretch (applied by forcibly extending the knee) and to vibration (applied to its tendon). The subject lay prone with the knee at a right angle and the leg pointing upwards. A strap round the leg was connected to the electromagnetic stretcher by a light chain. Same subject as in Fig. 2, and other details similar. (Obtained in collaboration with C. M. Pickup.)

though the long flexor is simultaneously giving the long-latency response that was previously presumed to be transcortical (Matthews, 1984b). A spatial segregation of the neural elements reflexly regulating two muscles that normally co-operate in their action would be so puzzling that the finding, of itself, raises doubt about the validity of the transcortical hypothesis. On the other hand, in the present state of knowledge there is no difficulty in confessing that one does not understand the factors that determine the balance of Ia and II action in producing a spinal reflex, and how far they are central or peripheral.

Recent experiments with C. M. Pickup, on the hamstring muscles, raise further doubts over the transcortical hypothesis; these have yet to be published in detail. In some subjects these muscles may give well-marked, long-latency responses that again appear attributable to group II action, on the basis of the same arguments as before. In other subjects, however, the stretch responses at both "on" and "off" may be dominated by short-latency effects. Fig. 5 shows an example of a long-latency "on" response to stretch, demonstrated by virtue of the fact that the response to vibration is very much more phasic than that to stretch. Again, it would be pressing matters to attempt to decide upon the precise latency of the postulated delayed excitation responsible for the maintenance of motor firing; the precise moment of commencement of the obvious second wave in the response might depend upon other factors than the first arrival of group II im-

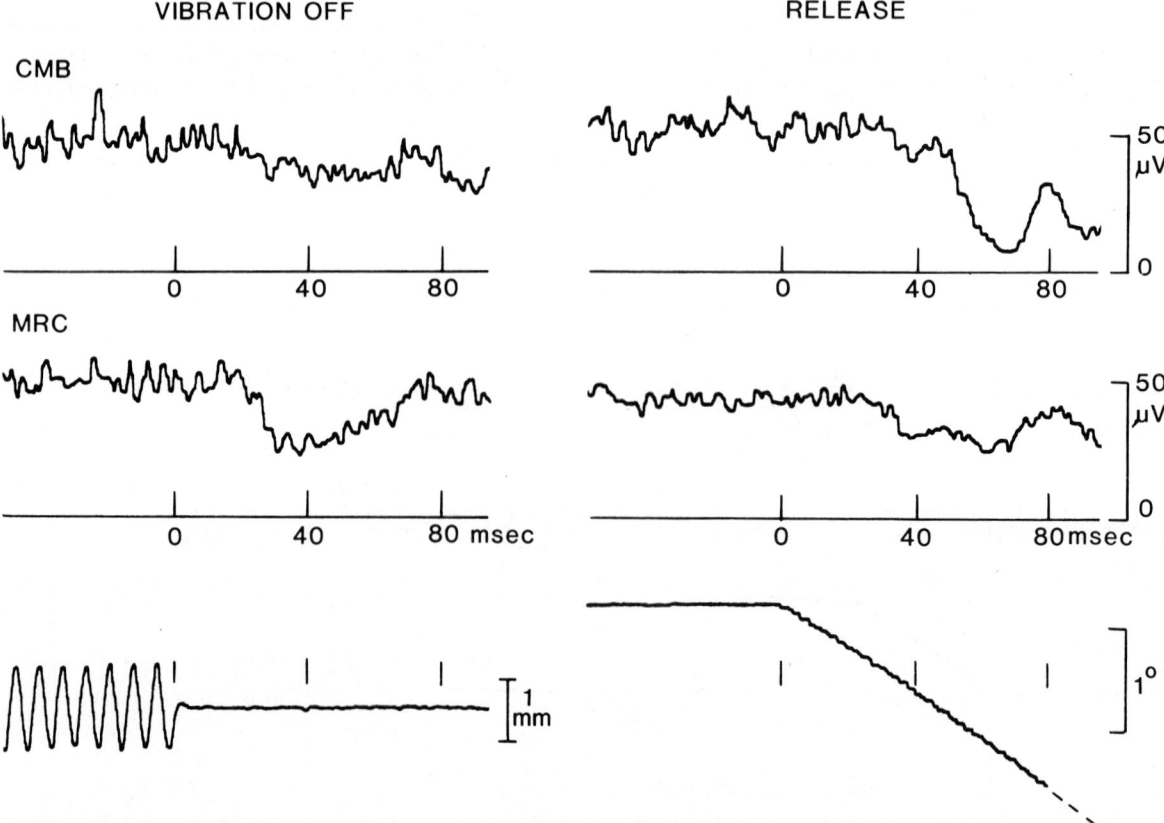

Fig. 6. The "off" responses of semitendinosus for two different subjects (C.M.B., M.R.C.). C.M.B.'s long-latency pathway seemed to be more potent than her short-latency pathway, whereas for M.R.C. the situation was reversed. The duration of the stimuli, preceding their termination, was 300 mseconds. (Obtained in collaboration with C. M. Pickup.)

pulses at the cord. However, the latency of the initial response of semitendinosus, about 30 mseconds, happens to be very similar to that for the long thumb flexor, so that any group II response of semitendinosus would also be expected to occur with a latency of 40 mseconds or above. It may be noted in passing that the semitendinosus short-latency response seems to be rather brisker than that of the long thumb flexor, since simply in terms of the rate of angular deflection of their respective joints the velocity of movement in Fig. 5 for semitendinosus is only about 15% of that in Fig. 2 for flexor pollicis longus.

Fig. 6 shows the "off" effects from two other subjects. C.M.B. (top) had a small short-latency "off" response that was only just detectable with either mode of stimulation. But she showed a clear, large, long-latency response with a latency of nearly 50 mseconds. Her long-latency "on" response to stretch (not illustrated) was appreciably more clearcut than that illustrated in Fig. 5. Subject M.R.C. (Fig. 6, bottom) had brisk short-latency responses and a questionable long-latency response. His "off" response to vibration was large and unequivocal and appears to consist simply of a short-latency component. His "off" response to stretch began with a quite definite short-latency component, much more so than that of C.M.B., and was followed by what may be presumed to be a small long-latency effect. The latter, however, was so weak that no significance could be attached to the downward deflection that it produces were it not for its similarity to C.M.B.'s response. Thus, by combining the data from the two subjects it is possible to recognise unequivocally both short- and long-latency "off" effects for stretch. The importance of this is that it eliminates the possibility that C.M.B.'s obvious delayed response on release of stretch was due merely to mechanical lags slowing the Ia afferent response; the inertia of the leg is much greater than that of the thumb and this might slow its response to stretch without affecting that to vibration, which was applied directly to its tendon. The two subjects were of similar physique, so unloading of their muscle spindles on release might be expected to be similar, even if the shortening of the muscle was an appreciably slowed version of that applied by the stretcher, which is what was recorded.

It is concluded that the group II afferents of semitendinosus, like those of flexor pollicis longus, can reflexly excite their own motoneurones and so produce a spinally mediated long-latency component of the stretch reflex. This extension of the group II hypothesis to cover another muscle is relatively unsurprising, and does little to strengthen the hypothesis per se since the same assumptions and indirect arguments about vibration are involved for both muscles. However, the findings are important in demonstrating that a muscle that is primarily involved in locomotion and posture may possess a distinct long-latency stretch reflex. For now, for such a muscle, the transcortical hypothesis looks distinctly unpromising. There seems no reason to suppose that the hamstrings are under particularly tight cortical control. Kicking backwards does not give one the impression of being an activity that one can control with fine discrimination, least of all in female subjects unaccustomed to using their feet in ball games, as was C.M.B. Thus, it seems implausible to suggest that a significant part of the stretch reflex of semitendinosus could usefully be translocated from the cord to the cortex for certain subjects.

Finally, it should be noted that although semitendinosus is a flexor of the knee it is an extensor of the hip, so it seems unlikely that the present long-latency response can be simply a response of "flexors". The extensors of the wrist have also long been considered to show good long-latency responses to stretch; although their response to vibration has yet to be studied, there can be little doubt that it would elicit the usual phasic response and so provide evidence for an excitatory group II action for these muscles also. Thus, the presently postulated group II autogenetic excitation is believed to be a specific reaction applicable to a wide variety of muscles and not just an example of a widespread FRA (flexor reflex afferent) action that group II afferents have been classically suggested to produce, irrespective of whether they arise in a flexor or an extensor muscle.

Discussion

The present work leads to two conclusions. First, various new findings strengthen the view that there is indeed a separate long-latency component to the stretch reflex of some human muscles that is quite distinct from short-latency Ia action. This has already been urged by others, but their evidence has not met with general satisfaction. Second, the simplest explanation for this response is that it is due to an autogenetic spinal excitatory action of the group II spindle afferents of the stretched muscle. This one assumption is sufficient to cover all the findings since the additional delay, over that of the initial Ia response, then occurs inevitably by virtue of the slower conduction of the group II afferents. Many of the details remain obscure, but no other single hypothesis will satisfactorily cover all the data. This is especially true of the transcortical hypothesis, which fails entirely to meet the findings with vibration. It would also seem to fall down when comparing just the stretch responses of different muscles, without referring to those to vibration. Large, long-latency responses may be found when cortical control might be expected to be weak (semitendinosus), and relatively weak late responses may be seen when cortical control might be expected to be strong (flexor pollicis brevis).

Thus, the transcortical hypothesis would seem to have become untenable as the unique explanation of the specific long-latency component of the stretch reflex. But granted that the spindle group II afferents do elicit such a response, the question arises as to whether the transcortical route provides a significant additional contribution to the stretch reflex of some muscles under some conditions, since the potential neural wiring exists. The present experiments are inevitably silent, and cannot exclude any such contribution, especially under conditions with a different neural set. It has been difficult enough to distinguish long-latency from short-latency responses when both may be contributing simultaneously to the overall motor discharge. To fractionate the long-latency response so as to separate off a small, or a yet longer-latency, cortical component would require more discriminating methods of analysis. Vibration, for example, provides no help in answering the question as to whether the group II afferents might perhaps produce a transcortical response.

However, it would now seem the turn of the protagonists of the transcortical route to produce evidence that it regularly operates in parallel with the spinal group II route to provide a normal component of what can usefully be called a "stretch reflex". The classical view of this reflex is that it is initiated by stretch of a given muscle and then excites the motoneurones of the stretched muscle and its close synergists, and inhibits those of its immediate antagonists. On release, the stretch reflex is rapidly turned off. Clearly, there are some deviations from such strict usage. But to use the term for any response evoked by muscle stretch, including those involving delayed co-activation of agonists and antagonists, is to shift too far and to risk confusing the issue. The same mechanisms are then unlikely to be involved and the functional significance of the response is inevitably quite different from that of a more localised response. For example, Cheney and Fetz's (1984) important demonstration that in the monkey certain recorded pyramidal tract discharges may underlie certain relatively rapid arm responses need not have anything to do with the "stretch reflex" as I would use the term. Long-latency excitation of a muscle was evoked equally by its release, and both agonists and antagonists contracted simultaneously, thereby stiffening the limb. This reaction may perhaps be part of some higher-level more integrated response which can take over from, and superimpose itself upon, the later components of a simpler spinal stretch reflex when the need arises.

Finally, there seems little point in using the machinery of the cerebral cortex to operate something as crude as the classical stretch reflex. Of course, it is useful to provide the higher motor centres with detailed muscle afferent information, and as fast as possible. And in some circumstances they may well use it to modify immediately the outgoing motor pattern. But the cortex must be expected to be doing something different from the spinal cord and performing a more detailed analysis to produce more complex modes of response, including modification of the motor programme before it is used again. The stretch reflex can surely be handled quite adequately by the spinal cord, which seems complex enough also to be contributing to more complex automatic reactions involving recognition of distributed patterns of afferent activity. The stretch reflex, as widely understood, provides an immediate short-term correction to the level of activity of a muscle that is already contracting when its mechanical behaviour deviates from that intended, whether by its shortening too much or too little during movement, or by changing its length when it should be still. To incorporate a spinal group II excitation into such a response would seem to adapt it even better to its purpose, since the receptor properties of the slower afferents complement those of the faster afferents. The initial reflex response to stretch is triggered at short latency by the dynamically sensitive Ia afferents with their high conduction velocity; but with their considerable non-linearity of response they are not well fitted to deal with a progressively increasing disturbance. A more prolonged back-up reflex response would be effectively produced after a slight delay by the slower group II afferents when, with their lower dynamic sensitivity, they signalled that the mechanical deviation from the intended situation was in fact of significant extent, and not just a passing accident which could be expected to have been successfully corrected by the initial Ia-evoked reflex discharge.

Summary

Some human muscles, notably the long flexor of the thumb, do possess a distinct long-latency stretch reflex that is quite separate from short-latency Ia action. However, contrary to much recent belief, this is suggested to be due to a spinal autogenetic excitatory action of the spindle group II afferents rather than to a transcortical action of the Ia afferents. This thesis is based on a comparison of the reflex effects of stretch with that of vibration; the latter fails to elicit appreciable long-latency responses although it powerfully excites the Ia afferents. Both the application and the removal of the stimuli were studied. The transcortical hypothesis is weakened further by comparing the reflex responses of various muscles to stretch.

References

Baldissera, F., Hultborn, H. and Illert, M. (1981) Integration in spinal neuronal systems. In V. B. Brooks (Ed.), The Nervous System, Vol. II, Motor Control, American Physiological Society, Bethesda, MD, pp. 509–595.

Cheney, P. D. and Fetz, E. E. (1984) Corticomotoneuronal cells contribute to long-latency stretch reflexes in the rhesus monkey. J. Physiol., 349: 249–272.

Desmedt, J. E. (Ed.) (1978) Cerebral Motor Control in Man: Long Loop Mechanisms. Progress in Clinical Neurophysiology, Vol. 4, Karger, Basel, 392 pp.

Evarts, E. V. (1981) Role of motor cortex in voluntary movements in primates. In V. B. Brooks (Ed.), The Nervous System, Vol. II, Motor Control, American Physiological Society, Bethesda, MD, pp. 1083–1119.

Marsden, C. D., Merton, P. A. and Morton, H. B. (1976) Servo action in the human thumb. J. Physiol., 257: 1–44.

Marsden, C. D., Merton, P. A., Morton, H. B., Adam, J. and

Hallett, M. (1978) Automatic and voluntary responses to muscle stretch in man. In J. E. Desmedt (Ed.), Cerebral Motor Control in Man: Long Loop Mechanisms, Progress in Clinical Neurophysiology, Vol. 4, Karger, Basel, pp. 167–177.

Marsden, C. D., Rothwell, J. C. and Day, B. L. (1983) Long-latency automatic responses to muscle stretch in man: origin and function. In J. E. Desmedt (Ed.). Motor Control Mechanisms in Health and Disease, Raven Press, New York, pp. 509–539.

Matthews, P. B. C. (1969) Evidence that the secondary as well as the primary endings of the muscle spindles may be responsible for the tonic stretch reflex of the decerebrate cat. J. Physiol., 204: 365–393.

Matthews, P. B. C. (1972) Mammalian Muscle Receptors and their Central Actions, Arnold, London.

Matthews, P. B. C. (1984a) Evidence from the use of vibration that the human long-latency stretch reflex depends upon spindle secondary afferents. J. Physiol., 348: 383–415.

Matthews, P. B. C. (1984b) The contrasting stretch reflex responses of the long and short flexor muscles of the human thumb. J. Physiol., 348: 545–558.

Matthews, P. B. C. (1948c) Observations on the time course of the electromyographic response reflexly elicited by muscle vibration in man. J. Physiol., 353: 447–461.

Matthews, P. B. C. (1985) Human long-latency stretch reflexes — A new role for the secondary ending of the muscle spindle? In W. J. P. Barnes and M. H. Gladden (Eds.), Feedback and Motor Control, Croom Helm, Beckenham, in press.

Wiesendanger, M. and Miles, T. S. (1982) Ascending pathway of low-threshold muscle afferents to the cerebral cortex and its possible role in motor control. Physiol. Rev., 62: 1234–1270.

Experimental evidence for the existence of a proprioceptive transcortical loop

Mario Wiesendanger

Institut de Physiologie, Université de Fribourg, CH-1700 Fribourg, Switzerland

Introduction

60 years after the classical description of the stretch reflex by Liddell and Sherrington (1924), there is still a continuing debate as to its precise nature and functional significance. The matter was complicated, as it was realized that the response to stretch is not limited to a monosynaptic excitation of the stretched muscle, but that a number of receptors other than spindle primaries are activated, that the central effects are not only monosynaptic and, finally, that the afferent volley evoked by stretch will also reach supraspinal targets, which in turn may generate a centrifugal volley transmitted down to the spinal cord. More specifically, it was found by a number of investigators that identified corticospinal neurones often exhibit a burst discharge at a short latency in response to the stretch stimulus. In view of these well documented observations, the notion of a transcortical loop imposed itself. Furthermore, it was reported that the stretch-induced burst of neurones in the motor cortex depended in its magnitude on the amount of stretch, and thus it was considered to be of a "reflex-like" nature. This then led to the idea of a "transcortical reflex" with the further assumption that the "transcortical reflex" might contribute to the later portion of the myotatic response.

In a recent review, we (Wiesendanger and Miles, 1982) have detailed the experimental results and the arguments which led to the concept of a transcortical loop. In that review, we also provided a critique to the concept of a transcortical load-compensating mechanism. The main arguments concern the middle-latency (M2) response to stretch. It was found that this response had too small a gain and occurred too late to account for an effective role in compensating unexpected load perturbations (e.g., Allum, 1975); that similar M2 responses were obtained in lesioned animals with interruption of the proposed transcortical loop (Ghez and Shinoda, 1978; Tracey et al., 1980; Miller and Brooks, 1981); and that muscle spindles often react with a double burst during load perturbations of human arm muscles, which could account for the double myographic response (Eklund et al., 1982a,b). To this we now have to add the results of Matthews (1984a,b,c and Section II), which indicate that muscle spindle secondaries are likely to produce the middle-latency EMG response in some of the distal muscles of the human arm.

We now face the situation that the transcortical servo loop as originally proposed by Phillips (1969) has come under a severe challenge. To cite Matthews (1984a): "Human work, it would appear, has as yet shown nothing that can be unequivocally attributed to a rapid transcortical servo-type reflex evoked by muscle stretch; but ... there seems no immediate prospect of excluding its existence". Although much has already been written about transcortical reflexes, I will try to take stock of the situation, especially from the viewpoint of results obtained in animal experiments. It is my conviction that it would be premature to bury the idea of a transcortical loop and that, on the contrary, further work on the transcortical loop might shed some light on more interesting functions of the muscle spindles than their role in producing spinal stretch reflexes. I will first summarize the main electro-anatomical evidence for the existence of a transcortical loop and then discuss its possible functional significance. I will provide grounds for my opinion that the transcortical loop is bound to provide some of the myotatic response, but that it is difficult to conceive the extent of this contribution and its functional meaning. I will further suggest (as others have done before) that the transcortical loop may play a more meaningful role as an adaptive controller engaged in non-reflex changes of motor commands imposed by the environment in a predictable situation.

There is a powerful projection of low-threshold proprioceptive afferents to the cerebral cortex

This projection has been reviewed in detail (Wiesendanger and Miles, 1982) and there is no need to recapitulate the extensive work done in different species. In brief, the primary cortical receiving area for group I afferents is situated in area 3a (area tenuigranularis) just caudal to the motor cortex and in the depth of the central fissure (Phillips et al., 1971). The system is characterized by rapid conduction, secure synaptic transmission and precise somatotopy. The thalamic relay was found to be localized in a rostral shell of the ventrobasal complex (Maendly et al., 1981). Most recently, we have explored also the first synaptic relay in the lower brainstem. Some of our preliminary results have been published (Wiesendanger and Hummelsheim, 1985). It was found that stretch-sensitive neurones were concentrated in an outer shell of pars rotunda of the main cuneate nucleus, and in the pars triangularis extending towards the external cuneate nucleus and of course also in the external cuneate nucleus proper. This localization fitted well with the extent of anterograde, transganglionic labeling with the marker horseradish peroxidase, which was applied to the deep radial nerve. Filling the cutaneous superficial branch labeled, in a patchy fashion, the core of pars rotunda of the cuneate nucleus (Hummelsheim et al., 1985). In the subcortical structures, the neuronal response properties were similar to those previously observed in cortical area 3a. It also appeared that at all levels the proprioceptive and cutaneous submodalities are spatially segregated. Step displacements of single forearm muscles very effectively excited 3a neurones at threshold amplitudes as small as 10 μm. The most effective stimuli were sinusoidal displacements, suggesting (together with the graded nerve stimulation) that muscle spindle primaries are involved. Of course, it is impossible to exclude the participation of Pacinian receptors, especially with the high-frequency vibratory stimuli, a difficulty encountered in all experiments of this sort, including those in humans (Matthews, 1984a). In a most recent study on neurones of area

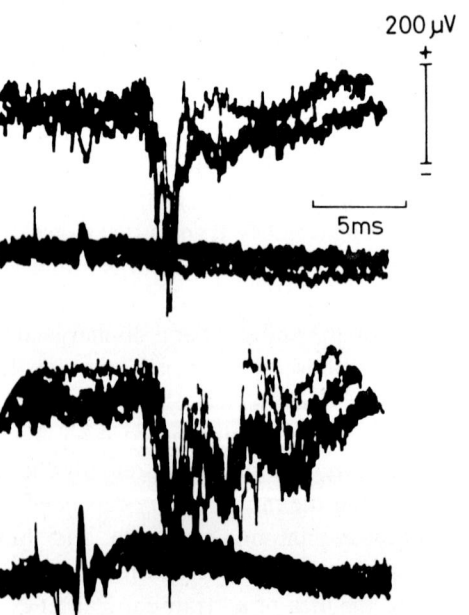

Fig. 1. Field potentials evoked in area 3a of the baboon's cortex (upper trace) by volleys in deep radial nerve. Incoming volley recorded in dorsal root entry zone (lower trace). Upper pair: responses to submaximal group I volley (about 30% of maximum). Lower pair: maximum responses to maximal group I volley + group II volley. Note addition of later cortical potentials (unpublished records from experiments of Phillips, Powell and Wiesendanger).

3a in cats, evidence was advanced that Golgi tendon organs are also likely to project to this area (McIntyre et al., 1984). Graded nerve stimulation in baboon revealed that augmentation of stimulus strength necessary to evoke a maximum group I volley and a subsequent later afferent volley also recruited a later component of the 3a-evoked field potential (Fig. 1). This is suggestive evidence that group II afferents may also influence 3a neurones (Phillips, Powell and Wiesendanger, unpublished observations).

Cortical neurones of the motor cortex are excited at short latency to load perturbations

The information reaching area 3a is further distributed to caudal somatosensory areas and also to the motor cortex. Possibly some proprioceptive input reaches the motor cortex also directly from the thalamus (for discussion of conflicting data, cf. Wiesendanger and Miles, 1982). There is no doubt, however, that motor cortex neurones do also respond to controlled stretch stimuli of single forearm muscles. An example is illustrated in Fig. 2, which is from an identified corticospinal neurone. Although it was noted that under anaesthesia the motor cortex neurones and particularly the output neurones were clearly less sensitive to the proprioceptive signals, later studies in several laboratories have now revealed that in the unanesthetized performing monkey, small load perturbations can indeed effectively excite motor cortex neurones. Wolpaw (1980) showed that discrete (25–50 μm) stretches of a single forearm muscle by an implanted electromagnetic device were likewise capable of evoking burst discharges of motor cortex cells (which included pyramidal tract neurones) at a peak latency of 25 mseconds. Unfortunately, participation of cutaneous receptors was not excluded in these experiments. Demonstration of a transcortical loop for low-threshold muscle afferents comes also from H-reflex experiments in monkeys (Chofflon et al., 1982). It was shown that conditioning stimulation of the popliteal nerve below threshold for the production of an H-reflex and a muscle twitch produced a late facilitation of a subsequent H-reflex at a latency compatible with a fast transcortical loop. This late facilitation was selectively suppressed during reversible cooling of the leg area of the motor cortex, without general depression of the excitability curve.

The most direct evidence for the existence of a transcortical loop was provided by the experiments of Cheney and Fetz (1984). The authors found that nearly all cells which produced a postspike facilitation of a target muscle ("corticomotoneuronal cells") also responded with a short latency burst when the target muscle was briefly stretched. The sum of the afferent transmission time (latency of cortical response to load pulse) and of the efferent transmission time (latency of postspike facilitation) corresponded to the transcortical loop time and was in the range of the M2 electromyographic response elicited by the load pulse. The case of causal relationship was further strengthened for some neurones: if the EMG averages were triggered selectively by those spikes evoked by the torque pulse, the amount of facilitation was larger than if com-

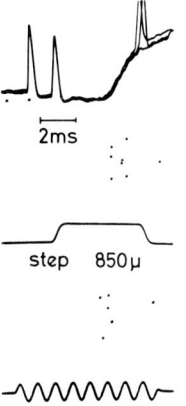

Fig. 2. Responses of identified corticospinal neurone recorded in precentral cortex of Cebus monkey. Above: antidromic response (and later transsynaptic response) elicited by a pair of electrical stimuli at 1-msecond interval (indicated by two dots) applied to the dorsolateral funiculus. Below are dot displays of the spike discharge to a step displacement and a brief train of vibration of the extensor digitorum communis muscle. Response latency about 25 mseconds. The arm was denervated, except for the deep radial nerve. Time calibration for dot rasters indicated by sinusoidal stretch. Adapted from Lucier et al. (1975).

puted with all spikes recorded during the conditioned movement. Furthermore, the perturbation-evoked spikes could also facilitate, at the same latency, a normally unfacilitated synergist. The distinct onset of facilitation was the chief argument which spoke against a non-causal facilitation by other neurones co-activated by the load pulse. Matthews (Section II) would not accept these observations as evidence for a "stretch reflex" partly mediated via the motor cortex because not only stretching of a muscle but sometimes also shortening produced a middle-latency (M2) EMG discharge. Nevertheless, the middle-latency responses observed by Cheney and Fetz (1984) and by many other investigators do have reflex-like properties (i.e., they are graded with the strength of perturbation) and it seems somewhat academic not to consider these responses as myotatic reflexes.

The problem with lesion experiments

The graded, reflex-like discharge of corticomotoneuronal cells must affect motoneuronal excitability. A totally different question is whether or not excitation via the motor cortex contributes significantly in counteracting a load perturbation. First, it should be noted that EMG output occurring at M2 latency, by virtue of its phasic nature, cannot have a servo action in the strict sense. However, it may contribute in the initial phase of compensation, but not complete the job. Furthermore, the effectiveness appears to depend on the size of the perturbation, being greater for small disturbances occurring during the active performance of motor tasks (e.g., Sanes and Evarts, 1983). Many have attempted to evaluate the role of supraspinal structures in the production of middle-latency responses (Tatton et al., 1975; Marsden et al., 1977a,b; Ghez and Shinoda, 1978; Miller and Brooks, 1981; Lenz et al., 1983). Unfortunately, all attempts to assess the role of the transcortical loop by lesions are not conclusive because it can always be argued that the lesions also changed the tonic descending influence exerted at spinal level. Thus, suppression of M2 responses may be due to lack of necessary tonic facilitation. Conversely, persistence of middle-latency responses may result from a disinhibition of other mechanisms operating at a latency similar to that of the transcortical loop. Nevertheless, and with this caveat in mind, the experiments of Noth et al. (1983) provide reasonable evidence for the presence of a transcortical myotatic response in man: in chorea patients, known to have cortical damage, the late component of the myotatic response was either lacking or strongly reduced, and this occurred together with an absent or diminished cortical potential evoked by the stretch stimulus. The possibility that this was due to a diminished descending facilitation was weakened by the finding that a second stretch stimulus applied with appropriate timing evoked a second EMG response at an interval of the normally occurring M2 response.

The hypothesis of an adaptive controller

That the extremely complex neural network of the cerebral cortex might operate also as a reflex centre was an irritating idea for many of us. In fact, it brings back the old doctrines of Sechenov (1965) and Pavlov (1960) about the existence of cortical reflexes. This argument was also brought forward by Matthews (Section II): "Finally, there seems little point in using the machinery of the cerebral cortex to operate something as crude as the classical stretch reflex".*

In 1970, Granit posed the question about the functional meaning of the muscle spindle feedback to the cerebral cortex: "Might not the purpose of the mechanism be to ensure within the cortex a proper balance of alpha and gamma output both, as such, and in relation to the extensor-flexor antagonism in movement?". A long time ago, Gellhorn and Hyde (1953) had found that the motor map could be changed radically with changing limb position. These observations and Granit's proposition

---

* To this, a discussant at the meeting remarked that one could also argue the other way round: namely, that the stretch reflex is too important to be left entirely to the spinal cord!

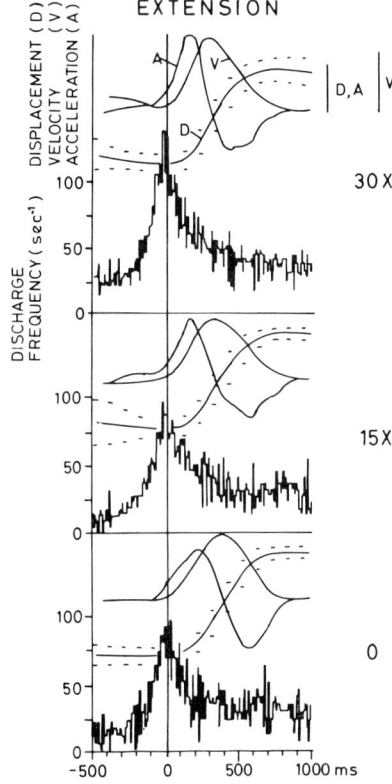

Fig. 3. Computer-averaged movement parameters and histograms of discharge of a precentral neurone co-varying with active elbow extension. Cebus monkey. "0" time indicates movement onset. Calibrations: 20° for displacement (D) and 500°/sec² for acceleration (A); 100°/sec for velocity (V). The self-paced extension movements were exerted against 30, 15 and 0 g of steady loads opposing elbow extension. Note increase of discharge frequency during both the initial "hold" phase and the phasic discharge preceding the movement. Adapted from Conrad et al. (1977).

suggest that proprioceptive feedback may influence motor cortex output in a non-reflex fashion.

There can be little doubt that one of the chief tasks of the motor cortex is to ensure that the motor command is always adapted to the ever changing environment. Much of this can occur in an open loop condition when the disturbances are predictable; this is a preprogrammed adaptation. But even in a predictable situation, a closed-loop adaptation might be useful. An example of such an adaptive change was observed in the experiments of Conrad et al. (1977). We trained monkeys to perform self-paced arm movements against or with steady loads. The loads were changed after blocks of 15–20 trials. (This was essentially also the paradigm used by Evarts (1968), on which Phillips (1969) partly based his transcortical hypothesis.) In this situation, discharge frequency of motor cortex cells increased with increasing load, both in the hold phase and in the move phase. In the latter, the motor cortex cells typically displayed a phasic peak discharge which increased with load. However, in many cells, this peak discharge occurred before movement onset (Fig. 3). The anticipatory phasic discharge was thus clearly preprogrammed and not reflex in nature.

Newell and Houk (1983) proposed a two-stage model of sensorimotor integration, as illustrated in Fig. 4. The important feature in this diagram is that besides the reflex pathways operating with continuous feedback, there is also inclusion of an adaptive controller capable of changing the degree of co-contraction, of changing the reflex gain and of reprogramming the motor command. All of these adaptive changes may help, on a longer time scale, to cope with load disturbances. What we would like to have in the scheme is a feedback (possibly a discontinuous one) to the adaptive controller, so that this controller acquires also self-adapting properties.

Asanuma and Arissian (1984) recently reported

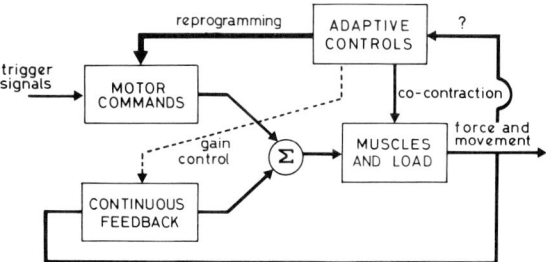

Fig. 4. Two-stage model of Newell and Houk (1983), with the addition of a possible proprioceptive feedback (?) to the adaptive controller. Adaptive changes in sensorimotor integration may be brought about by changes in the amount of co-contraction (cf. also Granit, 1970, p. 219), changes in the reflex gain (continuous feedback), and changes in reprogramming the motor command (which was considered to be triggered in the experimental situation described by Newell and Houk (1983)).

that if the motor cortex is deprived of its somatosensory input by combined postcentral and dorsal column lesions, the motor behaviour was severely disturbed. Initially, there was a paralysis of the hand. Then, disoriented hand movements occurred without target reaching. Finger manipulations were lost. This deficit did not improve markedly over the survival time of 4–5 weeks. These are drastic motor deficits which underline the importance of somatosensory feedback to the cortex for the execution especially of manipulatory tasks. Future experiments with smaller lesions or isolated lesions of the dorsal columns may reveal whether the capacity for the adaptive changes of the sort described in the experiments by Conrad et al. (1977) are impaired.

The non-reflex adaptive mechanisms subserved by proprioceptive feedback to the motor cortex may involve complicated circuits in the motor cortical fields, including premotor areas which are thought to participate in programming movements. We recently found that subpopulations of neurones in both the postarcuate region and the supplementary motor cortex were strikingly responsive to passive arm displacements imposed to the awake monkey (Wiesendanger et al., 1985). Therefore, it is conceivable that the supplementary motor area (SMA) and the premotor cortex act not only in the open-loop way by transmitting instructions to the motor cortex, but that neurones of these areas may already incorporate sensory cue signals in order to update a motor program.

Concluding remarks

The hypothesis of a transcortical servo-like mechanism, first put forward by Phillips (1969), had a remarkable influence in that it generated many experiments designed to test the validity of the hypothesis. Ironically, the hypothesis was refuted by Phillips et al. (1971) and Wiesendanger (1973), since it was found that in anesthetized baboons the cortical output cells to the spinal cord would not discharge to pure group I volleys. It later became apparent that motor cortical cells, including corticospinal neurones, do respond to stretch stimuli (Lucier et al., 1975; Sakai and Preston, 1978); and the sensitivity of motor cortex cells was found to be more pronounced in the fully awake monkey (e.g., Wolpaw, 1980; Cheney and Fetz, 1984). Thus, the idea of a transcortical reflex persisted and, as pointed out in the present account, it cannot be discarded. I have argued that the inherent difficulties to sort out a transcortical contribution from other, non-cortical mechanisms make the problem perhaps non-resolvable. Each theory which has been put forward to explain "late" components of the myotatic response rests on a number of assumptions and uncertainties; and this is also the case for the group II hypothesis of Matthews (Section II).

There are three main messages in this chapter which I would like to convey to the reader: (1) There is a powerful, rapid and somatotopically organized projection system, originating in stretch receptors, to the cerebral cortex, including the motor fields. (2) The descending output cells of the motor cortex may include in their command signal an "error signal" (provided by the muscle spindles). (3) There are behavioural data (Asanuma and Arissian, 1984) which show that if an otherwise intact motor cortex is deprived of its somatosensory input, the motor control, especially of hand manipulations, is strikingly disturbed. These findings, in my opinion, are a great challenge and warrant further studies on the nature of the transcortical loop, especially with respect to adaptive mechanisms.

Acknowledgements

The work of the author and his collaborators was supported by the Swiss National Science Foundation (grant No. 3.522-83), by the Swiss Multiple Sclerosis Society, and by the Stanley-Thomas-Johnson Foundation. I thank Mrs. S. Rossier for typing the manuscript.

References

Allum, J. H. J. (1975) Response to load disturbances in human shoulder muscles: the hypothesis that one component is a pulse test information signal. Exp. Brain Res., 22: 397–426.

Asanuma, H. and Arissian, K. (1984) Experiments on functional role of peripheral input to motor cortex during voluntary movements in the monkey. J. Neurophysiol., 52: 212–227.

Cheney, P. D. and Fetz, E. E. (1984) Corticomotoneuronal cells contribute to long-latency stretch reflexes in the Rhesus monkey. J. Physiol. (Lond.), 349: 249–272.

Chofflon, M., Lachat, J. M. and Rüegg, D. R. (1982) A transcortical loop demonstrated by stimulation of low-threshold muscle afferents in the awake monkey. J. Physiol. (Lond.), 323: 393–402.

Conrad, B., Wiesendanger, M., Matsunami, K. and Brooks, V. B. (1977) Precentral unit activity related to control of arm movements. Exp. Brain Res., 29: 85–95.

Eklund, G., Hagbarth, K.-E., Hägglund, J. V. and Wallin, E. U. (1982a) Mechanical oscillations contribution to the segmentation of the reflex electromyogram response to stretching human muscles. J. Physiol. (Lond.), 326: 65–77.

Eklund, G., Hagbarth, K.-E., Hägglund, J. V. and Wallin, E. U. (1982b) The "late" responses to muscle stretch: The "resonance hypothesis" versus the "long-loop hypothesis". J. Physiol. (Lond.), 326: 79-90.

Evarts, E. V. (1968) Relation of pyramidal tract activity to force exerted during voluntary movements. J. Physiol., 31: 14–27.

Gellhorn, E. and Hyde, J. (1953) Influence of proprioception on map of cortical responses. J. Physiol. (Lond.), 122: 371–385.

Ghez, C. and Shinoda, Y. (1978) Spinal mechanisms of the functional stretch reflex. Exp. Brain Res., 32: 55–68.

Granit, R. (1970) The Basis of Motor Control. Academic Press, London, New York, p. 219.

Hummelsheim, H., Wiesendanger, R., Wiesendanger, M. and Bianchetti, M. (1985) The projection of low-threshold muscle afferents of the forelimb to the main and external cuneate nuclei of the monkey. Neuroscience, in press.

Lenz, F. A., Tatton, W. G. and Tasker, R. R. (1983) The effect of cortical lesions on the electromyographic response to joint displacement in the squirrel monkey forelimb. J. Neurosci., 3: 795–805.

Liddell, E. G. T. and Sherrington, C. S. (1924) Reflexes in response to stretch (myotatic reflexes). Proc. Roy. Soc. B., 96: 212–242.

Lucier, G. E., Rüegg, D. G. and Wiesendanger, M. (1975) Responses of neurones in motor cortex and in area 3a to controlled stretches of forelimb muscles in Cebus monkeys. J. Physiol. (Lond.), 251: 833–853.

Maendly, E., Rüegg, D. G., Wiesendanger, M., Wiesendanger, R., Lagowska, J. and Hess, B. (1981) Thalamic relay for group I muscle afferents of forelimb nerves in the monkey. J. Neurophysiol., 46: 901–917.

Marsden, C. D., Merton, P. A., Morton, H. B. and Adam, J. (1977a) The effect of posterior column lesions on servo responses from the human long thumb flexor. Brain, 100: 185–200.

Marsden, C. D., Merton, P. A., Morton, H. B. and Adam, J. (1977b) The effect of lesions of the sensorimotor cortex and the capsular pathways on servo responses from the human long thumb flexor. Brain, 100: 503–526.

Matthews, P. B. C. (1984a) Evidence from the use of vibration that the human long-latency stretch reflex depends upon spindle secondary afferents. J. Physiol. (Lond.), 348: 383–415.

Matthews, P. B. C. (1984b) The contrasting stretch reflex responses of the long and short flexor muscles of the human thumb. J. Physiol. (Lond.), 348: 545–558.

Matthews, P. B. C. (1984c) Observations on the time course of the electromyographic response reflexly elicited by muscle vibration in man. J. Physiol. (Lond.), 353: 447–461.

McIntyre, A. K., Proske, U. and Rawson, J. A. (1984) Cortical projection of afferent information from tendon organs in the cat. J. Physiol. (Lond.), 354: 395–406.

Miller, A. D. and Brooks, V. B. (1981) Late muscular responses to arm perturbations persist during supraspinal dysfunction in monkeys. Exp. Brain Res., 41: 146–158.

Newell, K. M. and Houk, J. C. (1983) Speed and accuracy of compensatory responses to limb disturbances. J. Exp. Psychol., 9: 58–74.

Noth, J., Friedemann, H.-H., Podoll, K. and Lange, H. W. (1983) Absence of long-latency reflexes to imposed finger displacement in patients with Huntington's disease. Neurosci. Lett., 35: 97–100.

Pavlov, I. P. (translated by G. V. Anrep) (1960) Conditioned reflexes. An investigation of the physiological activity of the cerebral cortex. Dover Publishers Inc., New York.

Phillips, C. G. (1969) The Ferrier lecture: Motor apparatus of the baboon's hand. Proc. Roy. Soc. B., 173: 141–174.

Phillips, C. G., Powell, T. P. S. and Wiesendanger, M. (1971) Projection from low threshold muscle afferents of hand and forearm to area 3a of baboon's cortex. J. Physiol. (Lond.), 217: 419–446.

Sakai, T. and Preston, J. B. (1978) Evidence for a transcortical reflex: primate corticospinal tract neuron responses to ramp stretch of muscle. Brain Res., 159: 463–467.

Sanes, J. N. and Evarts, E. V. (1983) Effects of perturbations on accuracy of arm movements. J. Neurosci., 3: 977–986.

Sechenov, I. M. (translated by S. Belsky) (1965) Reflexes of the brain. An attempt to establish the physiological basis of psychological processes. MIT Press, Cambridge, MA.

Tatton, W. G., Forner, S. D., Gerskin, G. L., Chambers, W. W. and Liu, C. N. (1975) The effect of postcentral cortical lesions on motor responses to sudden upper limb displacements in monkeys. Brain Res., 96: 108–113.

Tracey, D. J., Walmsley, B. and Brinkman, J. (1980) "Longloop" reflexes can be obtained in spinal monkeys. Neurosci. Lett., 18: 59–65.

Wiesendanger, M. (1973) Input from muscles and cutaneous

nerves of the hand and forearm to neurones of the precentral gyrus of baboons and monkeys. J. Physiol. (Lond.), 228: 203–219.

Wiesendanger, M. and Hummelsheim, H. (1985) The medullary relay of activity from low-threshold proprioceptive afferents of forelimbs in the monkey. In M. J. Rowe and W. D. Willis (Eds.), Development, Organization and Processing in Somatosensory Pathways, Alan Liss Inc., New York, pp. 175–181.

Wiesendanger, M. and Miles, T. S. (1982) Ascending pathways of low-threshold muscle afferents to the cerebral cortex and its possible role in motor control. Physiol. Rev., 62: 1234–1280.

Wiesendanger, M., Hummelsheim, H. and Bianchetti, M. (1985) Sensory input to the motor fields of the agranular frontal cortex: a comparison of the precentral, supplementary motor, and premotor cortex. Behav. Brain Res., in press.

Wolpaw, J. R. (1980) Correlation between task-related activity and responses to perturbation in primate sensorimotor cortex. J. Neurophysiol., 44: 1122–1138.

Visual inputs relevant for the optokinetic nystagmus in mammals

K.-P. Hoffmann

Abteilung für Vergleichende Neurobiologie, Biologie IV, Universität Ulm, Oberer Eselsberg, 7900 Ulm, F.R.G.

Introduction

To write about visual input relevant for optokinetic nystagmus one can take a very simplistic view, maybe an oversimplistic one. Visual information relevant for optokinetic nystagmus (OKN) is to be found in the midbrain structures of the nucleus of the optic tract (NOT) and the terminal nuclei of the accessory optic tract. Information concerning these structures becomes more and more sparse in higher mammals, and we know surprisingly little about their role, especially their role in visually guided behaviour of monkey and man. Therefore, I am going to describe what we know so far about the visual input to the NOT in the cat, and present evidence that the output of the NOT is the visual input relevant for horizontal OKN (Grasse and Cynader, 1984; Hoffmann, 1983a).

As sources of visual input to structures involved in the generation of the optokinetic nystagmus we have to consider, first and naturally, the retina and, second, the visual cortex. Fig. 1 shows the input streams to the pretectum in the cat, and we can only speculate that it may be similar in the monkey. Basically, the organization of these input streams seems very similar to the retinal input to the superior colliculus. Two major conduction velocity groups project directly from the retina to the pretectum: fast Y-like and slow W-like axons. The influence of the X-like axons is weak. In addition, we find an indirect relay through visual cortex, which in the cat is certainly through several visual areas (Schoppmann and Hoffmann, 1979). More specific information is available about the relay involving complex cells in layer V of areas 17 and 18 (Schoppmann, 1981). These corticopretectal cells are activated directly and indirectly by Y-axons from the lateral geniculate nucleus and it is very probable that they are the same cells that project to the superior colliculus (Hoffmann and Stone, 1971; Hoffmann, 1973). If we consider only the structure in the pretectum involved in the optokinetic nystagmus, the visual input to the NOT is provided by W-axons from the

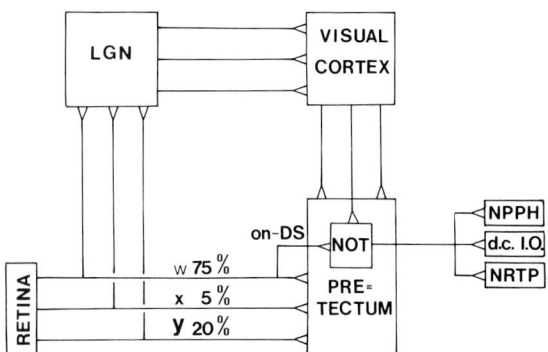

Fig. 1. Visual input to the pretectum of the cat. 75% of the cells in the pretectum are activated by slowly conducting retinofugal fibres of the W-cell class, 20% by the fast conducting fibres of the Y-cells, and only 5% by fibres of X-cells. The NOT receives a large proportion of its retinal input from W-cells with on-centre direction-selective receptive fields. The cortical input to the NOT originates from layer V pyramidal cells with "complex" receptive fields. The NOT projects to the nucleus prepositus hypoglossi (NPPH), the dorsal cap of the inferior olive (d.c. I.O.), and the nucleus reticularis tegmenti pontis (NRTP). LGN, lateral geniculate nucleus.

retina and by pyramidal cell axons from the visual cortex (Hoffmann, 1983a; Hoffmann and Schoppmann, 1981; Schoppmann, 1981). Why do we need a cortical input on top of the retinal input? Are both retinal and cortical visual input balanced or does one input play the dominant role? I would like to put forward the hypothesis that the visual input coming from visual cortex to the NOT strongly dominates the OKN. To develop the arguments to support this hypothesis I first have to describe the receptive field properties of cells in the NOT as the main relay structure for the horizontal OKN.

The visual receptive fields of neurons in the NOT are very large (up to 90° horizontal width) and they respond direction specifically over a very broad velocity spectrum (<0.1–$>100°/sec$). All cells in the left nucleus prefer movements to the left and all in the right nucleus prefer movements to the right in the visual world (Hoffmann and Schoppmann, 1981). The output of these neurons goes to, or at least near, three sites, i.e., the dorsal cap of the inferior olive, the nucleus prepositus hypoglossi and the area of the nucleus reticularis tegmenti pontis (Precht et al., 1980; Lannou et al., 1984). All these areas are involved in stabilizing reflexes of eyes, head or body. The evidence for a role of the output of neurons in the NOT of mammals in mediating OKN so far is indirect. Most of the evidence derives from the analysis of single cell responses to visual stimulation in the anaesthetized preparation and on the analysis of OKN in normal animals or in animals with pretectal or cortical lesions (Hoffmann, 1983a; Precht et al., 1980; Strong et al., 1984; Wood et al., 1973). We took the direct approach in recording from NOT neurons in awake cats with search coils implanted around their eyes to measure eye movements in a magnetic field during optokinetic stimulation. As in the NOT of anaesthetized cats, the cells preferred large area stimuli, responded well to very low velocities ($<1°/sec$), were direction specific for horizontal movement and were

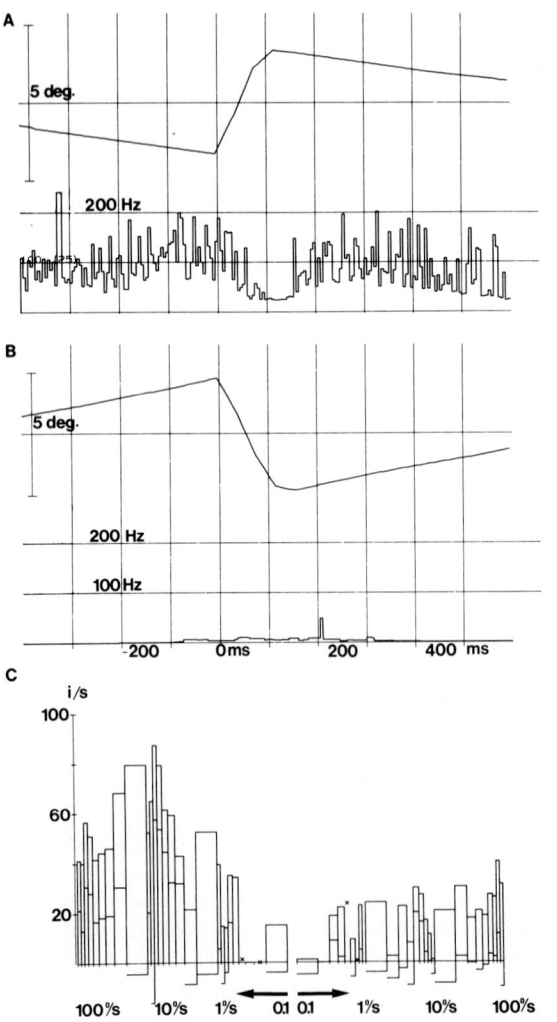

Fig. 2. Receptive field properties of cells in the nucleus of the optic tract. The upper traces in A and B show the eye position signal during OKN averaged from about 20 saccades. The lower traces show the averaged discharge frequency of NOT cells 400 mseconds before and 600 mseconds following the onset of the saccades. During smooth pursuit from right to left (A) the neuron shows an increased discharge due to the remaining retinal slip. During the saccades, the discharge frequency drops to the spontaneous level. During smooth pursuit from left to right (B) the neuron's discharge is completely suppressed, with a weak recovery during saccades. The neuron responds highly direction-specifically to retinal slip. C, discharge frequency (i/sec) on the ordinate is plotted versus slip during OKN (°/sec) on the abscissa. Discharge frequency increases with increasing slip velocities up to 20–30°/sec from right to left. Slip velocities during smooth pursuit from left to right have little influence on the discharge rate. The responses of several NOT cells have been pooled for this diagram. The relationship between slip and discharge rate has been calculated by a computer program from closed-loop OKN recordings.

mostly binocularly activated (see Fig. 2). So far, we have analysed the relationship to OKN in 36 cells from three animals. All cells responded to retinal slip over a range from less than 1°/sec to more than 100°/sec (best response at about 10–20°/sec). The discharge rate (spontaneous: 5–50 spikes/sec) was not modulated during optokinetic afternystagmus or during the vestibulo-ocular reflex in the dark. Electrical stimulation through the recording electrode (pulse width, 1 msecond; frequency, 60 Hz; maximal amplitude, 0.5 mA) elicited eye movements in a clear OKN pattern, as if the preferred stimulus had been presented to the cells.

Therefore, NOT cells provide a direction-selective signal about retinal slip during OKN. In a normal cat, slow-phase eye velocity during OKN was always slower than the stimulus velocity and cells in the left (right) NOT would discharge at a rate above spontaneous activity as long as the stimulus moved leftward (rightward) (Hoffmann and Huber, 1983).

The experimental method of identifying the specific input cells to the NOT has been the use of antidromic identification of retinal ganglion cells or corticofugal cells and the study of the receptive field properties of such antidromically identified cells.

Retinal output relevant for the optokinetic nystagmus

In a recent study (Hoffmann and Stone, 1985) we

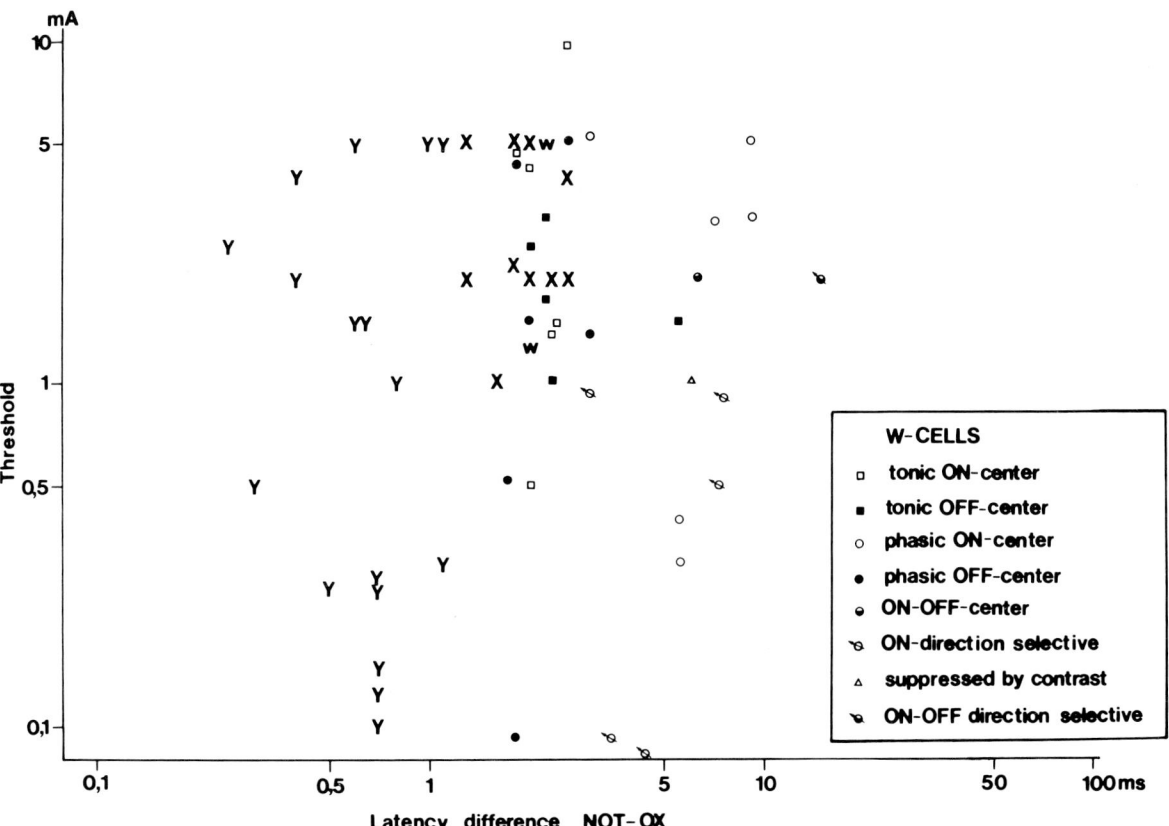

Fig. 3. This figure represents the relationship between threshold for antidromic stimulation from the NOT in mA and conduction time between the NOT and the optic chiasma (NOT-OX) in mseconds. Different ganglion cell classes are plotted by different symbols. Y, Y-cells; X, X-cells. The symbols representing W-cells are explained in the inset to Fig. 3. All on-centre direction-selective cells have a very low threshold, and by that probably project to the NOT. Many Y-cells have a low threshold too, but their latencies are too short to qualify as input to the NOT (for further explanations see text).

sought to identify the ganglion cells which project to the NOT by recording individual ganglion cells in the retina and by determining which could be activated antidromically and with weak stimulus currents by a stimulating electrode in the NOT. This allowed both a test of previous conclusions on retinal input and an assessment of the receptive field properties of the ganglion cells involved. In a population of 558 retinal ganglion cells 98 cells were activated antidromically from the NOT, including 43 Y-cells (35% out of 122), 21 X-cells (7% out of 310) and 34 W-cells (27% out of 126). These different ganglion cell classes were identified by their receptive field properties and the conduction veloc-

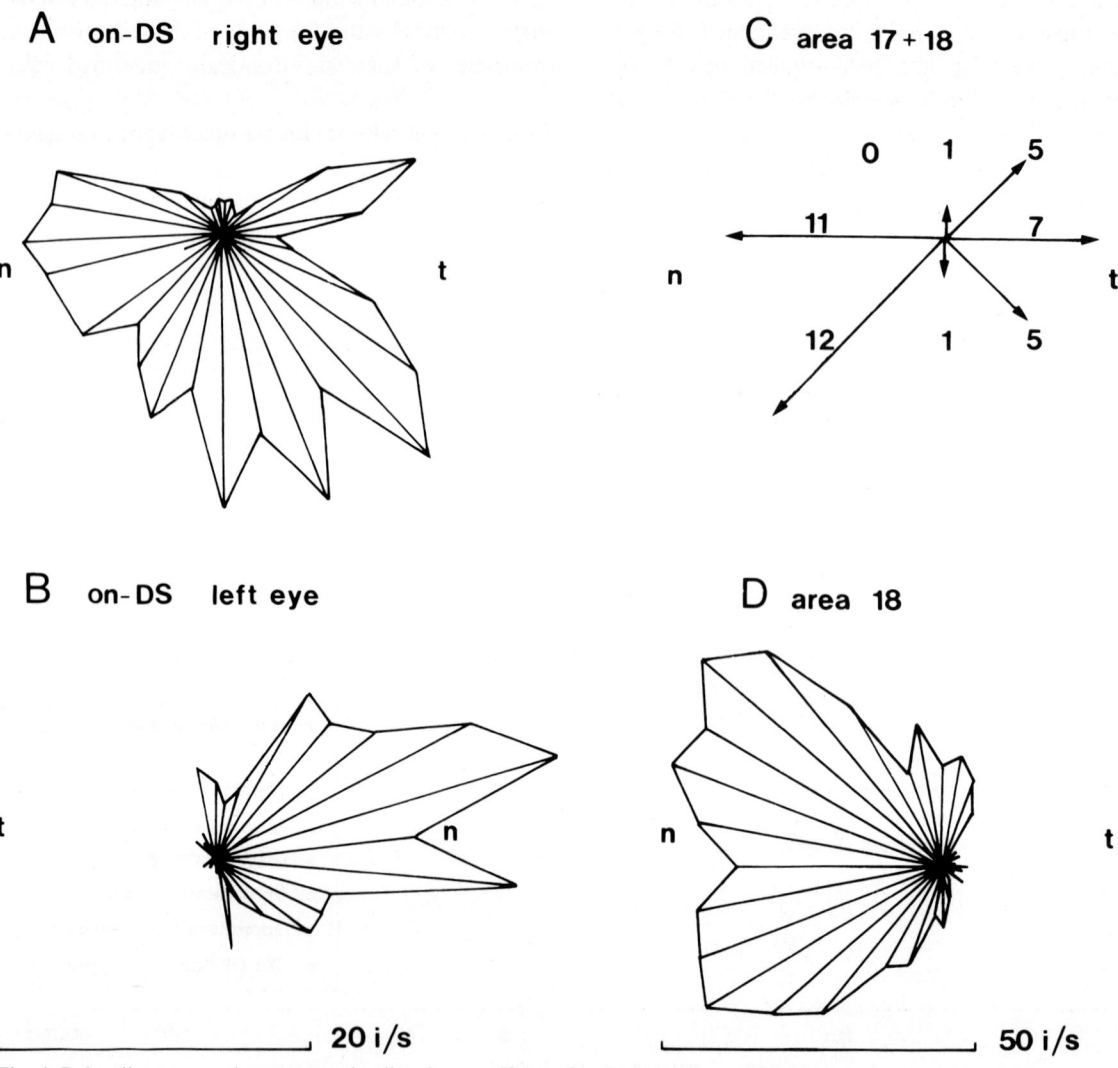

Fig. 4. Polar diagrams to demonstrate the direction specificity of retinal ganglion cells with on-centre receptive fields (A, B) and a cortical cell from area 18 (D) projecting to the NOT. Response strength to movement of a large area random dot pattern in different directions is presented by the length of the lines from the origin to the border of the polar diagram. t (temporal) and n (nasal) indicate the direction in visual space for the eye contralateral to the recorded NOT. Movements from temporal to nasal are preferred by cells in the NOT. In C, we present the frequency of preferred directions for cortical cells projecting to the NOT. This figure is taken from Schoppmann (1981).

ity of their axons. Y-cell axons have the highest conduction velocity and W-axons the lowest. Fig. 3 shows the relationship between latencies and threshold to electrical stimulation for the Y-, X- and W-cells. The different subclasses of W-cells are indicated with different symbols. The latencies shown on the X-axis are the differences between the cell's antidromic latency to NOT and to optic chiasm stimulation. This value is used for two reasons. It eliminates latency variations caused by differences between cells in their retinal location and allows comparisons with an earlier study of the conduction velocity of retinal afferents to the NOT cells (Hoffmann and Schoppman, 1981). That study indicated that the conduction time along retinal axons for the length from the chiasm to the NOT is 3–7 mseconds. This expected range of latencies indicates that Y-axons and most X-axons are too fast conducting and some W-axons are too slow conducting to contribute to the major retinal drive to NOT cells. Fig. 3 demonstrates that only Y-cells and W-cells could be activated at low threshold from the NOT electrode; thus, only W-cells meet two criteria of retinal afferents to the NOT, appropriate conduction velocity and low threshold of antidromic stimulation. This group of W-cells includes one or more example of the following subclasses of W-cells distinguished by Stone and Fukuda (1974): phasic (three cells), tonic (two cells), suppressed by contrast (one cell), and on-centre direction-selective (five cells). Of interest is the presence of five on-centre direction-selective cells among the 11 putative NOT afferent cells. This is much higher than the proportion of these cells among W-cells generally. The contribution made by these cells to the direction selectivity of NOT cells and by that to the OKN will be considered next. Among the five on-centre direction-selective cells activated from NOT at low threshold, the preferred directions of two were horizontal (temporal to nasal) and of three were oblique (one up and temporo-nasal, one up and naso-temporal, one down and naso-temporal). The directional tuning curves of two of these cells are depicted in Fig. 4A,B. Two more direction-selective on-centre cells were not activated from the NOT and had preferred directions downwards and temporo-nasal. Going into these experiments we had anticipated that the retinal input to the NOT might be formed principally or entirely by the on-centre direction-selective cells described by Stone and Fukuda (1964). We were influenced in that expectation by Oyster and Barlow's (1967) suggestion that direction-selective ganglion cells in the rabbit retina provide the error signal for stabilization of the retinal image. Their suggestion was developed by Oyster et al. (1972), Collewijn (1981) and Simpson (1984), with the idea that retinal slip direction is determined and coded by the accessory optic system. Two results indicate that this retinal direction selectivity is not sufficient to account for the marked preference of the NOT cells for stimuli moving horizontally from temporal to nasal in the visual field. First, the direction-selective ganglion cells were only a fraction of the W-cells activated at low threshold from the NOT (five out of 11); and second, in three of the five direction-selective cells the preferred direction was vertical rather than horizontal. Even so, the present results do not entirely preclude that direction-selective on-centre W-cells form a major part of the retinal input to the NOT. In comparing receptive field properties of NOT cells with those of the retinal on-centre direction-selective cells, some discrepancies have to be explained. The large size of NOT receptive fields can be made up by a lot of convergence of retinal ganglion cells. However, NOT cells in the adult cat respond to stimulus velocities up to 100°/sec whereas the direction-selective retinal input cells hardly respond to velocities above 20°/sec. Also, most NOT cells can be activated from both eyes whereas the retinal input seems to come almost exclusively from the contralateral eye (Hoffmann, 1983a; Ballas et al., 1981). As judged by the ontogeny of the optokinetic reflex, NOT neurons seem to be driven by the retinal input alone only during the first few months of life (Hoffmann, 1983a; Van Hof-Van Duin, 1978; Malach et al., 1981). After that, changes in the optokinetic reflex occur which can only be accounted for by a strong cortical input to the NOT cells. The functional role of the retinal input to NOT cells in the adult cat thus remains to be clarified by other methods.

Cortical output relevant for optokinetic nystagmus

As many anatomical and physiological studies show, layer V pyramidal cells provide the corticopretectal projection system. What are the response properties of these cells? Cortical cells projecting to the NOT were again identified by antidromic stimulation of the terminals of such cells in the NOT (Schoppmann, 1981). Antidromic latencies show a mean latency of 2.8 ± 1.5 mseconds, and the conduction velocity of corticopretectal fibres can thus be estimated to be approximately 13 m/sec. Response properties of cortical units activated antidromically from the NOT-stimulating electrode were very similar to the so-called corticotectal layer V pyramidal cells. All units have (for the visual cortex) quite large receptive fields, with up to 5° in diameter, and could be activated equally well by oriented light bars as by large area random dot patterns moved across their receptive field. By contrast, within the enitre cortical population tested only 48% of the recorded units could be activated by either of the two types of pattern. All the antidromically activated units preferred certain movement directions to others or were strongly direction-selective, with a preference for horizontal movements on the average (see Fig. 4C). Some units were studied in more detail for the velocity tuning and ocular dominance. With all the cells tested there was a peak response found for a stimulus velocity between 1 and 10°/sec in area 17 and the ve-

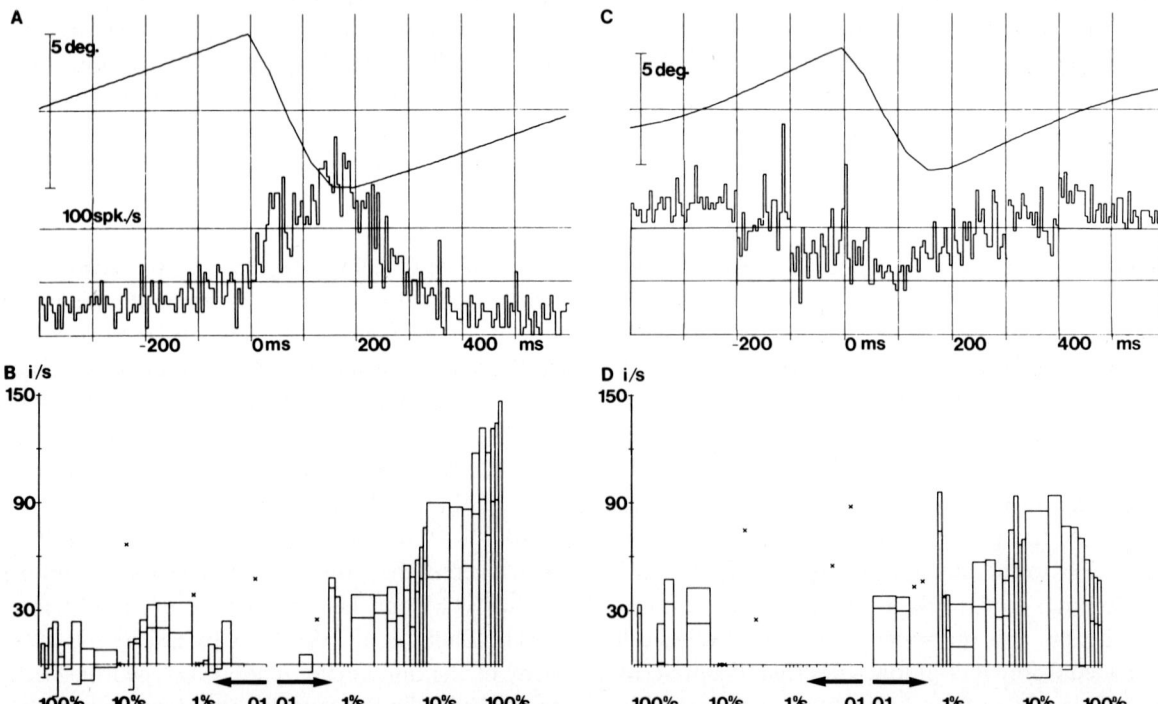

Fig. 5. Responses of area 18 cells in the awake cat during OKN. Presentation as in Fig. 2. A, B, cell prefers high stimulus velocities. C, D, cell tuned for moderate velocities (10–30°/sec). The cells' responses during OKN (A, C) can be explained by the velocity response profiles in B and D. A, C, upper traces represent eye position during OKN from left to right, which is the preferred direction of the cells; lower trace: averaged discharge rate before, during and after the saccades. Saccade onset at 0 mseconds. B, D, Averaged discharge frequency (i/sec) on the ordinate is plotted versus retinal slip velocity during OKN on the abscissa (°/sec). The neurons prefer movements from left to right.

locity response of area 18 cells was higher (see later). Generally, the velocity tuning of cortical cells was narrower than that of NOT cells recorded at the stimulation sites. The directional preference was found to be independent of the velocity of the stimulus. All cells but one were binocular and the responses were enhanced by binocular stimulation as compared to stimulation of either eye alone. In our study these corticopretectal cells could rarely be activated by electrical stimulation of the geniculocortical pathway. Nevertheless, from other studies on the input to layer V pyramidal cells projecting to the mesencephalon we can argue that such cells are most likely activated by Y-fibres from the geniculate (Singer et al., 1975). To get a more direct answer of the contribution of such corticopretectal cells to the optokinetic reflex we recorded neurons from area 18 simultaneously with eye movements in awake cats (Hoffmann et al., 1984). Figs. 4D and 5 show typical responses of such cells during optokinetic stimulation. In this study so far, there are only very few units responding clearly to eye movements in the dark. The interesting phenomena happen during the interaction between neuronal events signalling active eye movements and the information inflow from visual stimulation of the retina. Many cells in area 18 are capable of responding to both phases of the OKN, i.e., to the resultant retinal slip during the smooth pursuit and to the intermittent quick shifts induced by saccades (Fig. 5A, C). Regarding the retinal slip during smooth pursuit, there are cells specialized for the direction of the slip, with a response optimum at different values of the velocity range, or whose discharge frequency is directly related to the stimulus velocity at least up to 100°/sec (Fig. 5B, D). At least the paracentral and peripheral parts of area 18 thus appear to be involved preferentially in movement processing by different groups of cells tuned specifically for different directions and velocities of the stimulus. The relatively high proportion of retinal slip-encoding cells in layer V seems to be related to the control of the preoculomotor structures such as the NOT during those elements of the OKN, and it is especially the role of layer V complex cells for higher stimulus velocities which becomes important for the visual input to the OKN.

The activity bursts correlated with the quick retinal image displacements present themselves as a more complex phenomenon (see Fig. 5A, C). During the fast resetting phases eye velocities of more than 100°/sec appear for a short time in the opposite direction, as in the smooth pursuit phase. This leads to a high instantaneous acceleration in retinal image slip in the same direction as during smooth pursuit. Approximately 61% of the neurons respond with a short frequency increase (bursts). These bursts are dependent on slip velocity and are most evident for stimuli moving in the preferred direction of the cell, across the retina. A minority of neurons (about 9%) show temporary inhibition following the resetting saccades and 30% of the recorded neurons do not show any effects related to the saccadic eye movements. The latencies of bursting cells are more clearly determined and are mostly about 30–50 mseconds. These latencies are shorter than those induced by passive retinal image shifts. In all directions tested the bursts elicited by passive fast movements have considerably longer latencies than the saccade-related bursts, i.e., 57 ± 12 versus 39 ± 7.5 mseconds, respectively.

It is important to note here that the cells in the NOT tested under the same optokinetic condition do not respond with an activity increase during the resetting saccades of OKN. It seems that the characteristic response profiles to different velocities in cells of the NOT and the visual cortex entirely determine their behaviour during the slow and fast phases of OKN. The saccade-related bursts from corticopretectal cells must be eliminated by slow velocity-specific local circuits in the NOT or the cells of the NOT need such a high degree of convergence of many cells that the saccade-related bursts of some cells remain subthreshold. The problem remains unresolved in our current studies. The comparison of retinal and cortical input to the NOT very clearly shows that the typical response profile of the cells in the adult cat's NOT depends on a strong cortical input. As has been elaborated in a previous review (Hoffmann, 1983a), after early monocular deprivation or following lesions of the visual cortex in both hemispheres the remaining retinal input to the NOT leads to a much reduced modulation of the activity of these neurons and to the failure of these neurons to respond to velocities above 20°/sec (Hoffmann, 1979, 1983b). Concomitant changes can be seen in the OKN (Malach et al., 1984). Clearly, the new functional role of this cortical visual input on top of the retinal input consists in adding binocularity and response strength, particularly at higher stimulus velocities, to the visual input relevant for OKN.

What then remains as the contribution of the retinal input? To study this, one should be able to block selectively the retinal input to the NOT whereas the information flow through the visual cortex must remain functional. A lesion approach seems impossible because retinofugal fibres to the geniculate and to the pretectum are close together up to the geniculate. The corticofugal fibres join into the optic tract and brachium to the superior colliculus so that a lesion posterior to the geniculate also seems inappropriate. Recent studies by Schiller (1982), Bolz et al. (1984) and Slaughter and Miller (1981) have shown the possibility of blocking selectively the on-responses in the retina by injecting the drug 2-amino-4-phosphonobutyric acid (APB) into the vitreous body of the eye. As we have shown with our retinal recordings, the retinal input to the NOT is most probably made up to a large degree by the on-centre direction-selective cells. If we inject APB into the vitreous body these cells projecting to the NOT should be blocked whereas the off-cells projecting through the geniculate to the corticopretectal cells should remain functional. Sherk and Horton (1984) have shown that cortical cells retain their normal response characteristics, although at lower discharge rates after APB block of the on-channels. We have injected APB into the eye and then tested the OKN. Fig. 6 documents the gain of slow-phase eye velocity before and after the injection of APB. As can be seen, there is a slight but significant reduction in gain over the whole velocity range tested. Thus, the hypothesis that the retinal input may be particularly important at the low-velocity range, which would be optimal for the on-centre direction-selective cells, is not supported by this finding. Therefore, we have to assume that in the adult system the corticofugal influence on the cells in the NOT is strongly dominating their responses. And by that we can argue that the visual input relevant for the optokinetic nystagmus comes from the retina, not directly, but by way of the layer V pyramidal cells in the visual cortex. These cells most probably are activated by the Y-system. With respect to the retinal ganglion cell class providing the visual input to the OKN, it follows that the Y-cells are the most important candidates.

Another inference can be drawn from these studies. If one looks at the development of the relative strength of retinal and cortical contributions to OKN in man, there seems to be clear evidence that OKN is elicited through a retinofugal subcortical pathway during the first 6 months of life (Atkinson, 1979; Naegele and Held, 1982). Later, this pathway is substituted by binocular cortical cells. At present, it is unclear whether the cortical output for OKN is relayed through the NOT. Certainly this cortical

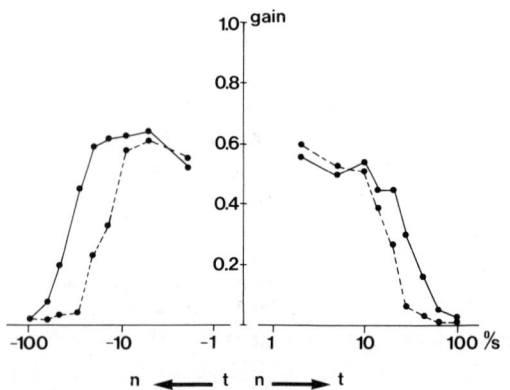

Fig. 6. Effect of APB on the gain of the OKN in the cat. Gain (eye velocity/stimulus velocity) is plotted on the ordinate, stimulus velocity in °/sec on the abscissa. OKN gain in response to temporo-nasal stimulus movement in the visual field is plotted to the left, and OKN gain in response to naso-temporal stimulation to the right. The same eye was tested before (continuous line) and 3–12 hours after the injection of APB (broken line). There is no selective decrease in gain at low stimulus velocities, which are optimal for the direct retinal input to the NOT.

output becomes very prominent, because in man with cortical lesions OKN can hardly be elicited. The retinal input to NOT in man may become replaced so completely by the cortical input that in the adult it has become non-functioning. A cortical lesion may thus lead to the wrong impression that the NOT does not exist in man. It is my hope that this paper will stimulate further research to identify the visual input relevant for OKN in primates, and in particular in man.

Conclusions

The visual input relevant for the horizontal OKN in the cat is relayed through neurons in the NOT and the dorsal terminal nucleus of the accessory optic tract. These neurons respond in a direction-selective manner to movements of large area stimuli over a broad velocity range (0.1–100°/sec). The discharge rate of all neurons in the left NOT increases with leftward movement, and vice versa. This makes these neurons optimally suited to code retinal slip during the slow phase of OKN. The visual input to these cells originates from W-cells in the retina and from complex cells in visual cortex. In the normal adult cat the receptive field properties of NOT neurons are determined by the cortical input which provides a binocular signal over the full velocity range. The retinal input is important during development and after visual deprivation or decortication. These pathways still await identification in primates.

Acknowledgement

This study was supported by DFG grant Ho 450/17.

References

Atkinson, J. (1979) Development of optokinetic nystagmus in the human infant and monkey infant: an analogue to development in kittens. In R. D. Freeman (Ed.), Developmental Neurobiology of Vision, NATO Advanced Study Institutes Series, Series A: Life Sciences, Vol. 27, Plenum Press, New York, pp. 277–287.

Ballas, I., Hoffmann, K.-P. and Wagner, H. J. (1981) Retinal projection to the nucleus of the optic tract in the cat as revealed by retrograde transport of horseradish peroxidase. Neurosci. Lett., 26: 197–202.

Bolz, J., Waessle, H. and Thier, P. (1984) Pharmacological modulation of on and off ganglion cells in the cat retina. J. Neurosci., 12: 875–885.

Collewijn, H. (1981) The oculomotor system of the rabbit and its plasticity. In H. B. Barlow, H. Bullock, E. Florey, O. J. Gruesser and H. Van der Loos (Eds.), Studies of Brain Function, Vol. 5, Springer-Verlag, Berlin, pp. 75–106.

Grasse, K. L. and Cynader, M. S. (1984) Electrophysiology of lateral and dorsal terminal nuclei of the cat accessory optic system. J. Neurophysiol., 51: 276–293.

Hoffmann, K.-P. (1973) Conduction velocity in pathways from retina to superior colliculus in the cat: A correlation with receptive field properties. J. Neurophysiol., 36: 409–424.

Hoffmann, K.-P. (1979) Optokinetic nystagmus and single-cell responses in the nucleus tractus opticus after early monocular deprivation in the cat. In R. D. Freeman (Ed.), Developmental Neurobiology of Vision, Plenum Press, New York, pp. 63–72.

Hoffmann, K.-P. (1983a) Control of the optokinetic reflex by the nucleus of the optic tract in the cat. In A. Hein and M. Jeannerod (Eds.), Spatially Oriented Behavior, Springer, New York, pp. 135–153.

Hoffmann, K.-P. (1983b) Effects of early monocular deprivation on visual input to cat nucleus of the optic tract. Exp. Brain Res., 51: 236–246.

Hoffmann, K.-P. and Huber, H. P. (1983) Responses to visual stimulation in single cells in the nucleus of the optic tract (NOT) during optokinetic nystagmus (OKN) in the awake cat. Soc. Neurosci. Abstr., 9: 1048.

Hoffmann, K.-P. and Schoppmann, A. (1981) A quantitative analysis of the direction-specific response of neurons in the cat's nucleus of the optic tract. Exp. Brain Res., 42: 146–157.

Hoffmann, K.-P. and Stone, J. (1971) Conduction velocity of afferents to cat visual cortex: a correlation with cortical receptive field properties. Brain Res., 32: 460–466.

Hoffmann, K.-P. and Stone, J. (1985) Retinal input to the nucleus of the optic tract of the cat assessed by antidromic activation of ganglion cells. Exp. Brain Res., 59: 395–403.

Hoffmann, K.-P., Bauer, R., Huber, H. P. and Mayr, M. (1984) Single cell activity in area 18 of the cat's visual cortex during optokinetic nystagmus. Exp. Brain Res., 57: 118–127.

Lannou, J., Cazin, L., Precht, W. and LeTaillanter, M. (1984) Responses of prepositus hypoglossi neurons to optokinetic and vestibular stimulations in the rat. Brain Res., 301: 39–45.

Malach, R., Strong, N. and Van Sluyters, R. C. (1981) Analysis of monocular optokinetic nystagmus in normal and visually deprived kittens. Brain Res., 210: 367–372.

Malach, R., Strong, N. P. and Van Sluyters, R. C. (1984) Horizontal optokinetic nystagmus in the cat: effects of longterm monocular deprivation. Behav. Brain Res., 13: 193–205.

Naegele, J. R. and Held, R. (1982) The postnatal development of monocular optokinetic nystagmus in infants. Vision Res., 22: 341–346.

Oyster, C. W. and Barlow, H. B. (1967) Direction-selective units in rabbit retina: distribution of preferred directions. Science, 155: 841–842.

Oyster, C. W., Takahishi, E. and Collewijn, H. (1972) Direction-selective retinal ganglion cells and control of optokinetic nystagmus in the rabbit. Vision Res., 12: 183–193.

Precht, W., Montarolo, P. G. and Strata, P. (1980) The role of the crossed and uncrossed retinal fibers in mediating the horizontal optokinetic nystagmus in the cat. Neurosci. Lett., 17: 39–42.

Schiller, P. H. (1982) Central connections of the retinal on and off pathways. Nature, 297: 580–583.

Schoppmann, A. (1981) Projections from areas 17 and 18 of the visual cortex to the nucleus of the optic tract. Brain Res., 223: 1–17.

Schoppmann, A. and Hoffmann, K.-P. (1979) A comparison of visual responses in two pretectal nuclei and in the superior colliculus of the cat. Exp. Brain Res., 35: 495–510.

Sherk, H. and Horton, J. C. (1984) Receptive field properties in the cat's area 17 in the absence of on-center geniculate input. J. Neurosci., 4: 381–393.

Simpson, J. I. (1984) The accessory optic system. Annu. Rev. Neurosci., 7: 13–41.

Singer, W., Tretter, F. and Cynader, M. (1975) Organization of cat striate cortex: a correlation of receptive field properties with afferent and efferent connections. J. Neurophysiol., 38: 1080–1098.

Slaughter, M. M. and Miller, R. F. (1981) 2-Amino-4-phosphonobutyric acid: a new pharmalogical tool for retinal research. Science, 211: 182–185.

Stone, J. and Fukuda, Y. (1974) Properties of cat retinal ganglion cells: a comparison of W-cells with X- and Y-cells. J. Neurophysiol., 37: 722–748.

Strong, N. P., Malach, R., Lee, P. and Van Sluyters, R. C. (1984) Horizontal optokinetic nystagmus in the cat: recovery from cortical lesions. Behav. Brain Res., 13: 179–192.

Van Hof-Van Duin, J. (1978) Direction preference of optokinetic response in monocularly tested normal kittens and light deprived cats. Arch. Ital. Biol., 116: 471–477.

Wood, C. C., Spear, R. D. and Braun, J. J. (1973) Direction-specific deficits in horizontal optokinetic nystagmus following removal of visual cortex in the cat. Brain Res., 60: 231–237.

Discussion

O.-J. Grüsser

Department of Physiology, Freie Universität, Arnimallee 22, 1000 Berlin 33, Germany

The lively discussion following Matthews' and Wiesendanger's contributions could be summarized as follows. Spinal and cortical long-latency mechanisms modifying the classical stretch reflex seem to coexist, but their relative contribution evidently depends on the experimental design. Matthews' interpretation, to attribute the late-latency reflex responses predominantly to spinal mechanisms depending heavily on group II proprioceptive afferents, is, according to his own discussion remarks, restricted to the classical Sherringtonian stretch reflex with the simultaneous agonist contraction and antagonist relaxation. Since Matthews did not question the empirical data described in Wiesendanger's contribution, he had found other teleological interpretations for the function of the cortical loop of proprioceptive signal processing, stating that the cortex probably does not control a mechanism "as trivial as the stretch reflex" but should be more involved in "high-level controlling" of spinal cord activity. One interesting additional argument in favour of the spinal cord hypothesis was mentioned by Matthews: In thumb movement the short flexor muscles only exhibit a short-latency stretch reflex response, while the long flexor muscles show a long-latency response predominantly. Why should one mechanism involve cortical and the other only spinal neurons?

Eccles questioned whether the 40-msecond delay differences for the short-latency and long-latency proprioceptive response could be attributed to spinal mechanisms, since conduction differences in the peripheral nerve are only 2 mseconds. Matthews attributed 15 mseconds to differences in the phase response properties of Ia and II afferents, and 15 mseconds for intraspinal processing of secondary muscle spindle signals.

Bizzi's questioned whether the spatial distribution of Ia signals evoked from a single muscle and reaching cortical area 3a and indirectly area 4 challenged the defenders of the cortical loop hypothesis. He asked: Are the cortical loop mechanisms restricted to muscles involved in the classical Sherringtonian reflex or is the proprioceptive input to cortex much more widely distributed and therefore less specific, i.e., more related to Matthews' higher level control mechanisms? Evidently, not enough experimental data are available to answer these questions precisely. It became clear from further discussion by Schomburg, Nashner and Hultborn that part of the controversy depends on how narrowly one defines the 'stretch reflex''. Hultborn's remark, to take an operative approach and not rest on classical reflex definitions, would facilitate research on the compromise mentioned above.

Grüsser proposed that since the frequency response properties of primary and secondary muscle spindle afferents are clearly different high-frequency (>150 Hz), low-amplitude (<20 μm) vibration might be used for selective Ia activation or low-frequency (30–50 Hz), large-amplitude (>100 μm) sine-wave stretch for activating group II afferents, or a combination of both. The data obtained in such studies might give some clues as to whether long-loop Ia or spinal cord II afferents signal processing dominates the long-latency responses.

In his concluding remarks, Wiesendanger pointed out that Eccles had been the first to propose the existence of long-loop modifications of the proprioceptive spinal stretch reflexes. Despite Matthews' arguments, the cortical loop via areas 3a and 4 still seems to be a candidate for this task. However, as Eccles noted, another long-loop mechanism is probably also involved, namely the spino-cerebello-spinal pathway.

SECTION III

Neuroanatomical Substrates of Premotor Centres

Anatomy of premotor centers in the reticular formation controlling oculomotor, skeletomotor and autonomic motor systems

Jean Büttner-Ennever[1] and Gert Holstege[2]

[1]*Brain Research Institute, University of Düsseldorf, D-4000 Düsseldorf, F.R.G., and* [2]*Department of Neuroanatomy, Medical Faculty, Erasmus University, Rotterdam, The Netherlands*

Introduction

In this article we will concentrate on the neuroanatomy of the reticular formation as a premotor relay for controlling the oculomotor, somatomotor and autonomic motor systems. An attempt is made to inter-relate these data and point out similarities and differences in their relation to the limbic system. The term reticular formation as used nowadays was coined by August Forel (1877) when he recognized the cytoarchitectural similarities of a column of neurons stretching from the spinal cord up to the meso-diencephalic junction. There are subtle variations in the cytoarchitecture of this enormous reticulum, or network, which have been meticulously described by Olszewski and co-workers (Meessen and Olszewski, 1949; Olszewski and Baxter, 1954). The reticular formation is taken here to include a lateral, medial and ventral region (Fig. 1), all of which are particularly clear at pontine and medullary levels. The midline raphe nuclei are included in the medial and ventral divisions. The reticular formation has been associated with a wide variety of functions, such as arousal (Moruzzi and Magoun, 1949), eye movement generation (Raphan and Cohen, 1978) and posture control (Kuypers, 1964).

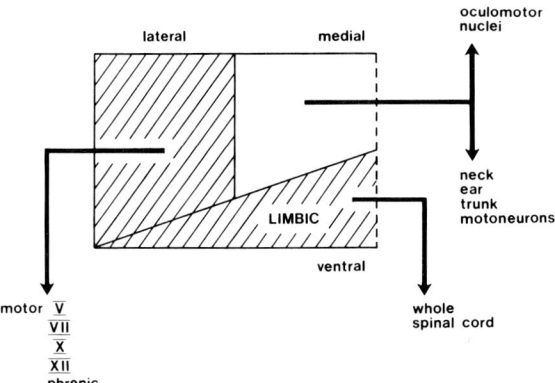

Fig. 1. The reticular formation of the caudal brain stem can be divided into three zones on the basis of its anatomical and physiological properties. Medial zone: oculomotor function related to saccade generation, directly premotor to motoneurons of extraocular and postural muscles. Lateral zone: directly premotor to lower cranial motor nuclei (other than III, IV and VI) and upper cervical motoneurons. Ventral zone: limbic function, projections to all spinal neurons. Shaded zones receive direct limbic afferents.

Oculomotor system

There are at least five different types of eye movement: 1, optokinetic responses (OKR); 2, vestibulo-ocular reflexes (VOR); 3, saccades; 4, smooth pursuit; 5, convergence.

Phylogenetically, the earliest types of eye movements are the vestibular and optokinetic responses: these are slow compensatory eye movements driven by a sensory input from the vestibular end-organs or the retina, respectively. Continuous vestibular or optokinetic stimulation produces nystagmus, during which the eyes are reset by fast eye movements. Such fast eye movements are included here in the term saccades. It is relevant for this article to remember that in some animals, for example, birds with long necks, the compensatory movements are mainly carried out by muscles of the head instead of the eyes. Cortical control of saccades, i.e., voluntary saccades, developed later phylogenetically, along with the appearance of retinal specializations such as the fovea (Walls, 1962). Smooth pursuit eye movements are used to follow small moving visual targets and can only be generated in the presence of visual targets. Therefore, the visual cortex is essential for smooth pursuit. This type of eye movement is not seen in rats and rabbits but is used by cats and primates to an increasing extent. For differences between optokinetic and smooth pursuit eye movements, see Büttner et al., Section IV-B. Phylogenetically, the most recently developed type of eye movement is convergence, which is used by frontal-eyed mammals to foveate a near object and establish stereoscopic vision.

Recent oculomotor studies indicate that the neural networks subserving these five types of eye movement are relatively independent of each other. For example, lesions in the pontine reticular formation may lead to deficits in the saccadic system but convergence remains unimpaired, while lesions in the cerebellum severely impair smooth pursuit, leaving saccades intact. Apparently the main pathways of the five types of eye movement remain functionally independent, although there are many interconnections between them. They are illustrated in Fig. 2. At present, the direct premotor inputs from the saccadic system onto motoneurons innervating eye muscles are thought to arise from neurons in the medial reticular formation only.

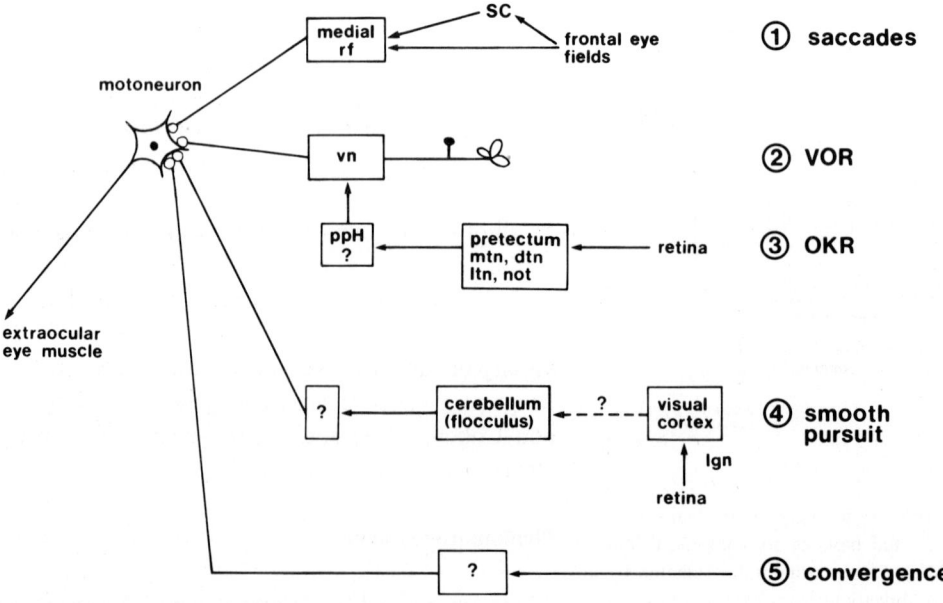

Fig. 2. Some basic structures involved in generation of the five types of eye movement. OKR and VOR are known to converge in the vestibular nuclei, before the level of the motoneuron. Many structures and connections are uncertain and here all cross-connections are omitted for simplicity. SC, superior colliculus; rf, reticular formation; vn, vestibular nuclei; ppH, prepositus hypoglossi; mtn, medial terminal nucleus; dtn, dorsal terminal nucleus; ltn, lateral terminal nucleus; not, nucleus of the optic tract; lgn, lateral geniculate nucleus.

Medial reticular formation in the generation of saccades

We will consider three specific regions of the medial reticular formation which have direct connections to the motoneurons of the extraocular eye muscles.

I. Specific cell groups in the paramedian pontine reticular formation (PPRF), such as long-lead bursters, short-lead bursters and omnipause neurons, are known to be essential for the generation of horizontal saccades (Raphan and Cohen, 1978; Fuchs et al., 1985). Monosynaptic inputs from neurons in the caudal part of this region into the abducens nucleus lead to activation of ipsilateral lateral rectus motoneurons in abducens nucleus, and, by way of the internuclear neurons, activate the contralateral medial rectus motoneurons in the oculomotor nucleus (Büttner-Ennever and Henn, 1976; Graybiel, 1977; Grantyn et al., 1980). In this way, activation of the PPRF can elicit horizontal conjugate eye movements. Lesion-degeneration and autoradiographic tracing and physiological studies (Nyberg-

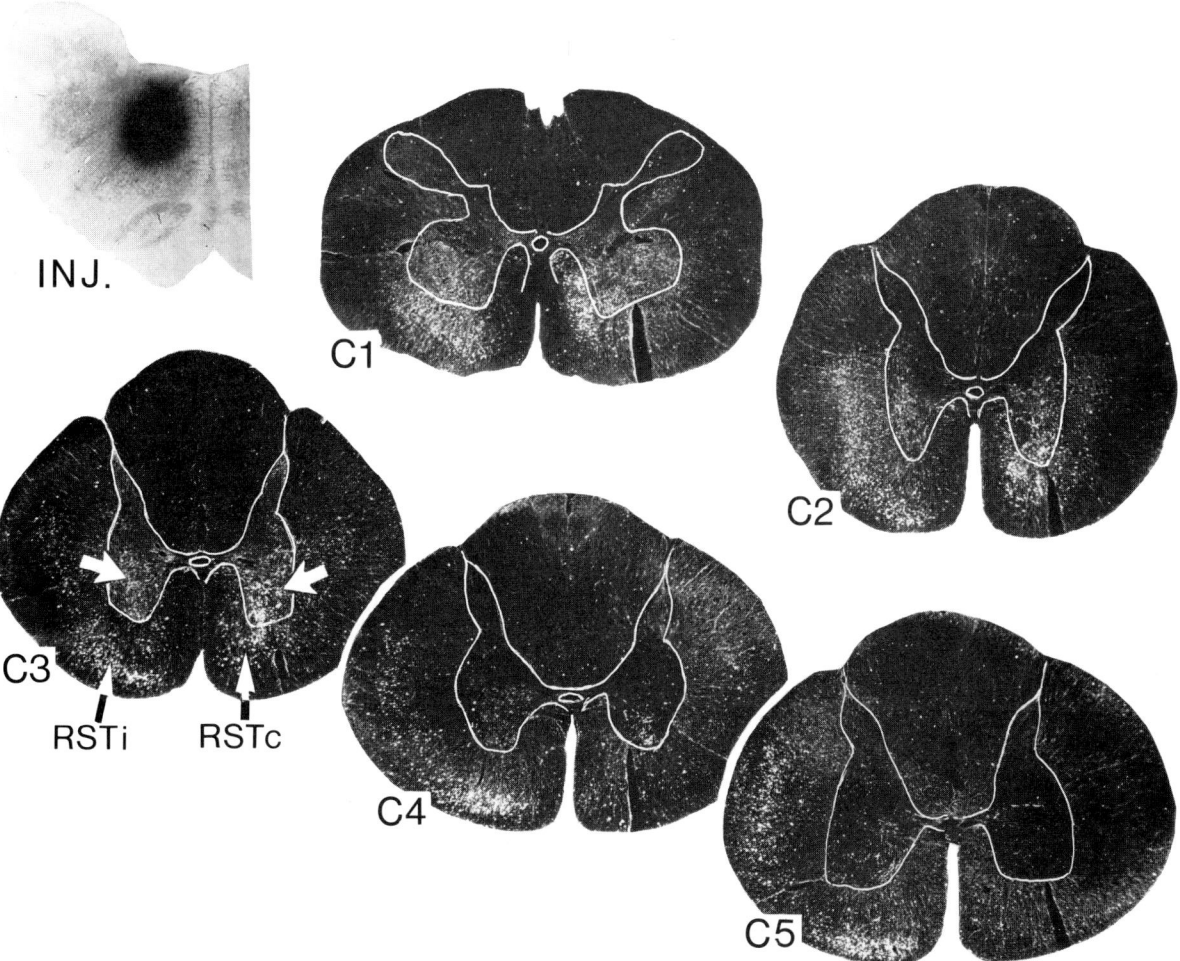

Fig. 3. Injection (inj) of tritiated leucine into the dorsomedial medullary reticular formation. Some tracer spread to the lateral zone but not to the PPRF. Note labeling of both contralateral (RSTc) and ipsilateral (RSTi) descending pathways (RST, reticulospinal tract). Direct labeling of the motoneuronal pool controlling neck musculature is seen on the contralateral side and marked with an arrow. The ipsilateral arrow indicates weaker labeling of the ventral horn.

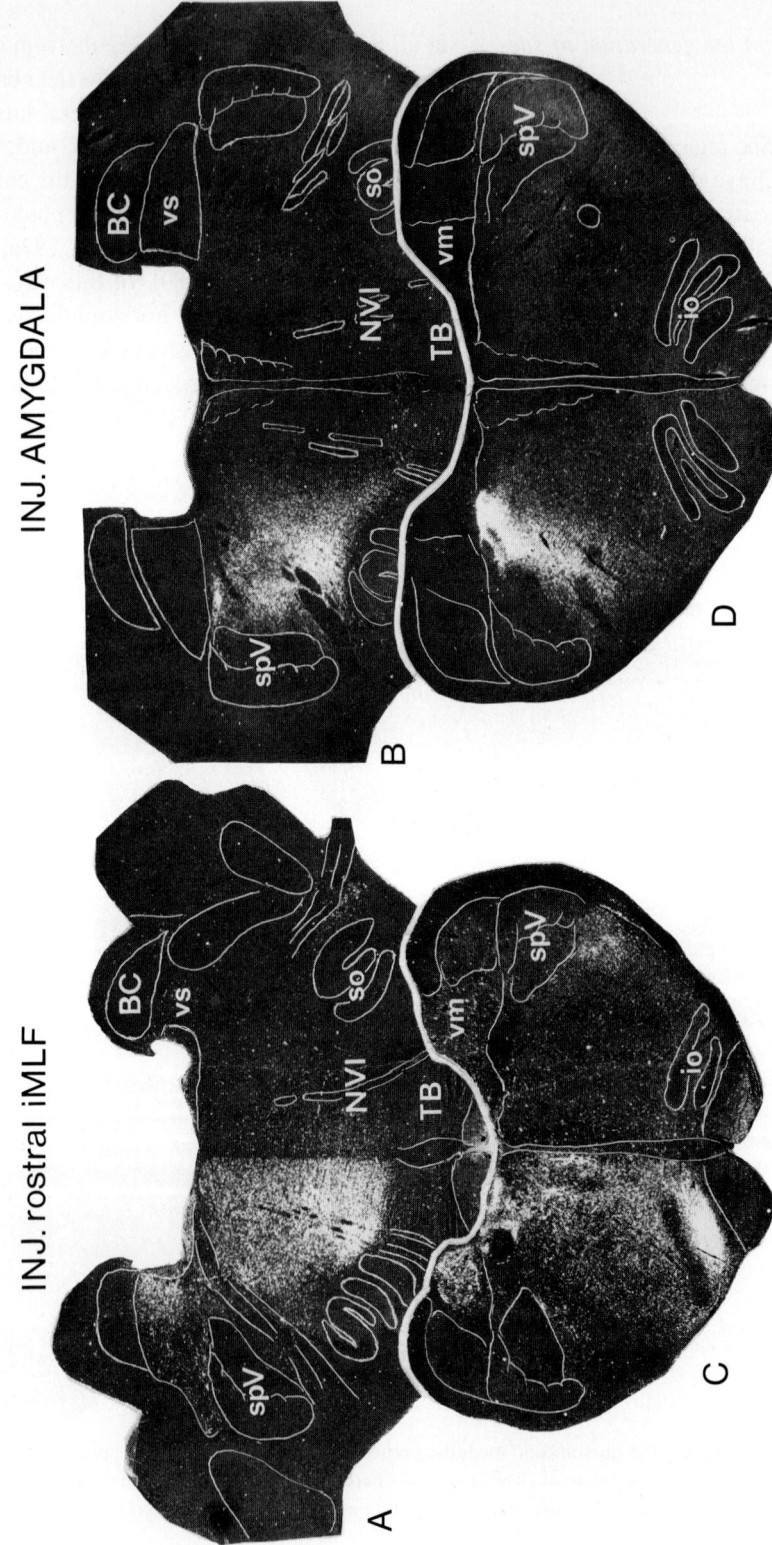

Fig. 4. A comparison of labeling after tritiated leucine injection on the left into an oculomotor-related structure (rostral iMLF, A and C) and a limbic structure (amygdala, B and D). Compare silver grain deposits in caudal pontine reticular formation in A and B, and the upper medullary reticular formation in C and D. Labeled afferents in the oculomotor case fill the medial reticular zone in A (around NVI) and C, but it is spared in B and D. In contrast, the lateral reticular zone, just medial to spinal trigeminal complex (spV), is heavily labeled in the limbic case (B and D), but not in the oculomotor case (A and C). BC, brachium conjunctivum; spV, spinal trigeminal complex; vs, superior vestibular nucleus; NVI, abducens rootlets; TB, trapezoid body; vm, medial vestibular nucleus; so, io, superior and inferior olives.

Hansen, 1965; Petras, 1967; Martin et al., 1979; Holstege and Kuypers, 1982) indicated that neurons in the PPRF area project ipsilaterally by way of the ventral funiculus to the medial part of the spinal intermediate zone (Rexed's laminae VIII and adjoining VII) throughout the length of the spinal cord. Possibly some of these fibers terminate directly on spinal motoneurons. The motoneurons in these areas would innervate mainly neck and proximal body muscles. Physiological studies by Peterson et al. (1980) confirmed these anatomical findings. It is possible that these reticulo-spinal neurons carry the horizontal saccade and/or eye position signal that can be recorded in neck muscles of the alert cat (Vidal et al., 1983). Lestienne et al. (1982) reported that in head free experiments different types of eye movement-related (burst) neurons can be found in the PPRF: those signalling only saccadic amplitude, and those encoding a combined eye-head signal. The PPRF area also projects bilaterally to the medial facial subnuclei, containing motoneurons innervating ear muscles (Holstege et al., 1977). Furthermore, recent studies using intracellular injection of horseradish peroxidase (Berthoz and Grantyn, Section V) show that some neurons, which receive the appropriate direct premotor activity for horizontal saccades, project to the abducens and facial nucleus and towards the spinal cord. It appears that all the eye movement-related (burst) neurons in the PPRF, whose axonal system has been reconstructed, have a descending axonal branch (Grantyn et al., 1980). However, it is not known if they all exert an influence at the spinal level.

II. The PPRF region is reciprocally interconnected with the dorsal part of the medullary medial reticular formation (Büttner-Ennever and Henn, 1976; Graybiel, 1977; Nakao et al., 1980; Langer and Kaneko, 1983). This part of the reticular formation is also involved in control of saccadic eye movements. Neurons here project to the contralateral abducens nucleus and inhibit lateral rectus motoneurons during an ipsilateral saccade (Hikosaka and Kawakami, 1977). The work of Yoshida et al. (1982) indicates that these same neurons may also have a contralaterally descending axon. In fact, injections of tritiated leucine in this part of the medullary reticular formation result in labeled fibers descending into the contralateral ventral funiculus of the cervical spinal cord, terminating on motoneurons innervating neck muscles (Fig. 3). In Fig. 3 an ipsilateral descending pathway is also shown to the ventral horn of C1 to C3.

III. PPRF also projects rostrally to specific areas of the mesencephalic reticular formation. One of these is the rostral interstitial nucleus of the medial longitudinal fasciculus (rostral iMLF) (Büttner-Ennever and Büttner, 1978) located at the meso-diencephalic junction. This region is involved in the generation of the vertical component of saccades (Büttner et al., 1977) and is the third region of the reticular formation with direct premotor inputs onto eye muscle motoneurons. It sends direct projections to trochlear and oculomotor nuclei, excluding the subgroups of medial rectus motoneurons (Büttner-Ennever and Büttner, 1978; Büttner-Ennever, 1981). The area of the rostral iMLF projects back to PPRF (Fig. 4A), the medial facial subnucleus (Holstege et al., 1984b) and the medial medullary reticular formation (Fig. 4C). A few fibers continued in the ventral funiculus of the spinal cord down to the level of the third lumbar segment, distributing fibers to Rexed's laminae VIII and adjoining VII (Holstege and Büttner-Ennever, unpublished results).

In summary, the oculomotor functions associated with the reticular formation are confined to the generation of saccades and not other eye movement types. There are three specific premotor areas known which directly innervate motoneurons of eye muscles. These three premotor regions all lie in the medial zone of the reticular formation in areas which are also known to have descending connections to ear, neck and trunk muscle motoneurons, i.e., postural musculature.

Somatomotor and autonomic motor system

Ventral part of the caudal pontine and medullary reticular formation

Until recently it was thought that the reticular formation maintained connections almost exclusively with those spinal neurons which control neck and trunk musculature: this was considered the major spinal influence of the reticular formation (Kuypers, 1964; Nyberg-Hansen, 1965; Petras, 1967; Martin et al., 1975). However, the introduction of fluorescence and autoradiographic tracing techniques into neuroanatomy revealed many additional reticulospinal projections. For example, the area of the nucleus raphe magnus and its directly adjoining reticular formation were shown recently to project densely to the dorsal horn throughout the length of the spinal cord and to the caudal spinal trigeminal nucleus (Basbaum et al., 1978; Martin et al., 1979; Holstege and Kuypers, 1982). More caudal parts of the reticular formation, i.e., the nucleus raphe pallidus and adjacent areas project to ventral parts of the spinal grey matter, i.e., the intermediate zone and the somatic motoneuronal areas, again throughout the length of the spinal cord (Holstege et al., 1979; Martin et al., 1979; Holstege and Kuypers, 1982). Thus, the medullary raphe nuclei and adjoining ventral reticular formation project to all laminae of the spinal grey matter throughout the whole length of the spinal cord. Nucleus raphe pallidus and adjacent reticular formation also project to brain stem somatic motor nuclei of the V, VII, X and XII cranial nerve, but *not* to the III, IV and VI motor nuclei* of the oculomotor system (Holstege, unpublished results). In addition, nucleus raphe magnus and pallidus and the adjoining reticular formation project densely to the sympathetic and parasympathetic motoneurons in the caudal brain stem and spinal cord (Basbaum et al., 1978; Holstege et al., 1979; Martin et al., 1979; Holstege and Kuypers, 1982).

---

* III, oculomotor; IV, trochlear; V, trigeminal; VI, abducens; VII, facial; X, vagal; XII, hypoglossal.

Many neurons in the nucleus raphe magnus and pallidus contain serotonin (Wiklund et al., 1981), substance P and Leu-enkephalin (Hokfelt et al., 1978, 1979). Bowker et al. (1982) in rat showed that many of these neurons project to the spinal cord. This indicates that part of these raphe-spinal projections contain serotonin, and probably also substance P and Leu-enkephalin, as neurotransmitters. It must be stressed, however, that not all of the spinal projecting neurons in these raphe nuclei and adjoining reticular formation contain serotonin (Bowker et al., 1982; Johannessen et al., 1984). Moreover, in cat virtually none of the neurons which descend through the dorsolateral funiculus of the spinal cord (Holstege et al., 1979; Holstege and Kuypers, 1982) contain serotonin (Johannessen et al., 1984).

Dorsolateral pontine reticular formation

Another brain stem area projecting to all parts of the spinal cord is the area of the nucleus subcoeruleus and nucleus Kölliker-Fuse, which are located in the dorsolateral pontine tegmentum and in some respects can be considered as specializations of the pontine reticular formation. Histofluorescent (Dahlström and Fuxe, 1964; Nygren and Olsson, 1977) and autoradiographical tracing studies (Holstege et al., 1979; Holstege and Kuypers, 1982) indicated that in the cat the nucleus subcoeruleus and nucleus Kölliker-Fuse project to the dorsal horn, intermediate zone and autonomic and somatic motor nuclei, throughout the length of the spinal cord. In addition, these dorsolateral tegmental nuclei project to the autonomic and somatic motor nuclei in the caudal brain stem, i.e., the motor nuclei V, VII, X and XII (Holstege et al., 1977). However, the nucleus subcoeruleus, like the raphe nuclei, does not project to the "oculomotor nuclei" of the III, IV and VI nerve (Holstege, unpublished results). In the nucleus subcoeruleus and nucleus Kölliker-Fuse many neurons contain noradrenaline as a neurotransmitter (Jones and Friedman, 1983). Dahlström and Fuxe (1965) demonstrated that noradrenaline-containing fibers and terminals are present in all parts of the spinal grey matter throughout its entire length. Nygren and Olsson (1977) showed that the noradrenaline-containing fibers in the spinal cord partly disappear after lesioning the nucleus subcoeruleus and Kölliker-Fuse bilaterally. This shows that part of the spinal projections derived from these nuclei, which have been traced using [^{3}H]leucine (Holstege et al., 1979; Martin et al., 1979; Holstege and Kuypers, 1982), are noradrenergic.

Lateral reticular formation of caudal pons and medulla

A completely different part of the reticular formation projecting to various parts of the spinal cord is the lateral reticular formation of caudal pons and medulla. Holstege et al. (1977) demonstrated that this part of the caudal brain stem projects densely to motoneuronal cell groups of the V, VII and XII nerves. Holstege and Kuypers (1982) showed that the lateral reticular formation also projects to the upper cervical cord, and they regarded this part of the reticular formation as a premotor relay for the caudal cranial nerve motor nuclei (V, VII, X and XII) and upper cervical motoneuronal cell groups, in the same way as the spinal intermediate zone serves as a premotor relay for the spinal motoneuronal cell groups (Sterling and Kuypers, 1968; Rustioni et al., 1971; Molenaar, 1978). Interneurons in the spinal intermediate zone project not only to the nearby located motoneurons but also to motoneurons located at larger distances (long propriospinal pathways). The same is true for interneurons in the lateral reticular formation of the medulla, because some of them project to motoneurons of the phrenic nerve, located in the C5–C6 spinal segments, and others at more caudal medullary levels to motoneurons innervating intercostal and abdominal muscles (Holstege et al., 1984a). These latter brain stem spinal pathways take part in the neuroanatomical framework of the respiratory control system and probably also of the system controlling swallowing and vomiting (Holstege et al., 1984a). The lateral reticular formation of the caudal brain stem does not project to the III, IV and VI "oculomotor nuclei".

Limbic afferents

Perhaps the projections from the ventral reticular structures and coeruleus complex may be involved in setting the level of all groups of motoneurons (cf. McCall and Aghajanian, 1979). Therefore, it is highly interesting that the major proportion of the afferents are derived from limbic structures, such as the periaqueductal gray matter (Gallager and Pert, 1978; Abols and Basbaum, 1981), lateral hypothalamus (Saper et al., 1976), amygdala (Hopkins and Holstege, 1978) and bed nucleus of the stria terminalis (Holstege et al., 1985). The sections selected for Fig. 4B and D do not show clearly the amygdala projection to the ventral reticular zone; in this experiment they are apparent at more caudal levels, e.g., at the level of the facial nucleus (Hopkins and Holstege, 1978). Maybe the ventral reticular zone should be regarded as the system by way of which these limbic areas control all spinal and many caudal brain stem neurons. This could explain the enormous effects of the emotional state on muscle tone and also pain perception. Various limbic areas, such as lateral hypothalamus (Saper et al., 1976), amygdala (Hopkins and Holstege, 1978) and bed nucleus of the stria terminalis (Holstege et al., 1985), project also to the lateral reticular zone also (Fig. 4B,D). These pathways together with the limbic projections to the ventral zone probably play an important role in the limbic control of respiration and blood pressure. In contrast, none of the limbic structures mentioned above seem to project to the medial reticular zone nor to the motoneurons of the III, IV and VI cranial nerves. In Fig. 4 the labeling in the caudal pontine and medullary reticular formation are compared after injections into an oculomotor structure (rostral iMLF) and a limbic structure (amygdala). Note that totally separate reticular zones are labeled (compare with Fig. 1).

Conclusions

On the basis of anatomical connections, the reticular formation can be subdivided into three zones (Fig. 1): medial, lateral and ventral. The medial region contains the premotor circuitry for the generation of fast eye movements or saccades. The same region and, in some cases, possibly the same neurons project not only to the motoneurons of the extraocular eye muscles but also to the spinal cord motoneurons innervating neck and trunk musculature; that is, the muscles involved in postural control. It may be that the control of postural muscles through the reticular formation comprises a basic motor programme and is independent of the pyramidal and extra-pyramidal systems which comprise voluntary motor programmes.

The lateral zone of the reticular formation contains interneurons innervating motoneurons of the motor nuclei of the trigeminal, facial, vagal, hypoglossal and phrenic nerves and can be regarded as the bulbar counterpart of the spinal intermediate zone.

The ventral zone projects to all parts of the spinal cord throughout its length. Afferents to the ventral zone are mainly derived from limbic areas, and therefore it may be regarded as part of the limbic system itself. Various limbic areas also project to the lateral reticular zone, but the medial zone seems to receive no limbic afferents. This suggests that the oculomotor and postural system, unlike the somatomotor or the autonomic motor system, are not under such direct limbic control and must be considered as unique in this respect.

Acknowledgements

The research work was supported by the Deutsche Forschungsgemeinschaft, SFB 200/A3, and by a European Science Foundation, ETP Twinning Grant, TW84/299. The authors wish to thank Miss Edith Klink for her excellent technical assistance.

References

Abols, I. A. and Basbaum, A. I. (1981) Afferent connections of the rostral medulla of the cat: a neural substrate for midbrain-medullary interactions in the modulation of pain. J. Comp. Neurol., 201: 285–297.

Basbaum, A. I., Clanton, C. H. and Fields, H. L. (1978) Three bulbospinal pathways from the rostral medulla of the cat: an autoradiographic study of pain modulating systems. J. Comp. Neurol., 178: 209–224.

Bowker, R. M., Westlund, K. N., Sullivan, M. C. and Coulter, J. D. (1982) Organization of descending serotonergic projections to the spinal cord. In H. G. J. M. Kuypers and G. F. Martin (Eds.), Progress in Brain Research, Vol. 57, Elsevier Biomedical Press, Amsterdam, pp. 239–266.

Büttner, U., Büttner-Ennever, J. A. and Henn, V. (1977) Vertical eye movement related unit activity in the rostral mesencephalic reticular formation of the alert monkey. Brain Res., 130: 239–252.

Büttner-Ennever, J. A. (1981) Anatomy of medial rectus subgroups in the oculomotor nucleus of the monkey. In A. F. Fuchs and W. Becker (Eds.), Progress in Oculomotor Research, Elsevier/North-Holland, pp. 247–252.

Büttner-Ennever, J. A. and Büttner, U. (1978) A cell group associated with vertical eye movements in the rostral mesencephalic reticular formation of the monkey. Brain Res., 151: 31–47.

Büttner-Ennever, J. A. and Henn, V. (1976). An autoradiographic study of the pathways from the pontine reticular formation involved in horizontal eye movements. Brain Res., 108: 155–164.

Dahlström, A. and Fuxe, K. (1964). Evidence for the existence of monoamine-containing neurons in the central nervous system. Acta Physiol. Scand., 72: 3–56.

Dahlström, A. and Fuxe, K. (1965) Evidence for the existence of monoamine neurons in the central nervous system. II. Experimentally induced changes in the intraneuronal amine levels of bulbospinal neuron systems. Acta Physiol. Scand., 64:7–35.

Forel, A. (1877) Untersuchungen über die Haubenregion und ihre oberen Verknupfungen im Gehirn des Menschen und einige Saugetiere, mit Beitragen zu den Methoden der Gehirn untersuchungen. Arch. Psychiat., 7: 393.

Fuchs, A. F., Kaneko, C. R. S. and Scudder, C. A. (1985) Brainstem control of saccadic eye movements. Annu. Rev. Neurosci., 8: 307–337.

Gallager, D. W. and Pert, A. (1978) Afferents to brain stem nuclei (brain stem raphe, nucleus reticular pontis caudalis and nucleus gigantocellularis) in the rat as demonstrated by microiontophoretically applied horseradish peroxidase. Brain Res., 144: 25–275.

Grantyn, R., Baker, R. and Grantyn, A. (1980). Morphological and physiological identification of excitatory pontine reticular neurons projecting to the cat abducens nucleus and spinal

cord. Brain Res., 198: 221–228.
Graybiel, A. M. (1977). Direct and indirect preoculomotor pathways of the brainstem: an autoradiographic study of the pontine reticular formation in the cat. J. Comp. Neurol., 175: 37–78.
Hikosaka, O. and Kawakami, T. (1977) Inhibitory reticular neurons related to the quick phase of vestibular nystagmus. Their location and projection. Exp. Brain Res., 27: 377–396.
Hokfelt, T., Ljungdahl, A., Steinbusch, H., Verhofstad, A., Nilson, G., Brodin, E., Pernow, B. and Goldstein, M. (1978). Immunohistochemical evidence of substance P-like immunoreactivity in some 5-hydroxytryptamine containing neurons in the rat central nervous system. Neuroscience, 3: 517–538.
Hokfelt, T., Terenius, T., Kuypers, H. G. J. M. and Dann, O. (1979) Evidence for enkephalin immunoreactivity neurons in the medulla oblongata projecting to the spinal cord. Neurosci. Lett., 14: 55–61.
Holstege, G. and Kuypers, H. G. J. M. (1982) The anatomy of brain stem pathways to the spinal cord in cat. In H. G. J. M. Kuypers and G. F. Martin (Eds.), Progress in Brain Research, Vol. 57, Elsevier Biomedical Press, Amsterdam, pp. 145–175.
Holstege, G., Kuypers, H. G. J. M. and Dekker, J. J. (1977) The organization of the bulbar fibre connections to the trigeminal, facial and hypoglossal motor nuclei. Brain 100: 265–286.
Holstege, G., Kuypers, H. G. J. M. and Boer, R. C. (1979) Anatomical evidence for direct brain stem projections to the somatic motoneuronal cell groups and autonomic preganglionic cell groups in cat spinal cord. Brain Res., 171: 329–333.
Holstege, G., Van Neerven, J. and Evertse, F. (1984a) Some anatomical observations on axonal connections from brain stem areas physiologically identified as related to respiration. Neurosci. Lett., Suppl. 18: S83.
Holstege, G., Tan, J., Van Ham, J. and Bos, A. (1984b) Mesencephalic projections to the facial nucleus in the cat. An autoradiographical tracing study. Brain Res., 311: 7–22.
Holstege, G., Meiners, L. and Tan, K. (1985) Projections of the bed nucleus of the stria terminalis to the mesencephalon, pons and medulla oblongata in the cat. Exp. Brain Res., 58: 379–391.
Hopkins, D. A. and Holstege, G. (1978) Amygdaloid projections to the mesencephalon, pons and medula oblongata in the cat. Exp. Brain Res., 32: 529–547.
Johannessen, J. N., Watkins, L. R. and Mayer, D. J. (1984) Non-serotonergic origins of the dorsolateral funiculus in the rat ventral medulla. J. Neurosci., 4: 757–766.
Jones, B. E. and Friedman, L. (1983) Atlas of catecholamine perikarya, varicosities and pathways in the brain stem of the cat. J. Comp. Neurol., 215: 382–396.
Kuypers, H. G. J. M. (1984) The descending pathways to the spinal cord, their anatomy and function. In J. C. Eccles and J. P. Schade (Eds.), Progress in Brain Research, Vol. 11, Elsevier, Amsterdam, pp. 178–200.
Langer, T. P. and Kaneko, C. R. S. (1983) Efferent projections of the cat oculomotor reticular omnipause neuron region: an autoradiographic study. J. Comp. Neurol., 217: 288–306.
Lestienne, F., Whittington, D. and Bizzi, E. (1982) Behaviour of pontine cells during eye-head coordination: evidence of gaze shift coding by preoculomotor bursters. In A. Roucoux and M. Crommelinck (Eds.), Physiological and Pathological Aspects of Eye Movements, Dr. W. Junk Publishers, The Hague, pp. 399–410.
Martin, G. F., Beattie, M.-S., Bresnahan, J. C., Henkel, C. K. and Hughes, H. C. (1975) Cortical and brain stem projections to the spinal cord of the American opossum (*Didelphis marsupialis virginiana*). Brain Behav. Evol., 12: 270–310.
Martin, G. F., Humbertson, A. O., Laxson, L. C., Panneton, W. M. and Tschiasmadia, I. (1979) Spinal projections from the mesencephalic and pontine reticular formation in the North American opossum: a study using axonal transport techniques. J. Comp. Neurol., 187: 373–401.
McCall, R. B. and Aghajanian, G. K. (1979) Serotonergic facilitation of facial motoneuron excitation. Brain Res., 169: 11–27.
Meessen, H. and Olszewski, J. (1949) Cytoarchitektonischer Atlas der Rautenhirn des Kaninchens, Karger, Basel.
Molenaar, I. (1978) The distribution of propriospinal neurons projecting to different motoneuronal cell groups in the cats brachial cord. Brain Res., 158: 203–206.
Moruzzi, G. and Magoun, H. W. (1949) Brain stem reticular formation and activation of the EEG. Electroenceph. Clin. Neurophysiol., 1: 455–473.
Nakao, S., Curthoys, I. S. and Markham, Ch. M. (1980) Direct inhibitory projection of pause neurons to nystagmus-related pontomedullary reticular burst neurons in the cat. Exp. Brain Res., 40: 283–293.
Nyberg-Hansen, R. (1965) Sites and mode of termination of reticulo-spinal fibers in the cat. An experimental study with silver impregnation methods. J. Comp. Neurol., 124: 71–100.
Nygren, L. G. and Olsson, L. (1977) A new projection from locus coeruleus: the main source of noradrenergic nerve terminals in the ventral and dorsal columns of the spinal cord. Brain Res., 132: 85–93.
Olszewski, J. and Baxter, D. (1954) Cytoarchitecture of the Human Brain Stem, Reinhardt, Basel.
Peterson, B. W., Fukushima, K., Hirai, N., Scher, R. H. and Wilson, V. J. (1980) Response of vestibulospinal and reticulospinal neurons to sinusoid vestibular stimulation. J. Neurophysiol., 43: 1236–1250.
Petras, J. M. (1967) Cortical, tectal and tegmental fiber connections in the spinal cord of the cat. Brain Res., 6: 275–324.
Raphan, T. and Cohen, B. (1978) Brain stem mechanisms for rapid and slow eye movements. Annu. Rev. Physiol., 40: 527–552.
Rustioni, A., Kuypers, H. G. J. M. and Holstege, G. (1971) Propriospinal projections from the ventral and lateral funiculi to the motoneurons of the lumbosacral cord of the cat. Brain Res., 35: 255–275.
Saper, C. B., Loewy, A. D., Swanson, L. W. and Cowan, W. M.

(1976) Direct hypothalamo-autonomic connections. Brain Res., 117: 305–312.

Sterling, P. and Kuypers, H. G. J. M. (1968) Anatomical organization of the brachial spinal cord in the cat. III. The propriospinal connections. Brain Res., 7: 419–443.

Vidal, P. P., Corvisier, J., and Berthoz, A. (1983) Eye and neck motor signals in periabducens reticular neurons of the alert cat. Exp. Brain Res., 53: 16–28.

Walls, G. L. (1962) The evolutionary history of eye movements. Vision Res., 2: 69–80.

Wiklund, L., Leger, L. and Persson, M. (1981) Monoamine cell distribution in the cat brain stem. A fluorescence histochemical study with quantification of indolaminergic and locus coeruleus cell groups. J. Comp. Neurol., 203: 613–647.

Yoshida, K., McCrea, R., Berthoz, A. and Vidal, P. P. (1982) Morphological and physiological characteristics of inhibitory burst neurons controlling horizontal rapid eye movements in the alert cat. J. Neurophysiol., 48: 761–784.

The organization of thalamic inputs to the "premotor" areas

Peter L. Strick

Research Service, V. A. Medical Center, Departments of Neurosurgery and Physiology, SUNY-Upstate Medical Center, Syracuse, NY 13210, U.S.A.

Introduction

One of the classical concepts concerning the cortical control of movement is that there are "premotor" areas in the frontal lobe which have direct access to the primary motor cortex. Although the function of these "premotor" areas has not been fully defined, they are thought to contribute to the preparation and structuring of skilled movement and the programming of motor cortex output (see Brinkman and Porter, 1979b; Humphrey, 1979; Wiesendanger, 1981; Weinrich and Wise, 1982, for recent reviews). In recent studies (Muakkassa and Strick, 1979) we have demonstrated that there are four spatially separate and somatotopically organized premotor areas which project directly to the motor cortex (Fig. 1) (see also Pandya and Kuypers, 1969; Jones and Powell, 1970; Pandya and Vignolo, 1971; Matsumura and Kubota, 1979; Godschalk et al., 1984). The densest projections originate from two of the premotor areas. One of these is the arcuate premotor area (APA), located laterally in area 6 around the caudal bank of the arcuate sulcus; and the other is the supplementary motor area (SMA), located medially in area 6 on the medial wall of the hemisphere (e.g., Woolsey et al., 1952). A third premotor area is located in the ventral bank of the cingulate sulcus and a fourth in the cortex surrounding the inferior and superior precentral sulci. In addition to projecting ipsilaterally, each of these premotor areas also projects to the contralateral motor cortex.

Based on the available anatomical and physiological evidence, we suggested that these premotor areas might represent elements in multiple parallel pathways which differentially control motor cortex output and/or motor behavior (Schell and Strick, 1984). In order to explore this hypothesis, we examined how two major subcortical motor systems, the cerebellum and the basal ganglia, project upon the premotor areas and motor cortex. Recent studies have shown that cerebellar, pallidal and nigral efferents project to the ventrolateral thalamus and that there is little overlap in the sites of termination of these systems (e.g., Mehler, 1971; Kuo and Carpenter, 1973; Carpenter et al., 1976; Kim et al., 1976; Percheron, 1977; Stanton, 1980; Kalil, 1981; DeVito and Anderson, 1982; Asanuma et al., 1983b). These studies have also suggested that, whereas cerebellar efferents terminate in thalamic regions which project to the primary motor cortex, efferents from the basal ganglia do not. However, the lack of precise information regarding the cortical projections of subdivisions of the ventrolateral thalamus has hampered attempts to link subcortical structures with particular cortical areas. Therefore, we employed retrograde transport of wheatgerm agglutinin-horseradish peroxidase (WGA-HRP) (Mesulam, 1982) to determine the origin of thalamic input to the two premotor areas with the densest projections to the motor cortex: the APA and the SMA. We observed that interconnections with the premotor areas originate from rather widespread regions of the thalamus. This chapter will focus on the organization of inputs from the ventrolateral thalamus. A complete presentation of the methods and results of this analysis has been published previously (Schell and Strick, 1984).

Results

Observations from two animals will be used to illustrate the projection from subdivisions of the ventrolateral thalamus upon the premotor areas. Thalamic labeling in a third animal, with injections into the motor cortex, will be presented for comparison. The injection sites in these animals are illustrated in Fig. 2.

Origin of thalamic input to the supplementary motor area (SMA)

In order to label the origin of thalamic input to the SMA, injection sites were placed along the medial wall of the hemisphere (Fig. 2B). The spread of WGA-HRP included the dorsal bank of the cingulate sulcus only caudally. At this point, reaction product was more than 8 mm from the level of the central sulcus. According to various maps of motor representation in the SMA (e.g., Woolsey et al., 1952; Brinkman and Porter, 1979b; Matsumura and Kubota, 1979; Muakkassa and Strick, 1979; Wise and Tanji, 1981; Tanji and Kurata, 1982), the spread of WGA-HRP included most of the "forelimb representation", and extended to parts of the "face representation", rostrally, and "hindlimb representation", caudally.

These SMA injections resulted in a slab of labeled neurons which was principally located in the thalamic subdivision termed nucleus ventralis lateralis pars oralis (VLo) by Olszewski (1952) (Fig. 3). The slab of labeled neurons was most extensive between Olszewski's levels A10.5 and A8.5, where VLo is most extensive. In many instances, changes in the location of labeled neurons paralleled cytoarchitectonic changes in VLo. For example, as VLo split into dorsal and ventral cell groups, la-

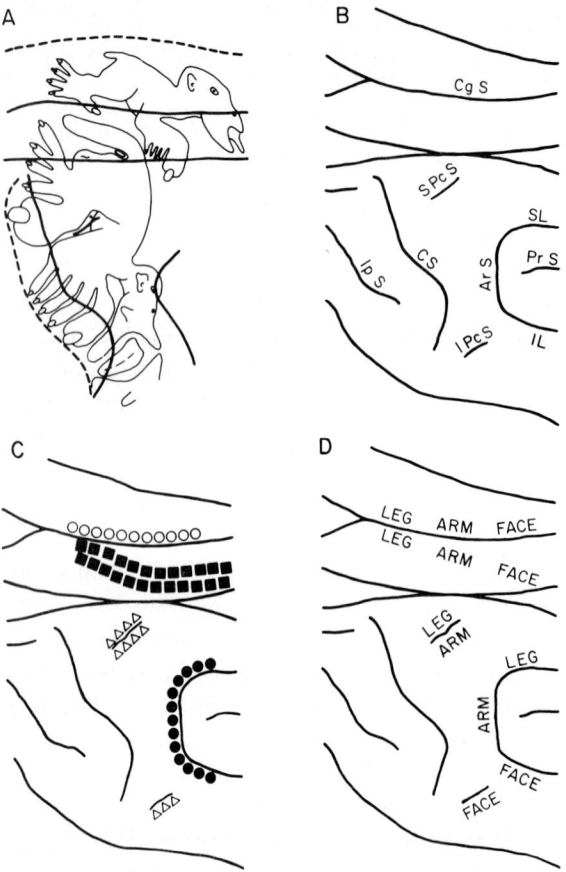

Fig. 1. Location and somatotopic organization of the four "premotor" areas. A. Body representation and the location of the primary (vertically oriented figurine) and supplementary (horizontally oriented figurine) motor areas in the rhesus monkey is illustrated according to Woolsey et al., (1952). The rostral bank of the central sulcus and the dorsal bank of the cingulate sulcus have been included (dashed lines) to illustrate the full extent of the two body maps. B. Sulci are labeled in the cortical region containing the premotor areas and the primary motor cortex. Neither the central sulcus nor the cingulate sulcus are opened in this view. C. The location and approximate spatial extent of the four premotor areas which project to the primary motor cortex are indicated by symbols: ●, the APA; ■, the SMA; △, the precentral sulci; ○, the cingulate sulcus. Note that the projection from the APA originates from its caudal bank and the projection from the cingulate sulcus originates from its ventral bank. D. Body representation in each of the four premotor areas is indicated by the words "face", "arm" and "leg". ArS, arcuate sulcus (IL, inferior limb; SL, superior limb); CS, central sulcus; CgS, cingulate sulcus; IPcS, inferior precentral sulcus; IpS, intraparietal sulcus; PrS, principal sulcus; SPcS, superior precentral sulcus. From Muakkassa and Strick (1979).

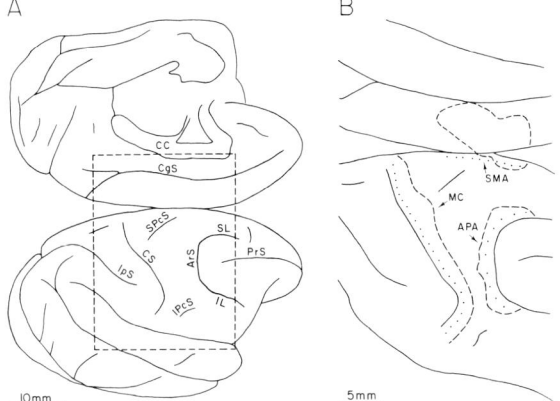

Fig. 2. Location of cortical injection sites. A. Two views of the cortical surface from the right hemisphere of a rhesus monkey. Lateral view (bottom) and medial view reflected upwards (top). B. Enlarged view of the cortical area included within the dashed rectangle of A. The cortical injection sites (small dots) and the spread of WGA-HRP reaction product (dashed lines) for the three animals are plotted on a single hemisphere. Motor cortex (MC): adjacent to the rostral bank of the central sulcus (CS). SMA: near the medial wall of the hemisphere. APA: adjacent to the caudal bank of the arcuate sulcus (ArS). CC, corpus callosum. Other abbreviations, see Fig. 1. From Schell and Strick (1984).

beled neurons also split into dorsal and ventral groups (Fig. 3, section 347).

The slab of labeled neurons extended outside of VLo into the most dorsal aspects of nucleus ventralis lateralis pars medialis (VLm) and the dorsal, parvocellular region just caudal to VLo (Fig. 3, section 372). Thalamic labeling extended as far caudally as A3.0, where a cluster of labeled neurons was found in the ventral portion of the nuclear subdivision termed pars postrema (VLps) (Olszewski, 1952). This labeling was located just dorsal to lateralis posterior (LP).

Origin of thalamic input to the arcuate premotor area (APA)

In order to label the origin of input to the APA, injection sites were placed 1 mm posterior to the caudal bank of the arcuate sulcus (Fig. 2B). WGA-HRP spread no more than 2 mm from any of the injection sites. Some reaction product was found in the caudal bank of the arcuate sulcus, but none was seen in the rostral bank. According to various maps of motor representation in the APA (e.g., Kubota and Hamada, 1978; Matsumura and Kubota, 1979; Muakkassa and Strick, 1979; Weinrich and Wise, 1982; Godschalk et al., 1984), the spread of WGA-HRP included most of the "forelimb representation" located around the spur of the arcuate sulcus, some of the "face representation" near the inferior limb of the sulcus, and some of the "hindlimb representation" near the superior limb of the sulcus.

These APA injections resulted in a slab of labeled neurons which was principally located in the thalamic subdivision termed "area X" by Olszewski

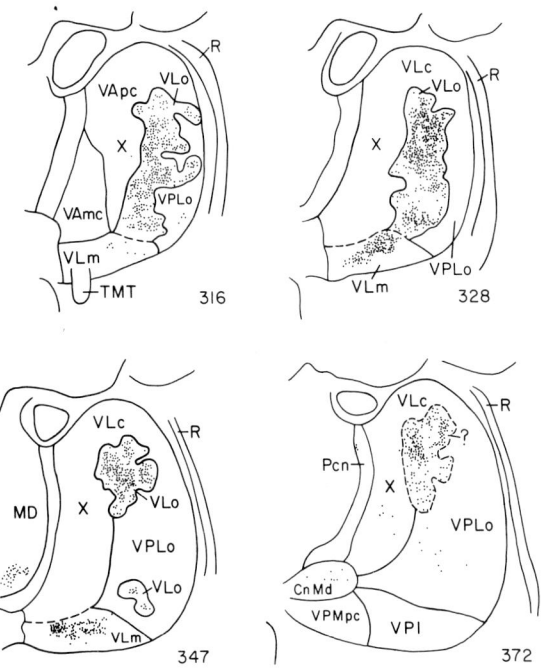

Fig. 3. Plots of labeled neurons resulting from WGA-HRP injections into the SMA. Labeled neurons found on single sections at different levels of the thalamus are indicated by small dots in Figs. 3–5. The injection sites in the SMA near the medial wall of the hemisphere are shown in Fig. 2B. Note that thalamic labeling is principally located in VLo. Labeling was also observed in nucleus medialis dorsalis (MD) and nucleus centralis lateralis (CL) at caudal levels of the ventrolateral thalamus, but is not illustrated in these plots. The thalamic nomenclature and the abbreviations used in Figs. 3–5 are according to Olszewski (1952), from Schell and Strick (1984).

(1952) (Fig. 4). The labeling in area X was just medial to the thalamic labeling which was seen after injections into the SMA. The slab of labeled neurons was most extensive between Olszewski's levels A9.5 and A7.5. Only the medial aspect of area X, adjacent to the internal medullary lamina, lacked substantial numbers of labeled neurons. Thalamic labeling also extended dorsally into contiguous areas of nucleus ventralis lateralis pars caudalis (VLc) and rostrally into the dorso-medial aspect of rostral VLm. Labeled neurons were found as far caudally as A3.0, where a small cluster of labeled neurons was seen in VLps. These labeled neurons were located just dorsal to the labeling seen after SMA injections.

Origin of input to the motor cortex from rostral regions of the ventrolateral thalamus

We also examined whether there is any overlap between the regions of the ventrolateral thalamus which project to the two premotor areas and the region which projects to the motor cortex. Since the preceding analysis had shown that the two premotor areas received their input from rostral parts of the ventrolateral thalamus we concentrated our analysis on this area. In order to label the origin of thalamic input to the motor cortex, injection sites were placed in the precentral cortex 1 mm rostral to the central sulcus (Fig. 2B). The rostral bank of the central sulcus (upper one-third) contained reaction product throughout its mediolateral extent. According to various maps of body representation in the motor cortex (e.g., Woolsey et al., 1952; Kwan et al., 1978), the spread of WGA-HRP involved largely the representation of distal limb parts and those parts of the "face and proximal body representations" which are adjacent to the central sulcus. In addition, reaction product spread into somatic sensory cortex in two regions: medially, where the "hindlimb representation" is located, and laterally, where the "face representation" is located.

These motor cortex injections resulted in labeling which at rostral levels was largely confined to the

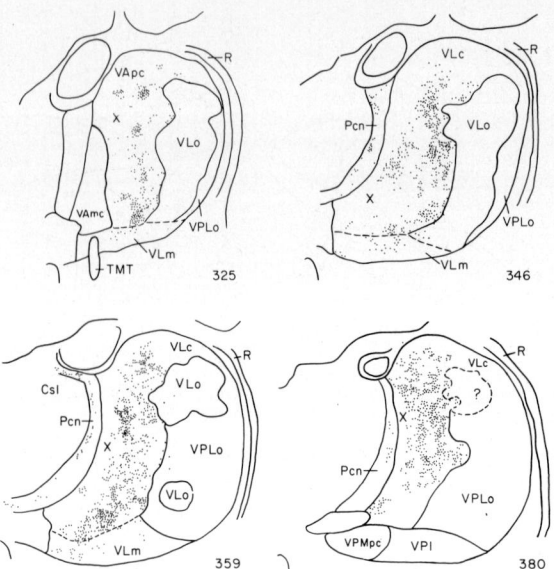

Fig. 4. Plots of labeled neurons resulting from injections into the APA. The injection sites in the APA near the caudal bank of the arcuate sulcus are shown in Fig. 2B. Note that thalamic labeling is principally located in area X. Labeling was also observed in MD and CL (not illustrated), but the regions labeled were different than those labeled after SMA injections. From Schell and Strick (1984).

thalamic subdivision termed nucleus ventralis posterior lateralis pars oralis (VPLo) by Olszewski (1952) (Fig. 5). The slab of labeled neurons filled VPLo and extended up to its borders with area X and VLo. No labeled neurons were found in area X or VLo following injections into the motor cortex. Scattered labeling extended across the ventral border of VPLo into the subdivision termed ventralis posterior inferior (VPI) by Olszewski (1952) (Fig. 5, section 400). Whether the labeling in VPI was the result of transport from the motor cortex or was due to spread of reaction product to adjacent somatic sensory cortex (see above) could not be determined from our studies.

Discussion

As noted in the Introduction, considerable information has recently become available regarding the differential patterns of cerebellar and pallido-nigral termination in subdivisions of the ventrolateral

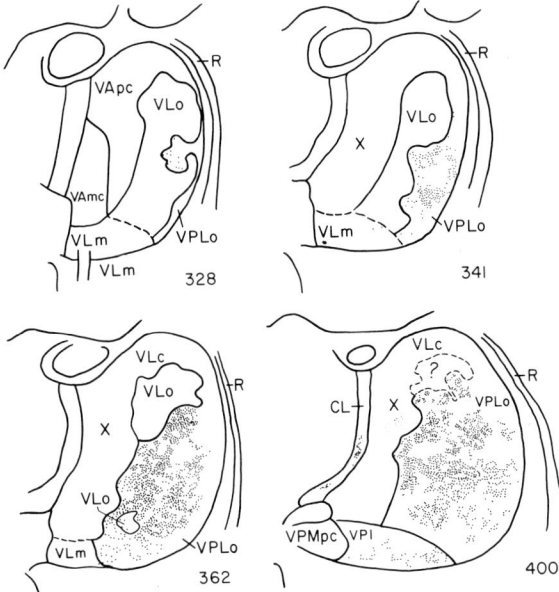

Fig. 5. Plots of labeled neurons resulting from injections into the motor cortex. The injection sites in the motor cortex near the rostral bank of the central sulcus are shown in Fig. 2B. Note that thalamic labeling is principally located in VPLo. Distinct regions of MD and CL also were labeled following motor cortex injections (not illustrated). From Schell and Strick (1984).

thalamus. The significance of these patterns of thalamic termination has not been completely understood because the precise cortical projection of each thalamic subdivision was previously unknown. In this chapter we have reviewed some of our evidence that the two premotor areas and the motor cortex each receive thalamic input from separate, cytoarchitectonically distinct subdivisions of the ventrolateral thalamus. Injections of WGA-HRP into the APA resulted in thalamic labeling which was most dense in area X. In contrast, injections into the SMA resulted in thalamic labeling which was most dense in VLo. As in previous studies (Strick, 1975, 1976; Kunzle, 1976; Kievit and Kuypers, 1977; Jones et al., 1979), VPLo was most densely labeled following injections into the motor cortex. In general, these findings are supported by the results of prior studies (e.g., SMA: DeVito and Smith, 1959; Wiesendanger et al., 1973; Kievit and Kuypers, 1977; Kalil, 1978; Kunzle, 1978; Bowker et al., 1979; Brinkman and Porter, 1979b. APA: Roberts and Akert, 1963; Akert, 1964; Kievit and Kuypers, 1977; Kunzle, 1978). In the remainder of this discussion we will review some of the recent primate studies on the sites of pallido-nigral and cerebellar termination in subdivisions of the ventrolateral

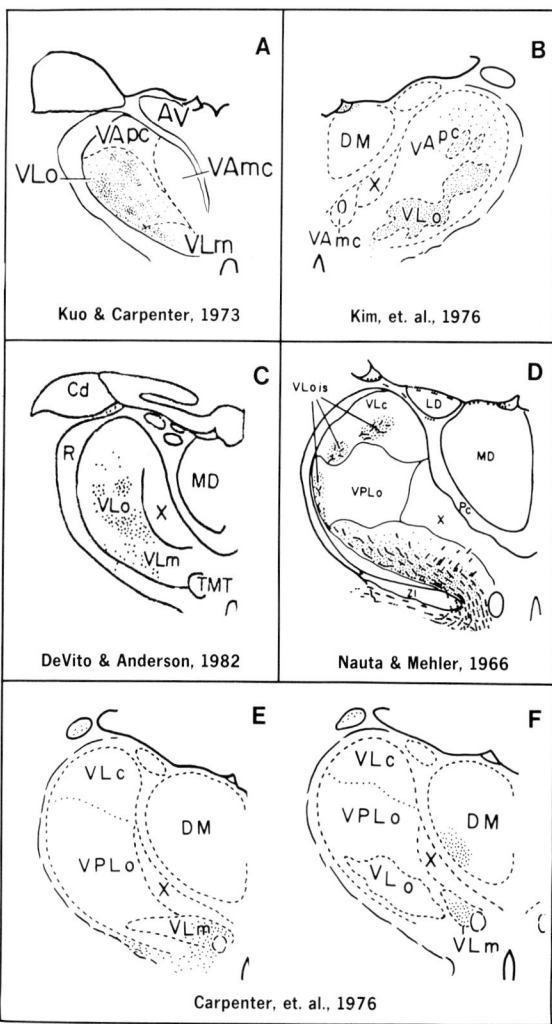

Fig. 6. Pattern of pallido-nigral termination in ventrolateral thalamus. Panels A–D represent the sites of termination for pallidal efferents in the ventrolateral thalamus taken from the studies of Kuo and Carpenter (1973), Kim et al. (1976), DeVito and Anderson (1982) and Nauta and Mehler (1966). Panels E and F represent the sites of termination for nigral efferents in the ventrolateral thalamus taken from the work of Carpenter et al. (1976). The levels of the sections chosen for illustration correspond as closely as possible to the levels of the experimental material illustrated in Figs. 3–5. From Schell and Strick (1984).

thalamus. We will then use this information to suggest how various thalamic subdivisions link subcortical motor nuclei with motor and premotor cortical areas.

Basal ganglia projections to the ventrolateral thalamus

The globus pallidus and the substantia nigra are the major output nuclei of the basal ganglia (for a complete review, see DeLong and Georgopoulos, 1981). Fig. 6 (A–D) illustrates some of the results of recent studies on the termination of pallido-thalamic efferents. Thalamic projections originate from the internal segment of the globus pallidus (GPi). Although there are some minor differences between studies, all emphasized that efferents from GPi project upon three subdivisions of the ventrolateral thalamus: VLo, parts of ventralis anterior pars parvocellularis (VApc) and VLm (Nauta and Mehler, 1966; Kuo and Carpenter, 1973; Kim et al., 1976; DeVito and Anderson, 1982).

The sites of termination of the substantia nigra in subdivisions of the ventrolateral thalamus have been extensively examined by Carpenter and his colleagues (Carpenter and McMasters, 1964; Carpenter and Strominger, 1967; Carpenter and Peter, 1972; Carpenter et al., 1976, 1981). The results of these studies are summarized in Fig. 6E and F. Thalamic projections originate from the pars reticulata segment of the nigra (SNpr) and terminate in two subdivisions of the ventrolateral thalamus: ventralis anterior pars magnocellularis (VAmc) and VLm. Additional projections also terminate in paralaminar medialis dorsalis (MD). The lack of overlap between nigral and pallidal sites of termination in the thalamus is evident in these figures.

These patterns of pallido-thalamic and nigrothalamic projections have been the basis for the generally accepted conclusion that the pallido-nigral system most directly influences areas 4, 6 and even prefrontal cortical areas (Brodal, 1981; De-Long and Georgopoulos, 1981). However, a comparison of our results with those of prior studies led us to suggest a different scheme of organization (Schell and Strick, 1984). Our observations indicate that part of the pallidal output is focused on subdivisions of the ventrolateral thalamus which project to the SMA (i.e., VLo and VLm). In addition, part of the nigral output also is focused on thalamic regions which project to the SMA (i.e., VLm and MD). Finally, neither pallidal nor nigral efferents appear to terminate in thalamic regions which project to the APA or the motor cortex.

In stating this scheme we do not mean to imply that all of the outputs from the pallido-nigral system are focused on the SMA. The cortical projections of VApc, which receives pallidal input, and VAmc, which receives nigral input, have not been well defined, but appear to project to cortical regions rostral to the premotor areas (Carmel, 1970; Kievit and Kuypers, 1977; Kunzle, 1978). Furthermore, the existence of eye movement-related neurons in SNpr suggests that there may be additional nigral efferents to thalamic regions which are concerned with oculomotor control (Hikosaka and Wurtz, 1983). However, our results indicate that of the cortical areas concerned with limb movement, the pallido-nigral system is most directly connected to the SMA.

Cerebellar projections to the ventrolateral thalamus

Cerebello-thalamic projections originate from all three deep cerebellar nuclei: dentate, interpositus and fastigial (see Brooks and Thach, 1981; Asanuma et al., 1983b,c, for recent reviews). Fig. 7 illustrates some of the results from recent studies on the termination of cerebello-thalamic efferents. Although studies differ in the nomenclature and borders applied to each nucleus, and in the techniques employed, they show remarkable agreement concerning the regions of ventrolateral thalamus which receive cerebellar input. The deep nuclei terminate in four subdivisions of the ventrolateral thalamus: VPLo, area X, VLc and VLps (Kusama et al., 1971; Mehler, 1971; Kievit and Kuypers, 1972; Batton et al., 1977; Chan-Palay, 1977; Percheron, 1977; Stanton, 1980; Kalil, 1981; Asanuma et al., 1983b,c). Some studies also report cerebellar terminations in

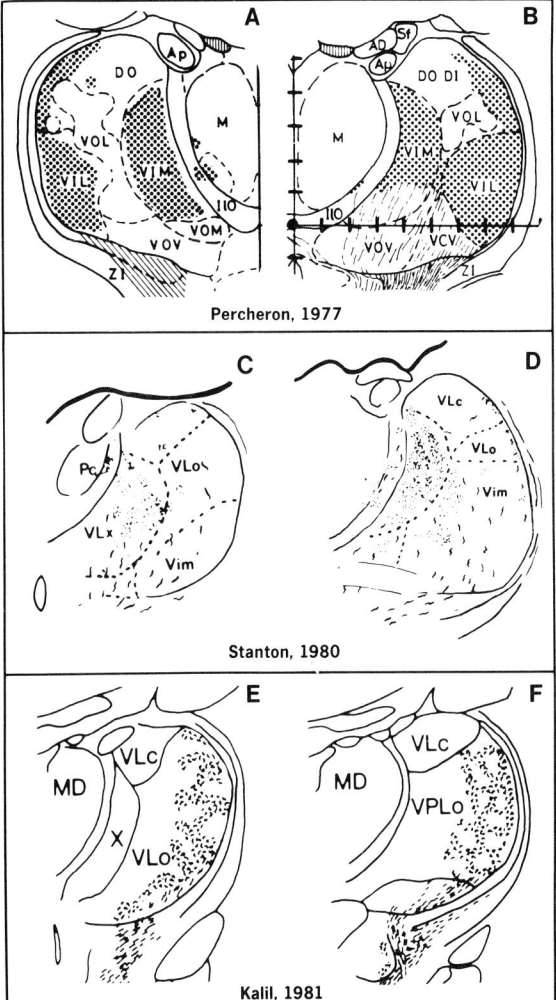

Fig. 7. Pattern of cerebello-thalamic termination in the ventrolateral thalamus. Panels A and B are taken from the work of Percheron (1977). They represent the combined sites of termination for efferents from all three deep cerebellar nuclei at two levels in the ventrolateral thalamus. Panels C and D are taken from the work of Stanton (1980). They represent the sites of termination of efferents from ventro-caudal portions of the dentate nucleus. Panels E and F are taken from the work of Kalil (1981). They represent the sites of termination of efferents from rostral portions of the dentate nucleus. The levels of the sections chosen for illustration correspond as closely as possible to the levels of the experimental material illustrated in Figs. 3–5. From Schell and Strick (1984).

VLo; however, this finding probably depends on differences in the delineation of nuclear borders and has not been supported by recent experiments (see Asanuma et al. (1983a–c) for a complete discussion on this issue). The lack of cerebellar terminations in VLo and VLm is particularly evident in degeneration studies where large portions of the deep nuclei were removed or the brachium conjunctivum was sectioned (see Fig. 7A and B, and Kievit and Kuypers, 1972; Percheron, 1977; however, see Stanton, 1980). Thus, Figs. 6 and 7 illustrate that cerebellar and pallido-nigral sites of termination do not overlap in the ventrolateral thalamus.

Studies of cerebellar projections also report that the origin of thalamic efferents from the deep nuclei is topographically organized. Projections from caudal regions of each deep cerebellar nucleus terminate medially in the ventrolateral thalamus in area X. In contrast, projections from rostral regions of each nucleus terminate more laterally in the ventrolateral thalamus in VPLo (see for illustration, Fig. 7C–F; Stanton, 1980; Kalil, 1981; Asanuma et al., 1983b,c).

Asanuma et al. (1983a,b) have suggested that the thalamic regions which receive cerebellar inputs (i.e., VPLo, VLc, area X and VLps) should be considered a common nucleus. They termed this nucleus the "cell-sparse zone", inferred that it projected to the motor cortex and concluded that "the cerebellum appears to influence only the primary motor area" (Asanuma et al., 1983b, p. 261). Furthermore, they inferred that the topographic organization of the cerebello-thalamic pathway reflects a somatotopic organization of the deep nuclei.

A comparison of our results with those of prior studies led us to propose an alternative interpretation of cerebello-thalamic topography (Schell and Strick, 1984). Our observations indicate that cerebello-thalamic projections are not limited to regions of the ventrolateral thalamus which project only to the motor cortex. In particular, our results indicate that area X, which receives efferents from the cerebellum, is the origin of inputs to the APA. We conclude that there are at least two separate cerebello-thalamic systems which originate from the deep nuclei. One system, located in rostral portions of the deep nuclei, projects largely to VPLo, and therefore most directly influences the motor cortex.

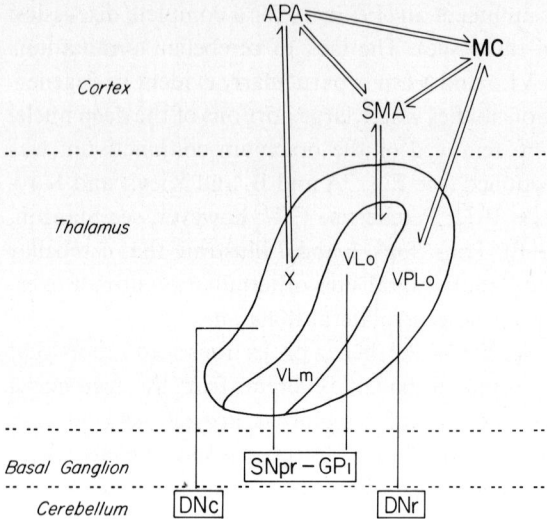

Fig. 8. Summary of anatomical relationships between cerebellar and basal ganglia efferents and motor and premotor cortical areas. This diagram illustrates: (1) the pathway from caudal portions of the deep cerebellar nuclei (DNc), to area X and the arcuate premotor area (APA), (2) the pathways from the pars reticulata of the substantia nigra (SNpr) and the internal segment of the globus pallidus (GPi), to VLm and VLo and the supplementary motor area (SMA), (3) the pathway from rostral portions of the deep cerebellar nuclei (DNr), to VPLo and the motor cortex (MC) and (4) the reciprocal connections between the MC, APA and SMA. See text for details. From Schell and Strick (1984).

A second system, located in caudal portions of the deep nuclei, projects largely to area X, and therefore most directly influences the APA. Additional support for these conclusions comes from physiological studies which report that cerebellar influences were directed to premotor, as well as motor cortical regions (Sasaki et al., 1976, 1979). The possibility that either or both of these systems might be somatotopically organized, as suggested by physiological observations (Brooks and Thach, 1981), remains to be examined.

Summary and speculation

The scheme of connections which results from our conclusions is diagrammatically represented in Fig. 8. Outputs from the cerebellum and basal ganglia supply three systems of subcortical afferents to the ventrolateral thalamus. These systems form parallel pathways to motor and premotor cortical areas. One parallel pathway originates in the caudal portions of the deep cerebellar nuclei and most directly influences the APA. A second pathway originates in SNpr and GPi and most directly influences the SMA. The third pathway originates in rostral portions of the deep cerebellar nuclei and most directly influences the motor cortex. Thus, each cortical area is the site of termination for a distinct subcortical system. Direct interactions between the three systems are largely limited to the cortical level, where the SMA, APA and motor cortex are reciprocally interconnected with one another. (Major interconnections between different subdivisions of the ventrolateral thalamus have not been described, although few studies have specifically examined this issue (Brodal, 1981).)

The present results suggest that the premotor areas may provide a major route by which subcortical motor nuclei influence motor cortex output. This suggestion may be particularly relevant to the basal ganglia which, unlike cerebellar nuclei, lack direct projections to thalamic regions which innervate area 4. These results are in line with the classical view that the premotor areas serve as "links in the chain of command to motor cortex" (see, for discussion, Brinkman and Porter, 1979b; Wiesendanger, 1981). On the other hand, the present results emphasize that the SMA, APA and motor cortex are anatomically and physiologically distinct cortical fields (see also Brinkman and Porter, 1979a,b; Matsumura and Kubota, 1979; Muakkassa and Strick, 1979; Roland et al., 1980a,b; Wise and Tanji, 1981; Weinrich and Wise, 1982). Furthermore, the premotor areas have direct projections to the spinal cord and to brainstem regions involved in motor control (see, e.g., Kuypers, 1960; Liu and Chambers, 1964; Kuypers and Lawrence, 1967; Biber et al., 1978; Murray and Coulter, 1981; for a recent review, see Kuypers, 1981). Thus, although the SMA and APA are interconnected with the motor cortex, it may be important to view the three cortical areas as components of functionally distinct efferent systems which are driven by largely separate subcortical nuclei.

Our conclusions may also have some important clinical implications. The anatomical relationship between the basal ganglia and the SMA suggests that some of the movement disorders associated with basal ganglia dysfunction might be mediated by the SMA. This suggestion is supported by clinical observations that some of the movement disorders associated with basal ganglia dysfunction are similar to the deficits caused by SMA damage. Akinesia, which Denny-Brown views as the primary deficit in human basal ganglia disorders (Denny-Brown, 1962; Denny-Brown and Yanagisawa, 1976), also is produced by lesions involving the SMA in humans (LaPlane et al., 1977; Damasio and Van Hoesen, 1980). It is also interesting to note the similarity between Marsden's suggestion that "the basal ganglia run a sequence of motor programs to achieve a motor plan" (Marsden, 1982), and studies that show selective increase in regional cerebral blood flow in the SMA of humans during the internal programming of motor sequences (Roland et al., 1980a).

The anatomical relationship between the cerebellum and the APA suggests the possibility of cerebellar involvement in the motor functions of the frontal lobe. Frontal lobe lesions in humans, in the region comparable to the APA, can result in a complex disorder of learned skilled movements termed apraxia (Geschwind, 1965; Heilman, 1979). Future studies might search for "apraxic-like" symptoms following lesions which involve caudal cerebellar efferent systems.

Acknowledgements

This work has been supported in part through funds from the Veterans Administration Medical Research Service, USPHS grant 02957 and the Department of Neurosurgery.

References

Akert, K. (1964) Comparative anatomy of frontal cortex and thalamofrontal connections. In J. M. Warren and K. Akert (Eds.), The Frontal Granular Cortex and Behavior, McGraw Hill, New York, pp. 372–394.

Asanuma, C., Thach, W. T. and Jones, E. G. (1983a) Cytoarchitectonic delineation of the ventral lateral thalamic region in the monkey. Brain Res. Rev., 5: 219–235.

Asanuma, C., Thach, W. T. and Jones, E. G. (1983b) Distribution of cerebellar terminations in the ventral lateral thalamic region of the monkey. Brain Res. Rev., 5: 237–265.

Asanuma, C., Thach, W. T. and Jones, E. G. (1983c) Anatomical evidence for segregated focal groupings of efferent cells and their terminal ramifications in the cerebellothalamic pathway of the monkey. Brain Res. Rev., 5: 267–297.

Batton, R. R., Jayaraman, A. III, Ruggiero, D. and Carpenter, M. B. (1977) Fastigial efferent projections in the monkey: an autoradiographic study. J. Comp. Neurol., 174: 281–306.

Biber, M. P., Kneisley, L. W. and LaVail, J. H. (1978) Cortical neurons projecting to the cervical and lumbar enlargements of the spinal cord in young and adult rhesus monkeys. Exp. Neurol., 59: 492–508.

Bowker, R. M., Murray, E. A. and Coulter, J. D. (1979) Intracortical and thalamic connections of the supplementary sensory and supplementary motor areas in the monkey. Neurosci. Abstr., 5: 704.

Brinkman, J. and Porter, R. (1979a) "Premotor" area of the monkey's cerebral cortex: Activity of neurons during performance of a learned motor task. Proc. Austr. Physiol. Pharmacol. Soc., 10: 198.

Brinkman, C. and Porter, R. (1979b) Supplementary motor area in the monkey: Activity of neurons during performance of a learned motor task. J. Neurophysiol., 42: 681–709.

Brodal, A. (1981) Neurological Anatomy In Relation to Clinical Medicine, Oxford University Press, New York.

Brooks, V. B. and Thach, W. T. (1981) Cerebellar control of posture and movement. In V. B. Brooks (Ed.), Handbook of Physiology. Section I: The Nervous System. Vol. II: Motor Control, American Physiological Society, Bethesda, pp. 877–946.

Carmel, P. W. (1970) Efferent projections of the ventral anterior nucleus of the thalamus in the monkey. Am. J. Anat., 128: 159–184.

Carpenter, M. B. and McMasters, R. E. (1964) Lesions of the substantia nigra in the rhesus monkey. Efferent fiber degeneration and behavioral observations. Am. J. Anat., 114: 293–320.

Carpenter, M. B. and Peter, P. (1972) Nigrostriatal and nigrothalamic fibers in the rhesus monkey. J. Comp. Neurol., 144: 93–116.

Carpenter, M. B. and Strominger, N. L. (1967) Efferent fiber projections of the subthalamic nucleus in the rhesus monkey. A comparison of the efferent projections of the subthalamic

nucleus, substantia nigra, and globus pallidus. Am. J. Anat., 121: 41–72.
Carpenter, M. B., Nakano, K. and Kim, R. (1976) Nigrothalamic projections in the monkey demonstrated by autoradiographic techniques. J. Comp. Neurol., 165: 401–416.
Carpenter, M. B., Carleton, S. C., Keller, J. T. and Conte, P. (1981) Connections of the subthalamic nucleus in the monkey. Brain Res., 224: 1–29.
Chan-Palay, V. (1977) Cerebellar Dentate Nucleus. Organization, Cytology and Transmitters, Springer Verlag, Berlin.
Damasio, A. R. and Van Hoesen, G. W. (1980) Structure and function of the supplementary motor area. Neurology, 30: 359.
DeLong, M. R. and Georgopoulos, A. P. (1981) Motor functions of the basal ganglia. In V. B. Brooks (Ed.), Handbook of Physiology. Section I: The Nervous System. Vol. II: Motor Control, American Physiological Society, Bethesda, pp. 1017–1061.
Denny-Brown, D. (1962) The Basal Ganglia and Their Relation to Disorders of Movement, Oxford University Press, London.
Denny-Brown, D. and Yanagisawa, N. (1976) The role of the basal ganglia in the initiation of movement. In M. D. Yahr (Ed.),The Basal Ganglia, Raven Press, New York, pp. 115–148.
DeVito, J. L. and Anderson, M. E. (1982) An autoradiographic study of efferent connections of the globus pallidus in *Macaca mulatta*. Exp. Brain Res., 46: 107–117.
DeVito, J. L. and Smith, O. A. Jr. (1959) Projections from the mesial frontal cortex (supplementary motor area) to the cerebral hemispheres and brain stem of the *Macaca mulatta*. J. Comp. Neurol., 111: 261–277.
Geschwind, W. (1965) Disconnection syndromes in animals and man II. Brain 88: 585–644.
Godschalk, M., Lemon, R. N., Kuypers, H. G. J. M. and Ronday, H. K. (1984) Cortical afferents and efferents of the monkey postarcuate area: an anatomical and electrophysiological study. Exp. Brain Res., 56: 410–424.
Heilman, K. M. (1979) Apraxia. In K. M. Heilman and E. Valenstein (Eds.), Clinical Neuropsychology, Oxford University Press, New York, pp. 159–185.
Hikosaka, O. and Wurtz, R. H. (1983) Visual and oculomotor functions of monkey substantia nigra pars reticulata. III. Memory-contingent visual and saccade responses. J. Neurophysiol., 49: 1268–1284.
Humphrey, D. R. (1979) On the cortical control of visually directed reaching: Contributions by nonprecentral motor areas. In R. E. Talbott and D. R. Humphrey (Eds.), Posture and Movement, Raven Press, New York, pp. 51–112.
Jones, E. G. and Powell, T. P. S. (1970) An anatomical study of converging sensory pathways within the cerebral cortex of the monkey. Brain, 93: 793–820.
Jones, E. G., Wise, S. P. and Coulter, J. D. (1979) Differential thalamic relationships of sensory-motor and parietal cortical fields in monkeys. J. Comp. Neurol., 183: 833–882.

Kalil, K. (1978) Neuroanatomical organization of the primate motor system: afferent and efferent connections of the ventral thalamic nuclei. In O. A. Otto (Ed.), Multidisciplinary Perspectives in Event-Related Brain Potential Research, U. S. Environmental Protection Agency, Washington, pp. 112–123.
Kalil, K. (1981) Projections of the cerebellar and dorsal column nuclei upon the thalamus of the rhesus monkey. J. Comp. Neurol., 195: 25–50.
Kievit, J. and Kuypers, H. G. J. M. (1972) Fastigial cerebellar projections to the ventrolateral nucleus of the thalamus and the organization of the descending pathways. In T. Frigyes, E. Rinvik and M. O. Yahr (Eds.), Corticothalamic Projections and Sensorimotor Activities, Raven Press, New York, pp. 91–114.
Kievit, J. and Kuypers, H. G. J. M. (1977) Organization of the thalamo- cortical connections to the frontal lobe in the rhesus monkey. Exp. Brain Res., 29: 299–322.
Kim, R., Nakano, K., Jayaraman, A. and Carpenter, M. B. (1976) Projections of the globus pallidus and adjacent structures: An autoradiographic study in the monkey. J. Comp. Neurol., 169: 263–289.
Kubota, K. and Hamada, I. (1978) Visual tracking and neuron activity in the post-arcuate area in monkeys. J. Physiol. (Paris), 74: 297–312.
Kunzle, H. (1976) Thalamic projections from the precentral motor cortex in *Macaca fascicularis*. Brain Res., 105: 253–267.
Kunzle, H. (1978) An autoradiographic analysis of the efferent connections from premotor and adjacent prefrontal regions (areas 6 and 9) in *Macaca fascicularis*. Brain Behav. Evol., 15: 185–234.
Kuo, J.-S. and Carpenter, M. B. (1973) Organization of pallidothalamic projections in rhesus monkey. J. Comp. Neurol., 151: 201–236.
Kusama, T., Mabuch, M. and Sumino, T. (1971) Cerebellar projections to the thalamic nuclei in monkeys. Proc. Jpn. Acad., 47: 505–510.
Kuypers, H. G. J. M. (1960) Central cortical projections to motor and somato-sensory cell groups. An experimental study in the rhesus monkey. Brain, 83: 161–184.
Kuypers, H. G. J. M. (1981) Anatomy of the descending pathways. In V. B. Brooks (Ed.), Handbook of Physiology. Section I: The Nervous System. Vol. II: Motor Control, part 1, American Physiological Society, Bethesda, pp. 597–666.
Kuypers, H. G. J. M. and Lawrence, D. G. (1967) Cortical projections to the red nucleus and the brain stem in the rhesus monkey. Brain Res., 4: 151–188.
Kwan, H. C., MacKay, W. A., Murphy, J. T. and Wong, Y. C. (1978) Spatial organization of precentral cortex in awake primates. II. Motor outputs. J. Neurophysiol., 41: 1120–1131.
LaPlane, D., Talairach, J., Meininger, V., Bancaud, J. and Orgogozo, J. M. (1977) Clinical consequences of corticectomies involving the supplementary motor area in man. J. Neurol. Sci., 34: 301–314.
Liu, C. N. and Chambers, W. W. (1964) An experimental study

of the corticospinal system in the monkey (*Macaca mulatta*). J. Comp. Neurol. 123: 257–284.

Marsden, C. D. (1982) The mysterious motor function of the basal ganglia: The Robert Wartenberg Lecture. Neurology, 32: 514–539.

Matsumura, M. and Kubota, K. (1979) Cortical projection to hand-arm motor area from post-arcuate in macaque monkeys: A histological study of retrograde transport of horseradish peroxidase. Neurosci. Lett., 11: 241–246.

Mehler, W. R. (1971) Idea of a new anatomy of the thalamus. J. Psychiat. Res., 8: 203–217.

Mesulam, M.-M. (1982) Tracing Neural Connections with Horseradish Peroxidase, John Wiley and Sons, New York.

Muakkassa, K. F. and Strick, P. L. (1979) Frontal lobe inputs to primate motor cortex: Evidence for four somatotopically organized "premotor" areas. Brain Res., 177: 176–182.

Murray, E. A. and Coulter, J. D. (1981) Organization of corticospinal neurons in the monkey. J. Comp. Neurol., 195: 339–365.

Nauta, W. J. H. and Mehler, W. R. (1966) Projections of the lentiform nucleus in the monkey. Brain Res., 1: 3–42.

Olszewski, J. (1952) The Thalamus of the *Macaca mulatta*. An Atlas for Use with the Stereotaxic Instrument, Karger, Basel.

Pandya, D. N. and Kuypers, H. G. J. M. (1969) Cortico-cortical connections in the rhesus monkey. Brain Res., 13: 13–36.

Pandya, D. N. and Vignolo, L. A. (1971) Intra- and inter-hemispheric projections of the precentral, premotor, and arcuate areas in the rhesus monkey. Brain Res., 26: 217–233.

Percheron, G. (1977) The thalamic territory of cerebellar afferents and the lateral region of the thalamus of the macaque in stereotaxic ventricular coordinates. J. Hirnforsch., 18: 375–400.

Roberts, T. S. and Akert, K. (1963) Thalamo-cortical connections and cytoarchitecture of opercular and insular cortex in *Macaca mulatta*. Schw. Arch. Neurol. Neurochir. Psychiat., 92: 1–43.

Roland, P. E., Larsen, B., Lassen, N. A. and Skinho, E. (1980a) Supplementary motor area and other cortical areas in organization of voluntary movements in man. J. Neurophysiol., 43: 118–136.

Roland, P. E., Shinho, E., Lassen, N. A. and Larsen, B. (1980b) Different cortical areas in man in organization of voluntary movements in extrapersonal space. J. Neurophysiol., 43: 137–150.

Sasaki, K., Kawaguchi, S., Oka, H., Sakai, M. and Mizuno, N. (1976) Electrophysiological studies on the cerebellocerebral projections in monkeys. Exp. Brain Res., 24: 495–507.

Sasaki, K., Jinnai, K., Gemba, H., Hashimoto, S. and Mizuno, N. (1979) Projection of the cerebellar dentate nucleus onto the frontal association cortex in monkeys. Exp. Brain Res., 37: 193–198.

Schell, G. R. and Strick, P. L. (1984) The origin of thalamic inputs to the arcuate premotor and supplementary motor areas. J. Neurosci., 4: 539–560.

Stanton, G. B. (1980) Topographical organization of ascending cerebellar projections from the dentate and interposed nuclei in *Macaca mulatta*: An anterograde degeneration study. J. Comp. Neurol., 190: 699–731.

Strick, P. L. (1975) Multiple sources of thalamic input to the primate motor cortex. Brain Res., 55: 1–24.

Strick, P. L. (1976) Anatomical analysis of ventrolateral thalamic input to primate motor cortex. J. Neurophysiol., 39: 1020–1031.

Tanji, J. and Kurata, K. (1982) Comparison of movement-related activity in two cortical motor areas of primates. J. Neurophysiol., 48: 633–653.

Weinrich, M. and Wise, S. P. (1982) The premotor cortex of the monkey. J. Neurosci., 9: 1329–1344.

Wiesendanger, M. (1981) Organization of secondary motor areas of cerebral cortex. In V. B. Brooks (Ed.), Handbook of Physiology. Section I: The Nervous System. Vol. II: Motor Control, part 2, American Physiological Society, Bethesda, pp. 1121–1147.

Wiesendanger, M., Seguin, J. J. and Kunzle, H. (1973) The supplementary motor area. A control system for posture? In R. B. Stein, K. C. Pearson, R. S. Smith and J. B. Bedford (Eds.), Advances in Behavioral Biology, Control of Posture and Locomotion. Vol. 7, Plenum, New York, pp. 331–346.

Wise, S. P. and Tanji, J. (1981) Supplementary and precentral motor cortex: Contrast in responsiveness to peripheral input in the hindlimb area of the unanesthetized monkey. J. Comp. Neurol., 195: 433–451.

Woolsey, C. W., Settlage, P. W., Meyer, D. R., Spencer, W. M., Hamuy, T. P. and Travis, A. M. (1952) Patterns of localization in precentral and "supplementary" motor areas and their relations to the concept of a premotor area. Res. Publ. Ass. Res. Nerv. Mental Dis., 30: 238–264.

Discussion

S. P. Wise

Laboratory of Neurophysiology, National Institute of Mental Health, Building 36, Room 2D-10, Bethesda, MD 20205, U.S.A.

In addition to the contributions presented in this volume, the session on premotor neural circuits included a lecture by H. G. J. M. Kuypers on "The Skeletomotor System". Unfortunately, it was impossible to include a paper by Dr. Kuypers in this section. However, his presentation closely followed an earlier review (Kuypers, 1981), and the reader is referred there for an indication of what transpired at the session. The discussion that followed the presentations by Kuypers, Büttner-Ennever and Strick focused on three main topics: (1) a comparison of cortical access to motor neurons in the eye- and limb-movement systems, (2) a consideration of putative phylogenetic changes in neural circuitry, and (3) localization of brain function.

Corticomotoneuronal connections

Kuypers has taught, for more than 15 years now, that the primate motor cortex and its main output pathway, the pyramidal tract, enable the independent control of skeletal muscles that usually work in concert and that monosynaptic cortical inputs to spinal motor neurons (see Fetz et al., Section IV-A) play a key role in this capability, termed movement fractionation. After his presentation, Kuypers was questioned about the possibility of direct cortical projections to oculomotoneurons and what role such connections might play in the cerebral control of eye movements. Although some investigators believe that there is at least a slight cortical projection to oculomotor nuclei (Leichnetz et al., 1984), it was the opinion of both Kuypers and Büttner-Ennever that the cerebral cortex does not project significantly to oculomotor neurons and that cerebral influences on eye movements are conducted through such structures as the paramedian pontine reticular formation (PPRF) and the superior colliculus. Kuypers suggested that the lack of direct cortical access to oculomotor neurons might reflect the absence of fractionation in eye movements. Since most eye movements are conjugate and the eye muscles always work in concert, there does not appear to be an eye-movement analogous to the movement fractionation seen in the limbs. Hence, one might predict a paucity of corticomotoneuronal connections upon oculomotor neurons and an abundance on skeletomotor neurons of species with a substantial repertoire of fractionated movements.

Brain evolution

The evolution of motor systems also served as the basis for discussion, most of which involved the view that there is a phylogenetic trend for the neocortex to become progressively more dominant in motor control during mammalian evolution. In her presentation, Büttner-Ennever argued that cats and monkeys, in that order, show progressively more cortical control of optokinetic nystagmus (OKN) than do rats. In a similar vein, Kuypers suggested that in an "ascending series" of mammals — commencing with opossums and continuing through cats, monkeys and chimpanzees to humans

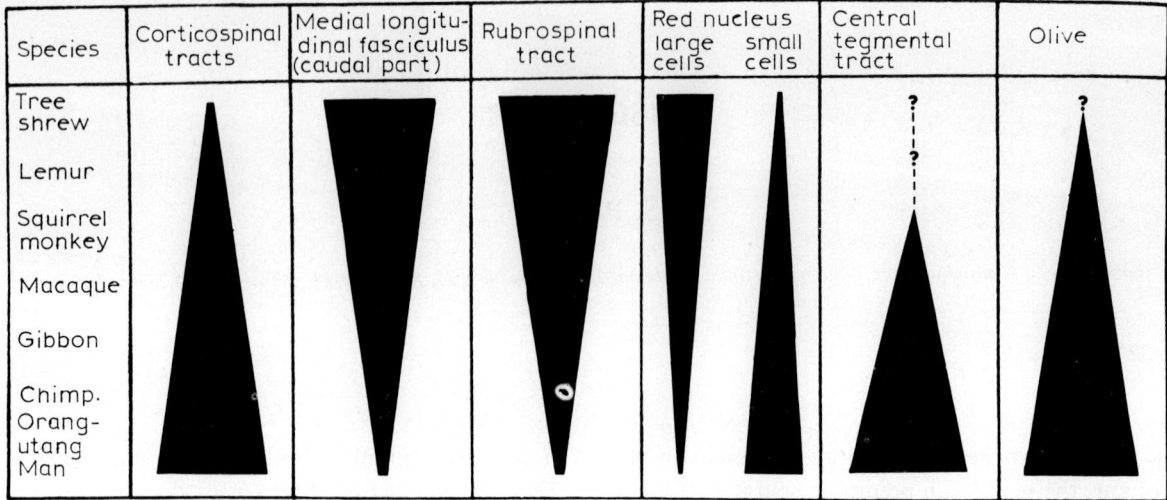

Fig. 1. Proposed "phylogenetic" trends for several motor-control structures and pathways. The relative size and importance of each structure and pathway is indicated by the width of the triangle at the "level" indicated by the species or genus listed in the left column. The authors propose that: "As the evolutionary scale is climbed, the parvocellular part of the red nucleus, the central tegmental tract and the olive all become larger and the magnocellular part of the red nucleus and the rubrospinal tract smaller." (Nathan and Smith (1982), p. 264, figure reproduced with permission.) Olive, inferior olivary complex of nuclei.

— the cortico-spinal fibers terminate progressively more ventrally, a morphological pattern that presumably indicates more direct cortical control over motor neurons (see Kuypers, 1981). The concept of cortical domination could be extended to the other two motor pathways discussed by Kuypers: the group A (largely reticulospinal) and group B (mainly rubrospinal) systems, each of which receives a major input from parts of the motor cortex in monkeys. Freund questioned the significance of the rubrospinal tract in man, since Nathan and Smith (1982), following earlier work, reported that the magnocellular red nucleus and rubrospinal tract are virtually absent in man. This would leave only two major corticofugal systems to the spinal cord: a direct corticospinal projection for control of fractionated distal movements and a premotor cortex-dominated group A pathway preferentially involved in the control of axial and proximal muscles. In reply, Kuypers suggested an evolutionary history of the magnocellular red nucleus that included a diffuse structure in primitive vertebrates, a more discrete and topographical organization in "lower" mammals, full development reflected by extant cats and monkeys, and a regression in chimpanzees and humans. Kuypers argued that concomitant with rubrospinal regression, the corticospinal system became completely dominant and elaborated a mechanism for movement fractionation. Fig. 1, taken from the work of Nathan and Smith (1982), summarizes current neurological thinking on this subject.

Baker objected to this entire mode of thought on the grounds that differences observed among extant species are better considered as examples of non-convergent evolution than of phylogenetic trends (see also Baker, Section IV-B). He averred that all extant species have their own long history of adaptation to their environment and that it is inappropriate to construct from these species a simple ladder of evolution (see Fig. 1 and its legend). As Gould (1976, p. 115) has expressed the problem: "... it seems as though comparative neurologists remain rooted to Lamarck's scala naturae — for they persist in studying a fish, a reptile, an insectivore, a tree shrew, a monkey, and a man and in drawing from such a comparison a set of conclusions about vertebrate evolution. The neuroanatomists speak of this sequence as though it represents phylogeny, which it manifestly does not."

Wise, who chaired this discussion, contended that in addition to theoretical problems concerning brain evolution, there is reason to question the validity of the data upon which certain proposed phylogenetic progressions are based. Both theoretical and practical problems can be discerned in studies of the corticospinal system. For example, domestic cats are sometimes treated as though they represent some sort of intermediate stage of corticospinal development along a path to man, and rats and opossums considered as though they possess a primitive corticospinal system. But, of course, carnivores are not intermediate, in any biologically meaningful sense, to rodents and marsupicarnivores, on the one hand, and primates on the other. Carnivores and primates have approximately 100 million years of separate evolution (Kielan-Jaworowska et al., 1979) and their most recent common ancestor did not resemble a modern cat. Accordingly, differences among these species are more likely to reveal specific adaptations in relation to their life history than to reflect a phylogenetic progression. As for the accuracy of the anatomical data upon which proposed phylogenetic progressions depend, Wise contended that much of it is unreliable. For example, older anatomical studies, using degeneration methods for tracing connections, tended to confirm the preconception that rats and opossums exhibited the supposedly primitive characteristic of a corticospinal system terminating mainly, if not exclusively, in the dorsal horn of the spinal gray matter, Rexed's laminae I-VI (Brown, 1971; Martin et al., 1975). However, subsequent studies have shown that the motor cortex of both the laboratory rat and the Virginia opossum projects extensively to intermediate layers of the spinal cord and contributes input to the ventral horn as well (Cabana and Martin, 1984; Wise and Donoghue, 1985). Since motor neuron dendrites branch extensively in the intermediate spinal gray matter (e.g., Valverde, 1966), there is, in these species, a clear possibility for the existence of corticomotoneuronal connections and, indeed, physiological evidence for such connections has been reported for rats (Elger et al., 1977). Thus, if it is assumed that the ancestral mammals lacked corticomotoneuronal connections, then rats, at least, do not appear to have a primitive corticospinal system. However, it seems evident that many assumptions about primitivity in mammalian brain organization need to be reassessed. To do so, a relatively large number of species, selected on the basis of sound biological principles, must be studied with modern neuroanatomical and neurophysiological methods.

Localization of function

Two additional points were raised in discussion, both related to the issue of functional localization in the brain. In development of Büttner-Ennever's thesis that the premotor circuits for each type of eye movement are largely separate, Noth argued that a single neural integrator is likely to be shared among each of these circuits.

Hepp inquired about the functional specializations of each motor cortical field listed by Strick. In his presentation, Strick emphasized the separation of at least four different motor cortical fields: the primary motor cortex, the supplementary motor cortex, an arcuate premotor area, and a ventral cingulate field immediately adjacent to the supplementary motor cortex. However, there was little discussion of the functional specializations of these different cortical fields. Similarly, the first presentation of the subsequent session, by Wise, was also devoted to the definition of a motor cortical field rather than any analysis of its specialized role in the cerebral control of movement. As Hepp's query points out, it remains one of the central problems in the fields of cerebral localization and motor physiology to define more precisely the functional specializations of each cortical field involved in the cerebral control of movement. More broadly, it will be of profound importance to develop a coherent understanding of the motor cortex as a whole, an understanding that must, ultimately, subsume both skeletomotor and oculomotor systems (see Goldberg and Bruce, Section IV-A). Of particular interest in this regard was the report, presented for the first time at this conference by Schlag-Rey and Schlag, that cells within the rostral part of the supplementary motor cortex, or immediately rostral to it, are related to the cerebral control of eye movement. It may be hoped that further physiological investigation of the oculomotor and skeletomotor cortex, much of which remains almost completely unexplored, will establish the foundation for a more general understanding of the cortical motor system.

References

Brown, L. T. (1971) Projections and terminations of the corticospinal tract in rodents. Exp. Brain Res., 13: 432–450.

Cabana, T. and Martin, G. F. (1984) The distribution of corticospinal projections in adult or pouch young opossums (*Didelphis virginiana*). Soc. Neurosci. Abstr., 10: 321.

Elger, C. E., Speckmann, E. J., Caspers, H. and Janzen, R. W. C. (1977) Corticospinal projections in the rat. I. Monosynaptic and polysynaptic responses of cervical motoneurons to epicortical stimulation. Exp. Brain Res., 28: 385–404.

Gould, S. J. (1976) Grades and clades revisited. In R. B. Masterton, W. Hodos and H. Jerison (Eds.), Evolution, Brain and Behavior: Persistent Problems, L. Erlbaum Associates, Hillsdale, NJ, pp. 115–122.

Kielan-Jaworowska, Z., Brown, T. M. and Lillegraven, J. A. (1979) Eutheria. In J. A. Lillegraven, Z. Kielan-Jaworowska and W. A. Clemens (Eds.), Mesozoic Mammals, University of California Press, Berkeley, pp. 221–258.

Kuypers, H. G. J. M. (1981) Anatomy of the descending pathways. In V. B. Brooks (Ed.), Handbook of Physiology, Section 1, The Nervous System, Vol. II, Motor Control, Part 1, American Physiological Society, Bethesda, MD, pp. 597–666.

Leichnetz, G., Spencer, P. F. and Smith, D. J. (1984) Cortical projections to nuclei adjacent to the oculomotor complex in the medial dien-mesencephalic tegmentum in the monkey. J. Comp. Neurol., 228: 359–387.

Martin, G. F., Beattie, M. S., Bresnahan, J. C., Henkel, C. K. and Hughes, H. C. (1975) Cortical and brain stem projections to the spinal cord of the American opossum (*Didelphis marsupialis virginiana*). Brain Behav. Evol., 12: 270–310.

Nathan, P. W. and Smith, M. C. (1982) The rubrospinal and central tegmental tracts in man. Brain, 105: 223–269.

Valverde, F. (1966) The pyramidal tract in rodents. A study of its relations with the posterior column nuclei, dorsolateral reticular formation of the medulla oblongata, and cervical spinal cord. Z. Zellforsch., 71: 297–363.

Wise, S. P. and Donoghue, J. P. (1985) Motor cortex of rodents. In E. G. Jones and A. Peters (Eds.), Cerebral Cortex, Vol. 3, Plenum Press, New York, in press.

… SECTION IV-A

Specialized Areas in Motor Control: Supratentorial

Movement-related activity in the premotor cortex of rhesus macaques

Steven P. Wise, Michael Weinrich and Karl-Heinz Mauritz

Laboratory of Neurophysiology, National Institute of Mental Health, Building 36, Room 2D-10, Bethesda, MD 20205, U.S.A.

Introduction

Several recent reports have held that the primate premotor cortex is a distinct cortical field that plays a specialized role in the cerebral control of movement (Roland et al., 1980; Wiesendanger, 1981; Weinrich and Wise, 1982; Halsband and Passingham, 1982; Brinkman and Porter, 1983; Freund and Hummelsheim, 1984). However, the definition of the premotor cortex has been the source of difficulty, and, as the premotor cortex is currently defined, its role in motor control has been questioned seriously (Woolsey et al., 1952; Travis, 1955).

One source of difficulty in understanding the premotor cortex can be traced to the difference between the modern and archaic usage of the term premotor cortex. Early investigators (Bucy, 1933; Fulton, 1935; Denny-Brown, 1966; Luria, 1980) considered the premotor cortex to be a single functional entity equivalent to area 6, despite the marked inconsistency in the architectonic delineation of that area (e.g., see Brodmann, 1909; Vogt and Vogt, 1919; Bucy, 1935; Von Bonin and Bailey, 1947; Denny-Brown and Botterell, 1948). However, it is now recognized that, as it is usually defined, area 6 consists of at least three functionally distinct parts. The most medial part of area 6 corresponds to the supplementary motor cortex (MII; Woolsey et al., 1952; Tanji and Kurata, 1982). The most caudal part of area 6 is best considered to be part of the primary motor cortex (MI), partly on the basis of the roughly somototopic representation revealed by intracortical microstimulation (Kwan et al., 1978). And a third part of "area 6", the part rostral to MI and lateral to MII, comprises the premotor cortex (PM).

Until recently, there has been little physiological evidence supporting a motor role for the premotor cortex. A fundamental contribution was made by Kubota and Hamada (1978). They observed single-unit activity in the premotor cortex that was closely related to visually guided limb movements. Two aspects of their data support the hypothesis that this neuronal activity was functionally related to the movement rather than the visuospatial cues that guided the movement: (1) the discharge rate of some of these neurons was correlated with limb velocity and acceleration, and (2) the onset of unit activity was generally (with the exception of 7% of the task-related units) better correlated, in time, with the onset of movement than with the visual cues that triggered the movement. Unfortunately, neither Kubota and Hamada nor later confirmatory reports (Weinrich and Wise, 1982; Brinkman and Porter, 1983) presented any quantitative documentation for this assertion (see Vicario et al., 1983). Accordingly, the temporal correlations between the changes in neuronal discharge, the presentation of the visual triggering cue, and the onset of movement were re-examined in the present study.

Another tactic for approaching the same hypothesis is to examine the activity of movement-related cells during "spontaneous" movements emitted in total darkness. This test would rule out the possibility that this activity actually reflects the visual aspects of limb movement or occlusion of visual stimuli during movement. We report here the activity of a small neuronal population during movements made in total darkness.

The evidence presented in this report supports the view that the movement-related discharge is functionally linked with the execution of movement, rather than any sensory stimuli. It must be emphasized, however, that not all neurons in the premotor cortex are movement related. Some cells appear to be responsive to the sensory signals that guide movement (Kubota and Hamada, 1978; Godschalk et al., 1981; Rizzolatti et al., 1981; Weinrich and Wise, 1982), others appear to reflect the animal's preparation for movement based on such sensory cues (Weinrich and Wise, 1982; Godschalk and Lemon, 1983), and still others appear to be modulated in anticipation of predictable environmental events or stimuli (Mauritz and Wise, 1985). For heuristic purposes, these patterns have been termed signal-related, set-related, and anticipatory, respectively. These activity patterns are not mutually exclusive, i.e., they are often combined in individual cells. One aspect of the combination of these activity patterns will be discussed in this report: the relationship between the directional specificity of the set-related activity and that for the movement-related activity when these patterns are combined in a single neuron.

Materials and methods

Four male rhesus monkeys (*Macaca mulatta*) were studied. The monkeys were seated in a primate chair in a dark room and operantly conditioned to perform a limb movement. Each monkey was allowed to work for as many juice rewards as it desired in the 2–4-hour sessions.

Two behavioral tasks were used in these experiments. Two monkeys, monkeys A and B, participated in the first task, reported in detail previously (Weinrich et al., 1984), in which the forearm was placed in a plastic brace coupled to a potentiometer. This procedure allowed the continuous monitoring of forelimb position and the movements of the forelimb around the elbow. The movements were guided by visual cues projected onto a tangent screen in front of the monkey. In brief, there were two small (0.3°) spots of light projected onto the tangent screen. One of these light spots reflected the position of the forelimb (the position light) and the other was controlled by a PDP 11/03 computer (the target light). The monkey's task was to align the position light with the target light to within 2°. After the monkey aligned these light spots the target light would "jump" to a different location on the screen. This target light jump indicated the direction and magnitude of the next limb movement to be executed, but the monkey was conditioned not to begin the movement until the target light dimmed slightly. The dimming of the target light served as a trigger stimulus and the monkey was then required to re-align the target and position lights in order to receive reinforcement. The neural activity associated with these visually guided movements could then be compared to activity associated with unconditioned, "spontaneous" movements made in total darkness. In each case the activity of neurons could be compared with the position and acceleration of the limb, all of which was recorded with an FM analog tape recorder for off-line analysis.

Two other monkeys, monkeys C and D, were the subjects of a second motor task, also described in detail elsewhere (Wise and Mauritz, 1985). In this task the monkey was seated within arm's reach of a panel of three illuminable switches (Fig. 1A). The monkey began each trial by depressing the central of the three target keys. After a period of time either the left or the right target key became illuminated. This event indicated which of the remaining two keys was to be the target on that particular trial, but, as in the experiment described above, the monkey was not allowed to execute the movement immediately. Instead, the monkey was conditioned to withhold movement until a light-emitting diode directly above the target key was illuminated. This served as the trigger stimulus for the monkey to

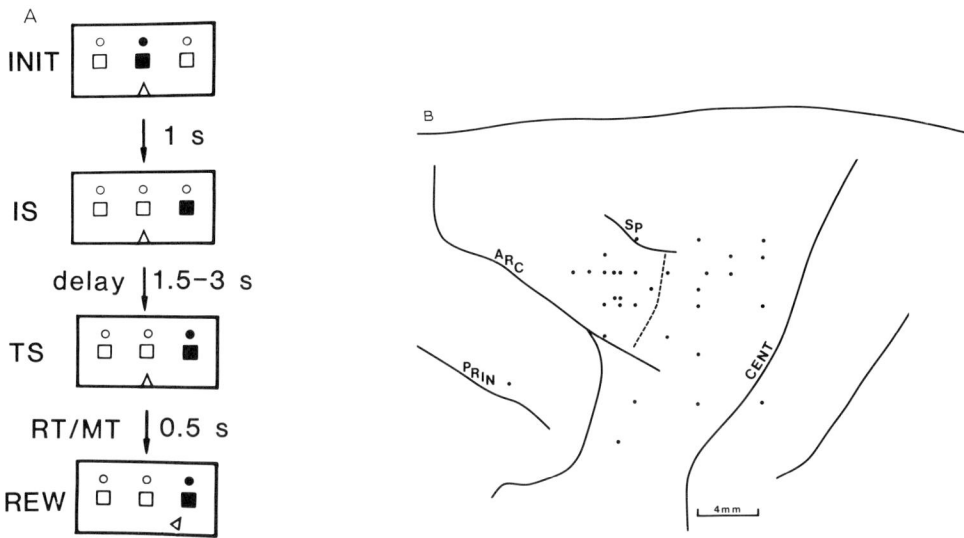

Fig. 1A. Behavioral paradigm. Each rectangle represents the panel in front of the monkey, and associated with each rectangle are: three squares, each representing a key, three circles, each representing a light-emitting diode (LED), and an open arrow, indicating the key depressed by the monkey at any given time. Filled symbols indicate illuminated keys or LEDs. To initiate (Init) each trial, the monkey depressed the central target key. After a brief period of time, one of the two remaining keys was illuminated to serve as an instruction stimulus (IS). After an instructed delay period, the LED was illuminated to serve as a trigger stimulus (TS) that signalled the monkey to begin a movement to the illuminated key. If the monkey completed the movement within a reaction time (RT) plus movement time (MT) limit of 500 mseconds, it received a juice reward. After another brief period of time, the central light became illuminated again and the cycle was repeated. B. Surface map of movement-related units in monkey C. Each dot indicates the approximate surface site of an electrode penetration in which movement-related neurons were found. The dashed line indicates the approximate boundary between the premotor and primary motor cortex as defined by intracortical microstimulation (see Weinrich and Wise, 1982).

begin a movement to depress the target key. If the monkey acquired the target within 500 mseconds of receiving the trigger stimulus, it received a reward. The onset of movement was approximated by the time the monkey lifted off of one of the keys to begin a movement toward another of the keys.

Recordings were obtained from transdurally inserted, platinum-iridium electrodes and the single-unit activity was amplified and discriminated by standard methods. The localization of penetration sites and histological analysis and the method for premotor cortex definition have been described previously (Weinrich et al., 1984; Wise and Mauritz, 1985). The cells described in this report as premotor cortex neurons were located within a zone of frontal agranular cortex rostral to the primary motor cortex as defined by intracortical microstimulation.

The premotor cortex cells were located within and slightly medial to the dorsomedial bank of the arcuate sulcus, from about the level of its genu laterally to the level of the superior precentral sulcus medially (Fig. 1B).

Results

Neuronal sample and cell classes

This report is based mainly upon a study of 176 premotor cortex neurons analysed in detail from two monkeys (C and D) that performed the task illustrated in Fig. 1A and 16 additional cells from two different monkeys (A and B) in which movements made in total darkness were monitored.

On the basis of their patterns of discharge during

TABLE I

Neuronal classification in premotor cortex

Activity pattern	Monkey group		
	Previous study[a]	Monkeys A & B	Monkeys C & D[b]
Movement-related	149 (73%)	185 (65%)	103 (58%)
Set-related	59 (29%)	97 (34%)	111 (63%)
Signal-related	89 (43%)	134 (47%)	101 (57%)
Anticipatory	0 (0%)	44 (15%)	49 (28%)

[a] Weinrich and Wise (1982).
[b] The neuronal sample for these two monkeys was intentionally biased toward set-related neurons.

a visually instructed movement that included an enforced, instructed delay period, the units were classed into four groups: signal-, set- and movement-related, and anticipatory. The criteria for classifying these cells have been reported in detail (Weinrich and Wise, 1982; Weinrich et al., 1984; Mauritz and Wise, 1985) and will be summarized briefly here. Cells were classed as movement-related if they altered their discharge rate immediately before or during the execution of the operantly conditioned limb movement. They were classed as signal-related if they showed a transient change in firing rate shortly after the presentation of a visuospatial instruction stimulus. And neurons were considered set-related if they showed sustained increases or decreases in discharge from a time shortly after the presentation of an instruction stimulus until about the beginning of the limb movement. Cells were considered to have anticipatory activity if discharge modulation preceded the presentation of the instruction stimulus (Mauritz and Wise, 1985). The relative proportions of neurons showing these patterns of activity are shown in Table I.

Movement-related activity

The movement-related activity observed in these monkeys was comparable to that reported previously (Weinrich and Wise, 1982). 25 movement-related neurons, from monkey C (see Table I), were selected for quantitative analysis. These cells began to increase neuronal discharge 124 ± 30 mseconds before the onset of movement, as detected by key release. This value is comparable to the mean of 130 ± 60 mseconds obtained in an earlier key-release task (Weinrich and Wise, 1982) and a mean of 137 ± 61 mseconds, taken from two monkeys (A and B) in which the onset of movement was detected by the initial limb acceleration (Weinrich et al., 1984). The 25 neurons discussed here reached a mean peak discharge rate of 106 ± 41 impulses/sec over a background activity of 11 ± 10 impulses/sec. Thus, a modulation of about 95 impulses/sec was observed in this selected sample of neurons. This value compares with means of 80 and 82 impulses/sec reported previously (Weinrich and Wise, 1982; Weinrich et al., 1984).

Movements in the dark

13 neurons that were clearly movement-related during visually guided movements were later tested while the monkeys made unrewarded movements in the dark. All of these cells were modulated during the execution of these "spontaneous" movements in total darkness. Ten of these cells were located in the premotor cortex of one monkey and three were from the premotor cortex of another. In addition, there were three cells tested with ambiguous results, but in these cells the movement-relationship during visually guided movements was also less clear than in the other 13 cells tested. For ten of the 13 cells clearly related to movement, it was possible to re-examine neuronal activity during a second phase of visually guided, rewarded movements after the period of unrewarded movements in the dark. This procedure ensured that the isolated cell had the same characteristics in the second phase of visually guided movements as in the first. The number of tested cell was small because the monkeys, having been momentarily deprived of the ability to work for rewards, often made movements of sufficient abruptness to cause cell isolation to be lost. Since the number of units tested in this condition is rather

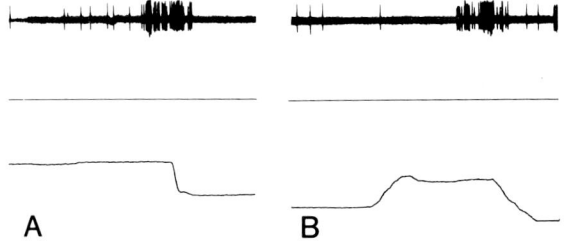

Fig. 2. Two traces showing neuronal activity during movement. Below each trace is a record of limb position. A. Movement made in response to and guided by visuospatial cues. B. "Spontaneous" movement made in total darkness. Downward deflections of the position trace indicate flexions around the elbow.

small, the results must be considered highly tentative. Nonetheless, the basic uniformity of the result makes it seem likely that the result is a general one.

Examples of two of these neurons are shown in Figs. 2 and 3. Both of these cells were excited before flexion movements of both the visually guided and "spontaneous" types. It must be emphasized that the parameters of movement were not identical for these different types of movements. Movements made in the dark tended to be of higher velocity and were often biphasic, i.e., the monkey reversed the direction of the forearm during the movement (e.g., Fig. 3B). Note that although the activity and the movements themselves are quantitatively different in these two situations, the direction of activity change before the movement is the same. Comparison with visually guided or "spontaneous" movements in the opposite direction show a decrease or no change in activity. Thus, movement-related activity of the premotor cortex does not depend on visual guidance or any visual stimulus that might occur during a movement.

Temporal correlation with the onset of movement

One tactic for determining whether the onset of neuronal discharge is more closely related, temporally, with the onset of movement or the presenta-

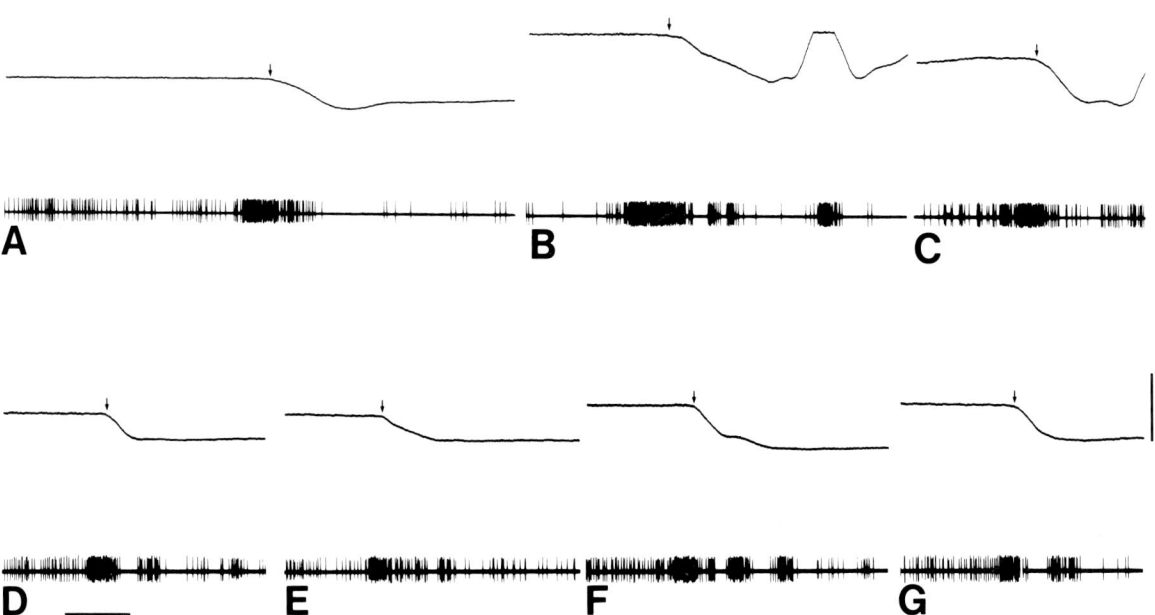

Fig. 3. Discriminated single-unit activity taken from the premotor cortex. In each pair of records the angle of the contralateral forelimb (elbow) is shown above the discriminated unit activity. A–C. Flexion movements made "spontaneously" in total darkness. D–G. Movements made in response to and guided by the visuospatial cues. In each case, limb flexion is preceded by a burst of discharge from the neuron, activity that is not seen during maintenance of a limb position or during limb extension (not shown). Time calibration (D), 1 second; limb position calibration (G), 50°.

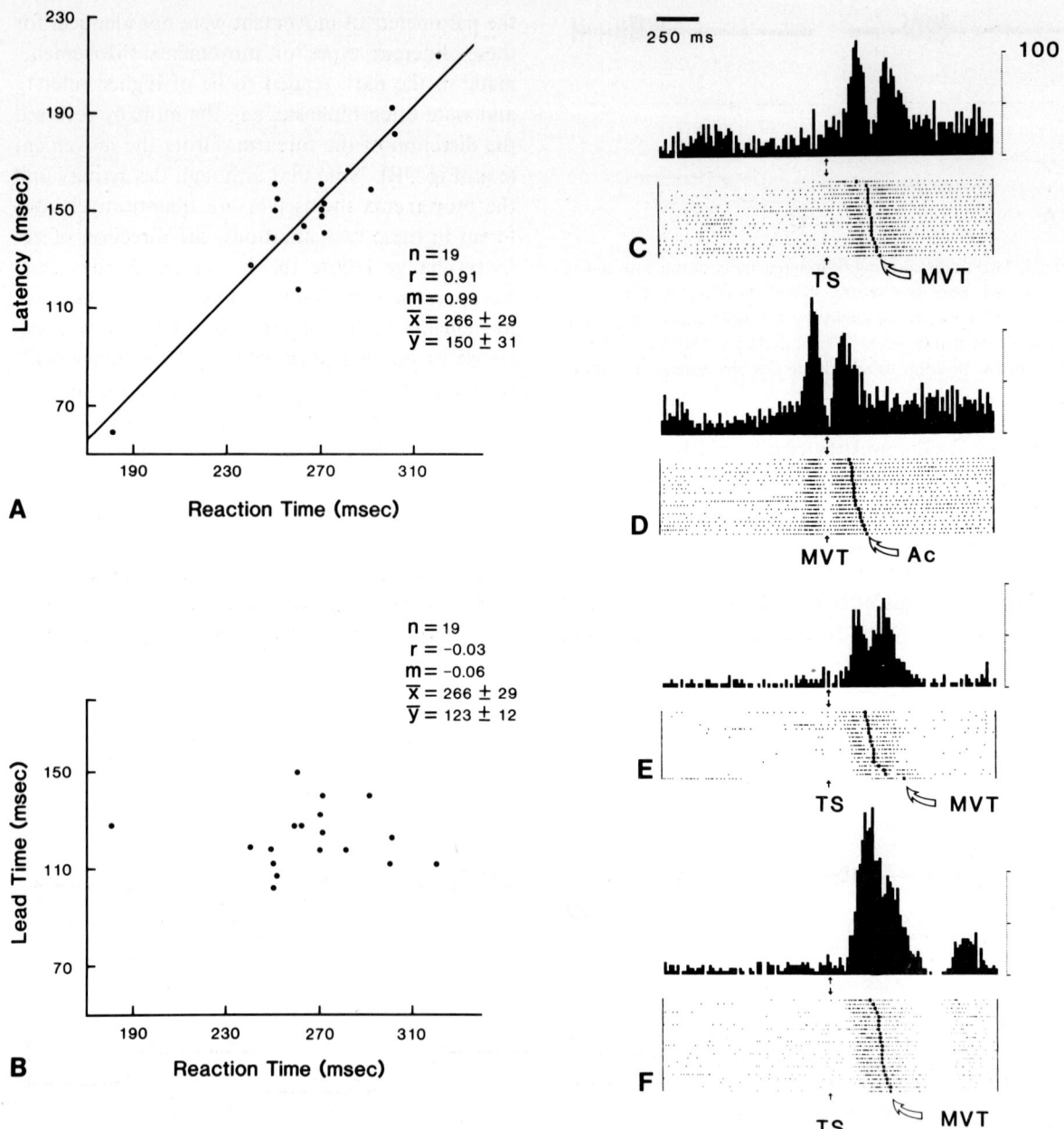

Fig. 4. Close correlation of unit discharge with the onset of movement (A) rather than the presentation of the trigger stimulus (B). Data for A and B were obtained with blind methods. A. Time, for each trial, from the trigger stimulus (TS) to the onset of a change in neuronal discharge rate ("latency") vs. the time, for the same trial, from the TS until the monkey lifted off of the central key (reaction time). These data are taken from the MI cell illustrated by the raster and histograms in C and D. These data are comparable to those observed in the premotor cortex. B. Time of the change in neuronal discharge rate until the approximate beginning of movement ("lead time") vs. reaction time for the same trials as in A. C. Raster and histogram of single-unit activity, centered on the presentation of the TS. This is the unit from which the data in A and B were taken. D. The same data as in C, centered instead on the onset of movement. E and F. Two different MI cortical neurons also showing a clear correlation of latency with reaction time, i.e., a close relationship of neuronal discharge with movement onset. The activity scale for all units (C–E) is the same and is expressed as impulses/sec. Abbreviations: n, number of trials; r, Pearson's correlation coefficient; m, slope of the linear regression; MVT, movement onset: Ac, Target acquisition. Histogram bin width, 15 mseconds.

tion of the visual cues that trigger a movement is to compare the correlation between the "latency" of activity change and the reaction time on a trial-by-trial basis. In this sense, the term latency is used to indicate the elapsed time from the presentation of a visual cue until the first change in unit activity. The reaction time is the elapsed time from the cue until the onset of movement. If these two parameters are highly correlated, then the unit activity can be said to be more closely related to the onset of movement than the visual cue. Alternatively, a close correlation between the "lead time" (i.e., the elapsed time from the onset of neural discharge until the beginning of movement) with reaction time indicates a close temporal relation with the visual cue. The graphs of Figs. 4A and B, based upon the data presented in Figs. 4C and D, show that the activity of this neuron is much more closely related to the onset of movement than to the presentation of the visual cue. Figs. 4E and F show two different single units that are also better correlated with the movement onset than with the visual cue.

Based on a qualitative evaluation of 70 movement-related cells in the premotor cortex of two monkeys, 54 neurons appeared to be more closely related to movement onset, whereas four (6%) appeared to be more closely correlated with the presentation of the visual trigger cue. A qualitative assessment was difficult in 12 of these neurons. A subpopulation of 23 cells was selected for quantitative analysis on the basis of their suitability for measurement of the onset of neuronal activity increases and their cortical location. These factors included a relatively low level of discharge and the lack of high-frequency activity bursts in the 1-second interval before the onset of movement, as well as an increase in activity before movement of greater than 33 impulses/sec. Of these 23 cells, 11 were located in the primary motor cortex and 12 in the premotor cortex. Since some cells were bidirectionally related to movement, their timing could be examined for both movement directions. In the premotor cortex, there were 15 significant correlations ($P<0.05$) between the reaction time and the latency of neuronal activity increase. In addition, there were four significant correlations between the reaction time and the "lead time". Since the former correlation represents a closer time-locking of neuronal modulations with the onset of movement and the latter with the visual cue, the premotor cortex activity clearly is more closely coupled with movement onset. In the primary motor cortex, neuronal activity was time-locked to movement in 13 instances and to the visual cue three times. Thus, our small primary motor cortex sample was comparable to that obtained in premotor cortex with regard to this feature of cell activity. Only two cells showed better correlations with the visual cue than movement onset, and these were both found within the premotor cortex. The significant correlations of reaction time and "latency" generally were between 0.70 and 0.92, and the distribution of the Pearson correlation moments in the premotor and primary motor cortex were comparable.

The qualitatively judged correlation between muscle activity and the onset of movement, in a broad sample of axial, proximal and distal muscles, was roughly comparable to that between unit activity and the onset of movement.

Directional specificity and neuronal cell classes

Of 77 movement-related premotor cortex units examined in detail, 40 (52%) were directionally specific. In 26 the directionally specific activity was absolutely so, i.e., the cell showed activity modulation only before movement of the limb in one of two opposite directions. Four of these directionally specific, movement-related neurons located in the premotor cortex are illustrated in Fig. 5. 14 cells were specific for leftward movement and 26 for rightward movement. These data are comparable to previously obtained neuronal samples in the premotor cortex (Weinrich et al., 1984).

Set- and signal-related activity can also display directional specificity. Fig. 6 compares a directionally specific (A) with a bidirectional (B) set-related cell. In the present sample, 63% of the set-related premotor cortex neurons and 56% of the signal-related neurons showed directional specificity.

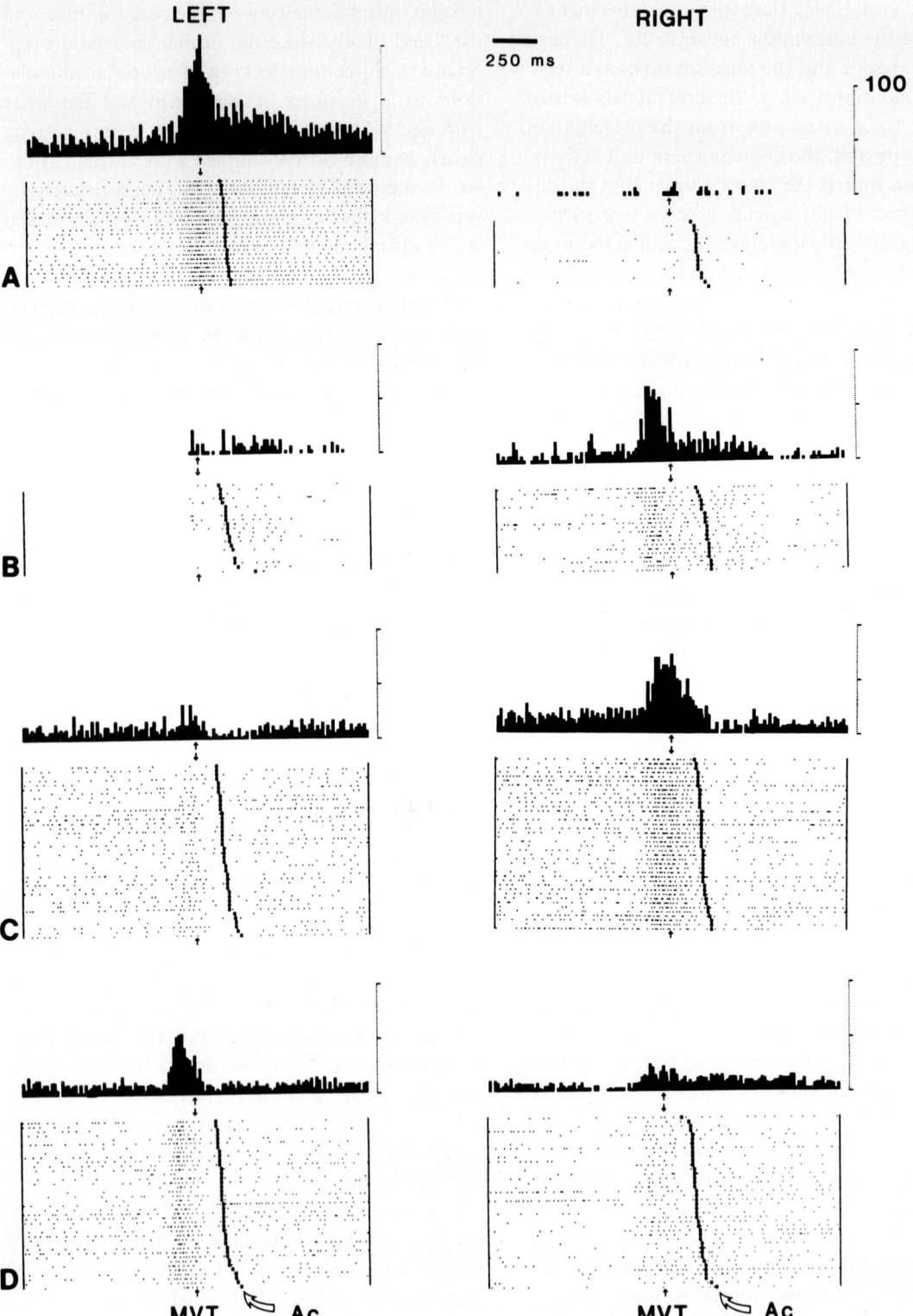

Fig. 5. Four premotor cortex cells, each of which is directionally specific. Each raster is centered on the onset of movement (MVT) and the square mark on each raster line indicates when the monkey acquired the target (Ac). The units shown in A and D are specific for movements to the left and those in B and C are specific for movements to the right. Bin width, 15 mseconds.

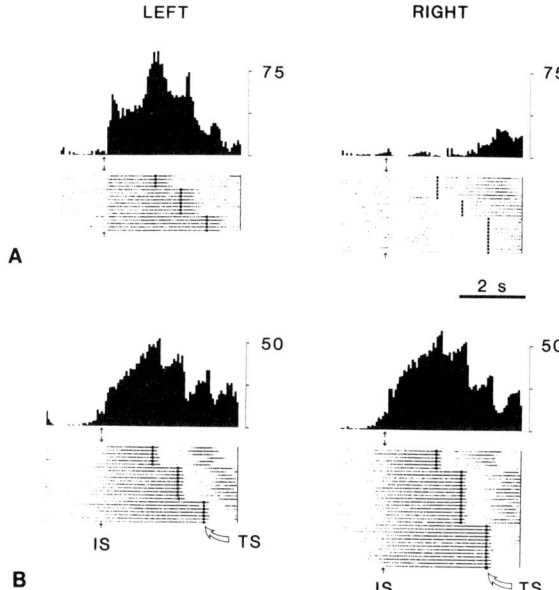

Fig. 6. Directionally specific and bidirectional set-related activity. A. A directionally specific, set-related premotor cortex neuron. B. A bidirectional, set-related premotor cortex neuron. All rasters are centered on the presentation of the instruction stimulus (IS) and the square on each raster line marks the time of the trigger stimulus (TS). The delay between the IS and TS was randomly chosen as one of the three possibilities shown here, but they are resorted according to the order of the delay.

Directional correspondence between set-related and movement-related activity in single cells

Many cells show both set- and movement-related activity (Figs. 7, 8 and 9). Fig. 10 shows the different combinations of unit-activity patterns that were observed in one of the monkeys examined in this study (monkey C) and indicates that 26% of that neuronal sample consisted of units combining set- and movement-related activity. Many cells show what might be termed a "directional correspondence" for set- and movement-related activity. In these cells, as exemplified by Fig. 7A, if the cell is specific for movement to the right, it also increases its activity during the set for rightward movements. However, not all set- and movement-related neurons show this sort of directional correspon-

dence. Several cells show the opposite pattern. Examples of the "non-corresponding" directional specificities are shown in Figs. 7B, 8 and 9. In these cells, the cell activity is modulated oppositely during the preparatory period and immediately prior to the execution of movement. For example, the neuron shown in Fig. 7B is inhibited during the preparatory period for movement to the right and excited in relation to the onset of rightward movement. Of a sample of 60 directionally specific set-related neurons taken from two monkeys, 33 (55%) were also related to movement. Of these 33 neurons, nine showed the corresponding pattern of movement- and set-relationships, 14 showed a non-corresponding combination, and in ten of these cells the movement-relationship was bidirectional.

Discussion

Movement-related activity

Several lines of evidence support the view that the discharge modulations occurring in the premotor cortex shortly before the onset of an operantly conditioned movement are related to the movement rather than the visuospatial cues that trigger the movement: (1) The changes in discharge rate are, in general, time-locked to the onset of movement and not to the visuospatial signals that trigger the movement (Kubota and Hamada, 1978; Weinrich and Wise, 1982; present study), (2) they depend upon the execution of a limb movement rather than the presentation of visual stimuli that trigger the movement (Weinrich et al., 1984), (3) they occur if movements are made "spontaneously" in total darkness (present study), and (4) the magnitude of this activity can be correlated with the movement parameters of velocity and acceleration of the limb in certain instances (Kubota and Hamada, 1978; Weinrich et al., 1984). The precise role of these movement-related discharges in the control of limb movements is unknown, although they fulfill one of the necessary prerequisites for playing a role in the control of movement execution: the onset of unit activity modulation precedes the earliest muscle ac-

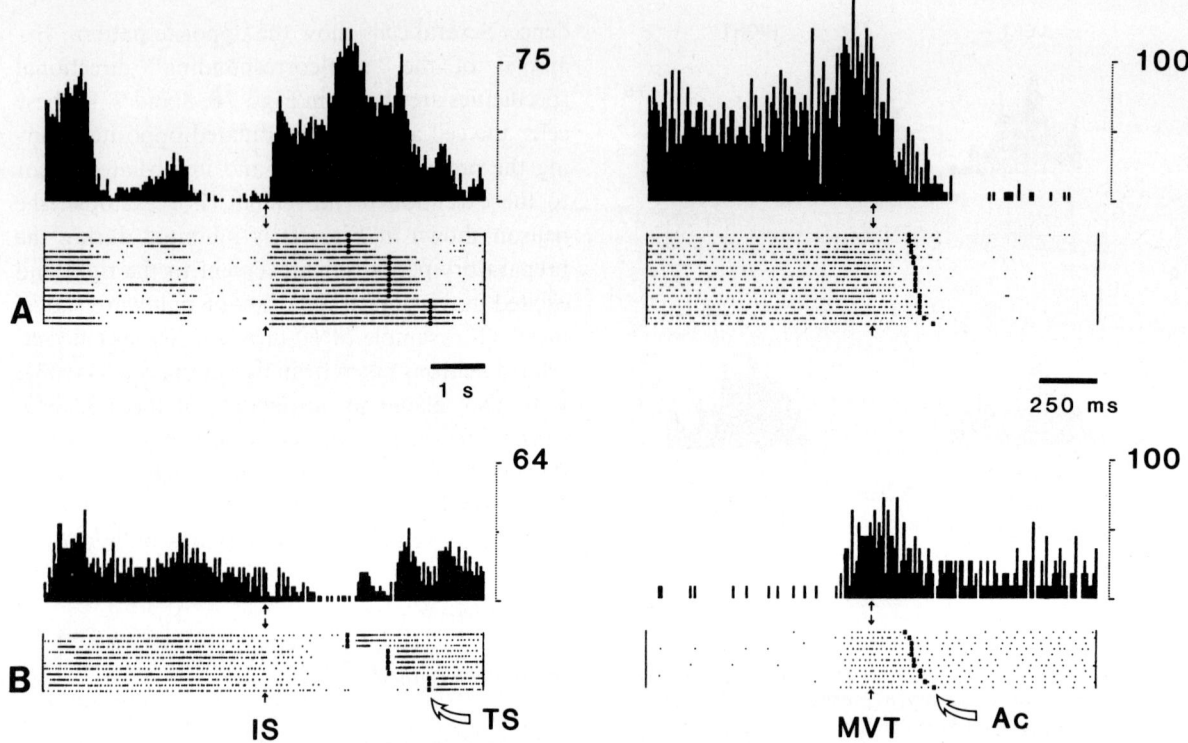

Fig. 7. A. A set-related premotor cortex neuron in which the directional specificity of the set-relationship corresponds to that of the movement relationship. B. A premotor cortex neuron with non-corresponding set- and movement-directional specificities. For both rows, the left and right columns show the same data, but the time scale is changed on the right to display better the movement-relationship. Left histograms: bin width, 40 mseconds; right histograms: bin width, 10 mseconds.

tivation. In our sample they do so by a mean of about 50 mseconds.

Although the properties cited above are also seen in the primary motor cortex, some features of premotor cortex movement-related activity contrast with those observed in the primary motor cortex. For example, Kurata and Tanji (personal communication) have recorded premotor cortex neurons with movement-related activity specific for the modality of the trigger stimulus. Another potential difference between premotor and primary motor cortex concerns the degree of somatotopy observed in each. Slow-wave potentials that occur before movements in the premotor cortex show much less somatotopy and lateralization than in the primary motor cortex (Hashimoto et al., 1981). If the slow-wave potentials observed by Hashimoto et al. reflect an underlying, non-topographical pattern of organization, it might be proposed that the premotor cortex is necessary for motor generalization, e.g., when a motor pattern learned for the forelimb is to be performed by the hindlimb. This proposition has not been adequately tested in either clinical or experimental settings, but is readily amenable to examination with behavioral methods. It must be noted, however, that studies of single-unit activity related to conditioned forelimb and hindlimb movements show more somatotopy in premotor cortex than do the slow-wave studies (Kurata and Tanji, personal communication) and are in agreement with neuroanatomical studies suggesting a topography in premotor cortex not unlike that seen in the primary motor cortex (Muakassa and Strick, 1978).

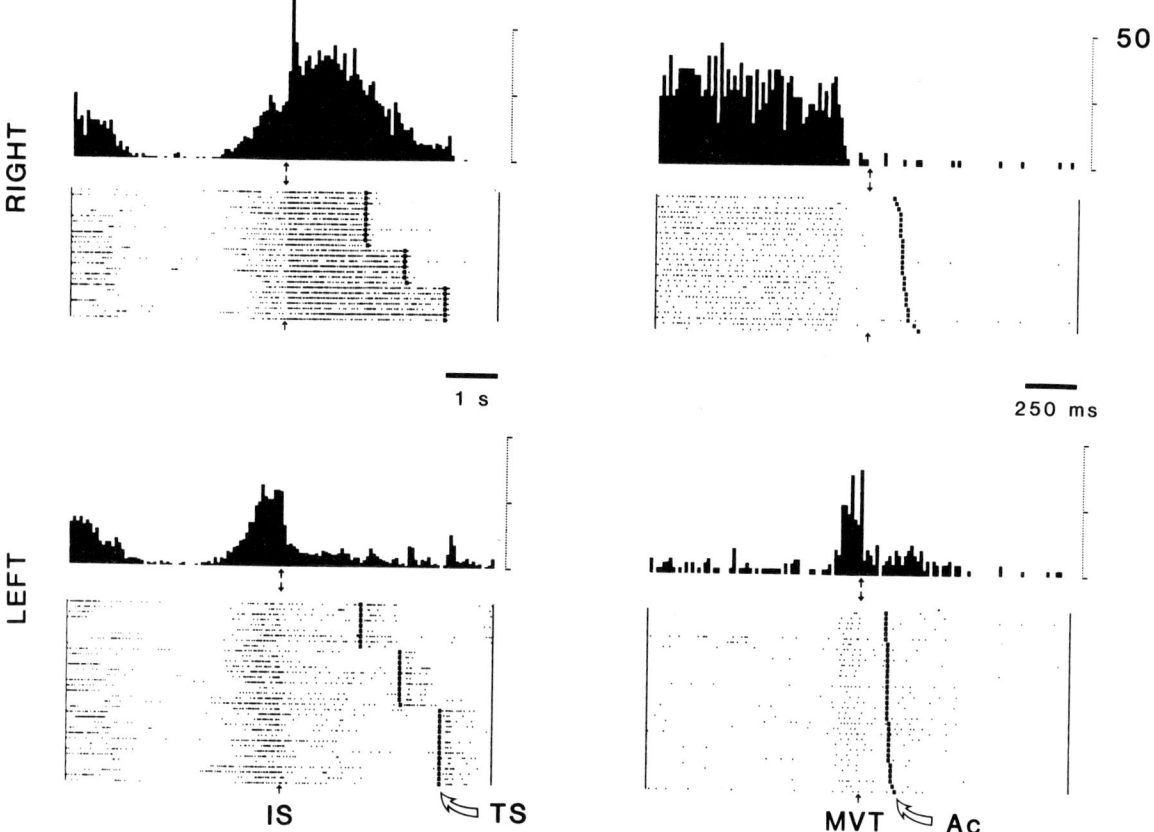

Fig. 8. Premotor cortex cell with non-corresponding directional specificities of set-related and movement-related activity. Note that the left and right column differ by time scale and the centering event. This cell is excited before movements to the left (bottom row) and during preparation for movements to the right (top row). Left histograms: bin width, 60 mseconds; right histograms: bin width, 15 mseconds.

Conditional movement relationships and comparison with posterior parietal cortex

It has been reported that neurons in the posterior parietal cortex (areas 5 and 7) are related to movements, but only those movements made "when the animal projects his arm or manipulates with his hand within immediate extràpersonal space to obtain an object he desires; e.g., food when he is hungry, or to touch a lighted switch he has learned means liquid when he is thirsty. These cells are not active during other movements in which the same muscles are utilized" (Mountcastle et al., 1975, p. 904). Thus, the movement-related activity of cells in the posterior parietal cortex could be said to be "conditional" for appetitively driven movements. Mountcastle et al. reported that the posterior parietal movement-related activity was largely independent of the direction and velocity of the limb movement and predicted that the premotor fields to which areas 5 and 7 project should show properties intermediate between those of the parietal cortex and the primary motor cortex, where neuronal activity is thought be more closely linked with the peripheral motor apparatus.

How do our results in the premotor cortex correspond to this prediction? Before discussing this question, it must be noted that any comparison between neuronal activity in different cortical fields raises a number of conceptual and methodological

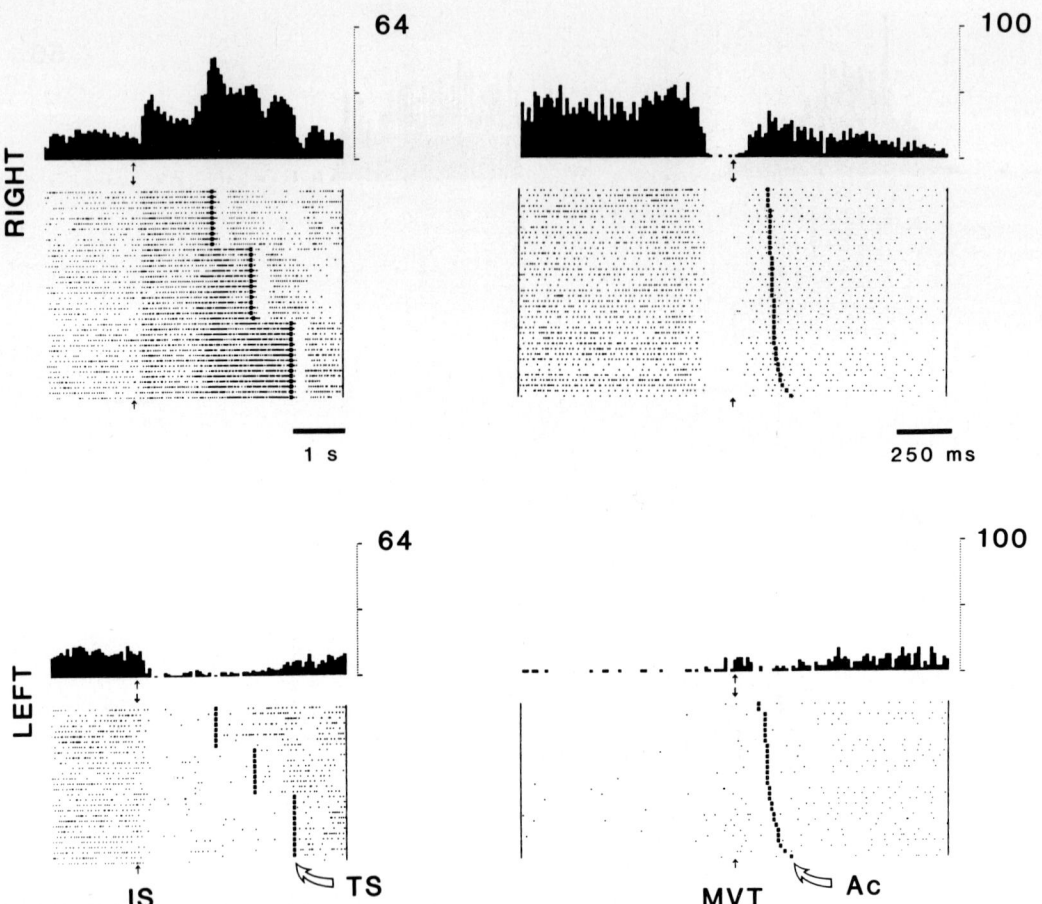

Fig. 9. Premotor cortex cell with non-corresponding directional specificities of set-related and movement-related activity. This cell is excited during preparation for movements to the right and inhibited before movements to the right (top row). Further, this cell is inhibited during preparation for movements to the left (bottom row). Left histograms: bin width, 60 mseconds; right histograms: bin width, 15 mseconds.

problems. One must be especially cautious in comparing activity observed in different experimental situations, different individual animals, and different species. Further, it is difficult, in an operantly conditioned monkey, to determine that precisely the same muscles are being employed for movements of the limb made in different behavioral contexts. An extensive EMG analysis of prime mover and other muscles should be performed to rule out the possibility that one or more muscle groups might be active in a well-controlled limb movement and inactive in a violent or undirected limb movement. Thus, a cell that appears to be movement-related only during appetitively driven movements might instead simply reflect the activity of some muscle groups that are active for relatively accurate limb movements and inactive for relatively uncontrolled movements of an aggressive or aversive nature.

These problems aside, the premotor cortex activity does not appear to display the same conditional properties reported for the posterior parietal cortex (Mountcastle et al., 1975). Premotor cortex neurons that have movement-related activity during appetitively driven movements in response to visual signals are also modulated in relation to unrewarded

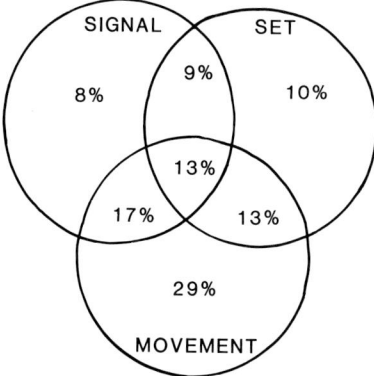

Fig. 10. Venn diagram of signal-, set- and movement-related activity patterns, and their combinations, in the premotor cortex of a rhesus monkey, $n = 99$.

movements made in total darkness. It must be stressed, however, that our tested sample is very small and we did not perform a "clinical" examination of the neuronal activity while the monkey performed uncontrolled movements. Instead, the monkey was placed in total darkness while we waited for the monkey to make movements of the forelimb "spontaneously". There is no way to determine the motivational objectives of these movements, so it is impossible to rule out unequivocally the possibility that the monkey was trying to guide his movements from memory to positions that had in the past yielded rewards. However, the behavior of the monkey during the "spontaneous" movements argues against this possibility: the monkey did not usually position the limb for extended periods of time and instead usually made violent movements to the extreme positions of the manipulandum. And although it is necessary that some of the same muscle groups were involved in the visually guided (rewarded) movements and the "spontaneous" (unrewarded) movements, there was no EMG analysis during the latter type of movements to determine the extent of similarity of recruited muscle groups. Nevertheless, the results indicate that cells increase their activity before movements made in the dark without reward and those made in response to visual cues for rewards.

In addition to lacking their conditional nature, some reports suggest that premotor cortex neurons may also be unlike posterior parietal neurons (Mountcastle et al., 1975) in that the former are often, indeed most often, specific for the direction of the limb movement and, occasionally, reflect the acceleration or velocity of limb movement (Kubota and Hamada, 1978; Weinrich et al., 1984). However, more recent studies of area 5 neurons have demonstrated directional specificity (Kalaska et al., 1983; Chapman et al., 1984) and a correlation with peak velocity (Chapman et al., 1984). Thus, the movement-related discharge in premotor cortex and posterior parietal cortex appears to be at least grossly comparable with respect to these properties. However, no static positional sensitivity, such as that seen in area 5 (Georgopoulos et al., 1984), has yet been observed in premotor cortex.

Directional specificity

Set-, signal- and movement-related activity in the premotor cortex is often specific for the direction of limb movement. When these patterns of activity are combined in individual neurons, it is observed that the directional specificities do not always correspond. That is, a cell (see Fig. 7A) activated during the preparatory period for rightward limb movements may be excited before rightward movements (a "corresponding" combination), whereas another cell (see Fig. 8) with the same sort of set-related activity may be excited before the opposite, leftward movement (a "non-corresponding" pattern).

These combinations of activity patterns may yield some clues about the functional organization of the premotor cortex and its role in the cerebral control of movement. For example, set-related neuronal activity has been proposed to be involved in the suppression of lower-order, brainstem-mediated circuits (see Wise and Mauritz, 1985). If these premotor cortex cells suppress activity in agonist flexor muscles, then such suppressive influences should be removed before the execution of the flexion movement. This pattern is seen in the top rows of Figs. 8 and 9. When the flexor muscles act as antagonists, they should be inhibited when the movement begins, and a cell involved in the suppression of its activity might also be expected to be activated just before an extensdion movement. This pattern is seen in the bottom row of Fig. 8. These two features comprise the "non-corresponding" combination of set-related directional specificities. Conversely, the "corresponding" combinations of set-related directional specificities might be expected for a cell involved in both the preparation of a movement driven by a synergistic muscle groups and its execution.

Summary

The premotor cortex of macaque monkeys contains neurons exhibiting changes of discharge rate 120–140 mseconds before the onset of operantly conditioned limb movements. Two observations reported here support the proposition that these changes are functionally related to the limb movement, rather than any concomitant sensory stimulus: (1) the changes of neuronal activity are more closely time-locked to the beginning of movement than to the visuospatial cues that trigger the movement, and (2) neuronal modulations occur when the limb is moved "spontaneously" in total darkness. Many of these "movement-related" cells also show activity following visuospatial cues that supply instructions for upcoming movements. This activity can be transient ("signal-related") or sustained until about the beginning of movement ("set-related"). Directional specificity is observed for all of these patterns of discharge. The directional preference of the set- and movement-related activity, when these two patterns are combined in a single neuron, do not always correspond, and this finding may yield clues about the functional specializations of these cells.

Acknowledgements

We appreciate the support and assistance of the late Dr. E. V. Evarts in all phases of this project. We also thank William Burris for his technical aid, Lori Budzinski for photography, and Betty Al-Aish for preparation of the manuscript. Karl Mauritz was supported by the Deutsche Forschungsgemeinschaft (Heisenberg Program).

References

Brinkman, J. and Porter, R. (1983) Supplementary motor area and premotor area of monkey cerebral cortex-functional organization and activities of single neurons during performance of a learned movement. Adv. Neurol., 39: 393–420.

Brodmann, K. (1909) Vergleichende Lokalizationlehre der grosshirnrinde in ihren Prinzipien dargestellt auf Grund des Zellenbaues, J. A. Barth, Leipzig.

Bucy, P. C. (1933) Electrical excitability and cyto-architecture of the premotor cortex in monkeys. Arch. Neurol. Psychiat., 30: 1205–1224.

Bucy, P. C. (1935) A comparative cytoarchitectonic study of the motor and premotor areas in the primate. J. Comp. Neurol., 62: 293–331.

Chapman, C. E., Spidalieri, G. and Lamarre, Y. (1984) Discharge properties of area 5 neurons during arm movements triggered by sensory stimuli in the monkey. Brain Res., 309: 63–77.

Denny-Brown, D. (1966) The Cerebral Control of Movement, Liverpool University Press, Liverpool.

Denny-Brown, D. and Botterell, E. H. (1948) The motor functions of the agranular frontal cortex. Res. Publ. Ass. Res. Nerv. Ment. Dis., 27: 235–345.

Freund, H.-J. and Hummelsheim, H. (1984) Premotor cortex in man: evidence for innervation of proximal limb muscles. Exp. Brain Res., 53: 479–482.

Fulton, J. F. (1935) Definition of the motor and premotor areas. Brain, 58: 311–316.

Georgopoulos, A. P., Caminiti, R. and Kalaska, J. F. (1984) Static spatial effects in motor cortex and area 5: Quantitative relations in a two-dimensional space. Exp. Brain Res., 54: 446–454.

Godschalk, M. and Lemon, R. N. (1983) Involvement of monkey premotor cortex in the preparation of arm movements. Exp. Brain Res., Suppl. 7: 114–119.

Godschalk, M., Lemon, R. N., Nijs, H. G. T. and Kuypers, H. G. J. M. (1981) Behavior of neurons in monkey peri-arcuate and precentral cortex before and during visually guided arm and hand movements. Exp. Brain Res., 44: 113–116.

Halsband, U. and Passingham, R. (1982) The role of premotor and parietal cortex in the direction of action. Brain Res.., 240: 368–372.

Hashimoto, S., Gemba, H. and Sasaki, K. (1981) Distribution of slow cortical potentials preceding self-paced hand and hindlimb movements in the premotor and motor areas of monkeys, Brain Res., 224: 247–259.

Kalaska, J. F., Caminiti, R. and Geogopoulos, A. P. (1983) Cortical mechanisms related to the direction of two-dimensional arm movements: Relations in parietal area 5 and comparison with motor cortex. Exp. Brain Res. 51: 247–260.

Kubota, K. and Hamada, I. (1978) Visual tracking and neuron activity in the postarcuate area in monkeys. J. Physiol. (Paris), 74: 297–312.

Kwan, H. C., Mackay, W. A., Murphy, J. T. and Wong, Y. C. (1978) Spatial organization of precentral cortex in awake primates. II. Motor outputs. J. Neurophysiol., 41: 1120–1131.

Luria, A. R. (1980) Higher Cortical Functions in Man, Basic Books, New York.

Mauritz, K.-H. and Wise, S. P. (1985) The premotor cortex of rhesus monkeys: Neuronal activity before predictable environmental events. Exp. Brain Res., in press.

Mountcastle, V. B., Lynch, J. C., Georgopoulos, A., Sakata, H. and Acuna, C. (1975) Posterior parietal association cortex of the monkey: Command functions for operations within extrapersonal space. J. Neurophysiol., 38: 871–908.

Muakassa, K. and Strick, P. L. (1978) Frontal lobe inputs to primate motor cortex: evidence for four somatotopically organized "premotor" areas. Brain Res. 177: 176–182.

Rizzolatti, G., Scandolara, C., Matelli, M. and Gentilucci, M. (1981) Afferent properties of periarcuate neurons in macaque monkeys. 2. Visual responses. Behav. Brain Res., 2: 147–163.

Roland, P. E., Skinhoj, E., Lassen, N. A. and Larsen, B. (1980) Different cortical areas in man in organization of voluntary movements in extrapersonal space. J. Neurophysiol., 43: 137–150.

Tanji, J. and Kurata, K. (1982) Comparison of movement-related activity in two cortical motor areas of primates. J. Neurophysiol., 48: 633–653.

Travis, A. M. (1955) Neurological deficiencies following supplementary motor area lesions in *Macaca mulatta*. Brain, 78: 174–198.

Vicario, D., Martin, J. H. and Ghez, C. (1983) Specialized subregions in the cat motor cortex: a single unit analysis in the behaving animal. Exp. Brain Res., 51: 351–367.

Vogt, O. and Vogt, C. (1919) Ergebisse unserer Hirnforschung. J. Psychol. Neurol. (Leipzig), 25: 277–462.

Von Bonin, G. and Bailey, P. (1947) The Neocortex of Macaca Mulatta, University of Illinois Press, Urbana, IL.

Weinrich, M. and Wise, S. P. (1982) The premotor cortex of the monkey. J. Neurosci., 2: 1329–1345.

Weinrich, M., Wise, S. P. and Mauritz, K.-H. (1984) A neurophysiological analysis of the premotor cortex of the monkey. Brain, 107: 385–414.

Wiesendanger, M. (1981) Organization of secondary motor areas of cerebral cortex. Handb. Physiol., 2: 1121–1147.

Wise, S. P. (1985) The primate premotor cortex: past, present and preparatory. Annu. Rev. Neurosci, 8: 1–19.

Wise, S. P. and Mauritz, K.-H. (1985) Set-related neuronal activity in the premotor cortex of rhesus monkeys: effects of changes in motor set. Proc. Roy. Soc. (Lond.), Series B, 223: 331–354.

Woolsey, C. N., Settlage, P. H., Meyer, D. R., Sencer, W., Pinto Hamuy, T. and Travis, A. M. (1952) Patterns of localization in precentral and "supplementary" motor areas and their relation to the concept of a premotor area. Res. Publ. Ass. Res. Nerv. Ment. Dis., 30: 238–264.

Activity of forelimb motor units and corticomotoneuronal cells during ramp-and-hold torque responses: comparisons with oculomotor cells

E. E. Fetz, P. D. Cheney and S. S. Palmer

Department of Physiology and Biophysics, and Regional Primate Research Center SJ-50, University of Washington, Seattle, WA 98195, U.S.A.

Introduction

To compare the functional organization of the somatomotor and oculomotor systems, it may be helpful to begin by comparing the response properties of their motoneurons and monosynaptically connected premotor neurons under behavioral conditions which are as comparable as possible. In the oculomotor system, the activity of ocular motoneurons and putative premotor neurons has been abundantly documented during saccadic eye movements (Baker and Berthoz, 1977; Fuchs and Becker, 1981; Fuchs et al., 1985). In the somatomotor system, the activity of single forelimb motor units and input cells from precentral motor cortex during ramp-and-hold torque responses has been sufficiently characterized to provide some basis for comparison. Such ramp-and-hold responses, alternating between flexion and extension target zones, were chosen to reveal the neural activity related to changes in force and to maintained static force; for purposes of discussion, these ramp-and-hold wrist responses may be considered analogous to saccadic eye movements followed by fixation. We here review the response properties and organization of somatic motor units and corticomotoneuronal (CM) cells, with brief comments on some interesting analogies with comparable oculomotor neurons.

Motoneurons

The responses of single motor units during generation of isometric ramp-and-hold torques have been studied in forelimb flexor and extensor muscles of the wrist and fingers (Palmer and Fetz, 1985a,b). Single motor units were recorded by a tripolar microelectrode positioned within the muscles through a remotely controlled microdrive, and the multiunit EMG activity of six flexors and six extensors was recorded simultaneously with permanently implanted wire electrodes. Thus, the parent muscle of each motor unit could be identified in motor unit-triggered averages of multiunit EMG activity. The response patterns of typical motor units during performance of moderate ramp-and-hold torque responses are illustrated in Fig. 1. Many of the forelimb motor units exhibited either tonic (33%) or phasic-tonic (23%) discharge patterns; their tonic activity was constant during the static hold period, and was proportional to the level of active force. Another 5% of the motor units exhibited only phasic discharge at onset of movement; however, the studies of Freund and co-workers (1975, 1983) suggest that these motor units would probably exhibit phasic-tonic firing at the highest force levels. In addition, another 39% of the motor units showed decrementing discharge during the main-

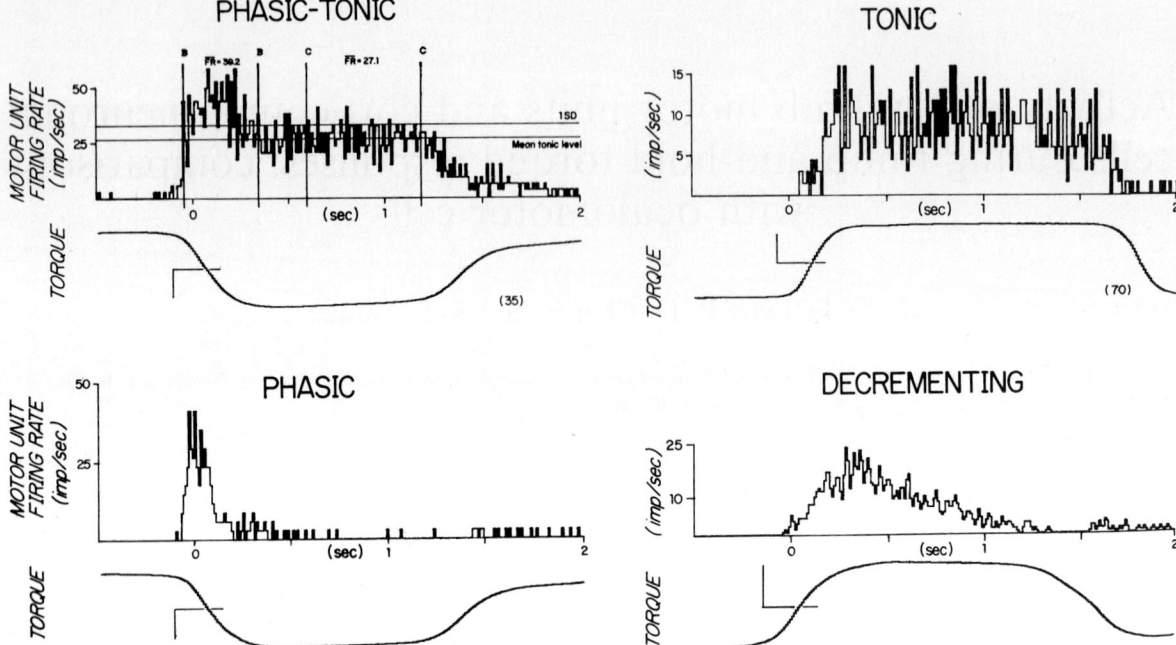

Fig. 1. Response patterns of forelimb motor units during isometric ramp-and-hold torque responses. Each set shows a time histogram of motor unit activity with the associated isometric torque about the wrist. The vertical torque calibration bar represents $6 \cdot 10^5$ dyne/cm and the horizontal bar indicates zero torque level. FR, mean firing rate between vertical bars (top left). From Palmer and Fetz (1985a,b), with permission.

tained static hold; different units showed varying rates of decline in firing rate. As yet, there is no definitive evidence concerning the physiological motor unit types (Burke, 1981) associated with these response patterns; nevertheless, these patterns appear to encompass all motor unit types.

By comparison, most ocular motoneurons appear to exhibit a burst-tonic discharge pattern during saccadic eye movements (Fuchs and Luschei, 1970; Henn and Cohen, 1973; Robinson, 1970). Other units recorded in ocular motoneuron pools exhibit predominantly tonic or purely phasic discharge (Henn and Cohen, 1973); assuming these are motoneurons, their activity would resemble that of corresponding somatic motor units. However, they appear to be in the minority compared with burst-tonic ocular motoneurons, whose discharge is well suited to dynamic requirements to generate saccades. The tonic discharge frequency of ocular motoneurons is proportional to eye position in the orbit, and therefore proportional to active force, since the fixated eye presents an elastic load. Ocular motoneurons, like their somatic counterparts, are recruited over a wide range of active muscle force but, unlike somatic motoneurons, the overlapping recruitment ranges of antagonist muscles assures that control of eye position normally involves co-contraction of antagonist muscles.

Premotor neurons

While the relation of motoneurons to muscle force is relatively direct, and essentially similar for somatomotor and oculomotor systems, the relation of premotor neurons to motoneurons is of more relevance to the central organization of the systems. (Here, we use the term "premotor neurons" to designate cells with monosynaptic input to motoneurons.) The input cells to forelimb motoneurons can be identified in behaving monkeys by spike-trig-

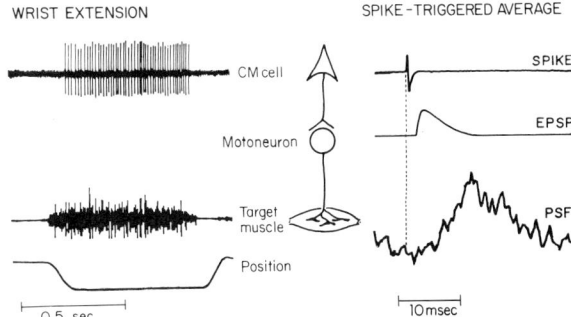

Fig. 2. Example of PSF used to identify CM cells. Left, record of extension-related CM cell and target muscle EMG. Right, spike-triggered average of unit and rectified EMG showing PSF. Drawing indicates intervening motoneuron with EPSP. From Cheney and Fetz (1984), with permission.

gered averaging of multi-unit EMG activity. The appearance of clear postspike facilitation (PSF) in spike-triggered averages of rectified EMG activity suggests the presence of sufficiently potent synaptic connections to mediate this correlational linkage (Fig. 2). For reasons discussed elsewhere (Fetz and Cheney, 1980), a clear and repeatable PSF may be interpreted as evidence of monosynaptic connections. Although averages of EMG activity do not provide a quantitative measure of postsynaptic effects, the PSF is useful to identify CM cells as well as their target muscles.

The response patterns of precentral CM cells during ramp-and-hold wrist responses fell into four categories, as illustrated in Fig. 3. The large majority (59%) fired with a phasic-tonic pattern; onset of the phasic burst usually preceded the onset of target muscle activity (by an average of 71 mseconds). Another 28% of CM cells showed tonic discharge, without any burst preceding the subsequent tonic firing level. For both types the tonic firing rates remained constant through the hold period and increased in proportion to the static force levels. The remaining CM cells showed a gradual increase in activity throughout the static hold period; some of these also exhibited a burst of discharge at onset of movement (Fig. 3, bottom left); others had only the ramp increase in discharge during the static hold.

These gradual "ramp" increases in firing rate during the steady hold resemble the inverse of the decrementing discharge exhibited by many motor units; indeed, the ramp and phasic-ramp CM cells may serve to overcome the tendency of motoneurons to accommodate to steady input (Kernell, 1965).

In the oculomotor system, the response patterns of candidate premotor cells include pure burst and pure tonic patterns, as well as burst-tonic patterns similar to those of ocular motoneurons (Luschei and Fuchs, 1972; Keller, 1974). The relative proportions of these premotor types remain uncertain. While the burst-tonic and tonic premotor neurons are clearly analogous to corresponding CM cells, the convergence of pure burst cells onto ocular motoneurons has no known correlate among CM cells. Many motor cortex cells do discharge phasically at onset of ramp-and-hold movements, but none of

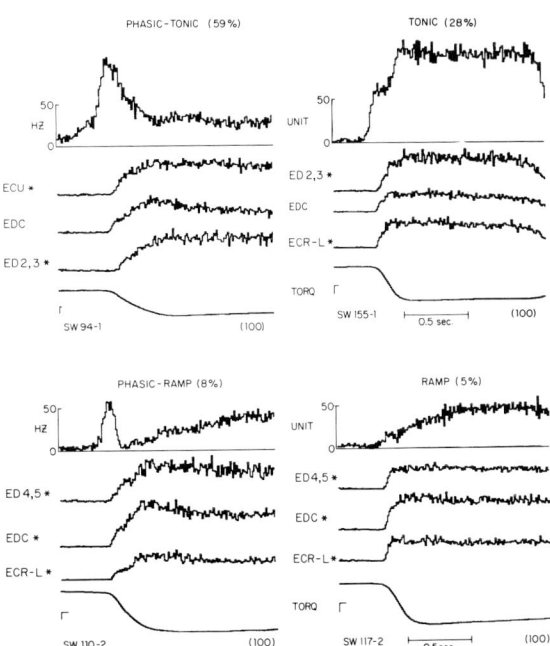

Fig. 3. Response patterns of CM cells during isometric ramp-and-hold torque responses. Each set shows a time histogram of CM cell activity, and average of synergist extensor muscles and isometric torque. Target muscles of the CM cells are indicated by an asterisk. From Cheney and Fetz (1980), with permission.

these has ever produced PSF in the agonist muscles. These phasic precentral cells may be located higher in the neural hierarchy preceding motor units (indeed, evidence of synaptic connections from phasic to CM cells would be of considerable interest).

Although the burst premotor cells in the oculomotor system have no counterpart among CM cells, an analogue may exist in other areas. Preliminary evidence suggests that some rubromotoneuronal cells (identified by PSF) may fire more in relation to the phasic onset of movement than to sustained force during the static hold (Cheney, 1980). Other regions, such as spinal cord and brain stem, also contain somatic premotor cells, whose response patterns remain to be documented.

What are the functional implications of these phasic and tonic patterns? They seem an obvious requirement for generating the muscle forces necessary to overcome inertial loads and to maintain tonic contractions. (Indeed, it is more surprising that the same patterns characterize responses of sensory system cells to ramp-and-hold stimuli (Fetz, 1984).) The significance of these response patterns for understanding the functional organization of motor systems depends not only on their existence, but also on their mode of generation. Understanding the genesis of this activity requires further information on the synaptic connections between the relevant cells. Our results suggest that these connections may not be readily deducible from the response patterns themselves. For example, the response histograms of most CM cells do not resemble the profile of net activity of their target muscles (Fig. 3): much of their phasic discharge is apparently utilized in bringing motoneurons to threshold. Thus, in addition to characterizing the response patterns of candidate cells, we need independent evidence of their correlational linkages to understand the functional organization of these systems.

Relation to active force

The tonic discharge of CM cells, like that of ocular premotor cells, increases with the active force generated by their target motoneurons (Cheney and Fetz, 1980). Most CM cells were found to be active at very small force levels: during ramp-and-hold movements they discharge tonically even with minimal muscle activity. In contrast, the forelimb motor units are recruited over a much wider range of forces. Thus, the CM cells contribute to increases in active force by increasing the firing rate of an active population rather than by sequential recruitment of CM cells into activity. Motor units, in contrast, generate increased force by both mechanisms: increased rates of active units and recruitment of higher threshold motor units (Burke, 1981; Clark et al., 1978; Milner-Brown et al., 1973). By comparison, the tonic premotor cells of the oculomotor system exhibit a range of recruitment levels that is quite similar to the recruitment range of ocular motoneurons (Luschei and Fuchs, 1972; Keller, 1974).

It should be noted that corticospinal cells are more strongly modulated with force during finely controlled movements than forceful or ballistic responses. Thus, pyramidal tract neurons (PTNs) were often more active during a precision tracking task than with rapid wrist movements (Fromm and Evarts, 1977). CM cells that discharged strongly during controlled ramp-and-hold movements were paradoxically inactive when the monkey generated vigorous ballistic movements, which involved even greater activity in their target muscles (Cheney and Fetz, 1980). Similarly, CM cells related to finger movements were more active during a precision grip than during a power grip (Muir and Lemon, 1983). This suggests that the somatomotor system utilizes different premotor cells for different types of movement. A comparable specialization exists for oculomotor pathways involved in saccadic and pursuit eye movements, as well as subsets of these evoked by different types of stimuli.

Organization of CM connections

In the somatomotor system, we have some information on the convergence and divergence of connections between CM cells and individual motoneurons. Intracellular recording of primate corticomotoneuronal excitatory postsynaptic potentials (CM-EPSPs) evoked by cortical stimulation has shown convergent connections onto single limb motoneurons from a "colony" of CM cells distributed over wide cortical areas (Phillips and Porter, 1964; Jankowska et al., 1975). Virtually every forelimb motoneuron in the baboon receives such monosynaptic input from motor cortex; maximal CM-EPSPs are comparable in magnitude to Ia-EPSPs evoked from Ia afferents of the limb muscles. The number of CM cells converging onto a given motoneuron is clearly greater for motoneurons of distal forelimb muscles than proximal muscles.

The existence of divergent connections from a single CM cell to many motoneurons is also characteristic. Anatomically, single corticospinal axons have been shown to ramify among many motoneurons (Shinoda et al., 1981); and electrophysiologically, single pyramidal tract neurons can be backfired from multiple motor nuclei (Asanuma et al., 1979). In chronic monkeys, spike-triggered averages from single CM cells typically reveal PSF in more than one of the synergistically activated muscles. The muscle field of CM cells ranges from one to all six muscles recorded; the number of facilitated muscles is, on the average, slightly larger for extensor CM cells than for flexor CM cells (Fetz and Cheney, 1980).

The effects of single intracortical microstimuli (S-ICMS) delivered near CM cells further suggest the convergence of many CM cells onto the same target motoneurons (Cheney and Fetz, 1985). The poststimulus facilitation evoked by 5–10-μA stimuli typically appeared in the CM cell's target muscles, and with the same relative amplitudes, but was several times greater than the PSF produced by the single CM cell. This would suggest that low-intensity S-ICMS recruits a group of CM cells with common target muscles, and that these are either clustered in the vicinity of the stimulating electrode or strongly interconnected. Spike-triggered averages from neighboring CM cells confirm that they usually have overlapping or identical muscle fields.

To resolve the distribution of effects within a motoneuron pool, the effect of S-ICMS on individual motor units has been documented by compiling poststimulus time histograms of motor unit activity (Palmer and Fetz, 1985a,b). 95% of the motor units recorded in muscles showing poststimulus facilitation of multiunit EMG were individually facilitated. S-ICMS at a single cortical site typically facilitated all four types of motor units. These results would suggest that CM cells may affect diverse groups of motoneurons, much like the Ia afferents. This remains to be confirmed by cross-correlating individual CM cells and single motor units.

In contrast to the divergent connections from single CM cells to multiple synergist limb muscles, the synaptic connections between premotor cells and ocular motoneurons appear to remain separately organized according to specific eye muscles. Thus, each ocular motoneuron pool has its separate set of premotor neurons, which remain anatomically segregated. Although terminals of single premotor cells may diverge within a target motoneuron pool, they do not appear to contact motoneurons of different muscles. Definitive evidence on this issue remains to be obtained, but the coordination of

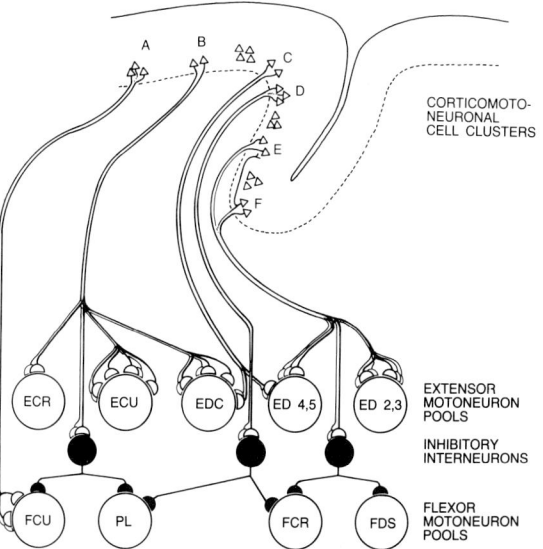

Fig. 4. Diagram of the simplest corticospinal connections that may mediate the correlational linkages observed in spike- and stimulus-triggered averages. From Cheney and Fetz (1985), with permission.

eye muscles synergistically activated in oblique movements is currently thought to involve cells at a higher level than the premotor neurons.

Reciprocal connections to antagonist muscles

The efficacy of agonist muscles in generating limb and eye movements is usually enhanced by simultaneous suppression of antagonist muscles. In the somatomotor system, such reciprocal inhibition is mediated by spinal cord interneurons, such as the Ia-inhibitory interneuron which receives input from Ia muscle afferents and corticospinal cells (Jankowska et al., 1976). Many CM cells not only facilitate their target muscles, but also suppress the antagonist muscles. Such reciprocal inhibition was demonstrated by S-ICMS delivered near CM cells; in addition to producing poststimulus facilitation of the cells' target muscles, S-ICMS also evoked poststimulus suppression of antagonists at a third of the cortical sites (Cheney et al., 1985a). Reciprocal inhibition was also demonstrated to be produced by single CM cells: using glutamate to generate trigger spikes during the phase of movement when the CM cell is normally silent, Kasser and Cheney (1985) compiled spike-triggered averages of the antagonists of the cells' target muscles. 40% of the extensor CM cells and 15% of the flexor CM cells produced reciprocal postspike suppression of antagonist muscles during alternating wrist movements. Thus, the discharge patterns of these reciprocal CM cells produce a proportional suppression of antagonists, simultaneous with facilitation of agonist target muscles.

Central commands generating eye movements also involve reciprocal inhibition of antagonist muscles. The inhibitory burst neuron (IBN) has been shown to produce monosynaptic inhibitory postsynaptic potentials in abducens motoneurons by spike-triggered averages (Hikosaka et al., 1978). The terminals of single IBNs were estimated to branch to approximately 60% of the motoneuron pool. Tonic inhibitory input to ocular motoneurons also seems probable during fixed gaze, but the relevant premotor cells remain to be characterized.

Purely inhibitory effects on limb muscles have also been observed from corticospinal cells (Cheney et al., 1985a,b). Both spike- and stimulus-triggered averages revealed suppression of certain muscles (usually flexors), but no facilitation of any other muscles. The response patterns of these inhibitory cells differed from CM cells and often included an intense burst as the inhibited muscles were shut off.

Fig. 4 schematically summarizes the main features of the organization of corticospinal connections to forelimb motoneurons suggested by our cross-correlation studies. This diagram illustrates the simplest synaptic connections underlying the observed postspike effects. Corticospinal cells with common target elements are shown clustered together, as evidenced by effects of S-ICMS and recordings from neighboring cells. The three basic patterns of cortical effects on forelimb muscles are facilitation of agonists with no effect on antagonists (A and C), facilitation of agonists with simultaneous suppression of antagonists (B, F), and suppression without observed facilitation (D).

Peripheral feedback

A major difference between somatomotor and oculomotor systems is the form of peripheral feedback used to guide movements. While the somatomotor system relies on proprioceptive feedback from muscle receptors to move the limbs accurately in the face of varying load conditions, the oculomotor system, presented with a predictable load, uses visual feedback to acquire visual targets, or vestibular input to compensate for head movements.

The effects of proprioceptive inputs to somatic motoneurons and premotor neurons have been abundantly documented (see Matthews, 1972). These effects are particularly well demonstrated when the inputs are synchronously activated by muscle stretch. Such a stimulus typically evokes a series of responses in the stretched muscle: the first (M1) appears to be segmentally mediated, while the mechanism mediating the second (M2) has been vigorously debated. A contribution to M2 via a transcortical loop now seems to have been proven,

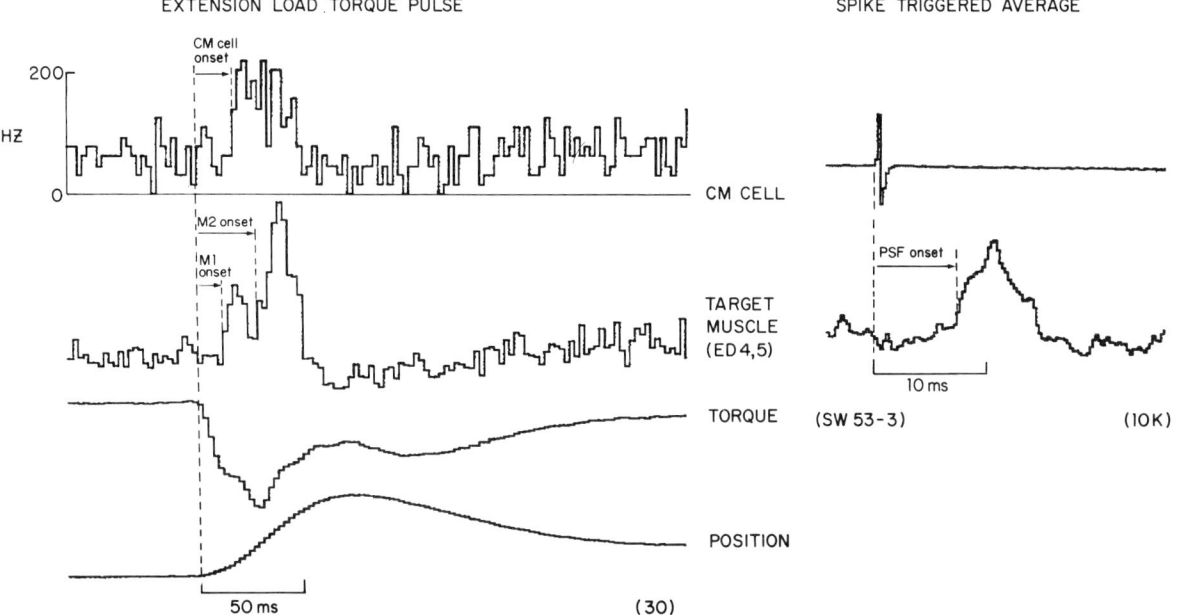

Fig. 5. Response of CM cell and target muscle to transient stretch of muscle. Left, response average for 30 flexion torque pulses delivered during active extension. From top: time histogram of CM cell, average of rectified EMG, torque perturbation and position (flexion up). Right, spike-triggered average showing PSF in target muscle. From Cheney and Fetz (1984), with permission.

since CM cells respond to muscle stretch at the appropriate time and this activity facilitates the muscles showing the M2 response (Cheney and Fetz, 1984). Fig. 5 illustrates the transient responses of an extensor CM cell and one of its target muscles to a brief flexion torque pulse. The PSF of this muscle (right) confirms the output effects of the CM cell, and provides the corticospinal conduction time. As for most CM cells tested, the latency of the M2 response agrees well with the transcortical loop time, namely, the sum of the afferent conduction time (CM cell onset latency) plus efferent conduction time (PSF latency).

While perturbations of the limb reveal the effects of inputs activated synchronously, the same inputs may also contribute during steady-state conditions. Thus, during the hold period of the ramp-and-hold movements, the tonic discharge of CM cells may well be sustained by continuous peripheral feedback. This kind of positive feedback would allow changes in movement to be triggered by phasic central commands, which reset the level of tonic reverberating discharge. In effect, a peripheral feedback loop would represent an integrator of phasic command signals. (The oculomotor system, in lieu of proprioceptive feedback, is thought to rely on a neural integrator (Robinson, 1975; Fuchs et al., 1985).) To what extent the tonic discharge of CM cells is sustained by peripheral versus central input remains to be tested.

Concluding comments

This brief review has touched on several points of comparison between the final elements of the somatomotor and oculomotor systems. In light of our current limited understanding, it may seem premature to contrast and compare these systems in search of common principles. Nevertheless, the exercise helps to identify some of the relevant missing information. For example, the observation of comparable response patterns in premotor and motor neurons would reflect a comparable organization only if their interconnections were also similar.

More information on the correlational linkages of the observed cells with their inputs and their targets would be helpful for understanding the source and consequences of their response properties. If our experience with CM cells is any guide, it may be hazardous to infer these connections only on the basis of anatomical location or response patterns. Independent correlational evidence seems necessary if we are to understand the functional organization of these networks and how they generate the patterns controlling movements.

Acknowledgments

We thank Ms. Kate Schmitt for editorial assistance and Drs. Chris Kaneko and Albert Fuchs for helpful discussions. This work was supported in part by NIH grants RR00166 and NS12542.

References

Asanuma, H., Zarzecki, P., Jankowska, E., Hongo, T. and Marcus, S. (1979) Projections of individual pyramidal tract neurons to lumbar motor nuclei of the monkey. Exp. Brain Res., 34: 73–89.

Baker, R. and Berthoz, A. (Eds.) (1977) Control of Gaze by Brainstem Neurons, Developments in Neuroscience, Vol. 1, Elsevier, Amsterdam.

Burke, R. E. (1981) Motor units: anatomy, physiology, and functional organization. In V. B. Brooks (Ed.), Handbook of Physiology, Section 1, Vol. II, Part 1, American Physiological Society, Bethesda, pp. 345–422.

Cheney, P. D. (1980) Response of rubromotoneuronal cells identified by spike-triggered averaging of EMG activity in awake monkeys. Neurosci. Lett., 17: 137–142.

Cheney, P. D. and Fetz, E. E. (1980) Functional classes of primate corticomotoneuronal cells and their relation to active force. J. Neurophysiol., 44: 773–791.

Cheney, P. D. and Fetz, E. E. (1984) Corticomotoneuronal cells contribute to long-latency stretch reflexes in the rhesus monkey. J. Physiol., 349: 249–272.

Cheney, P. D. and Fetz, E. E. (1985) Comparable patterns of muscle facilitation evoked by individual corticomotoneuronal (CM) cells and by single intracortical microstimuli in primates: evidence for functional groups of CM cells. J. Neurophysiol., 53: 786–804.

Cheney, P. D., Fetz, E. E. and Palmer, S. S. (1985a) Patterns of facilitation and suppression of antagonist forelimb muscles from motor cortex sites in the awake monkey. J. Neurophysiol., 53: 805–820.

Cheney, P. D., Kasser, R. J. and Fetz, E. E. (1985b) Motor and sensory properties of primate corticomotoneuronal cells. Exp. Brain Res., Suppl. 10: 211–231.

Clark, R. W., Luschei, E. S. and Hoffman, D. S. (1978) Recruitment order, contractile characteristics and firing patterns of motor units in the temporalis muscle of monkeys. Exp. Neurol., 61: 31–52.

Fetz, E. E. (1984) Functional organization of motor and sensory cortex: symmetries and parallels. In G. M. Edelman, W. E. Gall and W. M. Cowan (Eds.), Dynamic Aspects of Neocortical Function, John Wiley and Sons, New York, pp. 453–473.

Fetz, E. E. and Cheney, P. D. (1980) Postspike facilitation of forelimb muscle activity by primate corticomotoneuronal cells. J. Neurophysiol., 44: 751–772.

Freund, H. J. (1983) Motor unit and muscle activity in voluntary motor control. Physiol. Rev., 63: 387–436.

Freund, H. J., Büddingen, H. J. and Dietz, V. (1975) Activity of single motor units from human forearm muscles during voluntary isometric contractions. J. Neurophysiol., 38: 933–946.

Fromm, C. and Evarts, E. V. (1977) Relation of motor cortex neurons to precisely controlled and ballistic movements. Neurosci. Lett., 5: 259–266.

Fuchs, A. F. and Becker, W. (Eds.) (1981) Progress in Oculomotor Research, Developments in Neuroscience, Vol. 12, Elsevier/North-Holland, New York.

Fuchs, A. F. and Luschei, E. S. (1970) Firing patterns of abducens neurons of alert monkeys in relationship to horizontal eye movement. J. Neurophysiol., 33: 382–392.

Fuchs, A. F., Kaneko, C. R. S. and Scudder, C. A. (1985) Brainstem control of saccadic eye movements. Annu. Rev. Neurosci., 8: 307–337.

Henn, V. and Cohen, B. (1973) Quantitative analysis of activity in eye muscle motoneurons during saccadic eye movements and positions of fixation. J. Neurophysiol., 36: 115–126.

Hikosaka, O., Igusa, Y., Nakao, S. and Shimazu, H. (1978) Direct inhibitory synaptic linkage of pontomedullary reticular burst neurons with abducens motoneurons in the cat. Exp. Brain Res., 33: 337–352.

Jankowska, E., Padel, Y. and Tanaka, P. (1975) Projections of pyramidal tract cells to alpha motoneurones innervating hindlimb muscles in the monkey. J. Physiol., 249: 637–667.

Jankowska, E., Padel, Y. and Tanaka, P. (1976) Disynaptic inhibition of spinal motoneurones from the motor cortex in the monkey. J. Physiol., 258: 467–487.

Kasser, R.J. and Cheney, P. D. (1985) Characteristics of corticomotoneuronal postspike facilitation and reciprocal suppression of EMG activity in the monkey. J. Neurophysiol., 53: 959–978.

Keller, E. L. (1974) Participation of medial pontine reticular formation in eye movement generation in monkey. J. Neurophysiol., 37: 316–332.

Kernell, D. (1965) High frequency repetitive firing of cat lumbosacral motoneurons stimulated by long-lasting injected current. Acta Physiol. Scand., 65: 74–86.

Luschei, E. S. and Fuchs, A. F. (1972) Activity of brain stem neurons during eye movements of alert monkeys. J. Neurophysiol., 35: 445–461.

Matthews, P. B. C. (1972) Mammalian Muscle Spindles and Their Central Actions, Williams and Wilkins, Baltimore.

Milner-Brown, H. S., Stein, R. B. and Yemm, R. (1973) Changes in firing rate of human motor units during linearly changing voluntary contractions. J. Physiol. Lond., 230: 371–390.

Muir, R. B. and Lemon, R. N. (1983) Corticospinal neurones with a special role in precision grip. Brain Res., 261: 312–316.

Palmer, S. S. and Fetz, E. E. (1985a) Effects of single intracortical microstimuli in monkey motor cortex on activity of identified forelimb motor units. J. Neurophysiol., 54: 1194–1212.

Palmer, S. S. and Fetz, E. E. (1985b) Discharge properties of primate forearm motor units during isometric muscle activity. J. Neurophysiol., 54: 1178–1193.

Phillips, C. G. and Porter, R. (1964) The pyramidal projection to motoneurones of some muscle groups of baboon forelimb. Progr. Brain Res., 12: 222–245.

Robinson, D. A. (1970) Oculomotor unit behavior in the monkey. J. Neurophysiol., 33: 393–404.

Robinson, D. A. (1975) Oculomotor control signals. In G. Lennerstrand and P. Bach-y-Rita (Eds.), Basic Mechanisms of Ocular Motility and Their Clinical Implications, Pergamon, Oxford.

Shinoda, Y., Yokota, J.-L. and Futami, T. (1981) Divergent projection of individual corticospinal axons to motoneurons of multiple muscles in the monkey. Neurosci. Lett., 23: 7–12.

The role of the arcuate frontal eye fields in the generation of saccadic eye movements

Michael E. Goldberg[1,2] and Charles J. Bruce[1,2,3]

[1]Laboratory of Sensorimotor Research, National Eye Institute, National Institutes of Health, Bethesda, MD 20205, [2]Department of Neurology, Georgetown University School of Medicine, Washington, DC 20057, and [3]Section of Neuroanatomy, Yale University School of Medicine, New Haven, CT 06520, U.S.A.

Introduction

The arcuate frontal eye fields have been implicated in the generation of eye movements since the 19th century, when Ferrier (1874) discovered that electrical stimulation of this region evoked contraversive eye movements in the monkey. Subsequent stimulation experiments have clarified this finding (Robinson and Fuchs, 1969): electrical stimulation of the arcuate frontal eye fields of the awake monkey evokes saccades that do not differ in their amplitude-velocity relationship from saccades made naturally. This suggested the frontal eye fields played a role in the initiation of saccades, but the earliest single unit studies did not support the hypothesis. Bizzi (1968) recorded from a large number of arcuate frontal eye field neurons while monkeys made spontaneous saccades. He did not observe any consistent activity that preceded saccades, although he noted a small proportion of cells that discharged during and after saccades.

The first indication that neurons in the arcuate frontal eye fields might help generate saccades was the observation of Mohler et al. (1973) that many frontal eye field neurons have visual receptive fields. These results established that the arcuate frontal eye fields are active before visually guided saccades. Furthermore, the visual activity of these neurons is enhanced when the monkey makes saccades to stimuli in the cell's receptive field (Wurtz and Mohler, 1976). Such enhancement does not occur when the monkey uses the same stimuli in a peripheral attention task or a reaching task, but is forbidden to make saccades to these stimuli (Goldberg and Bushnell, 1981).

However, monkeys and humans can make purposive saccades using targeting information other than the visually derived location of the target. In the experiments described here we studied neurons in the monkey arcuate frontal eye fields in several paradigms designed to separate the visual responsiveness of neurons from their presaccadic activity. We conclude that there is significant neural activity in the monkey's frontal eye fields before purposive saccades, whether or not those saccades are made under direct visual guidance.

Methods

Rhesus monkeys were surgically prepared for eye position measurement with the implanted magnetic search coil technique (Robinson, 1963; Judge et al., 1980) and chronic single neuron recording using conventional methods which have been described elsewhere (Goldberg, 1983; Bruce and Goldberg, 1984). The monkeys were trained on four visuomotor tasks outlined in Fig. 1. The first task was the no-saccade task: The monkeys had to look at a spot of light and maintain fixation for a specified period of time, usually 1–3 seconds. If the monkeys broke fixation the trial was terminated. They learned not to break fixation if a peripheral stimulus appeared

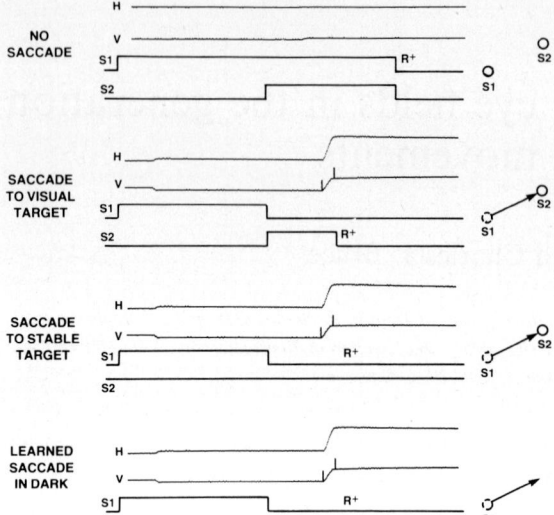

Fig. 1. Behavioral paradigms. Horizontal and vertical eye position (labeled H and V) and stimulus light traces (S1 and S2) are shown for each of four behavioral paradigms. In the no-saccade paradigm S1 appears and remains on. The monkey fixates S1 and does not break gaze to look at S2 when it appears (upward deflection in S2 trace) or disappears (downward deflection). The monkey receives a reward at R+ for either releasing a bar to signal a dimming of S1, or merely for maintaining the proper eye position. The figure on the right shows that no eye movement is made. In the saccade to the visual target, S1 disappears when S2 appears, and the monkey makes a saccade to fixate the target. The ticks at the beginning and end of saccade in the vertical trace are placed by the computer to signal the on-line recognition of saccade beginning and end. The arrow in the right-hand figure represents a saccade. In the saccade to stable target S1 is on all the time. The signal to make the saccade from S1 to S2 is the disappearance of S1, signaled by the downward deflection in the S1 trace. The right-hand figure shows the saccade from S1 to S2. In the learned saccade task the monkey makes a saccade to where S2 was in the previous visually guided saccade trial. The signal to make the eye movement is the disappearance of S1, after which the monkey remains in total darkness. The right-hand figure shows that the saccade is made in the absence of a target. Reproduced, with permission, from the Journal of Neurophysiology (Bruce and Goldberg, 1985).

on the screen, and this stimulus was used to study the visual receptive fields of neurons. The second task was the saccade task: The fixation point disappeared when a new stimulus appeared, and the monkey had to saccade to the new stimulus. The third task was the stable target task: In this task the second stimulus remained on the screen at all times, and the monkey learned to saccade to the stable target only when the fixation point disappeared. This task separated the response of a neuron to the stimulus' appearance from the neuron's activity before the saccade. The most difficult task was the learned saccade task: The monkey first practiced by making saccades to a very brief (25 mseconds) target. After the monkey reliably made saccades to the brief target, the target was eliminated altogether for half of the trials. The monkey was rewarded for continuing to make the same saccade on those trials lacking a target. This task separated a neuron's response before a purposive saccade from its response before a visually guided saccade of similar dimensions.

After training was completed, the activity of single neurons was recorded while the monkeys performed these tasks. Sites of interesting cells were marked with electrolytic lesions.

Results

We recorded 752 neurons in three monkeys. All neurons lay in the posterior portion of the arcuate sulcus, either in the anterior bank of the sulcus or on the cortical surface near the anterior lip. Over half of these neurons (409: 59%) discharged before visually guided saccades. 115 were studied exhaustively using the above paradigms. We found three different kinds of activity preceding visually guided saccades: 1. Visual activity: A discharge in response to visual stimulation even in the absence of eye movements. Cells with visual activity discharged in the no-saccade task. 2. Movement activity: A discharge preceding purposive saccades, even those made without visual targets. Cells with movement activity discharged in the learned saccade task, but usually were much less active before comparable spontaneous saccades made in the dark. 3. Anticipatory activity: An increased rate of background discharge when the monkey could predict the dimensions of the next saccade required. This activity occurred while the monkey was waiting to make a saccade, yet before either the saccade target or the cue to make the saccade had appeared. Anticipa-

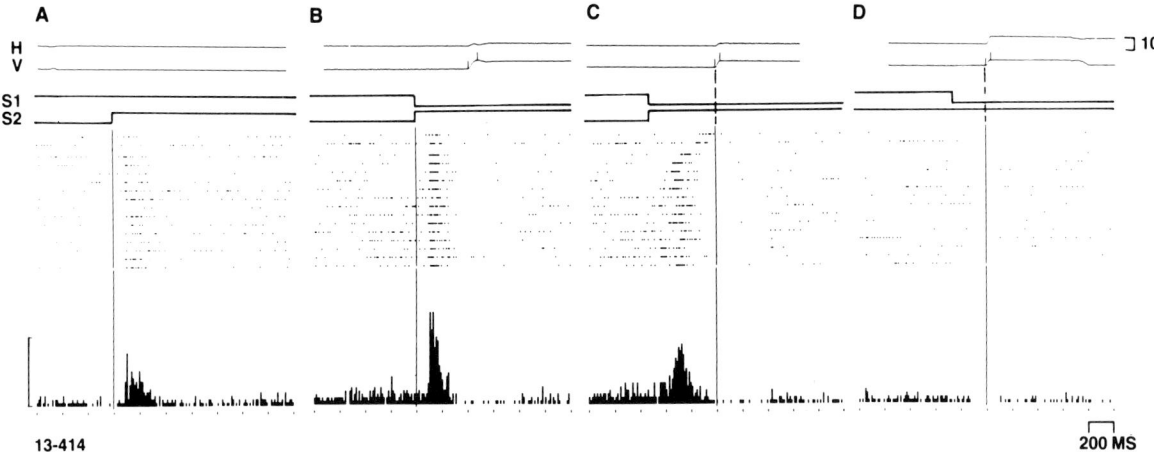

Fig. 2. Visual cell. A shows the response of the cell in the no-saccade task. Representative eye position and stimulus artifact traces are shown above each dot raster and histogram. In the dot raster each dot represents a cell action potential. Each line represents a 2-second epoch. Successive epochs are aligned on the onset of S1, which occurs at the vertical line. The histogram sums the lines of the raster above. The dots at the bottom of the histogram are spaced 200 mseconds apart. The calibration line of the histogram represents a discharge frequency of 100 impulses/sec. B shows the enhanced response of the stimulus in the saccade task, synchronized on the simultaneous offset of S1 and onset of S2. C shows the same trials now synchronized on the beginning of the saccade. D shows the absence of response in the stable target saccade task. Reproduced, with permission, from the Journal of Neurophysiology (Bruce and Goldberg, 1985).

tory activity did not occur on every trial, but rather developed over several trials, as described below.

These three activities were distributed differently in different neurons, and a given cell could have any or all of them. Based on the relative strength of their visual and movement activities, we divided presaccadic neurons into three different classes: visual, visuomovement, and movement cells.

40% of presaccadic cells were classified as visual cells because they had visual but not movement activity. These cells discharged in response to the onset of visual stimuli in the no-saccade task whether or not the monkey actually made saccades to the stimuli. Fig. 2 illustrates a visual cell. This cell gives a brisk, phasic response to the onset of a visual stimulus (A) which is enhanced when the monkey makes a saccade to the stimulus (B). The discharge cell is far better synchronized to the stimulus onset (B) than to the saccade beginning (C), and when the saccade is made in the context of the stable target task without the stimulus ever providing an on-response, the cell does not discharge (D). Therefore, the presaccadic activity of this cell is exclusively visual. Like the cell illustrated, half of the visual cells gave enhanced response to the visual stimulus when the monkey made a saccade to it. However, when the monkey made a learned saccade or a saccade to a stable target visual cells did not discharge.

20% of presaccadic cells were movement cells. These cells had similar activity before visually guided and learned saccades, but little or no visual activity. Fig. 3 shows a typical movement cell; it discharged similarly before saccades to a visual stimulus (A) and those made in the learned saccade task without a visual target (B). There was a very weak response in the no-saccade task (C).

A striking feature of movement cells is that they discharge much less before equivalent spontaneous saccades in the dark than before learned saccades. Roughly 40% of movement cells had no activity preceding spontaneous saccades in the dark. About 60% were active before spontaneous saccades, but for most such cells the activity preceding purposive saccades (both learned and visually guided) was substantially greater. Fig. 4 compares the activity of cells before learned saccades, visually guided saccades, spontaneous saccades in the dark, and in the no-saccade task. Note that even for these cells which discharged before spontaneous saccades the activity varied considerably, and did not correlate with the intensity of visual activity.

The remaining 40% of presaccadic neurons were classified as visuomovement cells because they had both visual and visuomovement activity. These cells discharged both in response to visual stimuli in the no-saccade task and before learned saccades. Their best discharge occurred before visually guided saccades. The discharge of the visuomovement cells frequently began in response to the stimulus to make the eye movement and continued through the reaction time period until the monkey actually made the saccade. Fig. 5 shows the activity of a visuomovement cell. The discharge began in response to stimulus appearance (A), preceded the saccade onset (B), and carried through past the saccade termination (C). It discharged, but less intensely, in response to the appearance of the visual stimulus in the no-saccade task (D), or before the saccade in either the learned saccade (E) or stable target task (F).

The visuomovement classification covers a spectrum of arcuate frontal eye field cells, with cells with predominantly visual activity and weak movement activity at one extreme, and cells with predominantly movement activity and weak visual activity at the other. Not surprisingly, all visuomovement cells responded more before visually guided saccades than before learned saccades or to visual stimuli that were not saccade targets. Presumably, the greater discharge in conjunction with visually guided saccades reflects the sum of a visual activity in response to the target together with a movement activity referable to the impending saccade.

For 15% of the arcuate frontal eye field movement and visuomovement neurons the background discharge rate varied as a function of the task. The rate was higher during blocks of trials in which the monkey made saccades into their movement fields than during blocks of trials in which the monkey

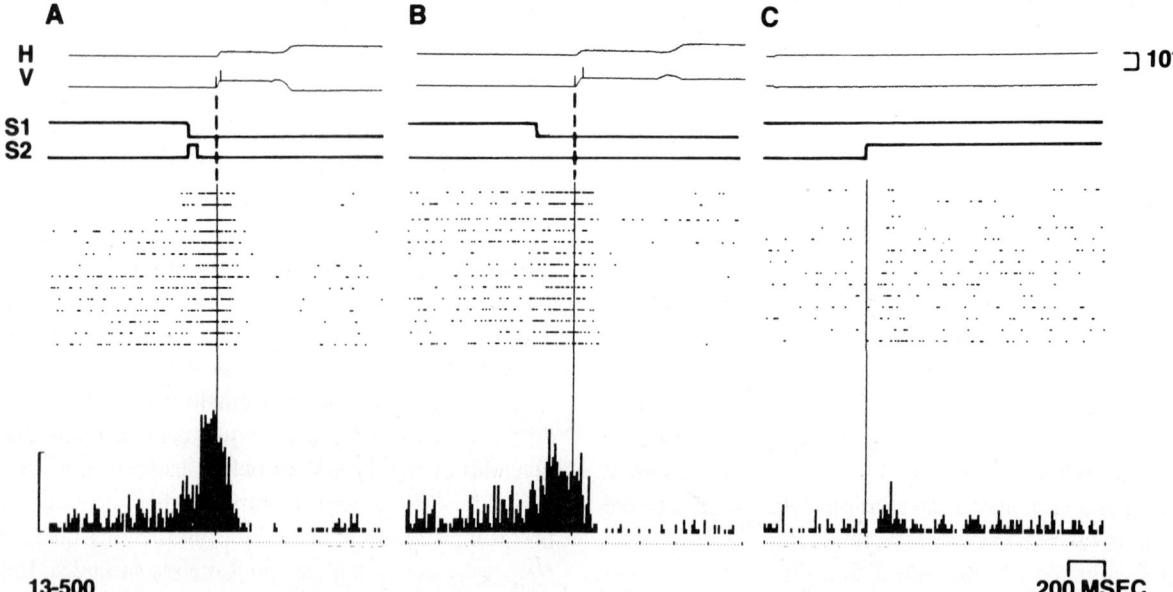

Fig. 3. Movement cell. A and B show the activity of the cell during a learned saccade experiment. A shows the activity in those trials in which the visual stimulus appeared. B shows the activity in those intermixed trials in which there was no visual stimulus. Trials in each raster are synchronized on the saccade onset. C shows the much weaker response of the cell to the visual stimulus in a subsequent no-saccade series. Trials in C are synchronized on the stimulus onset. Reproduced, with permission, from the Journal of Neurophysiology (Bruce and Goldberg, 1985).

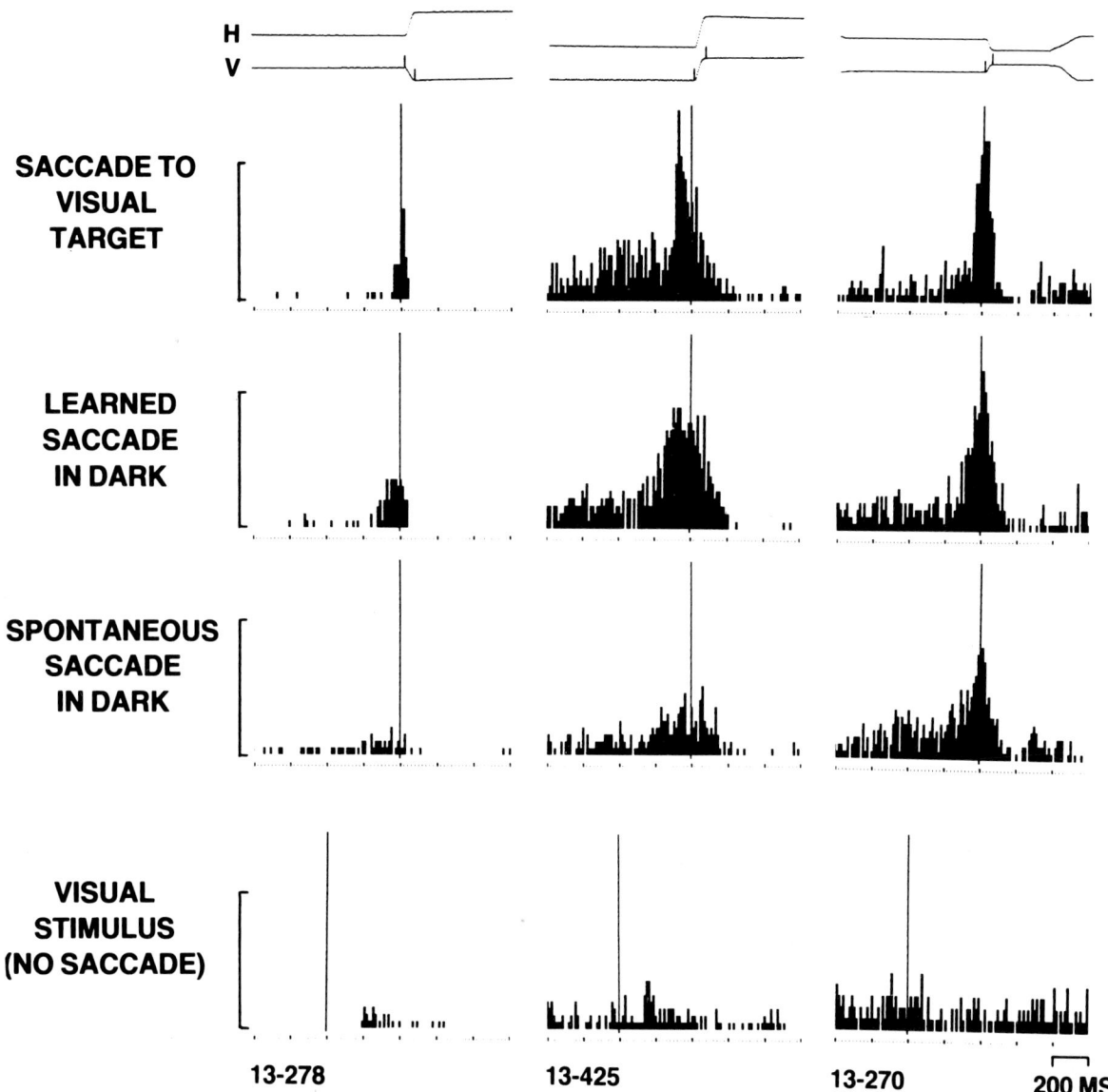

Fig. 4. Comparison of cell activity for visually guided, learned, and spontaneous saccades for cells with significant activity before spontaneous saccades. Each column shows the activity of a single cell in relationship to eye movements and visual stimuli. The eye movements at the top of the column show the optimum eye movement for the cell as determined in the visually guided saccade task. The first row shows histograms collected during visually guided saccades, synchronized on the onset of the saccade. In this and the subsequent two rows the vertical line signifies saccade onset. The second row shows histograms collected during learned saccades in the dark interspersed with the visually guided saccades in the first row. The third row shows spontaneous saccades of similar amplitude and direction collected during spontaneous eye movements in the dark. The fourth row shows activity during the no-saccade task synchronized on the onset of the same stimulus used to elicit the saccades in the first row, but here not used as the target for a saccade. The vertical line signifies stimulus onset. The calibration line at the left of the histogram corresponds to a discharge rate of 100 Hz. Reproduced, with permission, from the Journal of Neurophysiology (Bruce and Goldberg, 1985).

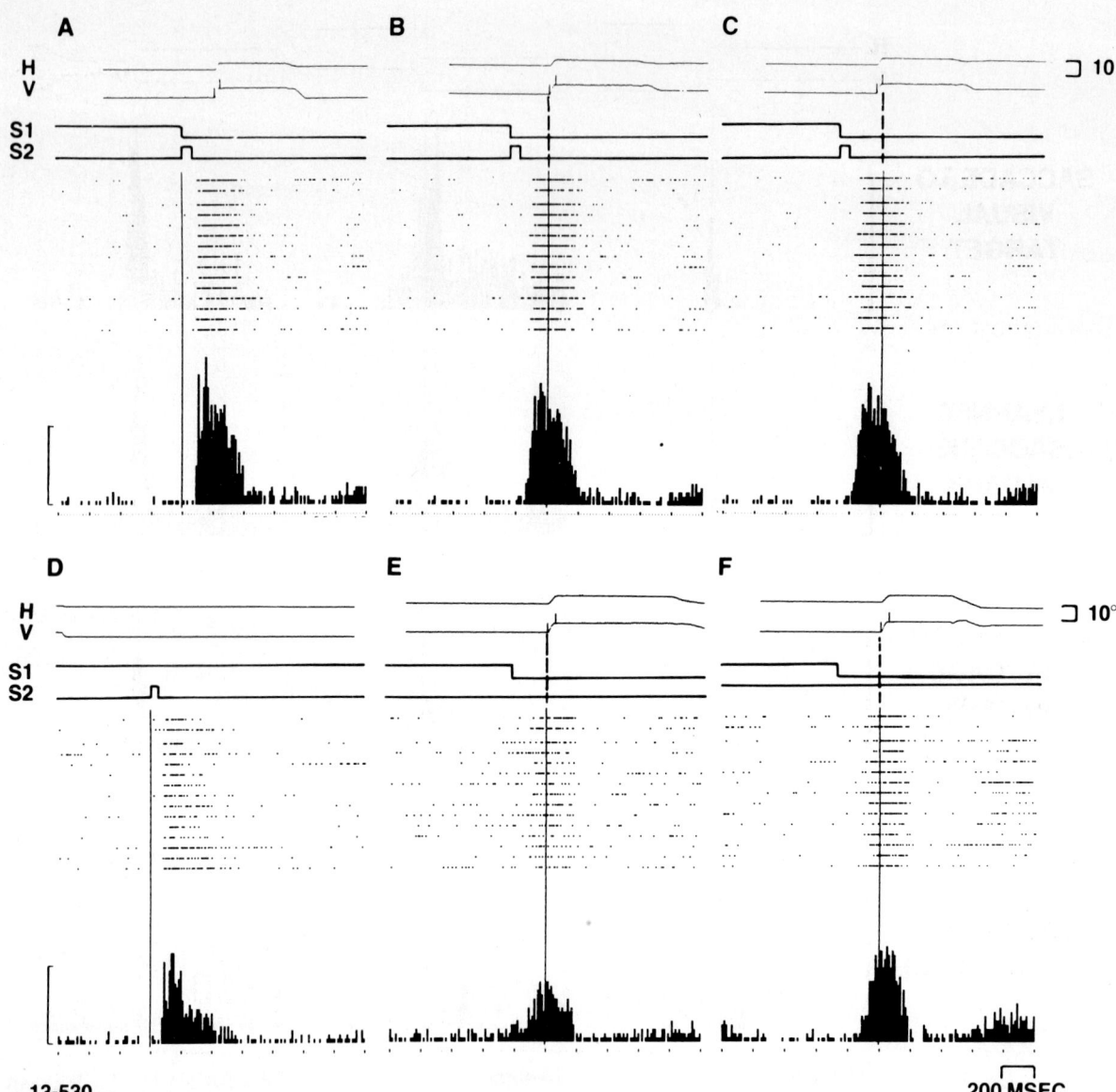

Fig. 5. Response of a visuomovement cell. A, B and C show the discharge of the cell in association with a visually guided saccade whose dimensions are shown in the records above each raster. The stimulus appeared on the screen for 50 mseconds and then disappeared, leaving the animal in total darkness. A shows activity synchronized on the onset of the visual stimulus, B shows the same activity synchronized on the beginning of the saccade, and C shows the same activity synchronized on the end of the saccade. The vertical lines denote the time of the synchronizing event. D shows the response of the cell to the same stimulus flashed during the no-saccade task. E shows the response of the cell before learned saccades interspersed with the visually guided saccades shown above. F shows the response of the cell in the stable target task. Note that the most vigorous response comes in the visually guided tasks. Reproduced, with permission, from the Journal of Neurophysiology (Bruce and Goldberg, 1985).

did not make saccades or made saccades outside of the movement field. This fluctuation of background rate can be seen in the movement cell illustrated in Fig. 3. In general, anticipatory activity required several saccade trials to become established and several no-saccade trials to disappear; the examples in Fig.

3 represent the stable activity obtained after such transition trials. Note that the cell begins to discharge well before the the saccade cue during the saccade trials (A), but not during a block of fixation trials (C).

Anticipatory activity was occasionally seen in cells without movement activity, as shown in Fig. 6. A learned saccade series is shown in the top three examples. Activity during visually guided trials in the learned saccade task are shown synchronized

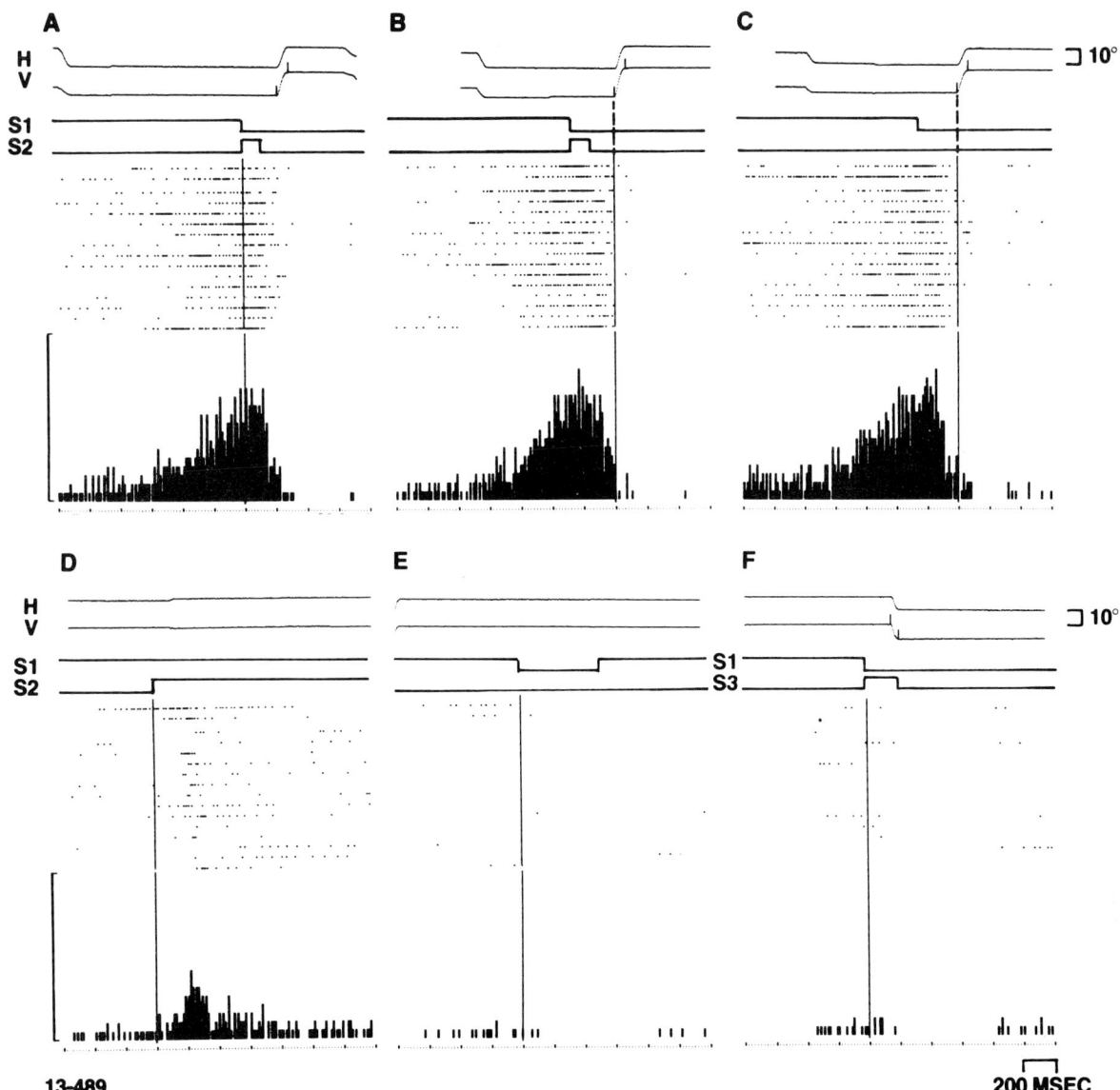

Fig. 6. Activity anticipatory of a saccade in a visual neuron. A shows the activity of the neuron synchronized on the onset of the stimulus to make an eye movement. B shows the same data synchronized on the beginning of the saccade. C shows the activity of the same neuron in learned saccade trials intermixed with the trials in A. D shows the activity in response to the same stimulus in fixation trials. E shows the response when the fixation point is blanked for 500 mseconds during a fixation trial. F shows the activity before a saccade to a visual target outside the receptive field (S3). The calibration line to the left of the histograms represents a discharge frequency of 100 Hz. Reproduced, with permission, from Vision Research (Goldberg and Bruce, 1985).

on the stimulus onset (A) and also on saccade (B). Note that the response began long before the cue to saccade. The histogram suggests that anticipatory activity builds up gradually before the saccade. However, examination of the individual trial records in the raster shows that the intensity of anticipatory discharge is fairly constant but the time of this discharge varies from trial to trial. Although in the visually guided trials the cell discharge overlaps the onset of the saccade (B), in the learned saccade trials, which have longer reaction times, the cell activity has ceased by the time the saccade begins (C). This cell had some visual activity in the no-saccade task (D). To see if the cell might really be anticipating the disappearance of the fixation point we used a modified no-saccade task in which the fixation point temporarily disappeared but the monkey had to maintain fixation. The cell did not respond in this task (E), nor did it discharge in anticipation of saccades to points outside the movement field of the anticipatory activity (F). Anticipatory activity usually took two or three trials to become established, and two or three trials to disappear. It occurred in 15% of visuomovement and visual cells, but in very few visual cells.

Both visual receptive fields and movement fields of frontal eye field neurons were organized in a retinotopic rather than a spatial or head-centered fashion. Neurons discharged before saccades of a particular direction and amplitude rather than be-

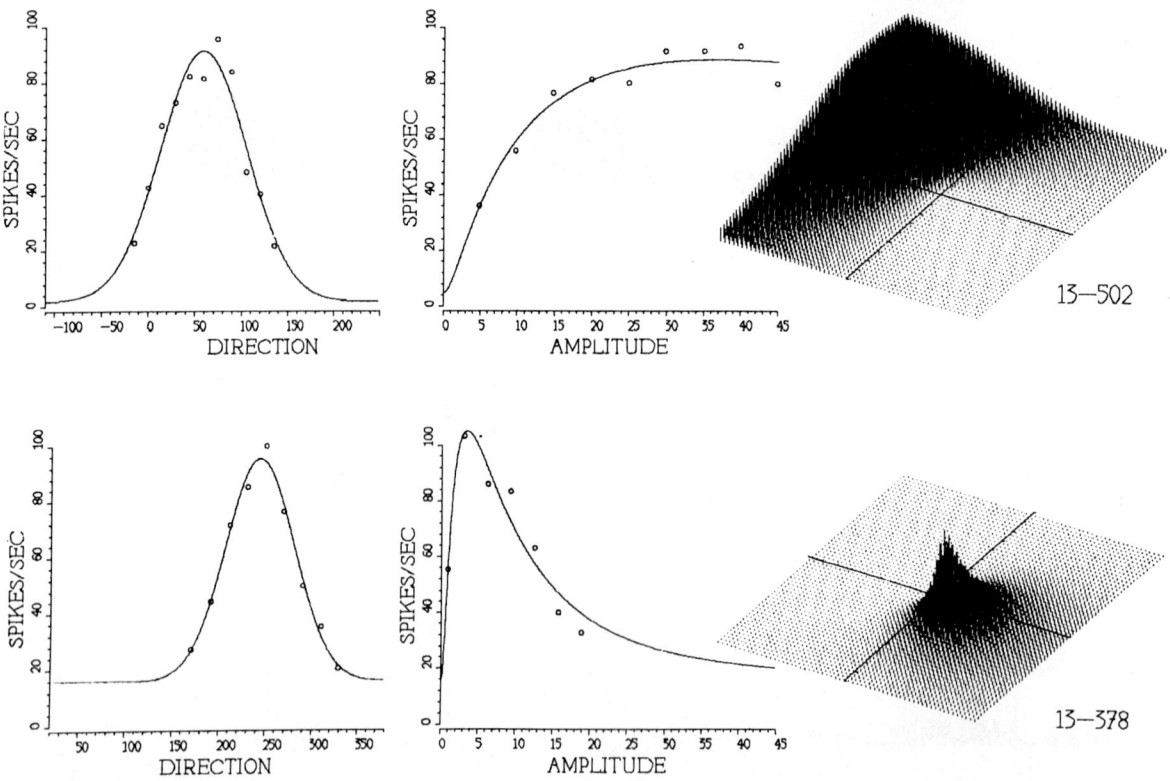

Fig. 7. Response fields of two movement neurons. Each row shows the quantitative response fields computed for a cell. The direction plots show discharge rates for various directions of saccades at an optimum amplitude, with a Gaussian function curve fit by the method of least-squares. The amplitude plots show discharge rates for various amplitudes of saccade in the optimum direction, with a log Gaussian function curve fit by the method of least-squares. The response surface is extrapolated by the computer from the amplitude and direction functions, with the plot arbitrarily rotated to provide the least obstructed view of the functions. Each point is the average of at least eight trials. The upper cell has a fairly eccentric movement field. The other (bottom) has a movement field near the fovea. Reproduced, with permission, from the Journal of Neurophysiology (Bruce and Goldberg, 1985).

fore saccades to a particular orbital position. We quantitatively studied these receptive fields and movement fields of neurons. After we manually estimated the optimal saccade for a large response, computer-controlled stimulus presentations varied the saccade direction at an optimum amplitude and the saccade amplitude at an optimum direction. Mean discharge rates per burst were plotted against saccade amplitude and direction.

Fig. 7 shows two plots for typical movement cells, one (top) preferring large saccades and the other (bottom) preferring small saccades. Neuronal discharge could be easily fit to a normal Gaussian function of saccade direction. Saccade amplitude could not be fit to such a symmetric function but rather required a log Gaussian distribution which could satisfy the requirement that the function was inevitably steeper for saccades to stimuli closer to the fovea than the optimum, and tailed off more gradually for longer saccades.

There were two different sorts of amplitude functions: for cells preferring small saccades the response was maximal for a particular saccade amplitude, and eventually disappeared for both larger and smaller saccades. However, for cells discharging best before large saccades, the presaccadic discharge frequently remained high for the largest saccades we could induce the the monkeys to make. The log Gaussian function could fit both the large and small amplitude-tuning curves.

The significance of the movement fields of frontal eye field neurons is clearly indicated by experiments that compare the activity of single neurons with the amplitude and direction of saccades evoked by electrical stimulation through the recording microelectrode at the site of those neurons (Goldberg and Bruce, 1983). Usually the optimal saccade for the movement or visuomovement cell predicted the saccade subsequently elicited by stimulating through the recording electrode. There were two exceptions to this rule: stimulation at the sites of cells with direction-tuning maxima near the vertical meridian resulted in saccades somewhat tilted toward the horizontal; sites with cells such as the one in Fig. 7 with amplitude-tuning curves with flat maxima resulted in saccades of the shortest amplitude associated with the maximum discharge. In general, the threshold for the electrical evocation of saccades was lower at the site of movement and visuomovement cells than at the site of visual cells that did not discharge before learned saccades in the dark.

Discussion

The results outlined here and in greater detail elsewhere (Bruce and Goldberg, 1985) show conclusively that activity in the arcuate frontal eye fields precedes purposive saccadic eye movements. This activity has three components: anticipatory, visual, and movement, and the discharge patterns of a given cell may have some or all of the three types of activity. Although more cells discharge before visually guided saccades than before any other type of saccadic eye movement, enough cells discharge before purposive saccades in the dark to establish that the arcuate frontal eye fields could play a significant role in the generation of non-visually guided purposive saccades.

Comparison with the superior colliculus

Like the arcuate frontal eye fields, the superior colliculus has a representation both of visual space and the eye movements required to achieve targets in that space. In both areas the eye movement or target position is coded by the anatomical location of the cell rather than a unique message in the discharge pattern or frequency. Visual activity in the frontal eye fields resembles that found in the superficial layers of the superior colliculus (Wurtz et al., 1980). The activity is enhanced when the monkey makes a saccade to a stimulus in the cell's receptive field, but not when the animal makes a saccade elsewhere or attends to the stimulus without making an eye movement (Goldberg and Bushnell, 1981). Movement activity resembles that found in the intermediate layers of the superior colliculus, with one major exception: in the superior colliculus eye movement-related activity occurs before all saccades, even the quick phases of nystagmus, whereas in the arcuate frontal eye fields this activity only occurs before purposive saccades. There are cells in the intermediate layers of the colliculus that resemble visuomovement cells in the arcuate frontal eye fields. These cells have both movement and visual activity (Wurtz et al., 1980), but unlike the frontal visuomovement cells the visual activity of the collicular cells is very independent of saccades. For example, collicular cells do not show enhancement of their visual responses before saccades to stimuli in their receptive fields. This is quite different from the arcuate frontal eye fields, whereas the visual activity of visuomovement cells often shows presaccadic enhancement.

These results suggest that in a normal monkey the superior colliculus participates in the generation of all saccades, whereas the frontal eye fields participate only in saccades germane to an animal's ongoing visual or task-related behavior. Spontaneous saccades unrelated to such critically important behavior have little antecedent activity in the arcuate frontal eye fields. Examples of these nonarcuate-frontal saccades would be spontaneous saccades in total darkness in the monkey, or the saccades a human might make while doing mental arithmetic.

The superior colliculus and the frontal eye fields are connected both directly through a projection from layer V of the cortex to the intermediate layers of the superior colliculus (Leichnetz, 1981), and indirectly via the projection from the arcuate frontal eye fields to the caudate nucleus, the caudate's projection to the substantia nigra, and the nigral projection to the intermediate layers of the colliculus (Wurtz and Hikosaka, Section IV-A). These projections suggest that the superior colliculus and the frontal eye field work in concert most of the time, although direct projections to the brainstem reticular formation (Leichnetz, 1981) allow the frontal eye fields to effect saccades independently of the colliculus. Indeed, stimulation of the arcuate frontal eye fields remains effective following colliculus lesions, whereas the ability of electrical stimulation of striate and posterior parietal cortex to elicit saccades is lost (Schiller, 1977). Similarly, removal of either the superior colliculus or the frontal eye fields alone does not eliminate visually guided saccades, but removal of both structures together does (Schiller et al., 1980).

Comparison with other cortical regions involved in saccades

Neurons in the posterior parietal cortex also discharge before visually guided saccades (Lynch et al., 1977), but the same cells discharge as vigorously in response to stimuli to which the monkeys attend, but do not saccade to (Bushnell et al., 1981). In contrast, enhancement in the frontal eye fields occurs only when the monkey makes saccades to a stimulus in the receptive field, and not when the monkey attends to the stimulus without making saccades to it (Goldberg and Bushnell, 1981). No activity related specifically to saccades as opposed to other sorts of attentive behavior has been found in the posterior parietal cortex (Robinson et al., 1978; Bushnell et al., 1981), but cells have not been studied there with paradigms such as the learned saccade task, in which the monkey makes a purposive saccade in the absence of a visual target.

Schlag and Schlag-Rey (1984) have recently described an area of the supplementary motor cortex which has cells discharging before saccades and from which saccades can be elicited by electrical stimulation at low currents. The most salient difference between this supplementary oculomotor cortex and the arcuate frontal eye fields is that in the arcuate frontal eye fields most movement activity occurs only before purposive saccades, and in the supplementary motor area the presaccadic activity always occurs before spontaneous saccades. Because combined lesions of the arcuate frontal eye fields and the superior colliculus render a monkey unable to initiate visually guided saccades, there must not be a direct path by which the supplementary motor cortical signal reaches the oculomotor system. Instead, its signal must pass through either the superior colliculus or the arcuate frontal eye fields.

Comparison with cortex involved in skeletal movement

The relationship of arcuate frontal activity to eye movement differs significantly from that of motor cortex to skeletal movement. Motor cortex projects directly to skeletal muscles (Fetz et al., Section IV-A), and the activity of many cortical neurons is related to muscular force rather than to parameters of the limb movement (Evarts, 1981). Conversely, the arcuate frontal eye field probably does not project monosynaptically to the extraoculomotor neurons, and the discharge of frontal eye field neurons specifies an amplitude and direction of saccade rather than discharge rate or muscular force of motor neurons. This may reflect the special nature of saccades and eye movements. The extraocular muscles have not significantly changed during evolution from simple vertebrates to primates. The same rapid eye movement which developed as the quick phase of vestibular nystagmus now serves the purpose of bringing a visual target to the fovea. The motor program is unchanged: what differs is the analysis that precedes the movement. The frontal eye fields, then, may have evolved to carry the results of cortical processing to the pre-existing rapid eye movement program in the brainstem. The motor cortex, on the other hand, has evolved along with the complexities of the distal musculature, and may be more intimately involved in creating the appropriate motor programs as well as triggering them. The responses of arcuate neurons may be more analogous to the responses of neurons in premotor cortex (Wise et al., Section IV-A), where there is also a significant sensory representation, and the discharge patterns of movement-related neurons appear unrelated to details such as force.

The results of lesion experiments also suggest that the frontal eye fields are more concerned with deciding which saccade to make rather than with the details of moving the eyes. Monkeys without frontal eye fields can make excellent visually guided saccades (Schiller et al., 1980), but they have impaired visual search (Crowne, 1983). Humans with frontal ablations for epilepsy which include the frontal eye fields have difficulty deliberately making saccades directed away from a visual target (Guitton et al., 1982). Recent work (Deng et al., 1984) suggests that monkeys with unilateral frontal eye field ablations have difficulty learning and performing saccades to remembered points, but not visually guided saccades. These lesion experiments all indicate that a frontal eye field lesion impairs the ability to move in eyes in a complex manner other than as a simple reflex to visual stimulation. The arcuate frontal eye fields may be the principal means by which the sophisticated information processing done in the cerebral cortex can be coordinated with an appropriate pattern of eye movements.

Acknowledgments

We are grateful to Messrs. Alvin Ziminsky and George Creswell and Misses Gerrie Snodgrass and Laurie Cooper for technical help, and to Mrs. Jean Steinberg for preparing the manuscript.

References

Bizzi, E. (1968) Discharge of frontal eye field neurons during saccadic and following eye movements in unanesthetized monkeys. Exp. Brain Res., 6: 69–80.

Bruce, C. J. and Goldberg, M. E. (1985) Primate frontal eye fields. I. Single neurons discharging before saccades. J. Neurophysiol., 53: 603–635.

Bushnell, M. C., Goldberg, M. E. and Robinson, D. L. (1981) Behavioral enhancement of visual responses in monkey cerebral cortex: I. Modulation in posterior parietal cortex related to selective attention. J. Neurophysiol., 46: 755–772.

Crowne, D. P. (1983) The frontal eye field and attention. Psychol. Bull., 93: 232–260.

Deng, S.-Y., Segraves, M. A., Ungerleider, L. G., Mishkin, M. and Goldberg, M. E. (1984) Unilateral frontal eye field lesions degrade saccadic performance in the rhesus monkey. Soc. Neurosci. Abstr., 10: 59.

Evarts, E. V. (1981) Role of motor cortex in voluntary movements in primates. In V. B. Brooks (Ed.), Handbook of Physiology Section 1: The Nervous System, Volume II. Motor Control, Part 2, pp. 1083–1120.

Ferrier, D. (1874) The localization of function in the brain. Proc. Roy. Soc., 22: 229–232.

Goldberg, M. E. (1983) Studying the neurophysiology of behavior: Methods for recording single neurons in awake behaving monkeys. In J. L. Barker and J. F. McKelvy (Eds.), Methods in Cellular Neurobiology, Vol. 3, John Wiley, New York, pp. 225–248.

Goldberg, M. E. and Bruce, C. J. (1983) The relationship of movement fields of frontal eye field neurons and the saccades evoked by electrical stimulation at the site of those neurons. Invest. Ophthalmol. Vis. Sci., 24 (Suppl): 272.

Goldberg, M. E. and Bruce, C. J. (1985) Cerebral cortical activity associated with the orientation of visual attention in the rhesus monkey. Vision Res., 25: 471–481.

Goldberg, M. E. and Bushnell, M. C. (1981) Behavioral enhancement of visual responses in monkey cerebral cortex. II. Modulation in frontal eye fields specifically related to saccades. J. Neurophysiol., 46: 773–787.

Guitton, D., Buchtel, H. A. and Douglas, R. M. (1982) Disturbances of voluntary saccadic eye movement mechanisms following discrete unilateral frontal lobe removals. In G. Lennerstrand, D. S. Zee and E. L. Keller (Eds.), Functional Basis of Ocular Motility Disorders, Pergamon Press, Oxford, pp. 497–500.

Judge, S. J., Richmond, B. J. and Chu, F. C. (1980) Implantation of magnetic search coils for measurement of eye position: an improved method. Vision Res., 20: 535–538.

Leichnetz, G. R. (1981) The prefrontal cortico-oculomotor trajectories in the monkey. A possible explanation for the effects of stimulation/lesion experiments on eye movements. J. Neurol. Sci., 49:387–396.

Lynch, J. C., Mountcastle, V. B., Talbot, W. H. and Yin, T. C. T. (1977) Parietal lobe mechanisms for directed visual attention. J. Neurophysiol., 40: 362–389.

Mohler, C. W., Goldberg, M. E. and Wurtz, R. H. (1973) Visual receptive fields of frontal eye field neurons. Brain Res., 61: 385–389.

Robinson, D. A. (1963) A method of measuring eye movement using a scleral search coil in a magnetic field. IEEE Trans. Biomed. Eng., 10: 137–145.

Robinson, D. A. and Fuchs, A. F. (1969) Eye movements evoked by stimulation of frontal eye fields. J. Neurophysiol., 32: 637–648.

Robinson, D. L., Goldberg, M. E. and Stanton, G. B.(1978) Parietal association cortex in the primate: Sensory mechanisms and behavioral modulations. J. Neurophysiol., 41: 910–932.

Schiller, P. H. (1977) The effect of superior colliculus ablation on saccades elicited by cortical stimulation. Brain Res., 122: 154–156.

Schiller, P. H., True, S. D. and Conway, J. L. (1980) Deficits in eye movements following frontal eye field and superior colliculus ablations. J. Neurophysiol., 44: 1175–1189.

Schlag, J. and Schlag-Rey, M. (1984) Visuo-motor units in frontal dorsomedial cortex of monkey. Soc. Neurosci. Abstr. 10: 989.

Wurtz, R. H. and Mohler, C. W. (1976) Enhancement of visual response in monkey striate cortex and frontal eye fields. J. Neurophysiol., 39: 766–772.

Wurtz, R. H., Goldberg, M. E. and Robinson, D. L. (1980) Behavioral modulation of visual responses in the monkey: stimulus selection for attention and movement. In J. M. Sprague and A. N. Epstein (Eds.), Progress in Psychobiology and Physiological Psychology, Vol. 9, Academic Press, New York, pp. 43–83.

Express saccades in man and monkey

B. Fischer

Department of Clinical Neurology and Neurophysiology, University of Freiburg, Hansastrasse 9, 7800 Freiburg, F.R.G.

Introduction

Under natural viewing conditions visual information is processed during periods of eye fixation interrupted by rapid changes of the direction of gaze that bring the centre of the fovea from one point of interest to the next. Since attentive fixation is an active process it must be interrupted before a saccade can be initiated. In addition, processes of directing attention to the next peripheral target, making a decision to move or not to move the eyes, and the computation of the horizontal and vertical coordinates (or size and amplitude) for the eye movement are among those processes that must be completed before the final motor command can go to the eye muscles.

During attempts to study the neural substrates of some of these processes in the monkey's visual association cortex (Fischer and Boch, 1981a, 1982) we used a paradigm where the fixation point was turned off some time before the peripheral saccade target was presented (gap paradigm). Looking at the time from the occurrence of the target to the actual beginning of the eye movement we observed surprisingly short and stable reaction times, on the order of 70 mseconds with standard errors in the order of ± 3 mseconds (Fischer and Boch, 1983). The corresponding saccades were called "express" saccades, because they reach the target so fast after its occurrence.

Several control experiments and the systematic changes of the reaction time of express saccades with changes of the physical and behavioural aspects of the task convinced us that the occurrence of the express saccades is not a consequence of any kind of artifact but a real phenomenon that reflects special aspects of the processes preceding visually guided saccades.

Here we present evidence for the existence of express saccades not only in the monkey but also in humans. We will argue on the basis of lesion experiments that the superior colliculus together with the primary visual cortex must be intact for the generation of correct express saccades, whereas the frontal eye fields are not needed (Sandell et al., 1984).

The existence of the express saccades offers a way to reduce the time of initiating eye movements by about 100 mseconds. We can also study other visually guided movements (such as reach movements) to determine whether or not the reaction times are influenced by the preceding eye movement.

Methods

Monkeys were trained to fixate a small (0.25°) central fixation point using a dimming paradigm: upon the appearance of the fixation point they had to press a lever, hold it for a randomly varying period of time (1–6 seconds) and release it when they detected a small decrease in luminance of the spot. Saccades were elicited by presenting the animal with a second peripheral stimulus. In this case the luminance of the target was decreased. Animals quickly learned to saccade to the peripheral target to facilitate perception of the decrease in luminance. Monkeys were never rewarded for making saccades, but rather for detecting the dimming within a reaction time of less than 700 mseconds.

Eye movements were recorded by an infrared light technique (Bach et al., 1983). The resolution was 0.1° in both horizontal and vertical directions. Saccadic reaction times were determined automatically by an electronic threshold detector that stopped a millisecond counter triggered by the onset of the target. Distributions of saccadic reaction times were constructed by a minicomputer using a bin width of 5 or 10 mseconds. Mean values and their standard errors were computed after inspection of the distributions.

Data collection and evaluation were essentially the same for monkey and human experiments. The task for human observers was the same as for monkeys, with the exception of the use of the dimming paradigm. Subjects were asked to fixate the central fixation spot and to look at the peripheral target as soon as possible after it had appeared. Target eccentricity was 4° in all experiments. Targets were 0.25° in size and 10 cd/m^2 in luminance superimposed on a moderate background of about 0.1 cd/m^2. The temporal gap between fixation point offset and target onset was 200 mseconds, unless stated otherwise. The presaccadic fixation period could be varied between 1 and 2 seconds.

Results

Existence of express saccades

Fig. 1 illustrates the basic observation in both monkey (upper part) and man (lower part). In the gap situation (left side) there are distributions of saccadic reaction times, with the first peak around 75 mseconds in monkey and around 100 mseconds in man. In man some saccades may also occur with reaction times of less than 75 mseconds from target onset. These are due to saccades initiated involuntarily at fixation point offset rather than target onset. They are of particular interest if one looks at their accuracy and the subsequent corrective saccades (see Fig. 2, below). The second peak occurs around 130 mseconds in monkey and around 140 mseconds in man. Saccades contributing to the first peak are called express saccades, those contributing to the second peak are called (fast) regular saccades.

For comparison we used the overlap paradigm in both species (right side): saccades were made to the same target, but the fixation point remained visible throughout the trial. The only difference between the gap and overlap trials was the absence or presence of the fixation point at the time of target occurrence. The corresponding distributions are also shown in Fig. 1 (right side): most saccadic reaction times were considerably longer (slow regular saccades) and exhibited a larger scatter than for the gap trials.

To our surprise, there was a bimodal distribution of saccadic reaction times even in overlap trials (see Fig. 1, right). The first peak, representing express saccades, emerged in monkeys, if they were trained for a number of days using only overlap trials, and if the dimming never occurred at the fixation point but always at the target. This was achieved by arranging the timing in such a way that the dimming never occurred before the target came on. The animals learned that the relevant stimulus was no

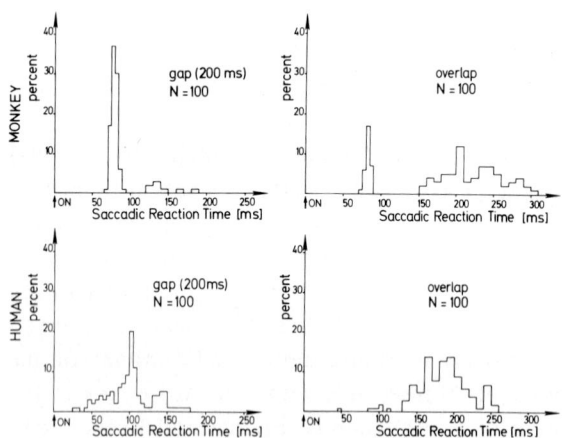

Fig. 1. Distributions of saccadic reaction times of monkey (upper) and man (lower) using the gap paradigm (left) and the overlap paradigm (right). Time from target onset is plotted horizontally, percent number of reaction times falling into each bin is plotted vertically. The express peak occurs at about 75 mseconds for the monkey and at about 100 mseconds for the human subject.

longer the fixation point and adopted a strategy whereby they would keep their eyes still while not actively fixating the spot. Therefore, by the time they saw the target, they did not have to "unfixate" their eyes. Consequently, their reaction times were about as short as on gap trials where there was no fixation point.

To elicit express saccades in man, we instructed the subjects to look at the central fixation point without fixating it attentively, although they should not move their eyes before target onset. This change in instruction set changed the distribution of their reaction time: there were more saccades with shorter reaction times than in the situation with attentive fixation, and eventually a small peak of express saccades appeared, as in Fig. 1 (lower right). We conclude from these observation that it is not the fixation point per se which inhibits express saccades, but rather the presence of active fixation.

Saslow (1967) and more recently Reulen (1984) used the gap and overlap paradigm for humans. Both authors have shown that saccadic reaction times were systematically reduced from above 200 mseconds to about 150 mseconds, if the delay between fixation point offset and target onset is changed from + 300 mseconds (overlap) to − 300 mseconds (gap). They did not report reaction times in the order of 100 mseconds, however, nor did they report bimodal distributions.

Control experiments

We controlled for the possibility that the monkey or the subject might have anticipated the onset of the target at the same location or at the same time by randomizing the parameters (Boch et al., 1984; Fischer et al., 1984). It became clear that the occurrence of express saccades and the reaction times depended on the amount of daily practice. It was also shown that the physical parameters of the target systematically influenced the reaction time of express saccades.

Similar control experiments have been conducted in man. When target positions of 4° to the right and left were randomized, there was a bimodal distribution, with the first peak occurring 120 mseconds and the second peak around 160 mseconds, and the very early reaction times (75 mseconds), observed with constant target location (Fig. 1, lower left), disappeared. The dip between express and regular saccades in the distribution was sometimes rather narrow and could be seen reliably only if the bin width used to construct them was below 20 mseconds. Randomization of the gap duration between 200 and 220 mseconds resulted in about the same distributions: the express peak occurred at the same position along the reaction time axis, showing that the saccades had been triggered by target onset rather than by fixation point offset.

As in the monkey, the relative number of human express saccades was increased as a consequence of daily practice, by about 20–30% depending on the subject.

Neural structures for express saccades

Neural structures involved in the generation of express saccades have been investigated in lesion experiments. Express saccades were still elicited after removal of the frontal eye fields (Sandell et al., 1984). However, when the superior colliculus was removed on one side, express saccades were abolished for contralateral but not for ipsilateral target locations.

Our preliminary studies show that a local lesion of striate cortex that produced a circumscribed scotoma in the contralateral visual field, leaving the foveal representation intact, caused a severe deficit in the generation of saccades into the blind part of the visual field. After more than 3 weeks of daily practice there were still no signs of correct express saccades: the reaction time distributions were unimodal, with a broad peak around 140 mseconds. More than 50% of the saccades — irrespective of their reaction time — missed the target by more than 10%.

Therefore, although the animal had improved its ability to make regular saccades considerably, there was no convincing evidence of the existence of express saccades after striate cortical lesions (compare also Mohler and Wurtz (1977)).

We believe, therefore, that express saccades are generated only by close collaboration of the striate cortex and superior colliculus. Whether or not this interaction takes place at the level of the colliculus or below is still unknown.

Corrective express saccades

As shown in the lower left part of Fig. 1, there were a number of reaction times less than 75 mseconds from target onset. Almost all of these saccades had wrong amplitudes, undershooting the target by more than 20%. We noticed that these saccades had an interesting feature: they were followed by corrective saccades, some of which occurred at a time when an express saccade would have been seen. Fig. 2 illustrates this phenomenon in two subjects (M.M. and M.G.). Traces were triggered by fixation point offset. The lower traces display target onset. For both subjects the two upper traces show express saccades with no (left) or a very small correction (right). The other traces show primary saccades occurring at different times and secondary or corrective saccades, always at the same time, as indicated by the vertical lines. This time was 94 mseconds from target onset for both subjects, a time that corresponds to the occurrence of their express saccades.

It should be noted that these observations were made only on those few trials where the subject anticipated the occurrence of the target, thereby initiating saccades that undershot the target. Of these, only a fraction were corrected at the express times, as shown in Fig. 2.

Despite the restricted number of cases we have seen, this pattern of two successive saccades shows that the primary saccade is programmed in parallel with the secondary or express saccade. Yet, the first saccade somehow and somewhere leaves a message of the retinal error that will remain after its execution. The next express saccade has access to this information and brings the fovea on target.

Coordinated eye and reach movements

The existence of saccades to a visual target after at least two clearly distinct reaction times differing by about 100 mseconds raised the question of whether or not a visually guided reaching movement of the hand, aimed from the fixation point to the same target, would follow the same reaction time as the eyes.

To study this a monkey was trained to touch the fixation point and move its hand to the target at the same visual command as the eye (i.e., target onset). We first trained the animal for stationary fixation. Then it practiced saccades and reach movements on gap trials until it produced express saccades exclusively. After that we put the animal in the overlap paradigm. During the first few sessions the animal produced only slow regular saccades, i.e., the saccadic reaction times were rather long and broadly scattered. The data of Fig. 3A were taken from the 6th session; each session consisted of 200 trials.

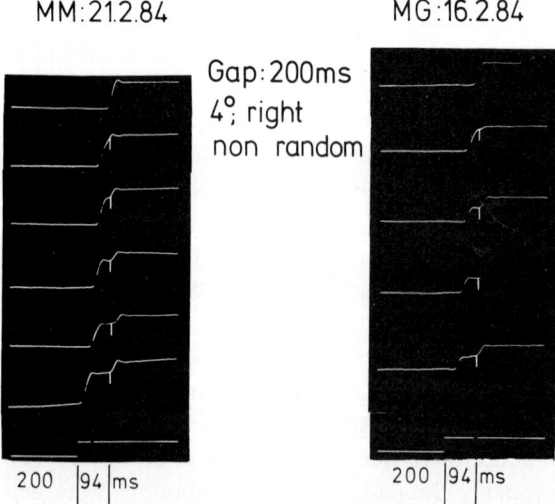

Fig. 2. Specimen records of eye movements from two subjects (M.M. and M.G.). Traces are triggered by fixation point offset. Target onset is indicated by the lowermost trace. Corrective (secondary) saccades, as indicated by a small vertical line, begin at about the same time (94 mseconds) after target onset. Primary saccades have reaction times below 75 mseconds. Depending on the onset of the primary saccade, the intersaccadic interval can be very short. Correct express saccades are shown in the uppermost traces.

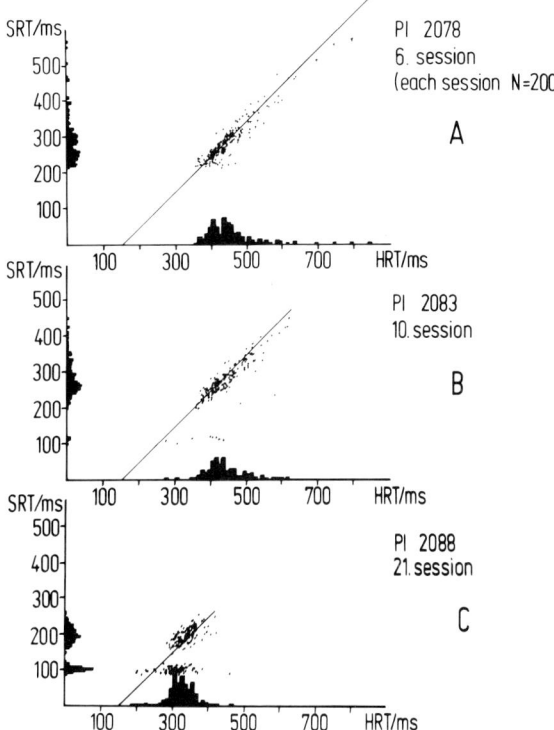

Fig. 3. Correlation between a monkey's saccadic reaction times (SRT, vertical) and reaction times of reach movements (HRT, horizontal) aimed at the same visual target using the overlap paradigm. Data in A were taken at the beginning of training, those in B in between, and those in C at the end. Before, the monkey was well trained for stationary fixation, for saccades — including express saccades — and for reach movements in the gap paradigm, not in the overlap paradigm. Bin width was 5 mseconds for saccadic reaction times and 10 mseconds for reach reaction times. As training goes on, one sees the development of two clearly distinct sets of data. Identical straight lines with a slope of 1 have been drawn through each of the plots.

During the next sessions the monkey began to produce a few express saccades (Fig. 3B), and finally, after many more sessions, a large number of express saccades occurred (Fig. 3C). As the amount of express saccades increased, the reaction time of the regular saccades decreased.

Fig. 3 shows the correlations between the reaction time of the eye (vertical axis) and the hand (horizontal axis) for the three sessions.

Fig. 3A shows a clear correlation between eye and hand reaction times, with the slope of a straight line through the data close to one. This implies that the difference between the individual reaction time is relatively constant and in the order of 150 mseconds. In other words, for slow regular saccades the hand follows the eye by a constant amount of time of about 150 mseconds, and, if the eye starts late, so does the hand.

As one looks at the population of express saccades (Fig. 3C) a different picture emerges. Even though there might be a correlation, the slope of a line through the data points would come close to zero. This means that if the eye moved early (express time) most of the time the hand could not follow 150 mseconds later, as it did in case of regular saccades. Nonetheless, the shortest reaction times of the hand were obtained if the preceding saccades were express saccades.

These observations suggest that the initiations of the eye and the hand movements are synchronized for slow regular saccades (Biguer et al., 1982) but not for express saccades. How this can be understood in relation to the processes of active fixation and relaxation of fixation remains a matter of discussion and experimentation. Of interest is that express saccades can be used to gain more insight into the coordination of visually guided movements.

Discussion

Our data show that in both monkey and man saccadic reaction times can change drastically depending on whether or not the subject is fixating a spot of light with the fovea at the time that a peripheral target occurs. If fixation is maintained until the target occurs, the time to "unfixate" the eye is included in the reaction time. If, on the other hand, the eye is already "unfixated", but still has not moved, the reaction time is correspondingly shorter. The existence of bimodal distribution, with the first peak presenting express saccades and the second peak fast regular saccades, shows that even if the eye is unfixated there are at least two more processes preceding the onset of eye movements: one may be identified with the computation of target position and the other with decision making (Fischer et al., 1984; Boch et al., 1984).

To clarify further the process of "unfixation" in the initiation of eye movements and coordinated reaching movements, one should take into account the neural mechanisms in the inferior parietal lobule, which is related to fixation, attention and manipulations within the monkey's immediate extrapersonal space (Lynch et al., 1977). For example, Shibutani et al. (1984) have shown that saccades elicited by electrical stimulation of the parietal association cortex are suppressed if the animal fixates actively. What happens in parietal neurons if visually guided reach movements are preceded by express saccades is still to be determined.

Summary

This chapter presents evidence for the existence of express saccades in man and monkey. Express saccades have short and stable reaction times of about 70 mseconds in monkey and 100 mseconds in man. They are obtained in gap trials in which the fixation point disappears at some time before the target occurs, as well as in overlap trials in which the fixation point remains on when the target occurs. Proper instruction to the observer and proper training for the animal also play a role.

Both the superior colliculus and the striate cortex are involved in the initiation of express saccades, whereas the frontal eye fields are not.

The reaction times of coordinated eye and reaching hand movements are closely correlated for regular saccades with long reaction times, but not for express saccades.

Acknowledgements

This work was supported by the Deutsche Forschungsgemeinschaft (DFG), Sonderforschungsbereich "Hirnforschung und Sinnesphysiologie" (SFB 70/Tp B7).

References

Bach, M., Bouis, D. and Fischer, B. (1983) An accurate and linear infrared oculometer. J. Neurosci. Methods, 9: 9–14.

Biguer, B., Jeannerod, M. and Prablanc, C. (1982) The coordination of eye, head, and arm movements during reaching at a single visual target. Exp. Brain Res., 46: 301–304.

Boch, R., Fischer, B. and Ramsperger, E. (1984) Express-saccades of the monkey: Reaction times versus intensity, size, duration, and eccentricity of their targets. Exp. Brain Res., 55: 223–231.

Fischer, B. and Boch, R. (1981a) Enhanced activation of neurons in prelunate cortex before visually guided saccades of trained rhesus monkeys. Exp. Brain Res., 44: 129–137.

Fischer, B. and Boch, R. (1981b) Selection of visual targets activates prelunate cortical cells in trained rhesus monkeys. Exp. Brain Res., 41: 431–433.

Fischer, B. and Boch, R. (1982) Modifications of presaccadic activation of neurons in the extrastriate cortex during prolonged training of rhesus monkeys in a visuo-oculomotor task, Neurosci. Lett., 30: 127–131.

Fischer, B. and Boch, R. (1983) Saccadic eye movements after extremely short reaction times in the monkey. Brain Res., 260: 21–26.

Fischer, B., Boch, R. and Ramsperger, E. (1984) Express-saccades of the monkey: Effects of daily training on probability of occurrence and reaction time. Exp. Brain Res., 55: 232–242.

Lynch, J. C., Mountcastle, V. B., Talbot, W. H. and Yin, T. C. T. (1977) Parietal lobe mechanisms for directed visual attention. J. Neurophysiol., 40: 362–389.

Mohler, C. W. and Wurtz, R. H. (1977) Role of striate cortex and superior colliculus in visual guidance of saccadic eye movements in monkeys. J. Neurophysiol., 40: 74–94.

Reulen, J. P. H. (1984) Latency of visually evoked saccadic eye movements. Biol. Cybern., 50: 251–262.

Sandell, J. H., Schiller, P. H. and Maunsell, J. H. R. (1984) The effect of superior colliculus and frontal eye field lesions on saccadic latency in the monkey. Perception, 13: A6.

Saslow, M. G. (1967) Effects of components of displacement-step stimuli upon latency of saccadic eye movements. J. Opt. Soc. Am., 57: 1024–1029.

Shibutani, H., Sakata, H. and Hyaerinen, J. (1984) Saccade and blinking evoked by microstimulation of the posterior parietal association cortex of the monkey. Exp. Brain Res., 55: 1–8.

The contribution of basal ganglia to limb control

M. R. DeLong, G. E. Alexander, S. J. Mitchell and R. T. Richardson

Departments of Neurology and Neuroscience, The Johns Hopkins University School of Medicine, Baltimore, MD 21205, U.S.A.

Introduction

This review is concerned primarily with the role of the basal ganglia in the control of limb movements. Data from recent anatomical and behavioral/neurophysiological studies in primates will be emphasized. For a more detailed review of these and related topics see DeLong and Georgopoulos (1981) and DeLong et al. (1984).

Functional organization

The overall anatomic relationships of the basal ganglia are summarized in Fig. 1. The striatum, the major "receptive" portion of the basal ganglia, receives inputs from the neocortex, the intralaminar nuclei of the thalamus, and the substantia nigra. Projections from the neocortex to the striatum are topographically organized (Goldman and Nauta, 1977; Kemp and Powell, 1971; Kunzle, 1975, 1978; Yeterian and Van Hoesen, 1978). Whereas the somatosensory, motor and premotor cortices project largely to the putamen, the "association" cortices project largely to the caudate. These anatomic relations suggest a division of the striatum into a sensorimotor portion involving largely the putamen and an "association" portion involving the caudate. Both anatomic (Kunzle, 1978) and physiologic studies (Crutcher and DeLong, 1984a; Liles, 1975, 1979) indicate a clear somatotopic organization within the putamen, as shown in Fig. 2.

The segregation of influences from "association" and sensorimotor cortices in the striatum appears

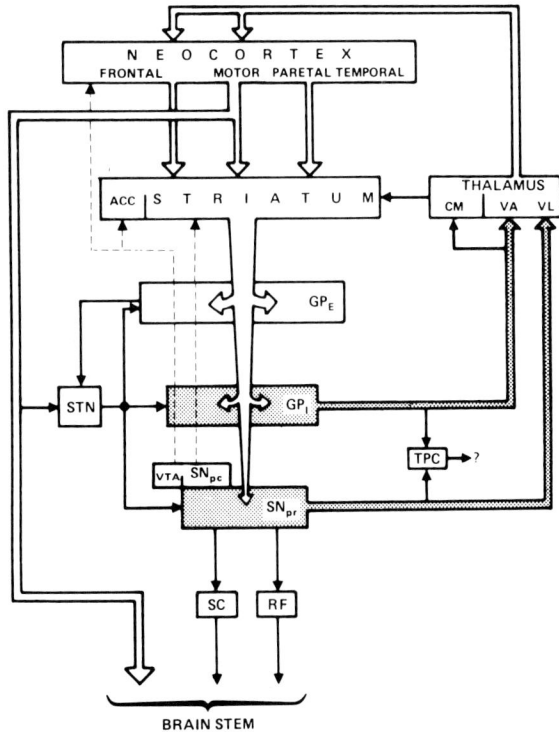

Fig. 1. Schematic diagram of principal intrinsic and extrinsic connections of basal ganglia. ACC, nucleus accumbens; GPe, external pallidal segment; GPi, internal pallidal segment; SNpr, substantia nigra pars reticulata; SNpc, substantia nigra pars compacta; STN, subthalamic nucleus; CM, center median; VL, n. ventralis lateralis; VA, n. ventralis anterior; SC, superior colliculus; RF, reticular formation; VTA, ventral tegmental area; TPC, n. tegmenti pedunculopontinus pars compacta. The dashed lines indicate dopamine pathways. Projections from the raphe to the striatum and substantia nigra have been omitted. Reproduced, with permission, from the American Physiological Society (DeLong and Georgopoulos, 1981).

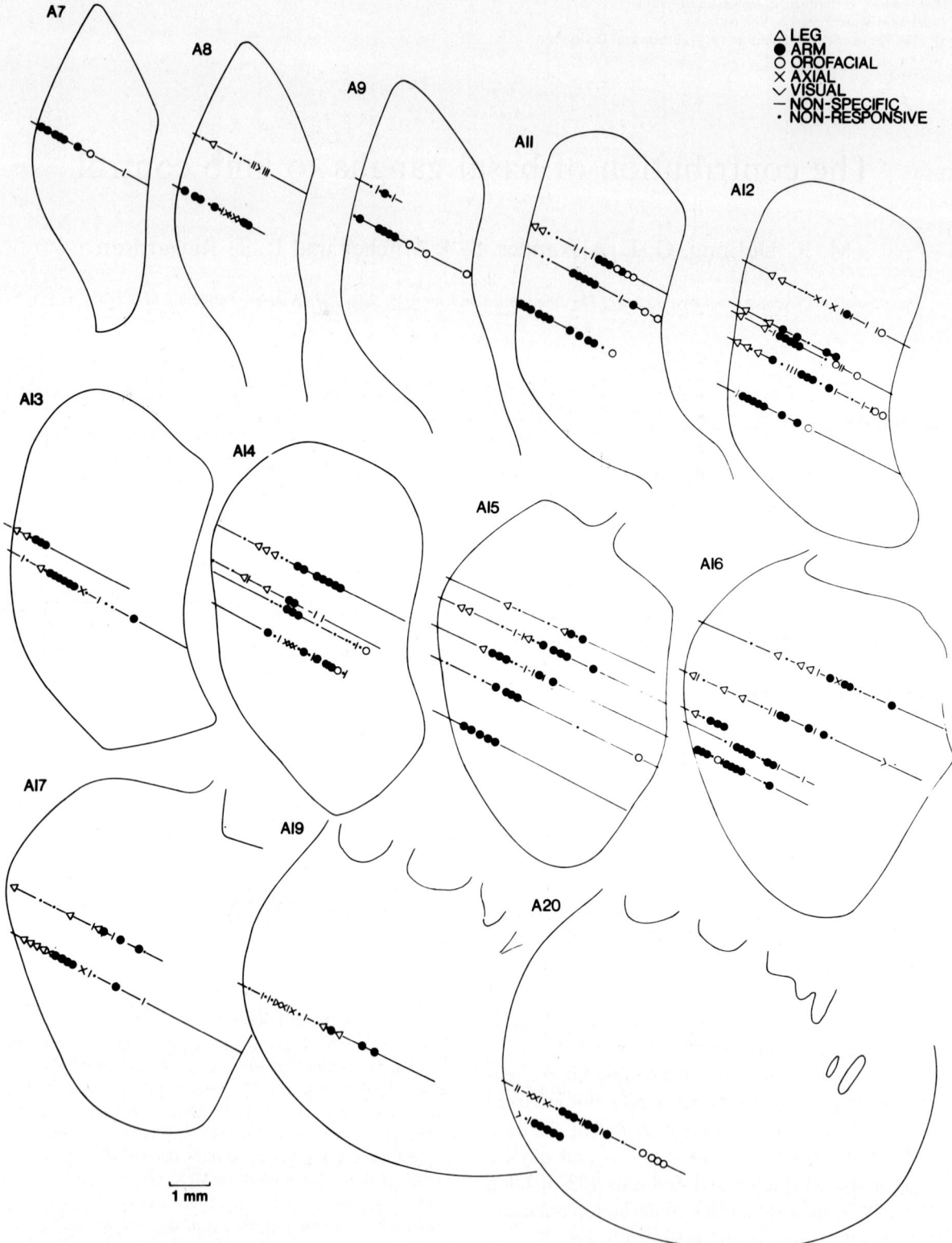

Fig. 2. Locations of putamen neurons related to movements of different body parts in one monkey. Data from both hemispheres are plotted on outline drawings of coronal sections of the left putamen. Each drawing shows the locations of all of the neurons studied within 0.5 mm of that anteroposterior level, ranging from anterior 7 (A7) to anterior 20 (A20). For each section, lateral is to the left. Reproduced, with permission, from Experimental Brain Research (Crutcher and DeLong, 1984a).

to be maintained at subsequent levels by topographically organized projections from the caudate and putamen (Johnson and Rosvold, 1971; Szabo, 1967, 1970) to separate regions of both segments of the globus pallidus (GP) and the pars reticulata of the substantia nigra (SNpr), the major sources of basal ganglia output. Within both the external (GPe) and internal (GPi) segments of the globus pallidus a somatotopically organized representation of movement-related neurons has been found, particularly in those portions which receive input from the putamen (DeLong, 1971; DeLong and Georgopoulos, 1979, 1981, DeLong et al., 1985). This is shown in Fig. 3.

The finding that specific neuronal relations to movements of individual body parts and a somatotopic organization are maintained in GP suggested that there exist segregated pathways through the basal ganglia for the control of different body parts and led us (DeLong and Georgopoulos, 1981) to question the widely held view that the basal ganglia serve as a "funnel" from association areas to the motor cortex (Evarts and Thach, 1969; Kemp and Powell, 1970). We concluded that the anatomic evidence was most consistent with the view that influences reaching the striatum from the sensorimotor and premotor cortices are ultimately directed upon premotor areas, whereas influences from the association areas are directed largely upon the prefrontal cortex. We thus proposed the existence of segregated, parallel cortico-subcortical loops subserving "motor" and "complex" functions, as shown schematically in Fig. 4. According to this scheme, just as the leg, arm and face representations remain segregated in the cerebral cortex, basal ganglia and thalamus, so are the influences from the

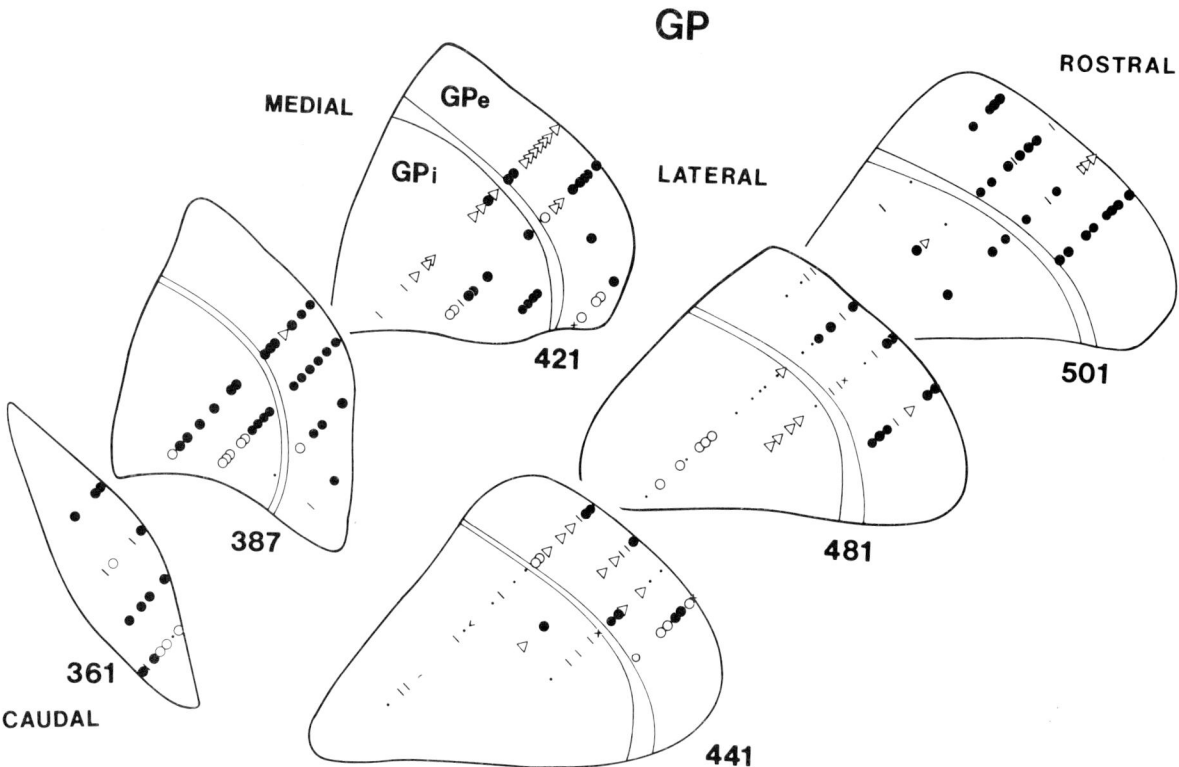

Fig. 3. Location of different cell types in GPe and GPi in one hemisphere. Symbols are as follows: △, leg; ●, arm; ○, orofacial; ×, axial; v, visual (or eye movements); −, non-specific; ·, non-responsive. Reproduced, with permission, from the American Physiological Society (DeLong et al., 1985).

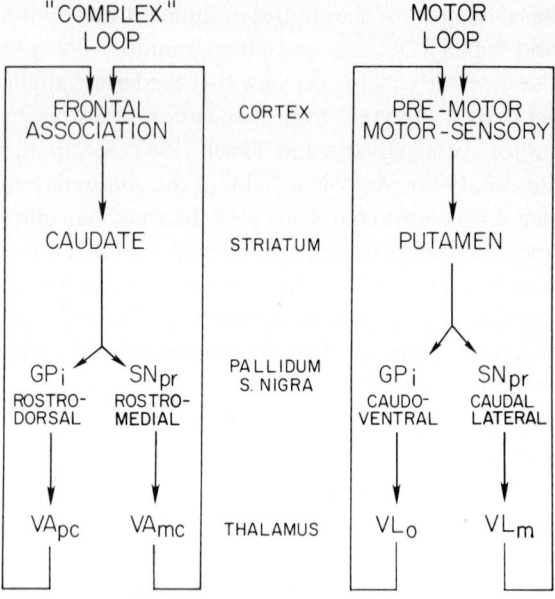

Fig. 4. Schematic depiction of the postulated segregation of pathways from the "association" (complex loop) and the sensorimotor areas (motor loop) through the basal ganglia and thalamus. Reproduced, with permission, from Experimental Brain Research (DeLong et al., 1983a).

cortical association areas separately routed through these subcortical nuclei by virtue of non-overlapping, topographically organized projections. This view of the functional organization of the basal ganglia provides a framework wherein disturbances not only in motor but also in more complex behavior may result separately from damage to different portions of these nuclei or their connections. This scheme is similar to that proposed by others (Divac, 1977) for the segregation of functions within the striatum, but differs significantly in proposing a maintained segregation, rather than an integration of influences from sensorimotor and association areas in the pallidum and thalamus.

The question of precisely which portions of the frontal lobe are influenced by basal ganglia output and the related issue of whether integration of basal ganglia and cerebellar output occurs at the thalamic or cortical level have recently been clarified. Several studies have shown that projections from the deep cerebellar nuclei, the globus pallidus and the substantia nigra terminate in separate parts of the thalamus (Asanuma et al., 1983; Carpenter et al., 1976; DeVito and Anderson, 1982; Kalil, 1981; Kuo and Carpenter, 1973; Mehler, 1971). In brief, these studies indicate that cerebellar efferents terminate in regions of the thalamus which project directly to the motor cortex, whereas basal ganglia efferents terminate in regions which project largely to pre-motor and prefrontal areas. A recent study by Schell and Strick (1984) indicates that whereas cerebellar output is directed to the motor cortex via the pars oralis subdivision of the nucleus ventralis posterior lateralis (VPLo), and to the arcuate premotor area (APA) via area X of the thalamus. According to this study, basal ganglia output is directed in large part to the supplemental motor area (SMA) via the pars oralis subdivision of ventralis lateralis (VLo). In addition, basal ganglia output can influence more rostral regions of the forebrain via projections from both the parvocellular and pars compacta portion of ventralis anterior (VA) and portions of medialis dorsalis (MD). Thus, basal ganglia and cerebellar influences appear to take separate pathways through the thalamus to the cortex, with basal ganglia output directed largely to the SMA and prefrontal cortex and cerebellar output to the motor cortex (area 4) and the APA.

Behavioral studies

Functional organization of movement-related neurons

In addition to the somatotopic grouping of movement-related neurons within the putamen, a clustering of neurons within the leg, arm and face areas with similar functional properties has been observed (Crutcher and DeLong, 1984b; Liles, 1978). As illustrated in Fig. 5, clusters of 2–5 neurons with similar relations to active movements or responses to somatosensory stimulation were typically encountered over a 100–500-μm distance along a given penetration. Different clusters of leg, arm and orofacial neurons were seen throughout most of the anteroposterior extent of the putamen. Some clus-

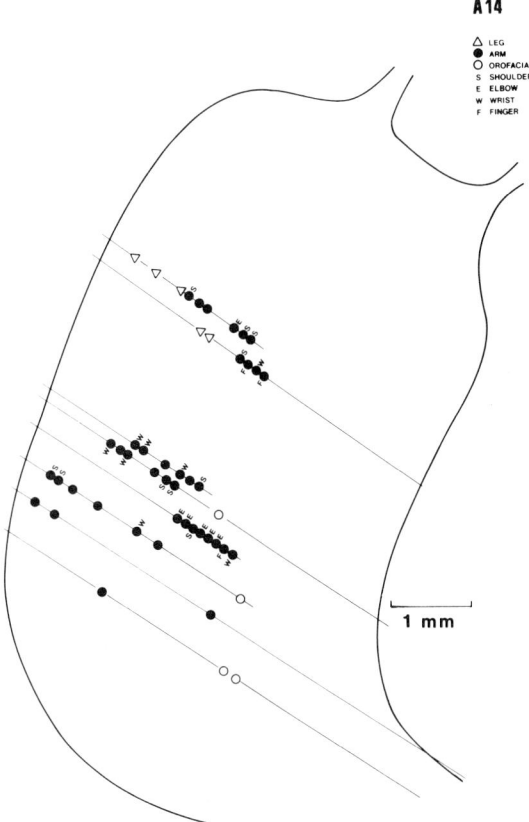

Additional evidence for a discontinuous representation of body parts within the putamen includes the recent demonstration of multiple discrete foci, striatal microexcitable zones (SMZ), from which motor responses can be evoked by microstimulation (Alexander and DeLong, 1983, 1985a,b). The functional properties of neurons within these low-threshold motor-response zones within the putamen correspond closely to the movements elicited by microstimulation. Moreover, the SMZs are organized somatotopically in accordance with the anatomical and physiologic data, as illustrated in Fig. 6 (Alexander and DeLong, 1985b).

How the functionally similar clusters of neurons in the putamen and SMZs correspond to the recently described anatomic compartments of the striatum, such as the patches of terminal label characteristic of corticostriate and thalamostriate projections (Goldman and Nauta, 1977; Jones et al., 1977), the cellular islands of the striatum (Goldman-Rakic, 1982) or the patterns of dopamine histofluorescence, acetylcholinesterase activity and enkephalin immunoreactivity (Graybiel et al., 1981; Graybiel and Hickey, 1982), remains to be deter-

Fig. 5. Locations of neurons related to active movements or passive manipulations of the leg (△), arm (●), mouth or face (○) at a single coronal lever (anterior 14) from one hemisphere. Arm symbols with adjacent letters indicate the locations of neurons responsive to passive manipulations of the shoulder (S), elbow (E), wrist (W) or fingers (F). Arm symbols without adjacent letters show the locations of neurons related to active, but not passive, arm movements. Lateral is to the left. Reproduced, with permission, from Experimental Brain Research (Crutcher and DeLong, 1984a).

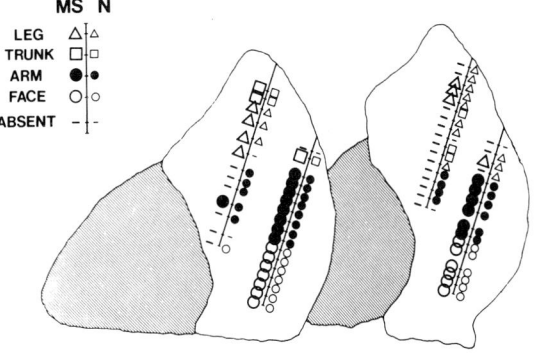

Fig. 6. Microelectrode penetrations through the putamen of one monkey at two anteroposterior levels (A16 and A14, left to right). To the right of each track are indicated the anatomic foci of the sensorimotor response areas of neurons (N) sampled at 250–500-μm intervals. The effects of microstimulation (MS) at each neuronal recording site are indicated for each site on the left side of each track. Note the dorsolateral-ventromedial gradient for sequential representation of leg-arm-face, both for the neuronal and the microstimulation maps. Reproduced, with permission from the American Physiological Society, from the Journal of Neurophysiology (Alexander and DeLong, 1985b).

ters contained neurons whose activity was related only to active arm movements while others contained neurons related to both passive and active arm movements. Clusters of neurons with sensory driving were organized by joints, i.e., all or most neurons in a cluster responded best to passive movements of the same joint. Within the "arm" area of the putamen there appear to be multiple clusters of neurons related to movements about individual joints.

mined. The results of single cell and microstimulation studies suggest that there may be a functional correlate to these anatomical subunits. Moreover, it is possible that the clusters of functionally similar neurons may represent the basic functional units of the striatum, analogous to the functional columns of the neocortex (Georgopoulos et al., 1983).

Somatosensory inputs

A significant proportion of movement-related neurons in the putamen and GP also respond to natural somatosensory stimulation (DeLong and Georgopoulos, 1979; Georgopoulos et al., 1983). For the putamen, 41% of arm movement-related cells responded to somatosensory stimuli. Essentially all parts of each limb are represented by ensembles of putamen neurons with response areas ranging in size from a single to several joints. Driving from the proximal portions of the arm was more commonly observed than from the distal. The preponderance of somatosensory responses in both putamen and GP was from deep rather than superficial structures and the majority (82%) responded to joint rotation. Only 5% of neurons in the putamen had cutaneous receptive fields on the glabrous skin of the hand and none responded to light touch of the hairy skin of the arm. The responses of neurons to controlled passive displacements of the elbow produced by application of load during a behavioral task were also studied. Of putamen neurons which responded to passive manipulations of the elbow or shoulder, 74% responded to load application at latencies between 25 and 50 mseconds; neuronal response latencies were somewhat later in GP (DeLong et al., 1985). Given the neuronal response latencies to perturbations observed in the sensory and motor cortices (Evarts, 1973) and the slow conduction velocity of corticostriatal axons (Liles, 1974), these short-latency responses are consistent with a "sensory" input to the putamen from the cortex. Neurons with short-latency, "sensory" responses typically exhibited highly specific directional and amplitude relations. These findings indicate that the putamen receives somatosensory information of a specific and spatially restricted nature and suggest that these inputs may be used to initiate, control or monitor ongoing movements.

These findings are in contrast to some earlier studies which indicated that striatal neurons have large receptive fields (Anderson et al., 1976; Harper and Lidsky, 1977; Sedgwick and Williams, 1967) or are responsive to polysensory stimuli (Albe-Fessard et al., 1960; Krauthamer, 1979; Sedgwick and Williams, 1967). These discrepancies may be due to the fact that most of the studies cited above were in the caudate nucleus of the cat, which receives major inputs from other areas of the cortex in addition to those from the sensorimotor cortex, whereas our study was carried out in that portion of the primate striatum which receives its major input from the sensorimotor cortex, i.e., the putamen. Species differences and anesthesia may also be significant factors.

The observation that more cells were related to the proximal than the distal arm is consistent with the prevalent view that the basal ganglia play a major role in the control of proximal musculature and posture (Martin, 1967). However, it should be emphasized that many neurons are clearly related to active movements and/or passive stimulation of the distal arm or leg. Moreover, recent studies in the putamen (Alexander and DeLong, 1985a,b) indicate a significant effect of microstimulation on distal arm and leg musculature. Clinically, as well, it is recognized that impairment of distal portions of the limbs in diseases such as Parkinsonism and Huntingtons Disease is as great as the proximal impairment. Together, these findings indicate that the basal ganglia are concerned with the control of distal, as well as proximal, limb musculature.

Initiation of movement

In reaction-time tasks it has been found that most changes in neuronal discharge in the basal ganglia begin after the first EMG changes (Aldridge et al., 1980; Crutcher and DeLong, 1984b; DeLong and Georgopoulos, 1981; Georgopoulos et al., 1983). Overall, changes in neuronal discharge occur later in the basal ganglia than in the motor cortex. In the putamen (Crutcher and DeLong, 1984b) changes in discharge rate occurred before the first EMG changes in about one-fourth of the cells. In GPe, GPi and subthalamic nucleus (STN) (Georgopoulos et al., 1983) the percentage was, respectively, 24, 11 and 29%. By comparing the results of studies in basal ganglia with those in motor cortex (Evarts, 1974; Thach, 1978), it appears that neuronal activation in the motor cortex may precede activation in the putamen and GP. It is noteworthy in this regard that lesions (Horak and Anderson, 1984a,b) and cooling (Beaubaton et al., 1981; Hore and Villis, 1980) of GP appear to have little effect on the timing of the onset of movement but have a significant effect on the speed of movement. It is interesting, in this respect, that microstimulation of the GP has been reported to slow limb movements when delivered after the first changes in EMG activity (Horak and Anderson, 1980). In fact, in the study by Beaubaton et al. reaction times were actually shortened. Taken together, these studies are consistent with the view that the basal ganglia in a reaction time task are more involved in the execution of the limb movement than in the timing of its initiation. A similar conclusion was reached from studies on Parkinsonism patients as well (Hallett and Khoshbin, 1980).

These findings do not rule out a role of the basal ganglia in the initiation of programming of movement per se. It is possible, for example, that the basal ganglia may play a role in the initiation of movement in other contexts, (e.g., self-initiated movements), or that different portions of the basal ganglia (e.g., the caudate or substantia nigra) may be involved more specifically in movement initiation. It is of interest that Neafsy et al. (1978) found a significant proportion of neurons in GP and entopedunculur nucleus of the cat that responded well before the first changes in EMG activity during self-initiated paw movements. In these studies, however, early changes occurred in the cortex and thalamus as well. Recently, Alexander (1984) has found that neurons in the primate putamen exhibit clear directionally selective changes in discharge following an instruction to prepare for a movement in a particular direction. Thus, the basal ganglia appear to play a role in the preparation for an upcoming movement as well as in its execution.

Movement parameters and muscle pattern

In order to evaluate further the finding (DeLong, 1971) of a relation of neural activity in basal ganglia neurons to the direction of arm movements and a possible relation of neural activity to the speed of movement (DeLong and Strick, 1974), the relation of neuronal discharge to movement parameters was studied in animals trained to perform a step-tracking task in which the amplitude, speed and direction of movement were varied (DeLong and Georgopoulos, 1979; DeLong et al., 1983b; Georgopoulos et al., 1983). Significant neuronal relations to both the direction and amplitude of movement were observed in GPe, GPi and STN during both the movement time (MT) and the initial premovement time (IPT), i.e., the 100 mseconds prior to the onset of movement, the period during which most of the changes in EMG began to occur. In general, the frequency of cell discharge was a linear function of the movement amplitude. The incidence of significant amplitude effects was highest in the MT, but the effects were also present in the IPT. The relations between cell discharge and peak velocity of movement in the step-tracking task were similar to those for the amplitude of movement.

The finding of significant directional effects in GP can be explained by the fact that neurons in both the putamen (Crutcher and DeLong, 1984b) and the STN (Georgopoulos et al., 1983), which both project to GP, show a strong relation to the direction of movement. The directional relations in the putamen and STN can, in turn, be accounted for by the inputs to these structures from the cerebral cortex, since both precentral and parietal neuron cells show significant relations to the direction of movement (Evarts, 1966; Georgopoulos et al., 1982; Schmidt et al., 1975).

In order to determine whether the activity of neurons in the basal ganglia is preferentially related to the direction of movement, per se, or to the underlying pattern of muscular activity, monkeys were trained in a separate study (Crutcher and DeLong, 1984b) to perform a visuomotor tracking task which required elbow flexion/extension movements with assisting and opposing loads. This task dissociated the direction of arm movement from the pattern of muscular activity. Of 120 arm movement-related neurons in the putamen 58% were related

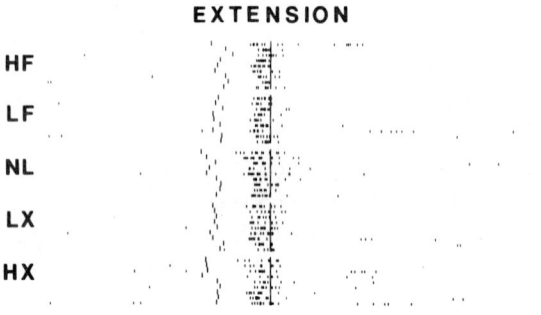

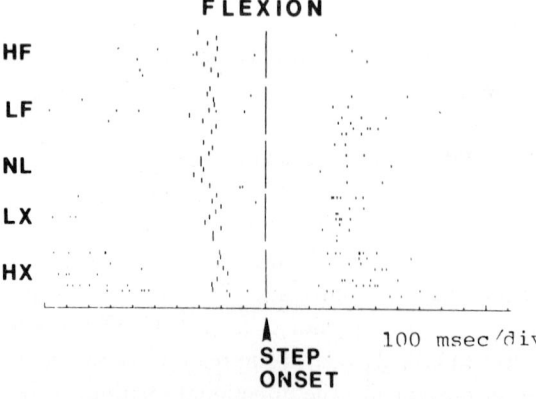

Fig. 7. Example of a neuron which was physically related to active elbow extension movements for each of five load conditions (HF, LF, NL, LX, HX). This neuron was inactive during elbow flexion movements. The dark vertical lines indicate the time of the onset of movement as determined from the first change in velocity. The dark vertical marks 200–300 mseconds prior to the onset of the step movement indicate the time of the stimulus to move for each trial. The time prior to these marks is the hold period. Reproduced, with permission, from Experimental Brain Research (Crutcher and DeLong, 1984b).

to the direction of arm movement whereas only 13% showed a pattern of activity "like muscle". A putamen neuron whose activity was related to direction is shown in Fig. 7. These results indicate that neurons in the putamen are predominantly related to the direction of movement, rather than to the activity of individual muscles. In an ongoing study in our laboratory similar relations to direction of movement have been found in GP (Mitchell et al., 1983). These results, together with those related to amplitude of movement (Georgopoulos et al., 1983), suggest that the basal ganglia may be involved in the control of parameters of movement rather than the selection of specific muscles. The significance of these directional effects is unclear, but it is of interest in this regard that Beaubaton et al. (1981) in a reaction time task found inaccuracies in movement produced by either reversible cooling or coagulation of GP. In fact, these workers suggested that movements were slowed because of these inaccuracies. The slowing of movements, however, appeared to be due to the loss of amplitude effects.

In a recent study of the effects of lesions of the GP on reaching movements in a reaction time task Horak and Anderson (1984a,b) reported that movements were slowed due to a generalized change in the amplitude and rate of rise of EMG activity in the muscles of the contralateral arm. In addition, microstimulation at different sites in GP produced either a speeding up or slowing of movement (Horak and Anderson, 1984b). With neither lesions nor microstimulation was the sequential activation of different muscles different from that of the controls. These findings are consistent with the data from single cell studies indicating a primary role of GP in modulating the amplitude of movement without effects on movement initiation or the pattern of muscular activity. It should be noted, however, that Hore and Villis (1980) reported increased co-contraction of agonist and antagonist muscles following cooling of the GP and putamen and suggested that the basal ganglia might play a role in the balance between agonists and antagonists for a particular motor act. Clearly, there is a need for further quantitative studies in primates of the effects of manipulations of basal ganglia output on motor performance.

In addition to the neuronal relations to movement amplitude and direction, several studies have shown a relation between the neuronal activity and force. In the putamen (Crutcher and DeLong, 1984b), for example, 44% of arm movement-related neurons had significant relations to the level of static load. Several previous studies in the basal ganglia have found relations of neuronal activity to steady force (Allum et al., 1983; Branch et al., 1980; DeLong, 1972; Liles, 1981, 1983). A significant proportion of neurons in the putamen also show significant dynamic load effects (Crutcher and DeLong, 1982; Liles, 1981, 1983), similar to those for neurons in the motor cortex (Cheney and Fetz, 1980; Conrad et al., 1977; Evarts, 1968).

The neuronal responses to movement may be regarded as the net result of various factors, including the direction and amplitude of movement. It is possible that a step change in cell discharge is related to movement direction, and that this step change is further modulated according to the amplitude of movement, as shown in Fig. 8. Direction and amplitude of movement may be separately controlled, since many neurons showed significant directional effects without amplitude effects, and others showed amplitude-related changes for only one direction of movement. These results may have implications for the broader issue of cerebral control of movement, since the observed neuronal relations in the putamen may largely reflect the nature of the inputs to this structure from the motor, pre-motor, and somatosensory cortices. Therefore, it is possible that similar neural relations to parameters of movement, independent of muscular activity, may also be found in these areas of cortex. In fact, a dissociation between muscular pattern and direction of intended movement was observed by Thach (1978) in the motor cortex and by Kalaska et al. (1984) in the parietal cortex. Therefore, the basal ganglia may function as a component of a more distributed system controlling parameters of movement.

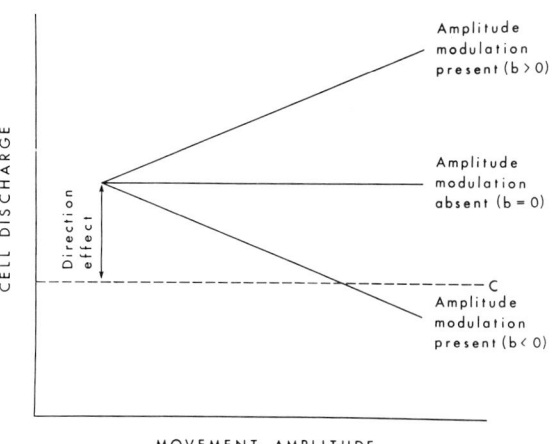

Fig. 8. Schematic diagram illustrating the hypothesis that single cell discharge in GP and STN may reflect both a movement direction-related step change and a superimposed movement amplitude-related modulation. Reproduced, with permission, from the Journal of Neuroscience (DeLong et al., 1983b).

These findings may be relevant to an understanding of the motor dysfunction in patients with basal ganglia disorders. Patients with Parkinson's disease, for example, frequently have difficulty in controlling the amplitude of their limb movements. Single-step, large-amplitude movements are impaired: these movements fall short of the target (Flowers, 1978), which is ultimately reached by a series of small-amplitude movements (Draper and Johns, 1964; Flowers, 1978). The mechanism of this phenomenon was partially elucidated recently by Hallett and Khoshbin (1980), who observed that Parkinsonian patients were unable to increase the amplitude of the agonist burst in step-tracking movements. Thus, large-amplitude movements were achieved by several small-amplitude steps. However, the duration of the EMG bursts were normal, as was the pattern of agonist and antagonist muscular activity. It is possible that loss of the pallidal output may account for the overall bradykinesia of Parkinsonian patients, whereas abnormal output may lead to the uncontrolled movements of patients with involuntary movements, such as chorea and hemiballismus.

How changes in basal ganglia output might influence movement more specifically may be considered in terms of the known patterns of neuronal activity and synaptic interactions along the pathway from putamen to the precentral motor fields. In the awake primate GPi/SNpr neurons exhibit a high tonic resting discharge (DeLong, 1971; Georgopoulos et al., 1983). By contrast, the spontaneous activity of putamen neurons is extremely low (Crutcher and DeLong, 1984b; DeLong and Strick, 1974). Since the projections from putamen to GPi and SNpr are largely inhibitory, with γ-amino butyric acid (GABA) as the primary neurotransmitter (Crossman et al., 1973; Fonnum et al., 1978; Kitai, 1981; Ohye et al., 1976; Yoshida et al., 1972) and, likewise, the projections from GPi and SNpr to the thalamus are GABAergic and inhibitory (Huffman et al., 1984; Kilpatrick et al., 1980; MacLeod et al., 1980; Penny and Young, 1981; Ueki et al., 1977; Uno and Yoshida, 1975), it is likely that the tonic inhibitory influence of GPi/SNpr on thalamic neurons is phasically decreased in association with increases in putamen inhibitory output during voluntary movement or microstimulation-evoked movements. It is noteworthy in this regard that phasic increases in neuronal activity in association with limb movement (Crutcher and DeLong, 1984a) are the rule in the putamen. Thus, the net effect of increased putamen output would be activation, through disinhibition, of the ventrolateral thalamus. This scheme is similar to that suggested previously by Kitai (1981) on the basis of a review of synaptic interactions in the basal ganglia.

Physiologic data in support of the hypothesis that a decrease in GPi/SNpr output may produce or facilitate movement have been obtained in the primate SNpr, where phasic decreases in discharge rate have been observed in association with saccadic eye movements (Hikosaka and Wurtz, 1983). Moreover, it has been shown that microinjections into the SNpr of the GABA agonist, muscimol, which reduces SNpr discharge, resulted in involuntary or irrepressible saccades (Hikosaka and Wurtz, 1985). It should be noted, however, that phasic increases as well as decreases in discharge rate have been observed in GPi neurons in association with conditioned limb movements (Georgopoulos et al., 1983). This may be accounted for behaviorally by the differences in requirements for control of limb and eye movements, such as the need for antagonist activity for the breaking of limb but not eye movements and the necessity of postural fixation of proximal joints for limb movements. Conceivably, input from the subthalamic nucleus might account for the phasic increases in GP discharge during movements.

In light of the aforementioned hypothesis, one might expect removal of GP tonic inhibitory influences upon thalamic neurons to result in dyskinesias or a facilitation of movement. In fact, slowing of movement has been most commonly observed following chronic lesions of GPi (Amato et al., 1978; DeLong and Coyle, 1979; Denny-Brown, 1962; Horak and Anderson, 1984b; Hore and Villis, 1980; Wilson, 1914). However, it remains to be determined whether acute reductions of GPi would evoke or facilitate limb movements, as is the case for eye movements following injection into SNpr. It is noteworthy that the converse test does not produce converse effects: injections of GABA antagonists into GPi, which should increase GPi output, do not result in involuntary limb movements in primates (Crossman et al., 1984).

The question of whether increased or decreased pallidal output results in movement has been addressed by Horak and Anderson (1984b), who have proposed, on the basis of their studies of the effects of lesions and electrical stimulation in and around the globus pallidus in monkeys, that increased, rather than decreased, pallidal outflow enables or facilitates rapid arm movements. As discussed previously, they found that movement times in a reaching task were permanently slowed opposite two of five hemispheres with kainic acid lesions that involved GPe, including one hemisphere in which the lesion involved both GPe and GPi (Horak and Anderson, 1984b). It is noteworthy, however, that in both of these animals the lesions included substantial portions of the putamen, making the interpretation somewhat uncertain. Moreover, from their stimulation studies Horak and Anderson (1984b) concluded that "movements were speeded primarily by stimulation at points in GPi". However, their data indicate that slowing of movement was seen at more GPi stimulation sites than was speeding of movement (20/77 vs. 26/77). Thus, these results do not seem to provide decisive support for either hypothesis with respect to the functional significance of increased pallidal outflow.

Summary

The results of recent neurophysiologic studies in trained primates suggest that basal ganglia output may play a role in scaling the amplitude of step movements by its effects on the magnitude of agonist EMG activity but that it is not primarily involved in the initiation of limb movement in a reaction time task or in the selection of specific muscles. These studies are generally consistent with the available data on limb movements in patients with Parkinson's disease, which likewise indicates a major deficit in the control of movement amplitude in step-tracking tasks, with little or no impairment of reaction time (DeLong and Georgopoulos, 1981; Neafsy et al., 1978) or disruption of the pattern of muscular activity. Evidence for a role of the basal ganglia in the preparation for movements has recently been determined. A role in other aspects of movement, such as motor programming and "complex" behavior, appears likely on the basis of both anatomical and physiological data (DeLong and Georgopoulos, 1981; Marsden, 1982; Divac, 1977, 1984; Oberg and Divac, 1979).

Acknowledgements

This work was supported by grants NS15417 and NS17678.

References

Albe-Fessard, D., Rocha-Miranda, C. and Oswaldo-Cruz, E. (1960) Activites evoquees dans le noyau caude du chat en response a des types divers d'afferences. II. Etude microphysiologique. Electroencephal. Clin. Neurophysiol., 12: 649–661.

Aldridge, J. W., Anderson, R. J. and Murphy, J. T. (1980) The role of the basal ganglia in controlling a movement initiated by visually presented cue. Brain Res., 192: 3–16.

Alexander, G. E. (1984) Instruction-dependent neuronal activity in primate putamen. Soc. Neurosci. Abstr., 10: 515.

Alexander, G. E. and DeLong, M. R. (1983) Motor responses to microstimulation of the putamen in the awake monkey. Soc. Neurosci. Abs., 9: 16.

Alexander, G. E. and DeLong, M. R. (1985a) Microstimulation of the primate neostriatum: I. Physiological properties of striatal microexcitable zones. J. Neurophysiol., 53: 1401–1416.

Alexander, G. E. and DeLong, M. R. (1985b) Microstimulation of the primate neostriatum: II. Somatotopic organization of striatal microexcitable zones and their relation to neuronal response properties. J. Neurophysiol., 53: 1417–1430.

Allum, J. H. J., Anner-Baratti, R. E. C. and Hepp-Raymond, M. C. (1983) Activity of neurons in the motor thalamus and globus pallidus during the control of isometric finger force in the monkey. In M. J. Paillard, W. Schultz and M. Wiesendanger (Eds.), Neural Coding of Motor Performance, Springer-Verlag, New York, pp. 194–203.

Amato, G., Trouche, E., Beaubaton, D. and Grangetto, A. (1978) The role of internal pallidal segment on the initiation of a goal-directed movement. Neurosci Lett., 9: 159–163.

Anderson, R. J., Aldridge, J. W. and Murphy, J. T. (1976) Somatic and visual feedback to monkey caudate nucleus during a central motor program. Soc. Neurosci. Abstr., 2: 59.

Asanuma, C., Thach, T. and Jones, E. G. (1983) Distribution of cerebellar terminations in the ventral lateral thalamic region of the monkey. Brain Res. Rev., 5: 237–265.

Beaubaton, D., Trouche, E., Amato, G. and Legallet, E. (1981) Perturbations du declenchement et de l'execution d'un mouvement visuellement guidé chez le babouin, au cours du refroidissement vu apres lesion du segment interne du globus pallidus. J. Physiol. Paris, 77: 107–118.

Branch, M. H., Crutcher, M. D. and DeLong, M. R. (1980) Globus pallidus: neuronal responses to arm loading. Soc. Neurosci. Abstr., 6: 272.

Carpenter, M. B., Nakano, K. and Kim, R. (1976) Nigrothalamic projections in the monkey demonstrated by autoradiographic technics. J. Comp. Neurol., 165: 401–416.

Cheney, P. D. and Fetz, E. E. (1980) Functional classes of primate corticomotoneuronal cells and their relation to active force. J. Neurophysiol., 44: 773–791.

Conrad, B., Wiesendanger, M., Matsunami, K. and Brooks, V. B. (1977) Precentral unit activity related to control of arm movements. Exp. Brain Res., 29: 85–95.

Crossman, A. R., Walker, R. J. and Woodruff, G. N. (1973) Picrotoxin antagonism of gamma-aminobutyric acid inhibitory responses and synaptic inhibition in the rat substantia nigra. Br. J. Pharmacol. Chemother., 49: 696–698.

Crossman, A. R., Sambrook, M. A. and Jackson, A. (1984) Experimental hemichorea/hemiballismus in the monkey. Study

on the intracerebral site of action in a drug-induced dyskinesia. Brain, 107: 579–596.
Crutcher, M. D. and DeLong, M. R. (1982) Functional organization of the primate putamen. Neurosci. Abstr., 8: 960.
Crutcher, M. D. and DeLong, M. R. (1984a) Single cell studies of the primate putamen. I. Functional organization. Exp. Brain Res., 53: 233–243.
Crutcher, M. D. and DeLong, M. R. (1984b) Single cell studies of the primate putamen. II. Relations to direction of movements and pattern of muscular activity. Exp. Brain Res., 53: 244–258.
DeLong, M. R. (1971) Activity of pallidal neurons during movement. J. Neurophysiol., 34: 414–427.
DeLong, M. R. (1972) Activity of basal ganglia neurons during movement. Brain Res., 40: 127–135.
DeLong, M. R. and Strick, P. L. (1974) Relation of basal ganglia, cerebellum, and motor cortex units to ramp and ballistic limb movements. Brain Res., 71: 327–335.
DeLong, M. R. and Coyle, J. T. (1979) Globus pallidus lesions in the monkey produced by kainic acid: histologic and behavioral effects. Appl. Neurophysiol., 42: 95–97.
DeLong, M. R. and Georgopoulos, A. P. (1979) Motor functions of the basal ganglia as revealed by studies of single cell activity in the behaving primate. In L. J. Poirier, T. L. Sourkes, and P. J. Bedard (Eds.), Advances in Neurology, Raven Press, New York, pp. 131–140.
DeLong, M. R. and Georgopoulos, A. (1981) Motor functions of the basal ganglia. In J. M. Brookhart, V. B. Mountcastle and V. B. Brooks (Eds.), Handbook of Physiology, The Nervous System, American Physiological Society, Bethesda, pp. 1017–1061.
DeLong, M. R., Georgopoulos, A. P. and Crutcher, M. D. (1983a) Cortico-basal ganglia relations and coding of motor performance. Exp. Brain Res., Suppl. 7: 30–40.
DeLong, M. R., Crutcher, M. D. and Georgopoulos, A. P. (1983b) Relations between movement and single cell discharge in the substantia nigra of the behaving monkey. J. Neurosci., 3: 1599–1606.
DeLong, M. R., Alexander, G. E., Georgopoulos, A. P., Crutcher, M. D., Mitchell, S. J. and Richardson, R. T. (1984) Role of basal ganglia in limb movements. Human Neurobiol., 2: 235–244.
DeLong, M. R., Crutcher, M. D. and Georgopoulos, A. P. (1985) The primate globus pallidus and subthalamic nucleus: functional organization. J. Neurophysiol., 53: 530–543.
Denny-Brown, D. (1962) The Basal Ganglia and their Relation to Disorders of Movement, Oxford University Press, London.
DeVito, J. L. and Anderson, M. E. (1982) An autoradiographic study of efferent connections of the globus pallidus. Exp. Brain Res., 46: 107–117.
Divac, I. (1977) Does the neostriatum operate as a functional entity?. In A. R. Cools, A. H. M. Lohman and J. H. L. Van den Bercken (Eds.), Psychobiology of the Striatum, Elsevier, Amsterdam, pp. 21–30.
Divac, I. (1984) Ciba Foundation Symposium 107: Functions of the Basal Ganglia, Pitman Press, London, pp. 201–215.
Draper, I. T. and Johns, R. J. (1964) The disordered movement in parkinsonism and the effect of drug treatment. Bull. Johns Hopkins Hosp., 115: 465–480.
Evarts, E. V. (1966) Pyramidal tract activity associated with a conditioned hand movement in the monkey. J. Neurophysiol., 29: 1011–1027.
Evarts, E. V. (1968) Relation of pyramidal tract activity to force exerted during voluntary movement. J. Neurophysiol., 31: 14–27.
Evarts, E. V. (1973) Motor cortex reflexes associated with learned movement. Science, 179: 501–503.
Evarts, E. V. (1974) Precentral and postcentral cortical activity in association with visually triggered movement. J. Neurophysiol., 37: 373–381.
Evarts, E. V. and Thach, W. T. (1969) Motor mechanisms of the CNS: cerebrocerebellar interrelations. Annu. Rev. Physiol., 31: 451–498.
Flowers, K. (1978) Some frequency response characteristics of Parkinsonism on pursuit tracking. Brain, 101: 19–34.
Fonnum, F., Gottesfeld, Z. and Grofova, I. (1978) Distribution of glutamate decarboxylase, choline acetyltransferase and aromatic amino acid decarboxylase in the basal ganglia of normal and operated rats. Evidence for striatopallidal, striatoentopeduncular and striatonigral GABAergic fibres. Brain Res., 143: 125–138.
Georgopoulos, A. P., Kalaska, J. F., Caminiti, R. and Massey, J. T. (1982) On the relations between the direction of two-dimensional arm movements and cell discharge in primate motor cortex. J. Neurosci., 2: 1527–1537.
Georgopoulos, A. P., DeLong, M. R. and Crutcher, M. D. (1983) Relations between parameters of step-tracking movements and single cell discharge in the globus pallidus and subthalamic nucleus of the behaving monkey. J. Neurosci., 3: 1586–1598.
Goldman-Rakic, P. S. (1982) Cytoarchitectonic heterogeneity of the primate neostriatum: Subdivision into Island and Matrix cellular compartments. J. Comp. Neurol., 205: 398–413.
Goldman, P. S. and Nauta, W. J. H. (1977) An intricately patterned prefronto-caudate projection in the rhesus monkey. J. Comp. Neurol., 171: 369–386.
Graybiel, A. M. and Hickey, T. L. (1982) Chemospecificity of ontogenetic units in the striatum: Demonstration by combining ^{3}H-thymidine neuronography and histochemical staining. Proc. Natl. Acad. Sci. U.S.A., 79: 198–202.
Graybiel, A. M., Pickel, V. M., Joh, T. H., Reis, D. J. and Ragsdale, C. W. Jr. (1981) Direct demonstration of a correspondence between the dopamine islands and acetylcholinesterase patches in the developing striatum. Proc. Natl. Acad. Sci. U.S.A., 78: 5871–5875.
Hallett, M. and Khoshbin, S. (1980) A physiological mechanism of bradykinesia. Brain, 103: 301–314.
Harper, J. A. and Lidsky, T. I. (1977) Trigeminal influences on

caudate and substantia nigra units. Soc. Neurosci. Abstr., 3: 38.

Hikosaka, O. and Wurtz, R. H. (1983) Visuomotor functions of monkey substantia nigra I: relation of sensory responses to saccades. J. Neurophysiol., 49: 1230–1240.

Hikosaka, O. and Wurtz, R. H. (1985) Modification of saccadic eye movements by GABA-related substances. II. Effects of muscimol in the monkey substantia nigra pars reticulata. J. Neurophysiol., 53: 292–308.

Horak, F. B. and Anderson, M. E. (1980) Effects of the globus pallidus on rapid arm movement in monkeys. Soc. Neurosci. Abstr., 6: 565.

Horak, F. V. and Anderson, M. E. (1984a) Influence of globus pallidus on arm movements in monkeys. I. Effects of kainic acid-induced lesions. J. Neurophysiol. 52: 290–304.

Horak, F. V. and Anderson, M. E. (1984b) Influence of globus pallidus on arm movements in monkeys. II. Effects of stimulation. J. Neurophysiol., 52: 305–322.

Hore, J. and Villis, T. (1080) Arm movement performance during reversible basal ganglia lesions in the monkey. Exp. Brain Res., 39: 217–228.

Huffman, R. D., Felpel, L. P. and Lum, J. (1984) An extracellular microelectrode study of globus pallidus and cerebellar projections to the thalamus in the monkey. Soc. Neurosci. Abstr., 10: 180.

Johnson, T. N. and Rosvold, H. E. (1971) Topographic projections on the globus pallidus and the substantia nigra of selectively placed lesions in the precommissural caudate nucleus and putamen in the monkey. Exp. Neurol., 33: 584–596.

Jones, E. G., Coulter, J. D., Burton, H. and Porter, R. (1977) Cells of origin and terminal distribution of corticostriatal fibers arising in the sensory-motor cortex of monkeys. J. Comp. Neurol., 173: 53–80.

Kalaska, J. F., Hyde, M. L. and Wechsler, R. (1984) Relative effect of movement direction vs direction of applied load. Soc. Neurosci. Abstr., 10: 738.

Kalil, K. (1981) Projections of the cerebellar and dorsal column nuclei upon the thalamus of the rhesus monkey. J. Comp. Neurol., 195: 25–50.

Kemp, J. M. and Powell, T. P. S. (1970) The corticostriate projection in the monkey. Brain, 93: 525–546.

Kemp, J. M. and Powell, T. P. S. (1971) The structure of the caudate nucleus of the cat: light and electron microscopy. Phil. Trans. R. Soc. Lond. B., 262: 383–401.

Kilpatrick, I. C., Starr, M. S., Fletcher, A., James, T. A. and MacLeod, N. K. (1980) Evidence for a GABAergic nigrothalamic pathway in the rat. I. Behavioral and biochemical studies. Exp. Brain Res., 40: 45–54.

Kitai, S. T. (1981) Electrophysiology of the corpus striatum and brain stem integrating systems. In J. M. Brookhart, V. B. Mountcastle and V. B. Brooks (Eds.), Handbook of Physiology: The Nervous System, American Physiological Society, Bethesda, pp. 997–1016.

Krauthamer, G. M. (1979) Sensory functions of the neostriatum. In I. Divac and R. G. E. Oberg (Eds.), The Neostriatum, Pergamon Press, Oxford, pp. 263–290.

Kunzle, H. (1975) Bilateral projections from precentral motor cortex to the putamen and other parts of the basal ganglia. An autoradiographic study in *Macaca fascicularis*. Brain Res., 88: 195–209.

Kunzle, H. (1978) An autoradiographic analysis of the efferent connections from premotor and adjacent prefrontal regions (areas 6 and 9) in *Macaca fascicularis*. Brain Behav. Evol., 15: 185–234.

Kuo, J. S. and Carpenter, M. B. (1973) Organization of pallidothalamic projections in the rhesus monkey. J. Comp. Neurol., 151: 201–236.

Liles, S. L. (1974) Single-unit responses of caudate neurons to stimulation of frontal cortex, substantia nigra and entopeduncular nucleus in cats. J. Neurophysiol., 37: 254–265.

Liles, S. L. (1975) Cortico-striatal evoked potentials in the monkey (*Macaca mulatta*). Electroencephal. Clin. Neurophys., 38: 121–129.

Liles, S. L. (1978) Unit activity in the putamen associated with conditioned arm movements: Topographic organization. Fed. Proc., 27: 396.

Liles, S. L. (1979) Topographic organization of neurons related to arm movement in the putamen. In T. N. Chase, N. S. Wexler and A. Barbeau (Eds.), Advances in Neurology, Raven Press, New York, pp. 155–162.

Liles, S. L. (1981) Activity of neurons in the putamen during movement and postural fixation of the arm against external loads. Soc. Neurosci. Abstr., 7: 778.

Liles, S. L. (1983) Activity of neurons in the putamen associated with wrist movements in the monkey. Brain Res., 263: 156–161.

MacLeod, N. K., James, T. A., Kilpatrick, I. C. and Starr, M. S. (1980) Evidence for a GABAergic nigrothalamic pathway in the rat. II. Electrophysiological studies. Exp. Brain Res., 40: 55–61.

Marsden, C. D. (1982) The mysterious motor function of the basal ganglia: the Robert Wartenberg Lecture. Neurology, 32: 514–539.

Martin, J. P. (1967) The Basal Ganglia and Posture, Pitman, London.

Mehler, W. R. (1971) Idea of a new anatomy of the thalamus. J. Psychiatr. Res., 8: 203.

Mitchell, S. J., Richardson, R. T., Baker, F. H. and DeLong, M. R. (1983) Activity of neurons in the globus pallidus in relation to direction of movement or pattern of muscular activity. Soc. Neurosci. Abstr., 9: 951.

Neafsy, E. J., Hull, C. D. and Buchwald, N. A. (1978) Preparation of movement in the cat. II. Unit activity in the basal ganglia and thalamus. Electroencephal. Clin. Neurophysiol., 44: 714–723.

Oberg, R. G. E. and Divac, I. (1979) "Cognitive" functions of the neostriatum. In R. G. E. Oberg (Ed.), The Neostriatum, Pergamon Press, New York, pp. 291–313.

Ohye, C., Le Guyander, C. and Feger, J. (1976) Responses of subthalamic and pallidal neurons to striatal stimulation: an extracellular study on awake monkeys. Brain Res., 111: 241–252.

Penny, J. B. Jr. and Young, A. B. (1981) GABA as the pallidothalamic neurotransmitter: implications for basal ganglia function. Brain Res., 207: 195–199.

Schell, G. R. and Strick, P. L. (1984) The origin of thalamic inputs to the arcuate premotor and supplementary motor areas. J. Neurosci., 4: 539–560.

Schmidt, E. M., Jost, R. G. and Davis, K. K. (1975) Reexamination of the force relationship of cortical cell discharge patterns with conditioned wrist movements. Brain Res., 83: 213–223.

Sedgwick, E. M. and Williams, T. D. (1967) The response of single units in the caudate nucleus to peripheral stimulation. J. Physiol., 189: 281–298.

Szabo, J. (1967) The efferent projections of the putamen in the monkey. Exp. Neurol., 19: 463–476.

Szabo, J. (1970) Projections from the body of the caudate nucleus in the rhesus monkey. Exp. Neurol., 27: 1–15.

Thach, W. T. (1978) Correlation of neural discharge with pattern and force of muscular activity, joint position and direction of intended next movement in motor cortex and cerebellum. J. Neurophysiol., 41: 654–676.

Ueki, A., Uno, M., Anderson, A. and Yoshida, M. (1977) Monosynaptic inhibition of thalamic neurons produced by stimulation of the substantia nigra. Esperientia, 33: 1480–1482.

Uno, M. and Yoshida, M. (1975) Monosynaptic inhibition of thalamic neurons produced by stimulation of the pallidal nucleus in cats. Brain Res., 99: 377–380.

Wilson, S. A. K. (1914) An experimental research into the anatomy and physiology of the corpus striatum. Brain, 36: 427–492.

Yeterian, E. H. and Van Hoesen, G. W. (1978) Cortico-striate projections in the rhesus monkey: The organization of certain corticocaudate connections. Brain Res., 139: 43–63.

Yoshida, M., Rabin, A. and Anderson, M. (1972) Monosynaptic inhibition of pallidal neurons by axon collaterals of caudatonigral fibers. Exp. Brain Res., 15: 333–347.

Role of the basal ganglia in the initiation of saccadic eye movements

Robert H. Wurtz and Okihide Hikosaka

Laboratory of Sensorimotor Research, National Eye Institute, National Institutes of Health, Bethesda, MD 20205, U.S.A.

Introduction

The impetus for the study of the basal ganglia in relation to vision and eye movements comes from what we now know about the connection of this structure to the superior colliculus (SC), a structure recognized as a critical station for the initiation of saccadic eye movements (Sparks et al., 1976; Wurtz and Albano, 1980). One output pathway of the basal ganglia, the pars reticulata of the substantia nigra (SNr), projects to the intermediate layers of the SC (Graybiel, 1978; Jayaraman et al., 1977), as shown schematically in Fig. 1. These cells in the intermediate layers discharge before saccadic eye movements when those eye movements are directed to one region of the visual field, the movement field of the cells. Stimulation of these intermediate layer cells leads to initiation of saccadic eye movements to the area of the movement field of the adjacent cells. Finally, cells in the intermediate layers of the SC have direct projections to the brainstem areas (mesencephalic reticular formation, MRF; paramedian pontine reticular formation, PPRF) where pre-oculomotor neurons are located, as is illustrated in Fig. 1.

The SNr projection to the SC represents one of the most prominent inputs to the intermediate layers of the SC. Furthermore, as indicated in Fig. 1, the SNr is not an isolated structure but can be regarded as part of a pathway that extends from the frontal cortex (probably including the frontal eye fields — FEF) through the caudate nucleus (C) within the basal ganglia, to the SC. The SNr also projects to thalamic nuclei that in turn project back upon the frontal cortex so that the frontal cortex and basal ganglia are intimately connected (Graybiel and Ragsdale, 1979). The FEF also projects directly to the intermediate layers of the SC (Leichnetz et al., 1982) and this cortical structure rep-

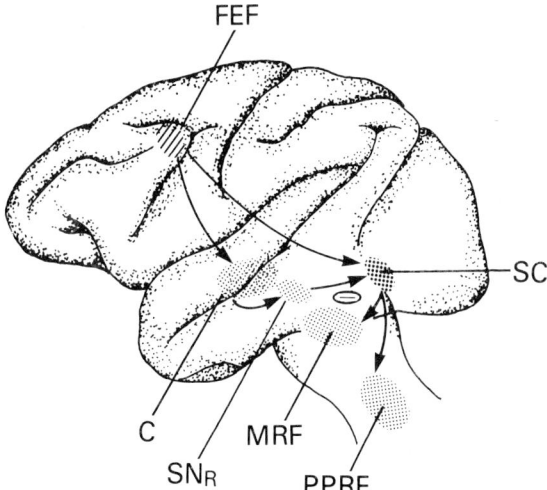

Fig. 1. Location of SNr in the pathway for the initiation of saccadic eye movements. The substantia nigra is one of the two most prominent inputs to the superior colliculus (SC), the other being from the frontal eye field (FEF). The superior colliculus in turn projects to brainstem areas concerned with horizontal (PPRF) and vertical (MRF) saccadic eye movements. The substantia nigra probably also receives input via the caudate (C) from frontal cortex, including the frontal eye field. The SNr action on the SC is probably inhibitory, as indicated by the minus sign.

resents a second prominent input to these layers (Fig. 1). Previous investigations of possible inputs to the intermediate layers of the SC have concentrated on the FEF, particularly those cells whose response to visual stimuli is modified by saccadic eye movements (Mohler et al., 1973; Goldberg and Bruce, 1985).

In a recent series of experiments (Hikosaka and Wurtz, 1983a,b,c,d,e, 1985a,b) we have investigated the relation of cells in the SNr to visual stimulation and the initiation of saccadic eye movements. This report is intended to summarize those aspects of the experiments that are related to the initiation of saccadic eye movements. After describing the general characteristics of cells in the SNr, we will consider a particular type of cell that discharges in relation to the initiation of saccades made to remembered targets. We will then summarize experiments showing the relation of the SNr to the SC as demonstrated both by antidromic stimulation and by altering the action of the presumed transmitter, γ-amino butyric acid (GABA), between the SNr and the SC. This series of experiments on visual-oculomotor functions of the basal ganglia leads us to conclude that the SNr conveys a signal to the SC by a pause in a tonic inhibitory drive and that this signal is probably most important for the initiation of saccades made in the absence of direct sensory control of which saccades to remembered targets is an example. These conclusions may have implications for understanding the function of the basal ganglia in the initiation of skeletal movements as well as for the initiation of saccadic eye movements.

Characteristics of substantia nigra neurons

Substantia nigra neurons were studied in awake, behaving Rhesus monkeys using the general procedures described previously (Wurtz, 1969). The behavioral methods used allowed analysis of the sensory properties of the cells within the SNr and the relation of the discharge of these cells to the initiation of saccadic eye movements. We trained the monkey to fixate on a small spot of light for several seconds and, while he did so, a second spot of light was projected onto the screen in front of him. This second spot was used to analyze the receptive field of a particular cell. Alternatively, if the fixation spot was switched off, as the second spot of light came on, this spot could be used as the target for a saccadic eye movement. In either case, on successive trials the monkey was asked to fixate or make saccades consistently, thus allowing analysis of the particular cell under study. The detailed methods used for single cell recording, recording eye movements, and control of behavior, have been described previously (Hikosaka and Wurtz, 1983a).

All cells studied were in the SNr. These neurons are presumed to be GABAergic, in contrast to the neurons of the SN pars compacta whose neurons are dopaminergic and project primarily back onto the striatum. Even within the SNr, the area where cell discharge is related to visual stimulation or saccadic eye movements is limited to a lateral subregion that lies adjacent to the cerebral peduncle. It is this lateral region that on anatomical grounds (Beckstead et al., 1981) has been indicated as the location of cells projecting to the SC in the monkey.

The salient characteristic of cells studied within the SNr is a high rate of discharge, frequently 80–100 spikes/sec, as can be seen in the histogram of Fig. 2A. The signal conveyed by these cells is always a decrease in the discharge rate, whether the change is related to a visual stimulus or the initiation of an eye movement. The response of one of these cells, a decrease in the discharge rate, is shown in Fig. 2B. Here, the onset of a spot of light in one part of the visual field is accompanied by a pause in the discharge rate of the SNr neuron.

One further characteristic of these SNr cells should be emphasized: their change in discharge rate is rarely related to just one event, but instead their response may be different as the experimental conditions vary. We therefore refer to the response of a cell not to the cell itself, and we have observed at least ten different types of responses (Hikosaka and Wurtz, 1983a). For example, the same cell might have a response to a visual stimulus as well as a change in discharge with a saccade made to a visual stimulus. Thus, in contrast to primary visual

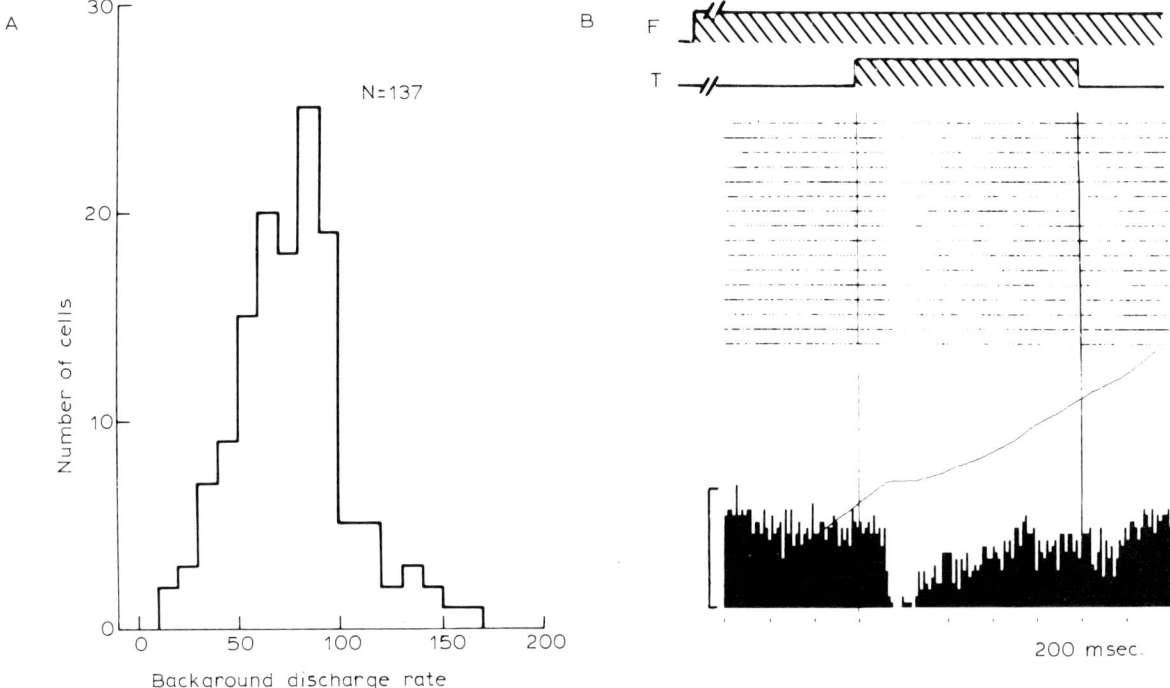

Fig. 2. Characteristics of SNr cells. A. High rate of discharge shown in this histogram was obtained while the monkey was alert but before he began to fixate. B. The signal conveyed by cells in the substantia nigra is a pause in activity shown here in response to the onset of a visual stimulus. In this and subsequent figures each cell discharge is indicated by a dot, successive presentations of stimuli or eye movements by successive lines, and the sum of these individual discharges is shown on the time histogram and the cumulative time histogram. Calibration for the histogram is 100 discharges/sec/trial; bin width is 12 mseconds. Time between scale marks is indicated in the lower right corner; cell number is in the lower left corner. Subsequent figures use the same conventions. After Hikosaka and Wurtz (1983a).

areas, or premotor areas, these SNr cells cannot be named by the occurrence of just one response. We will not dwell further on this multiple response relationship, but it is present in almost all cells to be described and must be a critical feature of SNr organization.

Saccades to remembered targets

Those SNr cells that discharge in relation to saccadic eye movements differed from most SC cells in a fundamental way. While most cells in the intermediate layers of the SC show a change of discharge before the onset of saccades made spontaneously in the light or dark, cells in the SNr do not. We did not encounter cells that discharged before such spontaneous eye movements. Instead, many SNr cells change their discharge only before saccades made to visual targets, as is the case for some cells in the SC (Mohler and Wurtz, 1976; Mays and Sparks, 1980). Still other cells have a striking characteristic that has not been described in the SC and only occasionally in the FEF (Bruce and Goldberg, 1985). These cells show a discharge in relation to a target that is no longer present but whose location must be remembered as the target for a saccade (Hikosaka and Wurtz, 1983c).

Fig. 3A shows an example of such a response and the experimental paradigm used to demonstrate the characteristics of this neural response. In this task, while the monkey fixated, a small spot of light flashed at one point on the screen in front of him.

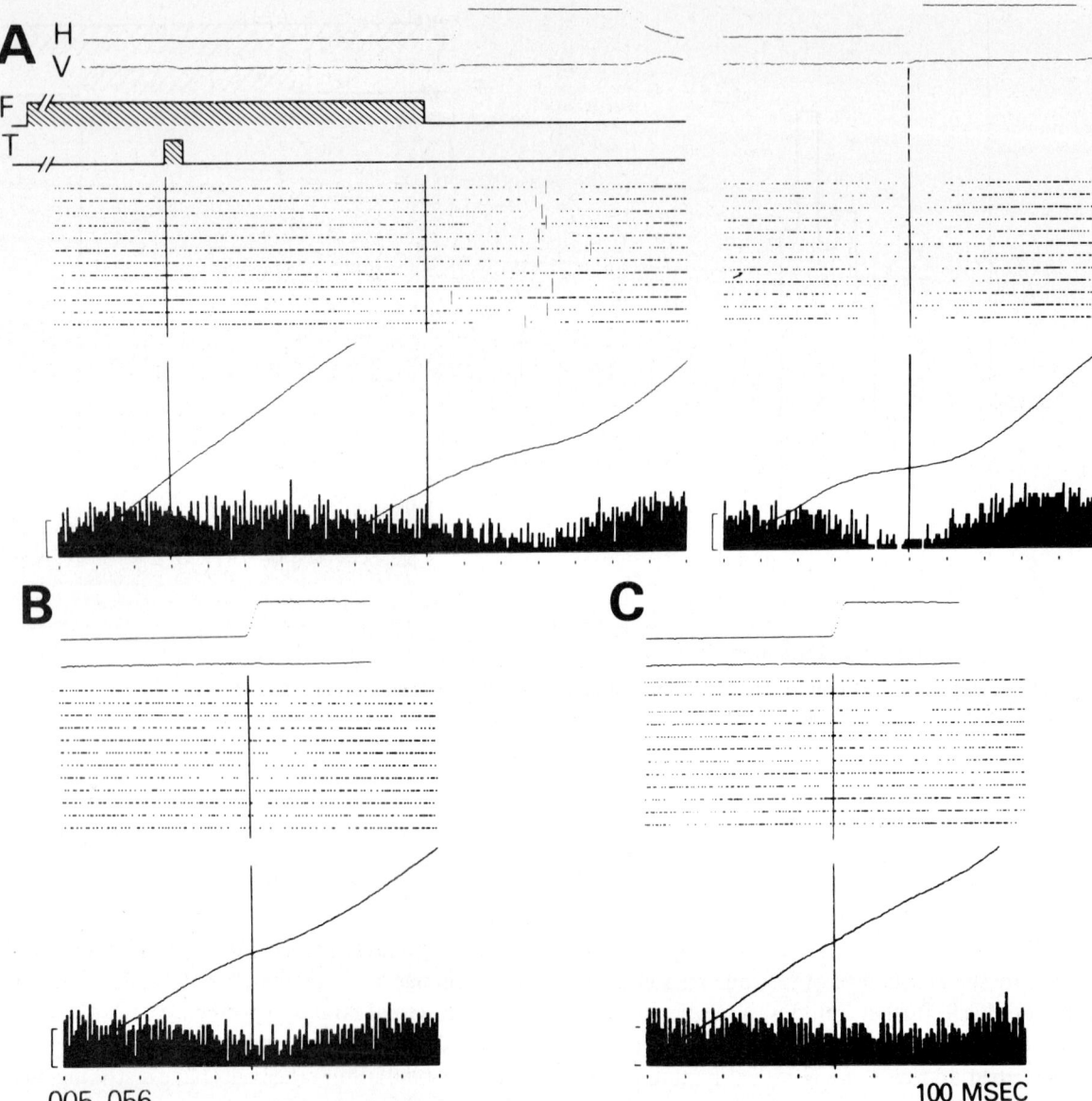

Fig. 3. Change in discharge of a substantia nigra cell with saccades to a remembered visual target. A. The schematic drawing shows the sequence of stimuli and saccadic eye movements in this experimental task. A flash of light (T) during the fixation period (F) identified the location to which the monkey was required to make a saccadic eye movement after the fixation point went off. The monkey obtained a reward if he was near the target since he could then detect the return of the target and its subsequent dim (not shown in the figure). The eye movement to the target location was not permitted until after the fixation point went off. Sample horizontal (H) and vertical (V) eye movements are shown. The time at which the monkey made the saccade to the stimulus on each trial is indicated by the tick marks on the dot pattern on the left. On the right the same records, which are aligned on the offset of the fixation point on the left, are lined up on the onset of the saccade. The cell showed a decrease in discharge rate when the monkey made saccades to the remembered target. B. For the same cell, saccades to a visual target at the same location as the flashed target in A produced no such clear decrease in discharge rate. C. Saccades made spontaneously in the dark also were not accompanied by a decrease in discharge rate. The eye movement trace in C is used as an example to indicate the onset of the saccade, not its amplitude. After Hikosaka and Wurtz (1983c).

The monkey was required to continue fixating until the fixation point went off, at which time he was allowed to make a saccade. If the saccade was made to the location of the briefly flashed spot, the monkey was able to detect the reappearance of the spot and its subsequent dimming (not shown in the figure) in order to obtain a reward. For the type of cell shown in Fig. 3A, when the monkey made this saccade to the remembered target, there was a decrease in the discharge rate of the cell associated with the saccade (indicated by the tick marks in the dot pattern on the left of Fig. 3A). This decrease in discharge is shown more clearly if the same single cell activity shown in Fig. 3A on the left is realigned on the onset of the saccadic eye movement, as is the case in Fig. 3A, right. In this paradigm, then, the monkey had to remember the location of the visual target and make a subsequent saccade to that target, and in this case the cell showed a decrease in activity related to that saccade.

Fig. 3B shows that if the monkey was required to make a saccade to the same target used in Fig. 3A while it was actually present, there was no such change in discharge rate. In this paradigm, used to elicit saccades to visual targets, the visual target came on as the fixation point went off. Fig. 3C shows that this type of cell does not respond with spontaneous eye movements made in the dark. In this case, an eye movement made in the dark was not associated with any consistent decrease in discharge rate even though if the same saccade had been made to a remembered target there would have been such a decrease in discharge rate.

Other cells in the SNr show a decrease in discharge rate not in relation to saccades made to the remembered location of a target, but in relation to the onset of the visual stimulus that gives this remembered target information (Hikosaka and Wurtz, 1983c). Still other cells show a persisting change in activity between the time of the flashed target to be remembered and the saccade initiation to the target location. Fig. 4 shows such a change in discharge rate using the same paradigm as that used in Fig. 3. Now the discharge rate of the cell decreases after the flashed target is presented (Fig. 4, left) and stays at a lower level until the monkey

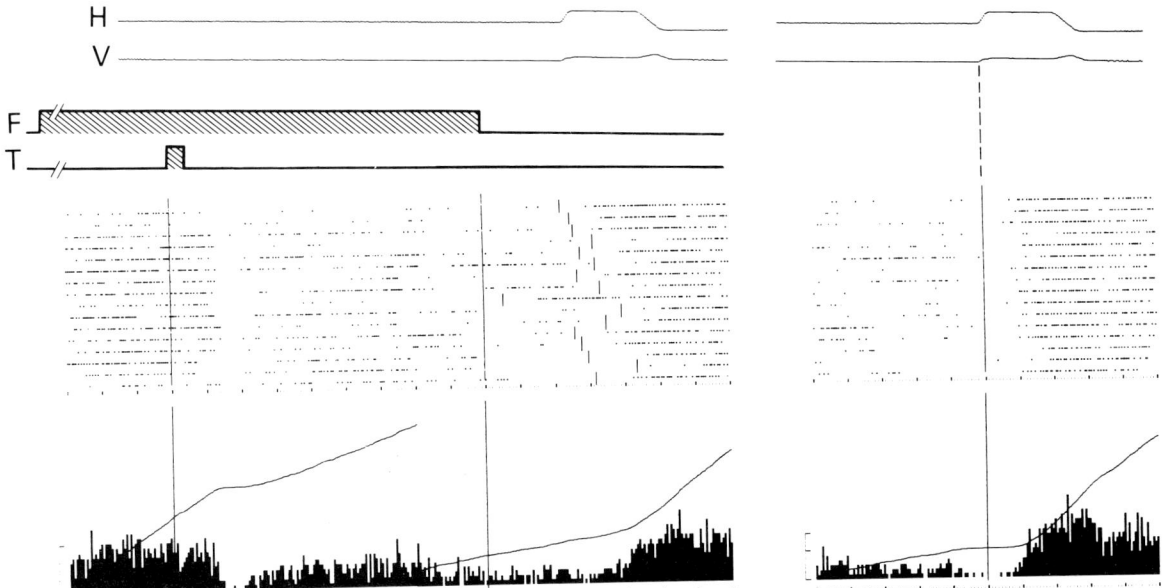

Fig. 4. Neural response persisting from onset of the flashed visual target until the saccade is made to the location of the remembered visual target. Onset of the 50 msecond target is indicated by T; onset of the saccade by the vertical tick mark on each line in the dot pattern on the left. On the right, the same records are aligned on the onset of the saccade made to the remembered visual target.

makes a saccade to the location of the flashed visual target (Fig. 4, right). This cell is an excellent candidate for the mechanism that might be preserving the information about the location of the briefly presented visual stimulus. The continuing change of discharge until the saccade is made is also reminiscent of quasi-visual cells described in the SC by Mays and Sparks (1980).

Inhibitory connection between substantia nigra and superior colliculus

The next step in our analysis was to determine whether the cells studied in the SNr that have a relation to visual and oculomotor activity were those that projected to the SC. While the anatomical studies cited previously suggest that this is the case, we had no way of knowing whether the particular cells we examined were those that projected to the SC. To try to determine how these cells in the SNr might project to the SC we electrically stimulated the SC and attempted to antidromically activate cells recorded in SNr. To do this, we recorded from the SNr, and at the same time recorded with a microelectrode inserted through a guide tube directed at the SC. This microelectrode in the SC allowed study of the response of cells to visual stimuli and their relation to saccadic eye movements so that the location of the electrode within the layers of the SC could be functionally established (Hikosaka and Wurtz, 1983d). We then stimulated within the SC and found that many cells in the SNr could be driven antidromically. In addition, we found that on a given penetration through the SC the threshold stimulation required to produce antidromic stimulation was usually lowest among cells typical of the intermediate collicular layers. There were several peaks in this curve as the electrode advanced through the presumed intermediate layers, possibly indicating separate groupings of axon terminals or axons of passage, but this profile has not been consistent from penetration to penetration. What was consistent was a drop in threshold as the electrode entered the intermediate layers. We concluded from these experiments that many of the cells in the SNr we have studied do indeed project to the intermediate layers of the SC.

These antidromic stimulation experiments also graphically illustrate the reciprocal change in discharge rate occurring within the SNr and the SC before the onset of saccadic eye movements, as illustrated in Fig. 5. The decrease in discharge rate of an SNr cell preceding a saccadic eye movement (Fig. 5, top) can be compared to the increase in discharge rate of an SC cell (Fig. 5, bottom). The

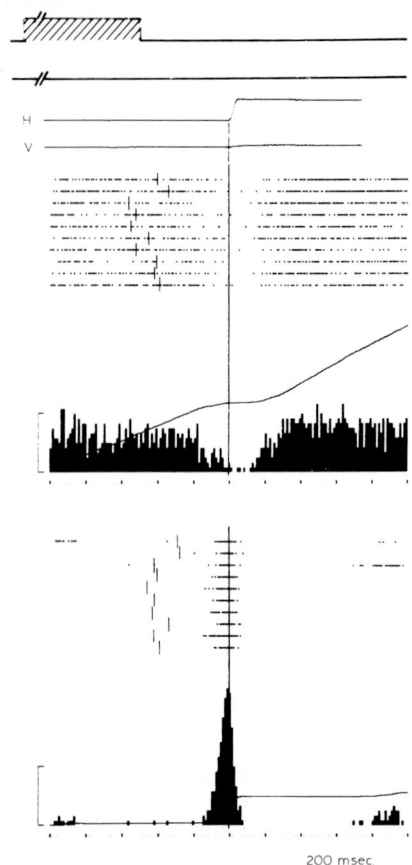

Fig. 5. Comparison of the discharge rate of a **substantia nigra** cell (top dot pattern and histograms) with that of a superior colliculus cell (bottom dot pattern and histograms) made as the monkey made saccades to a remembered visual target. The superior colliculus cell was recorded at the point in the superior colliculus where the substantia nigra cell could be antidromically activated by stimulation of the superior colliculus. The superior colliculus cell was one that discharged before saccades made under any condition. After Hikosaka and Wurtz (1983d).

SNr cell was antidromically activated by stimulation at the point where the SC cell was isolated. This does not mean that these cells are directly connected, nor does the figure show the simultaneous recording of SNr and SC activity since the data were gathered with saccades when the cells were studied separately. What Fig. 5 does illustrate is that the change in activity is the opposite in the SNr and the SC before the onset of a saccadic eye movement.

The hypothesis we developed about the relationship between these two structures is that the SNr produces a tonic inhibition upon the SC and that the pause in activity in the SNr either permits or facilitates the burst of discharge in the SC. This inhibitory connection between the two structures is consistent with observations made in the rat that have demonstrated that the transmitter action between the SNr and SC is inhibitory and that the transmitter itself is almost certainly GABA (see Hikosaka and Wurtz, 1985a, for references and discussion). While such confidence about the neural transmitter does not exist for the monkey, the comparatively high concentration of GABA present in the monkey SC (Fahn and Cote, 1968) suggests that the transmitter might be the same in the monkey. In any case, the variety of characteristics that we have studied directly in the monkey suggests that exploration of this hypothesis of an inhibitory mechanism might reveal both the nature of the connection between the SNr and the SC, and, more importantly, the functional system of which the SNr collicular pathway is a part.

Manipulation of GABA in superior colliculus

To alter the effect of the SNr on the SC, we injected a GABA agonist (muscimol) locally into the SC. The effect of muscimol should be to enhance artificially the inhibition that is normally exerted by the SNr and to reduce the efficiency of saccade initiation. The effect of an injection of a GABA antagonist (bicuculline) should be to block the inhibitory effects of the SNr acting on the SC and to increase efficiency of saccade initiation. In both cases it should be possible to determine whether the SNr connection to the SC is particularly important for saccades to remembered targets as opposed to those to visual targets.

In these experiments we first determined the area of the visual field to which single cells in the intermediate layers of the SC were related. We then implanted a guide tube which allowed us at a subsequent time to introduce a pipette into the SC. This pipette allowed injection of the muscimol agonist or antagonist and also carried a thin microelectrode that allowed us to identify again the area of the SC in which the electrode tip was located. By recording the movement fields of the cells at the tip of the electrode and by stimulating through the electrode to produce saccadic eye movements, we located the part of the visual field to which these cells in the intermediate layers were related. Following this localization, the monkey made saccades to a series of points throughout the visual field so that the latency, amplitude and velocity of the saccades could be determined. Saccades were made using both the paradigms already described that elicited saccades to visual targets or to the location of remembered targets. We then pressure injected between 1 and 5 μl of muscimol or bicuculline and determined the monkey's ability to make saccadic eye movements to the same set of targets. Details of these experiments are described in Hikosaka and Wurtz (1985a).

The effect of an injection of muscimol into the right SC is shown in Fig. 6. In A, the amplitude of the saccades evoked by electrical stimulation in the right SC both before and after the injection is indicated. The evoked saccades were horizontal and to the left; they did not change substantially after the injection of the muscimol, which is consistent with the expectation that the drug acts primarily on the GABA receptors of the SC cells, not on their axons, which should be activated by the electrical stimulation. The left visual field should be maximally affected by any injection near these cells in the right SC. Fig. 6B, PRE shows that saccades to visual targets located 5, 10 and 20° on the left and right horizontal meridian were comparable in la-

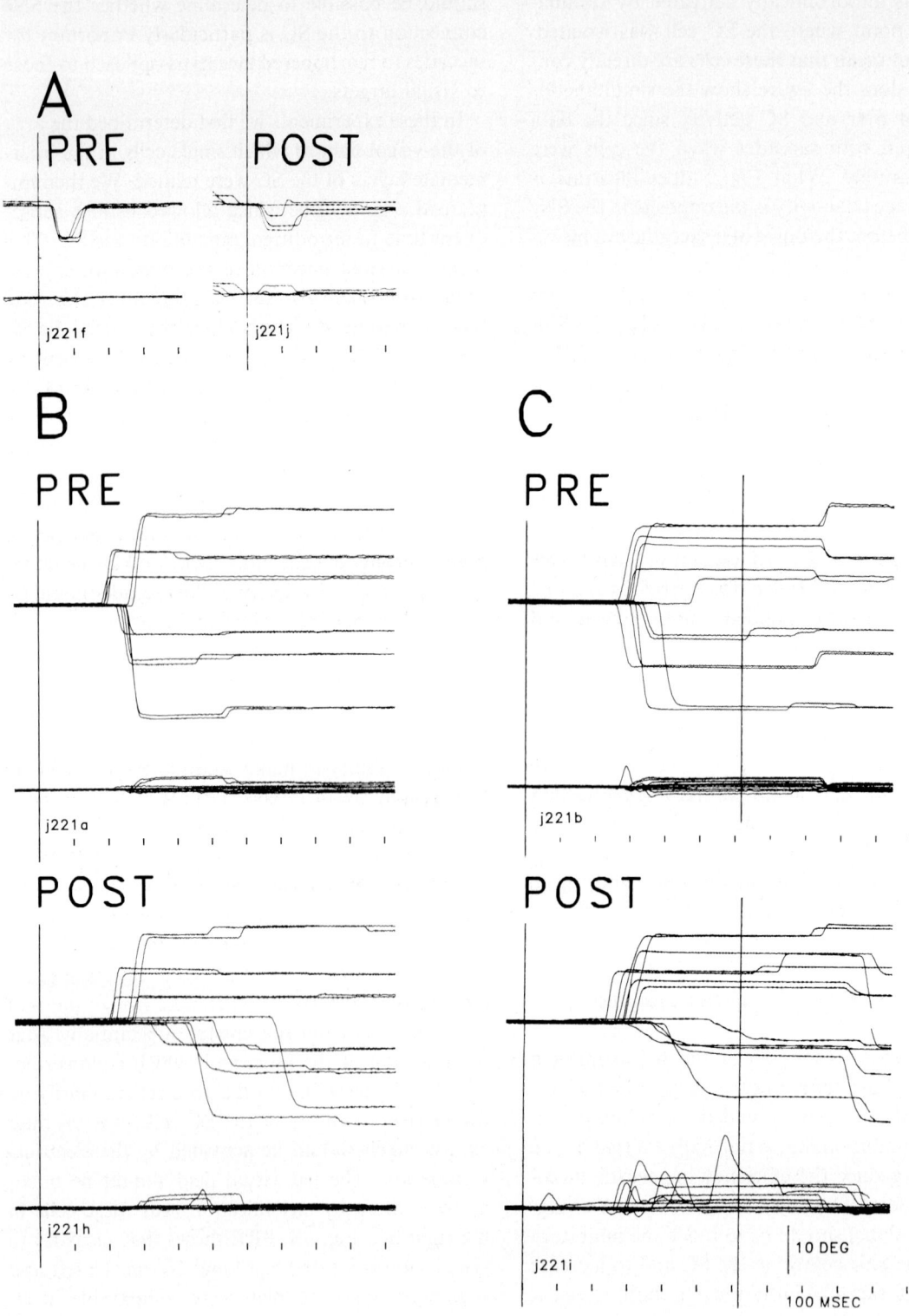

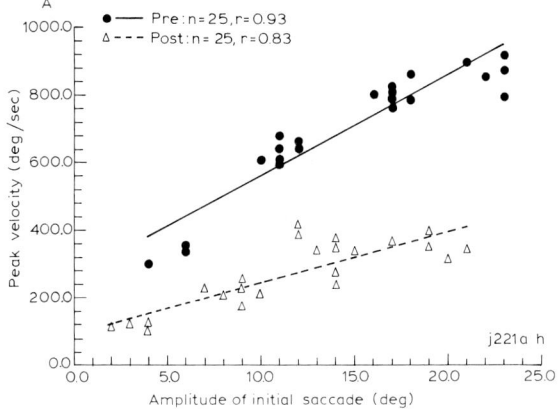

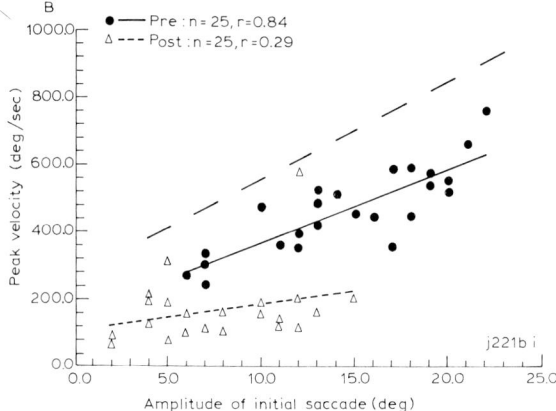

Fig. 7. Peak velocities of saccades to the contralateral side before (●) and after (△) injection of muscimol. Saccades to visual targets in A and saccades to remembered targets in B. Saccades were those made toward targets in the visual field most affected by the injection (between 135° and 225° polar angle in A, and between 157° and 225° in B: 0°, right; 180°, left). Amplitude and peak velocity of the saccade are determined using both horizontal and vertical components. Long dashed line in B is for saccades to visual targets before injection to allow comparison between saccades to visual and remembered targets. From Hikosaka and Wurtz (1985a).

tency, velocity and amplitude. Following an injection of muscimol (Fig. 6B, POST) the saccades to the right remain comparable to the preinjection saccades but the saccades to the left show an increase in latency, a decrease in velocity, but only slightly altered accuracy. The monkey could still get to the visual target even though his arrival on the target was delayed.

Fig. 7A shows a quantitative measure of the decrease in peak velocity following injection of muscimol. In this figure, the peak velocity of the first saccade made to the target is plotted against the amplitude of that saccade. The velocity for saccades to the affected left visual field area frequently became less than half the preinjection velocity.

Fig. 6C shows the effect on saccades to remembered targets before (PRE) and after (POST) the same injection of muscimol. Saccades to remembered targets were more severely disrupted than were saccades to the visual targets. Saccades to the location of previously present visual targets on the right and the left (at 5, 10 and 20°) had increased latencies and lower velocities, as was the case for saccades to visual targets, when the target was in the area of the left visual field affected by the injection. The peak velocity of the saccades to the remembered targets was reduced, as shown in Fig. 7B. However, since the velocity of saccades to remembered targets before the injection is lower than that to visual targets, the difference is comparatively small. The most striking effect of muscimol on saccades to remembered targets was the reduced accuracy of the saccades. The first saccades usually fell far short of target positions, as indicated by the large saccades correcting eye position after the targets reappeared. These corrective saccades were vis-

Fig. 6. Effects on saccades following injection of muscimol into the right superior colliculus. A. Saccades evoked by electrical stimulation in the right superior colliculus before (left, 22 μamp threshold) and after (right, 32 μamp threshold) injection while the monkey was looking at the fixation point. Stimulation was a train of biphasic, negative-positive pulses (200 Hz, 50 mseconds) with each pulse 0.2 msecond long. The vertical line indicates onset of stimulation. B. Saccades to visual targets before (PRE) and 6 minutes after (POST) injection of muscimol. Records for saccades to each of three different points on the right horizontal meridian (5°, 10°, 20°) and three on the left horizontal meridian are superimposed. Upper traces are horizontal eye positions (right is upward, left, downward) and lower traces are vertical eye positions (up is upward, down, downward). The vertical line indicates the time at which the fixation point went off and the target point came on. C. Saccades to remembered targets before (PRE) and 11 minutes after (POST) the same injection of muscimol into the right superior colliculus. The same saccade targets were used as in B and the left vertical line indicates offset of the fixation point and the right vertical line the onset of the target point. From Hikosaka and Wurtz (1985a).

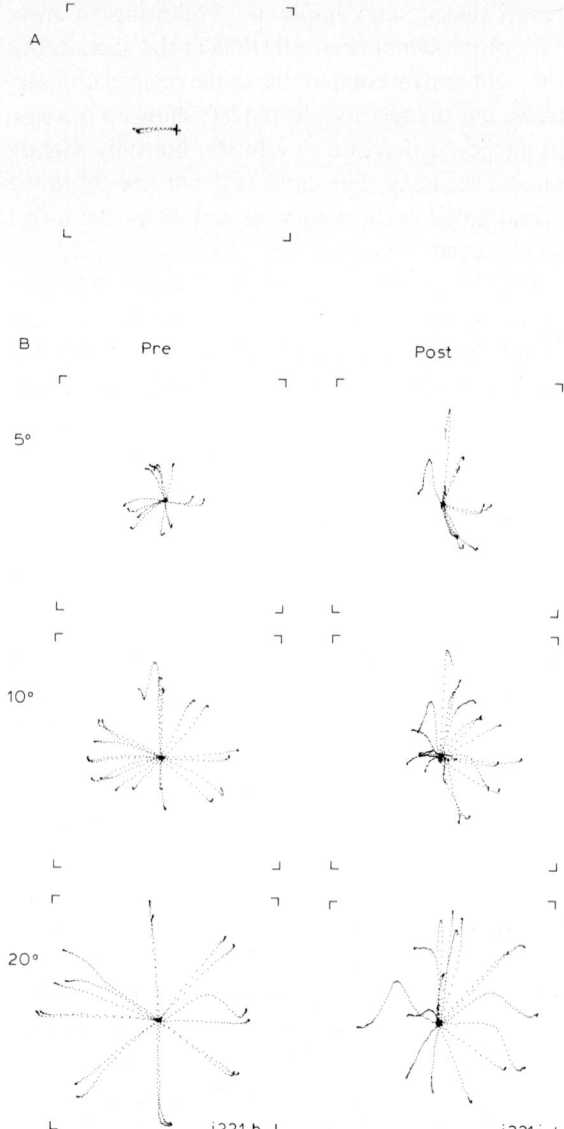

Fig. 8. Trajectories of saccades to remembered targets before (Pre) and after (Post) the injection of muscimol in the right superior colliculus shown on a vector diagram. A. Saccades evoked by electrical stimulation before injection — same stimulation records as in Fig. 6. B. Saccades to remembered targets with eccentricities of 5, 10 and 20° before (Pre) and after (Post) the injection. Length of each side of the square is 40°. Time interval between the dots is 2 mseconds. Eye positions are displayed for the period from the offset of the fixation point to the end of the first saccade. Two saccades are superimposed for each target point but only the first saccade attempted to the given target is shown. Closer spacing of the dots after the injection indicates lower saccadic velocities. From Hikosaka and Wurtz (1985a).

ually evoked, however, and had higher velocities than the just preceding saccades to remembered targets. In Fig. 8 the trajectory of the saccades to targets is shown on an x–y plot. Fig. 8A shows the trajectory of saccades following the stimulation described previously, and Fig. 8B shows the trajectories of the first saccade made after offset of the fixation point to points 5, 10 and 20° in various directions. Two saccades are shown to each of these targets. After the injection (Fig. 8B, POST) the saccades became distorted, as if they were compressed from the left side. Leftward saccades were fewer in number, short, and slow, or curved upwards. Vertical saccades tended to curve to the right side. In contrast, saccades made to visual targets before the muscimol injections were only slightly curved and ended near the target. Thus, following an injection of muscimol into the SC, saccades to remembered targets were affected more severely than were saccades to visual targets.

Spontaneous eye movements were also affected by muscimol injection, but these effects became evident at a later time after the injection than the effects described above. The primary effect was a deviation of the eye in the direction opposite to the direction of saccades evoked by electrical stimulation at the injection site. Thus, for the injection of muscimol described, the eye moved in a small area on the right, and the direction of gaze rarely crossed midline towards the left. Furthermore, leftward saccades were less frequent and much slower than rightward saccades. A nystagmus followed several hours after the injection with a quick phase to the right and a slow phase to the left.

In contrast to muscimol, injection of bicuculline into the SC facilitated the initiation of saccades. A successful injection of bicuculline was followed by stereotyped and apparently irrepressible saccades made to the area of the movement field of the SC cells near the injection site. These irrepressible saccades occurred both during the task that required the monkey to make saccades to visual targets and in the task where the monkey made saccades to remembered targets. An example of these irrepressible saccades during the long period of fixation in

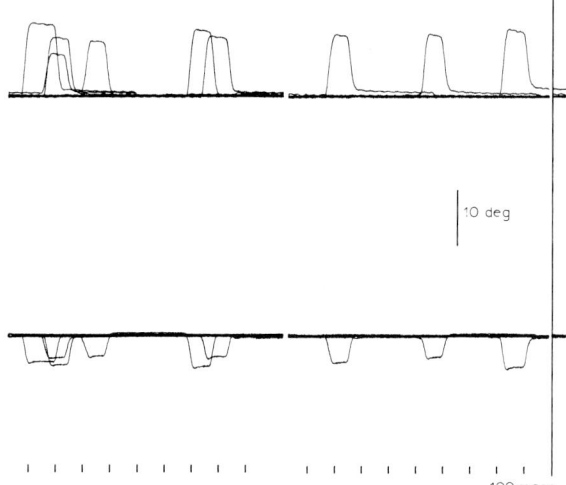

Fig. 9. Irrepressible saccades during the fixation period following injection of bicuculline into the left SC. Superimposed traces of eye position during the fixation period of eight trials of a delayed saccade task. Traces start after the target was flashed and end at offset of the fixation point. Upper traces are horizontal and lower lines are vertical eye positions. Target eccentricity was 20°. From Hikosaka and Wurtz (1985a).

the target task for saccades to remembered targets is shown in Fig. 9. The irrepressible saccadic jerks were very similar to the direction of evoked eye movements generated by electrical stimulation before the injection. The effect on saccades to targets, either visual or remembered, was to increase the velocity of saccades made to the affected area, or to eliminate the saccade to the target area if it were away from the area related to the injection. Spontaneous eye movement tended to be toward the direction of the affected area and the eye moved towards that side of the visual field, away from the side of the injection. Thus, the effect of bicuculline was to increase the monkey's tendency to make a saccade to one part of the visual field, and this tendency was at the expense of saccades to the other visual field whether those saccades were made spontaneously, to a visual target, or to a remembered target.

Our logic in using GABAergic agents in the SC was to intensify or reduce artificially the presumed GABA-mediated inhibitory inputs from the SN pars reticulata acting on the SC. It is possible, however, that other afferent connections to the SC or other neurons within the SC itself also use GABA as a neurotransmitter. Muscimol and bicuculline might then act on these synapses rather than, or in addition to, the SNr-SC synapses. An obvious way to resolve this issue was to alter transmitter release by the SNr neurons by manipulating activity of cells within the SNr itself rather than their terminals within the SC. Such manipulation is possible because one projection to the SNr itself is presumed to use GABA as a transmitter. If our hypothesis is correct about the effect of SNr on SC, injection of muscimol in the SNr should have the same effect as injection of bicuculline in the SC. To test our hypothesis we injected muscimol into the SNr of the monkey using techniques largely similar to those used for injecting muscimol and bicuculline into the SC (Hikosaka and Wurtz, 1985b). What we found was that muscimol injected into the SNr had largely the same effect as bicuculline injected into the SC: the generation of irrepressible saccades to the contralateral visual field. We conclude that a substantial portion of the action of GABA produced in the SC must result from the terminals originating in the SNr.

Function of substantia nigra in saccade initiation

These pharmacological experiments and the previous physiological and anatomical experiments allow us to draw two general conclusions about the role of the SNr in the control of saccadic eye movements.

The first conclusion is that the SNr exerts tonic inhibition on SC cells, that the signal conveyed is a pause in this inhibition, and that this inhibition is mediated by GABA. We have shown that cells in the SNr discharge rapidly but decrease their discharge rate before appropriate saccades. Furthermore, as demonstrated by antidromic stimulation, these cells in the SNr project to the layers within the SC where cells discharge in relation to saccades. The projection from SNr to SC is selective, so that there is a match between the movement fields of the

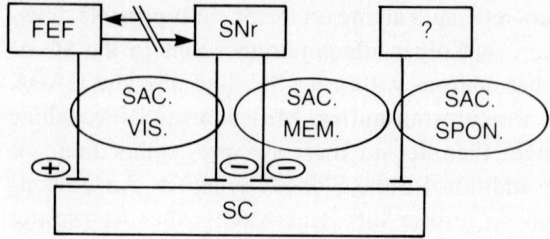

Fig. 10. Hypothetical convergence of saccade-related inputs onto SC. Inputs to the intermediate layers of the SC are not the same when saccades are made to visual targets (SAC/VIS), to remembered targets (SAC/MEM), or spontaneously (SAC/SPON). Inputs shown are from the FEF, the SNr, and an unknown source.

SNr cells and the movement fields of the SC cells. The response of the cells preceding a saccade in the SNr and the SC is reciprocal: the SNr cells pause as the SC cells burst.

If the tonic inhibition is mediated by GABA, a GABA agonist, muscimol, injected into the SC should act to increase the tonic inhibition on cells adjacent to the injection. These cells should require greater synaptic drive to activate them than do cells related to other parts of the visual field. The reduction in the number of evoked and spontaneous saccades made to the affected area of the visual field and the slowing of saccades that we have observed are consistent with such an increase in inhibition. Muscimol should also block any phasic changes, largely eliminating the pauses in inhibition related to initiation of saccades.

On the other hand, a GABA antagonist, bicuculline, can be regarded as either reducing the tonic inhibition from SNr or as artificially producing a pause in inhibition that could be taken as a signal for a saccade. The effect in either case might be likened to a "phosphene", but a motor one rather than a sensory one. This phosphene at the site of the injection competes with the activity in other areas of the colliculus related to other saccade-related inputs. The phosphene clearly is more powerful than the signals related to remembered targets, to many visual targets, and competes with visual fixation, as indicated by the saccadic jerks occurring in all these cases.

The second major conclusion from these experiments is that the SNr plays an important role in the initiation of saccadic eye movements made contingent upon behavioral conditions. Thus, some cells show a pause in activity before saccades to visual targets, and some before saccades to remembered targets. Cells do not show a change in discharge before saccades made spontaneously in the light or the dark.

Activity in the SNr might be particularly related to saccades made to remembered visual stimuli. Cells related to saccades to remembered targets have not been reported in the SC although, as noted above, certain types of SNr responses bear some similarity to "quasi-visual" responses reported by Mays and Sparks (1980). The relationship between saccades to remembered targets and the SNr to SC connection is supported by the observation that injecting muscimol into the SC affects saccades to remembered targets more markedly than it does saccades to visual targets.

We have described the saccades made in the absence of a visual target as saccades to remembered targets with the intention of providing an operational description of the experiment. Another way of looking at these saccades, however, is that they are movements made in the absence of direct sensory control. Since many eye movements are made under these conditions, that is, neither to a particular sensory target nor spontaneously, this function would be an important one in normal oculomotor control of saccadic eye movement. Furthermore, this identification of the relation of movements in the absence of direct sensory guidance is consistent with the possibility that the SNr is part of the system beginning in the frontal cortex and extending to the SC, as indicated in Fig. 1.

Function of superior colliculus in saccade initiation

Our observations on the relation of the SNr to the SC also raise several points related to the function of the SC in the initiation of saccadic eye movements.

The first point is that in normal behavior the intermediate layers of the SC are a common pathway for the initiation of saccades made under a variety of behavioral conditions, and this conjecture is shown schematically in Fig. 10. This diagram considers only the major direct inputs to the intermediate layers of the SC, those from the FEF and SNr. In the case of saccades to visual targets, there are inputs from both the FEF and the SNr. Thus, removal of the SNr input (as in the case of a muscimol injection) would not be expected to eliminate saccades to visual targets, and it does not. Furthermore, the input for saccades to visual targets is "push-pull": both a decrease in inhibition and (making the assumption that the input from FEF is excitatory) an increase in excitation, and this is consistent with the observations that the saccades to visual targets have the highest velocity of any saccades we observe. In contrast, saccades to remembered targets might have an input primarily via the SNr, even though the SNr itself is interconnected with the FEF. The consequence of this is that the injection of muscimol should have a more pronounced effect on saccades to remembered targets, and it does, and that saccades to remembered targets, with only one input, might be expected to have lower velocity, and they do.

The "spontaneous" saccades, those made in the light or dark in the absence of sensory targets or explicit behavioral instructions, probably are related to inputs from neither the SNr nor FEF since cells in neither structure discharge in relation to such saccades. While drawn as an input in Fig. 10, these saccades may be generated within the SC. Modulation of spontaneous saccades following muscimol injection would result not because of disruption of the input signal but because of a change in the tonic inhibition affecting all SC function.

The second point is the relation of damage to the SC to the initiation of saccades made to visual targets. In previous studies the effects of such damage was slight, particularly in those studies from our laboratory (as summarized in Hikosaka and Wurtz, 1985a). Increase in latency (Wurtz and Goldberg, 1972; Mohler and Wurtz, 1977; Schiller et al., 1980; Albano and Wurtz, 1982; Albano et al., 1982) decrease in frequency of spontaneous saccades (Albano et al., 1982), some change in velocity (Wurtz and Goldberg, 1972; Schiller et al., 1980), and slight changes in amplitude have been indicated by an increase in the number of corrective saccades (Mohler and Wurtz, 1977). Our injections of muscimol into SC should act in some ways like a surgical ablation, though briefly and reversibly, because they reduce the effectiveness of synaptic inputs to one set of SC neurons. Unlike the previous surgical or electrolytic lesions, however, muscimol produced more severe deficits in eye movements, and the difference in the two experimental approaches might be explained by the ability of the brain to compensate over time for a partial dysfunction. In all of the previous studies, the SC was damaged physically, and oculomotor behavior was tested usually after a lapse of a day, and frequently a week. Deficits such as the lower saccadic velocity may not have been observed because over time other brain areas compensated for some deficits in SC function, as we have discussed previously (Hikosaka and Wurtz, 1985a). An increase in latency was more severe in the present experiments with muscimol, and was so severe in one less well-trained monkey that he did not make saccades toward a visual target. This suggests that the SC might be more important for a naive monkey to initiate saccades to visual targets, and that other brain areas, such as the FEF (Schiller et al., 1980), cannot immediately substitute for the SC. The SC is probably a more critical station for saccade-related signals destined for the brainstem oculomotor system than previous ablation experiments of SC have indicated, but one for which substantial compensation for loss can be made.

Finally, one of the most surprising findings of these experiments with respect to the SC is that following injections of muscimol into the SC, saccadic velocity is substantially reduced (Hikosaka and Wurtz, 1985a). The SC has generally been considered to control the vector of a saccade but not its time course (Sparks et al., 1976; Wurtz and Albano, 1980). Saccadic velocity is well correlated with discharge frequency of burst neurons (Keller, 1974; King and Fuchs, 1979; Van Gisbergen et al.,

1981; Yoshida et al., 1982), and in order to alter velocity muscimol in the SC must lead to a lowering of this spike frequency. How this might occur at this point is a matter of speculation (Hikosaka and Wurtz, 1985a), but this relation of SC to saccade velocity might provide an additional clue as to how the retinotopic spatial map of the SC is transformed into the temporal burst patterns of MRF and PPRF neurons.

Comparison of basal ganglia function in oculomotor and skeletal motor control

Our experiments have shown that one part of the SNr, an output pathway of the basal ganglia, plays a significant role in the control of saccadic eye movements. The other major output of the basal ganglia, the internal segment of the globus pallidus, is clearly related to skeletal movements, as summarized by DeLong and co-workers (1981, 1984). This parallel organization of the two structures raises the question of how similar a role they might play in the initiation of movement, either oculomotor or skeletal. It would be premature to draw inferences about the skeletal system based on these oculomotor experiments, but a number of parallel observations are worth pointing out.

As in the SNr, many cells in the globus pallidus discharge rapidly and change their discharge rate in relation to movements of the limb, including many (but not all) that decrease their discharge rate (see DeLong et al., 1984). Furthermore, just as the SNr cells produce inhibition in the SC, pallidal cells monosynaptically inhibit neurons in the medial thalamus (Uno and Yoshida, 1975). These findings related to the globus pallidus suggest a scheme for basal ganglia function that relies on release of a target structure from inhibition, be it the SC in relation to eye movements or the thalamus in relation to skeletal movements. What is also clear from the studies on the globus pallidus is that a uniform population as in the SNr does not exist. For one subpopulation, however, it is worth entertaining the hypothesis that there is a high rate of discharge producing a tonic inhibition, that the signal conveyed is a release of this inhibition, and that this principle applies both to a subset of globus pallidus neurons that modulates skeletal movement, and to a subset of SNr neurons that modulates oculomotor movements, specifically saccades.

There is also some indication that the relation of the globus pallidus to movement might be dependent upon the condition under which skeletal movements are made, as is the case for the SNr and eye movements. Inactivation of the globus pallidus of the monkey by cooling disrupted self-paced elbow movements but use of a visual display improved performance (Hore et al., 1977). These results have some similarity to our observation that memory-evoked saccades were disrupted more severely than were those made to visual targets following inactivation of SNr cells by muscimol. Furthermore, cooling or ablation of the globus pallidus has been shown to reduce the reaction time for contralateral hand movements in the baboon (Amato et al., 1978), and these observations may be similar to the reduced latency for saccade initiation following muscimol injections into the SNr or bicuculline into SC. Finally, recent experiments by Kimura et al. (1984) have demonstrated that neurons in the putamen that have a high rate of discharge show a pause in discharge rate in response to auditory stimulation, but only when that stimulation is a trigger for movement. A similar set-dependent response was seen in the globus pallidus. These behaviorally contingent auditory responses in both putamen and globus pallidus are similar to the visual responses in SNr that are contingent upon use of stimuli as targets for saccades to remembered targets.

Thus, the two major conclusions we have drawn on the relation of the SNr to eye movements also might be taken to apply to skeletal movements. First, the basal ganglia contribute to the initiation of both eye and skeletal movements by a release of the target structure, SC or thalamus, from tonic inhibition. Second, this mechanism is particularly critical if these movements are based on stored or remembered information which is not currently available as incoming sensory signals.

References

Albano, J. E. and Wurtz, R. H. (1982) Deficits in eye position following ablation of monkey superior colliculus, pretectum, and posterior-medial thalamus. J. Neurophysiol., 48: 318–337.

Albano, J. E., Mishkin, M., Westbrook, L. E. and Wurtz, R. H. (1982) Visuomotor deficits following ablation of monkey superior colliculus. J. Neurophysiol., 48: 338–351.

Amato, G., Trouche, E., Beaubaton, D. and Grangetto, A. (1978) The role of internal pallidal segment on the initiation of a goal directed movement. Neurosci. Lett., 9: 159–163.

Beckstead, R. M., Edwards, S. B. and Frankfurter, A. (1981) A comparison of the intranigral distribution of nigrotectal neurons labeled with horseradish peroxidase in the monkey, cat, and rat. J. Neurosci., 1: 121–125.

Bruce, C. J. and Goldberg, M. E. (1985) Primate frontal eye fields: I. Single neurons discharging before saccades. J. Neurophysiol., 53: 603–635.

DeLong, M. R. and Georgopoulos, A. P. (1981) Motor functions of the basal ganglia. In V. B. Brooks (Ed.), Handbook of Physiology, The Nervous System II, American Physiological Society, Bethesda, Sect. 1, Part 2, Vol. II, Ch. 21, pp.1017–1061.

DeLong, M. R., Alexander, G. E., Georgopoulos, A. P., Crutcher, M. D., Mitchell, S. J. and Richardson, R. T. (1984) Role of basal ganglia in limb movements. Human Neurobiol., 2: 235–244.

Fahn, S. and Cote, L. J. (1968) Regional distribution of γ-aminobutyric acid (GABA) in brain of the rhesus monkey. J. Neurochem., 15: 209–213.

Goldberg, M. E. and Bruce, C. J. (1985) Cerebral cortical activity associated with the orientation of visual attention in the rhesus monkey. Vision Res., 25: 471–481.

Graybiel, A. M. (1978) Organization of the nigrotectal connection: an experimental tracer study in the cat. Brain Res., 143: 339–348.

Graybiel, A. M. and Ragsdale, C. W. Jr. (1979) Fiber connections of the basal ganglia. In M. Cuenod, G. W. Kreutzberg and F. E. Bloom (Eds.), Development and Chemical Specificity of Neurons, Elsevier, Amsterdam, pp. 239–283.

Hikosaka, O. and Wurtz, R. H. (1983a) Visual and oculomotor functions of monkey substantia nigra pars reticulata. I. Relation of visual and auditory responses to saccades. J. Neurophysiol., 49: 1230–1253.

Hikosaka, O. and Wurtz, R. H. (1983b) Visual and oculomotor functions of monkey substantia nigra pars reticulata. II. Visual responses related to fixation of gaze. J. Neurophysiol., 49: 1254–1267.

Hikosaka, O. and Wurtz, R. H. (1983c) Visual and oculomotor functions of monkey substantia nigra pars reticulata. III. Memory-contingent visual and saccade responses. J. Neurophysiol., 49: 1268–1284.

Hikosaka, O. and Wurtz, R. H. (1983d) Visual and oculomotor functions of monkey substantia nigra pars reticulata. IV. Relation of substantia nigra to superior colliculus. J. Neurophysiol., 49: 1285–1301.

Hikosaka, O. and Wurtz, R. H. (1983e) Effects on eye movements of a GABA agonist and antagonist injected into monkey superior colliculus. Brain Res., 272: 368–372.

Hikosaka, O. and Wurtz, R. H. (1985a) Modification of saccadic eye movements by GABA-related substances. I. Effect of muscimol and bicuculline in the monkey superior colliculus. J. Neurophysiol., 53: 266–291.

Hikosaka, O. and Wurtz, R. H. (1985b) Modification of saccadic eye movements by GABA-related substances. II. Effects of muscimol in the monkey substantia nigra pars reticulata. J. Neurophysiol., 53: 292–308.

Hore, J., Meyer-Lohman, J. and Brooks, V. B. (1977) Basal ganglia cooling disables learned arm movements of monkeys in the absence of visual guidance. Science, 195: 584–586.

Jayaraman, A., Batton, R. R., III and Carpenter, M. B. (1977) Nigrotectal projections in the monkey: an autoradiographic study. Brain Res., 135: 147–152.

Keller, E. L. (1974) Participation of medial pontine reticular formation in eye movement generation in monkey. J. Neurophysiol., 37: 316–332.

Kimura, M., Rajkowski, J. and Evarts, E. (1984) Tonically discharging putamen neurons exhibit set-dependent responses. Proc. Natl. Acad. Sci. U.S.A., 81: 4998–5001.

King, W. M. and Fuchs, A. F. (1979) Reticular control of vertical saccadic eye movements by mesencephalic burst neurons. J. Neurophysiol. 42: 861–876.

Leichnetz, G. R., Spencer, R. F., Hardy, S. G. P. and Astruc, J. (1982) The prefrontal cortico-tectal projection in the monkey. An anterograde and retrograde horseradish peroxidase study. J. Neurosci., 2: 1023–1041.

Mays, L. E. and Sparks, D. L. (1980) Dissociation of visual and saccade-related responses in superior colliculus neurons. J. Neurophysiol., 43: 207–232.

Mohler, C. W. and Wurtz, R. H. (1976) Organization of monkey superior colliculus: intermediate layer cells discharging before eye movements. J. Neurophysiol., 39: 722–744.

Mohler, C. W. and Wurtz, R. H. (1977) Role of striate cortex and superior colliculus in visual guidance of saccadic eye movements in monkeys. J. Neurophysiol., 40: 74–94.

Mohler, C. W., Goldberg, M. E. and Wurtz, R. H. (1973) Visual receptive fields of frontal eye field neurons. Brain Res., 61: 385–389.

Schiller, P. H., True, S. D. and Conway, J. L. (1980) Deficits in eye movements following frontal eye field and superior colliculus ablations. J. Neurophysiol., 44: 1175–1189.

Sparks, D. L., Holland, R. and Guthrie, B. L. (1976) Size and distribution of movement fields in the monkey superior colliculus. Brain Res., 113: 21–34.

Uno, M. and Yoshida, M. (1975) Monosynaptic inhibition of thalamic neurons produced by stimulation of the pallidal nucleus in cats. Brain Res., 99: 377–380.

Van Gisbergen, J. A. M., Robinson, D. A. and Gielen, S. (1981) A quantitative analysis of generation of saccadic eye movements for burst neurons. J. Neurophysiol., 45: 417–442.

Wurtz, R. H. (1969) Visual receptive fields of striate cortex neurons in awake monkeys. J. Neurophysiol., 32: 727–742.

Wurtz, R. H. and Albano, J. E. (1980) Visual-motor function of the primate superior colliculus. Annu. Rev. Neurosci., 3: 189–226.

Wurtz, R. H. and Goldberg, M. E. (1972) Activity of superior colliculus in behaving monkey: IV. Effects of lesions on eye movements. J. Neurophysiol., 35: 587–596.

Yoshida, K., McCrea, R., Berthoz, A. and Vidal, P. P. (1982) Morphological and physiological characteristics of inhibitory burst neurons controlling horizontal rapid eye movements in the alert cat. J. Neurophysiol., 48: 761–784.

Role of the central thalamus in gaze control

John Schlag and Madeleine Schlag-Rey

Department of Anatomy and Brain Research Institute, University of California, Los Angeles, CA 90024, U.S.A.

Introduction

Classically, the sector of the cerebral frontal lobes concerned with the movement of the eyes is known to lie rostrally, somewhat apart from the aligned representation of movements of the other body parts. Similarly, the sources of afferents to the oculomotor and skeletomotor cortical areas are separated in the thalamus. Whereas the frontal eye field (area 8) receives its projections from an external crescent of nucleus medialis dorsalis (Scollo-Lavizzari and Akert, 1963), the motor and premotor strips (areas 4 and 6) receive theirs from several nuclei of the ventrolateral group (see Strick, Section III in this volume). The separation is accented by the interposition of a thick fiber layer: the thalamic internal medullary lamina or IML.

In this chapter, we shall present evidence based on stimulation, lesion, and unit recording experiments that intralaminar cells in the central thalamus are playing a role in gaze shifts and gaze fixation. Guided by the known anatomy of this region and by assumptions on the ultimate destination of the neural signals recorded there, we shall examine how these signals can be utilized. The working hypothesis is that this part of the thalamus operates as a central controller.

Stimulation, lesion, unit recording in the IML of cats

Contraversive saccades were evoked by electrical stimulation from the cat central thalamus as easily as from the cat frontal eye fields. The most effective points (lowest threshold and shortest latency) were centered in the upper wing of the IML (Schlag and Schlag-Rey, 1971). Conversely, the destruction of this region resulted in a syndrome of contralateral visual neglect (Orem et al., 1973). This has now been corroborated by clinical observations in man (Watson and Heilman, 1979). Perhaps stimulations and lesions were effective because they involved not only nucleus medialis dorsalis itself, but also its efferents running within the IML. Another possibility was that neurons within the lamina — the so-called intralaminar nuclei — are themselves responsible for the results obtained.

Unit recording verified this last hypothesis. The recordings were made in alert cats trained to anticipate and acquire small visual targets (Schlag et al., 1974; Schlag-Rey and Schlag, 1977). Units were found which shared many properties with three types commonly encountered in the brain stem: discharging with saccades, pausing with saccades, or firing at a rate depending on eye position in orbit. Although some of these neurons were located in the paralamellar part of nucleus medialis dorsalis, most of them clearly lay within the territory of the IML. In recent experiments on cats which could move their head horizontally (Maldonado and Schlag, 1984), IML units were found discharging in relation to gaze shifts effected by any combination of eye and head movements.

In the same region many units gave visual responses (Schlag-Rey and Schlag, 1977). Largely unaffected by stimulus brightness, contrast, size, shape or color, these units seemed to provide information only on stimulus location, although usually in a crude way (i.e., large receptive fields). Remarkably, in the cat most saccadic neurons themselves (65%) yielded visual responses. The cat is an animal with an independent mind (and not a favored subject for conditioning experiments). It does not readily orient toward bright stimuli that it can see without looking at them. Eventually, it will orient toward dim stimuli, especially if they appear novel in shape, timing or location. Then, the cat will make targeting saccades, possibly delayed by a second or more. Such conditions were ideal to verify that, consistently, the same neurons gave a stimulus time-locked on-response and, later on again, gave a presaccadic burst time-locked to the eye movement. Both stimulus-evoked and movement-linked firing patterns were related in their directionality: a cell which had a preferred direction for movement (e.g., contraversive) responded only to stimuli (e.g., contralateral) attracting the eye in that direction. This principle of directionality always held true, even in more complicated experiments in which attempts were made, with moving targets, to dissociate stimulus location and saccade direction (Schlag and Schlag-Rey, 1982, 1983a).

Two main conclusions could already be drawn from these initial studies. First, the cell population investigated contains units very likely involved in gaze mechanisms since their activity was related not only to the various aspects of eye and head movements, but also to the occurrence of external events inducing such movements. Second, most of the neurons of this cell population were truly intralaminar rather than belonging to either nucleus medialis dorsalis or nucleus ventralis lateralis. Thus, a quite specific role could be given to a region considered and labelled unspecific.

Are the saccade-related neurons projecting upstream or downstream?

A major uncertainty had to be resolved before attempting to progress further in understanding the role of the central thalamus in the control of eye movements. IML presaccadic units had all the characteristics expected from neurons emitting a motor command. Since IML electrical stimulation still evoked saccades in chronically decorticated cats (Schlag and Schlag-Rey, 1971), could it be that IML neurons send oculomotor commands directly downstream to the brain stem? The idea of descending thalamic projections runs against traditional views of the thalamus position in the forebrain circuitry, but it had some support from Golgi observations in neonate animals, concerning precisely the intralaminar nuclei (Scheibel and Scheibel, 1967). To test this hypothesis, ibotenic acid lesions were made around the tip of a stimulating electrode in the central thalamus of cats. Saccades were produced at high-frequency stimulation (250 Hz) and cortical recruiting responses at low-frequency stimulation (10 Hz) from the same site, as a control before the lesion. After the lesion, saccades could still readily be evoked but the threshold for cortical recruitment increased considerably (Merker and Schlag, 1985). Since saccades are elicitable either after decortication destroying the trans-thalamic corticofugal pathway revealed by Leichnetz (1980) or after local destruction of thalamic cell bodies by ibotenic acid injection, it ought to be assumed that they result from antidromic invasion of projections to the IML. Such projections are known to exist, in particular, from the paramedian pontine reticular formation (Büttner-Ennever and Henn, 1976) and deep layers of the superior colliculus (Graham and Berman, 1981). As for the elicitation of paw movements from nucleus ventralis lateralis under similar conditions (Asanuma and Hunsperger, 1975), the existence of ascending projections to the IML can account for the effects of stimulation. Thus, there is no longer any argument to question the view that intralaminar neurons, like most — if not all — dorsal thalamic neurons, send their signals rostrally.

To discuss the significance of these signals, let us now turn to results obtained in monkeys, which will allow us to integrate our data with those collected in other structures, particularly, in this species.

Overview of the discharge properties of the IML neurons in monkeys

More than 300 units related to eye movements, visual stimuli or both have been recorded in the IML region in ten monkeys (*Macaca nemestrina*) trained in two visual fixation tasks. In the first task, trials were initiated by the monkey, who pressed a panel, turning on a 1°-annulus of dim light on a tangent screen, and released the panel when the circle became a square, in order to obtain a drop of juice. Continuous and accurate fixation of the target (1–10 seconds) was also enforced. In the second task, reward depended on visual fixation only and the trials were initiated by the experimenter. The target could be presented stationary or moving, at a particular location on the screen or at a particular distance from the instantaneous point of fixation of the gaze. During smooth pursuit trials, the moving target often was simply a dot (< 20 minutes of arc). In addition to the data collected during the performance of the tasks, the spontaneous eye move-

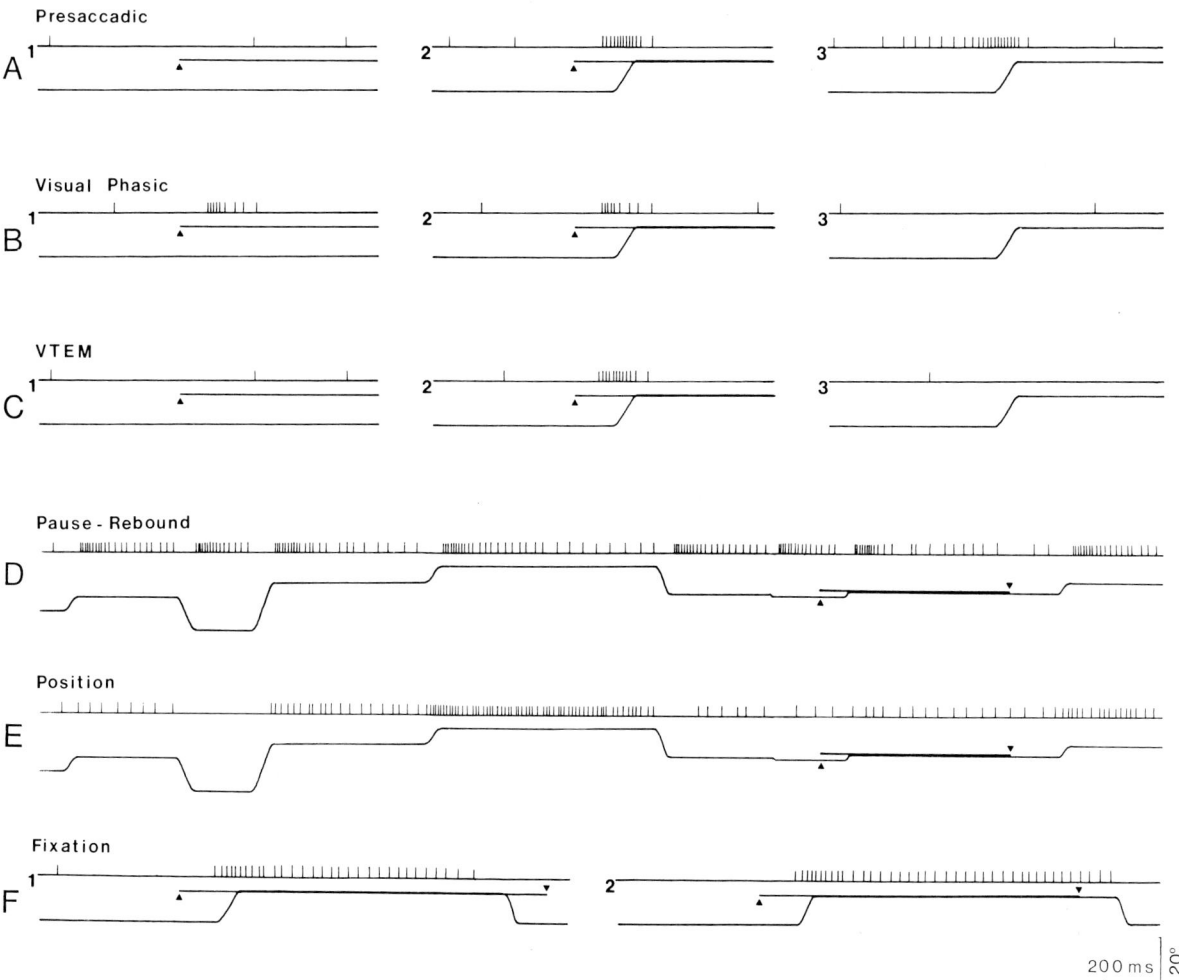

Fig. 1. Schematic representation of the typical firing patterns of five types of IML units in monkey. Drawings based on actual records in Schlag-Rey and Schlag (1984) and Schlag and Schlag-Rey (1984a). Onset and offset of visual stimulus marked by triangle with tip upward and downward, respectively. Lower trace in each case represents displacement of eye position in direction relevant to cell activity. Other explanations in the text. VTEM, visually triggered eye movements.

ments of the animals between trials were continuously recorded and analyzed off-line.

Thalamic IML units in monkey showed essentially the same characteristics as in cat. Roughly, they can be divided into categories of long-lead presaccadic burst, pause-rebound, eye-position, visually phasic, and visual tonic or fixation units. As a summary of the detailed analysis of their properties (Schlag-Rey and Schlag, 1984; Schlag and Schlag-Rey, 1984a), Fig. 1 shows the critical patterns of activity used to distinguish various types of units. It should be stressed that particular types were not necessarily recognizable by their firing patterns or response latency in a single behavioral circumstance; their identity emerged from the comparison of their activity under several conditions. For instance, the types illustrated in Fig. 1A, B and C became clearly distinguishable only when observed under three conditions: (1) when a visual stimulus was presented and the animal's gaze did not move, (2) when a stimulus elicited a targeting saccade and (3) when a spontaneous saccade occurred in the absence of stimulus. In all cases illustrated in Fig. 1, it is assumed that the conditions were optimal for the unit considered (i.e., stimuli were placed within the receptive field and eye movements were in the preferred direction).

Presaccadic units

Long-lead presaccadic bursters ($n=82$) were active with saccades in a preferred direction, usually contraversive, whether such saccades were self-initiated in light or dark (Fig. 1A–3) or visually triggered (Fig. 1A–2). In the first case, their prelude was quite variable in duration; it could anticipate the movement sometimes by 400 mseconds or more. With visually triggered saccades, the lead time depended on the reaction time. Its start was time-locked to stimulus onset, thereby giving the impression of a constant latency (80–100 mseconds).

Pause-rebound units

Pause units ($n=70$) were silent during all saccades and fired in bursts afterwards (Fig. 1D). For those that had no spontaneous activity the rebound often was the most conspicuous feature. In some cells, the pause duration was linearly related to saccade duration and the start of the rebound was time-locked to saccade offset. In other cells, the pause duration was fixed and, therefore, the start of the rebound was time-locked to saccade onset. Among all IML cell types, pause-rebound units were those which showed the greater consistency in their firing patterns whatever the saccade size. For most of these units the rebound was pandirectional. When all lights were turned off, some pause-rebound units progressively stopped firing as if they were ceasing to function when nothing was left to be seen. But the long time-course (more than 10 seconds) of this extinction as well as the absence of extinction in other pause cells made it impossible to attribute such rebounds to self-induced visual stimulation originating with eye movements in light.

Eye-position units

The frequency of discharge of eye-position units

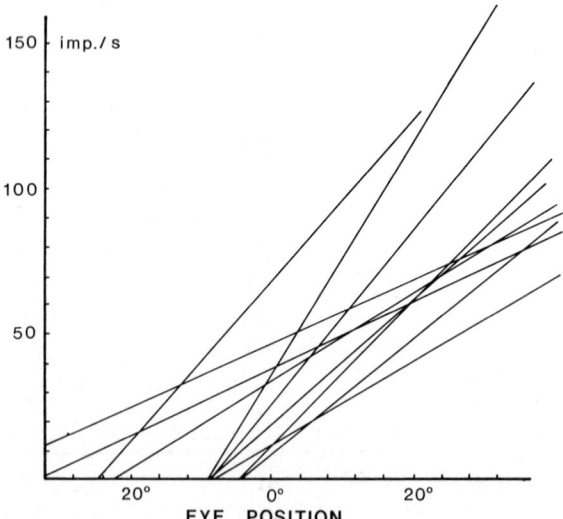

Fig. 2. Rate-position relation of ten IML eye-position units. Ordinate: firing rate measured in 500 mseconds epochs. Abscissa: eye position stable for at least 1400 mseconds along unit's preferred direction. Coefficients of correlation ranged between 0.96 and 0.76. imp./s, impulses/sec.

($n = 56$) depended on the eccentricity of the eye in orbit (Fig. 1E). Fig. 2 shows typical rate-position curves obtained from plots of firing rate as a function of gaze deviation in the unit preferred direction. The results were the same in light and in dark.

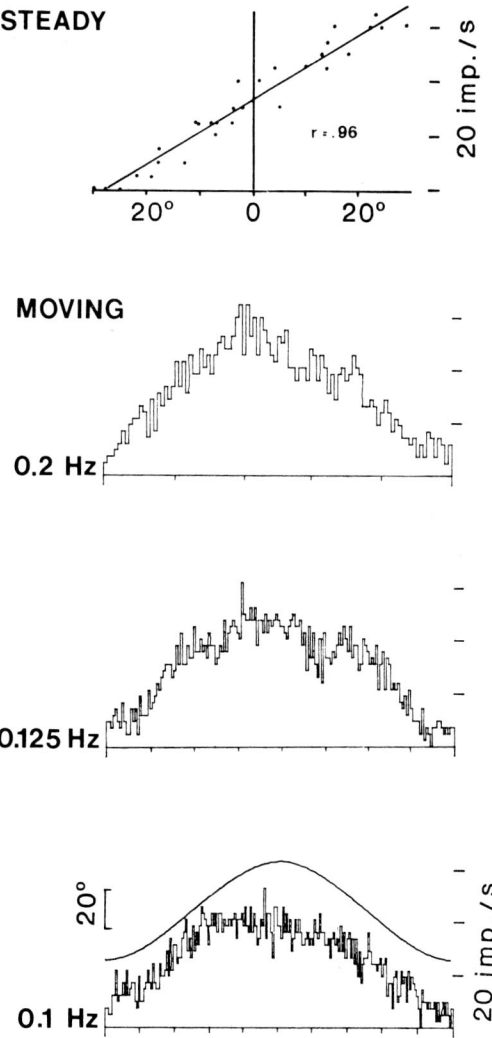

Fig. 3. Rate-position relation of an eye-position unit tested with moving stimuli. Upper plot (STEADY) concerns spontaneous eye positions (no stimulus); r = coefficient of correlation. Lower plots (MOVING) are rate averages during eight cycles of eye pursuit of stimulus sinusoidally moving at frequencies indicated on the left. Stimulus displacement was 50° peak to peak along the unit's preferred axis.

Recently, measurements were made during pursuit of targets sinusoidally moving at different frequencies (Fig. 3). The firing rate was found to be dependent on eye position, with little influence of eye velocity. During the execution of a saccade, the change of frequency started promptly, sometimes at or before saccade onset, implying that the causal factor could not be proprioceptive.

Are thalamic eye position signals related to eye, head, or gaze?

In three monkeys, a search coil was imbedded in the skull pedestal, to measure head rotations in the magnetic field. This coil was placed right above and in the same plane as the eye coil, in order to maximize the accuracy of measurements of eye signals obtained by subtracting head from gaze signals. During experiments with the head totally unrestrained, the monkey's body was immobilized by a harness. Microelectrodes were stereotaxically driven by a light-weight microdrive. When an eye-position unit was isolated, it was first studied in the head-fixed condition, then the head was released.

The results were more complex than expected. Modulation of firing rate related to eye position in orbit occurred when the head was immobile, though free to move. Thus, there are, in the IML, genuine eye position signals that cannot be construed as signals related to attempted head movements when the head is fixed. On the other hand, some of the eye-position units did also modulate their firing rate when the head moved in the on or off direction of the cell while the eyes remained centered in orbit. A typical instance of such complex behavior is illustrated in Fig. 4 for one unit which had a horizontal on direction. Below the two spike-traces (the top one shows the firing rate × 1/5), the multiplexed trace simultaneously represents head position (heavy solid line), eye in the head (no teeth = centered, teeth up = right, teeth down = left), and gaze (tips of the teeth). In A, the head was fixed, in B–D, it was free. The firing rate was clearly modulated by eye position when the head was fixed (A) or still (B), by head position when the eyes were centered (C) and by both (D), thus encoding gaze position.

Visual phasic units

The visual phasic units ($n = 72$) gave on-responses (Fig. 1B) to stimuli in their receptive field. The fields were usually very large (i.e., whole fields or hemifields for the majority). If horizontally asymmetrical, they always extended to the opposite side but included the center of fixation. Some visual phasic units also gave off-responses and post-saccadic responses. Six visual phasic units were also presaccadic in the dark (a much smaller proportion than observed in cat).

Visually triggered eye movement units (VTEM)

Comprised in the group of visually responding cells because their activity depended on the presence of a visual stimulus were 12 cells responding more strongly when a targeting saccade was made (enhancement, see Goldberg and Wurtz, 1972) and nine cells responding only when such a saccade was made. These cells were called VTEM (visually triggered eye movement, see Fig. 1C).

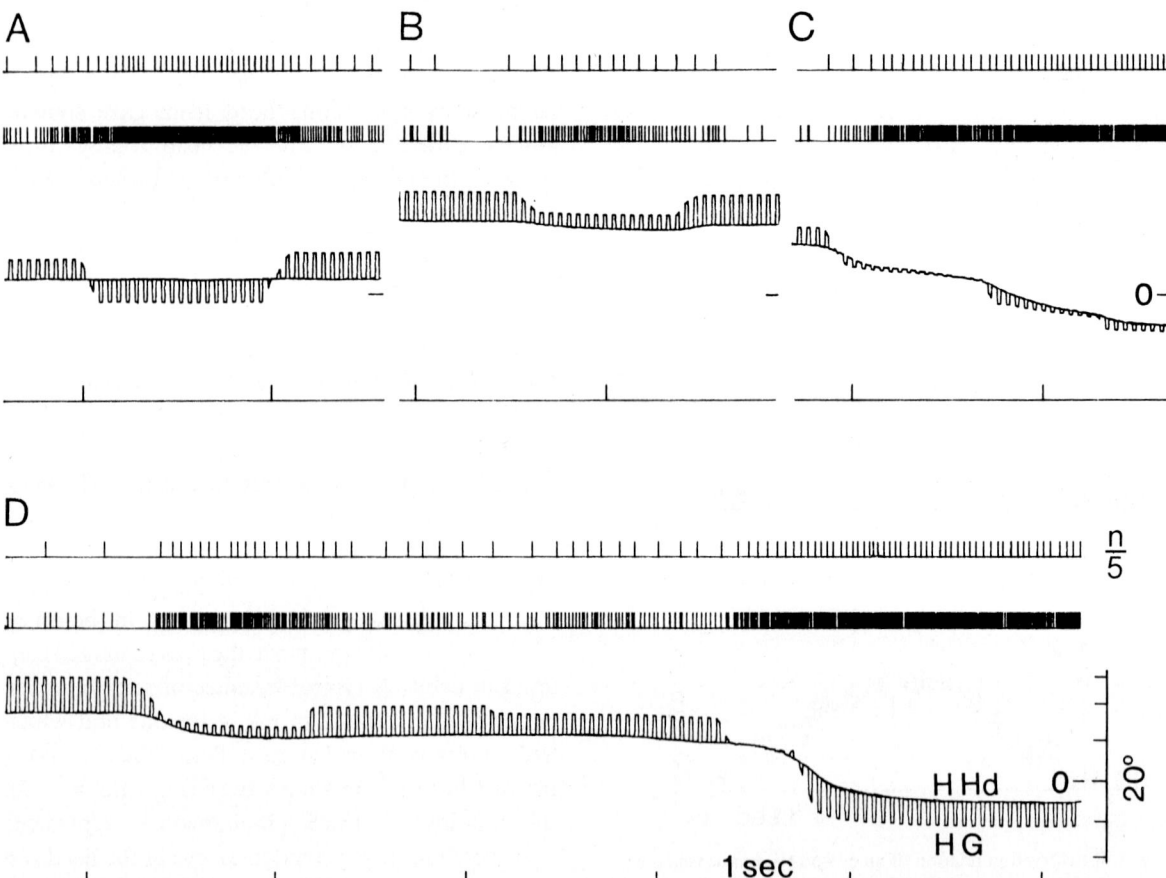

Fig. 4. Records of an eye-position unit head fixed and head free. Each record includes an upper trace showing one out of five impulses to facilitate the reading of the second trace representing the actual high-frequency discharge rate; multiplexed display of horizontal head and gaze positions (continuous line indicates head position (HHd), ends of excursions correspond to gaze position (HG), length of excursions indicates position of eye in orbit); lower trace is time. A, head fixed; B, head free but almost still; C, head shift with eyes little deviated in orbit; D, two head shifts with larger eye deviations in orbit. Midline alignment marked 0.

The comparison of the records schematized in Fig. 1A–C shows that clearly different types of units could give very similar patterns of firing under the same condition (e.g., column 2). As pointed out earlier, the unit type could nevertheless be recognized by its behavior under other conditions (e.g., columns 1 and 3).

Fixation units

All visual tonic units ($n=62$) showed a change of activity when a target was fixated anywhere on the screen (Fig. 1F). The direction of the gaze during fixation did not matter. Therefore, they were called fixation units: specifically Fix+ when the response consisted of an increase of firing and Fix– when it consisted of a decrease. Except for this change of sign, the properties of all fixation units were the same. Careful measurements of the timing of the changes of activity showed that they could not be due to passive visual effects. Fix+ and Fix– patterns started before the eye landed on a target, terminated before the eye moved away (1 in Fig. 1F), but persisted if the target was turned off during fixation (2 in Fig. 1F).

The fixation units showed their characteristic activity with foveal pursuit of moving targets as well as fixation of stationary ones. In the IML, no units were selectively active for smooth pursuit, as were the visual tracking neurons of the inferior parietal lobule (Mountcastle et al., 1975).

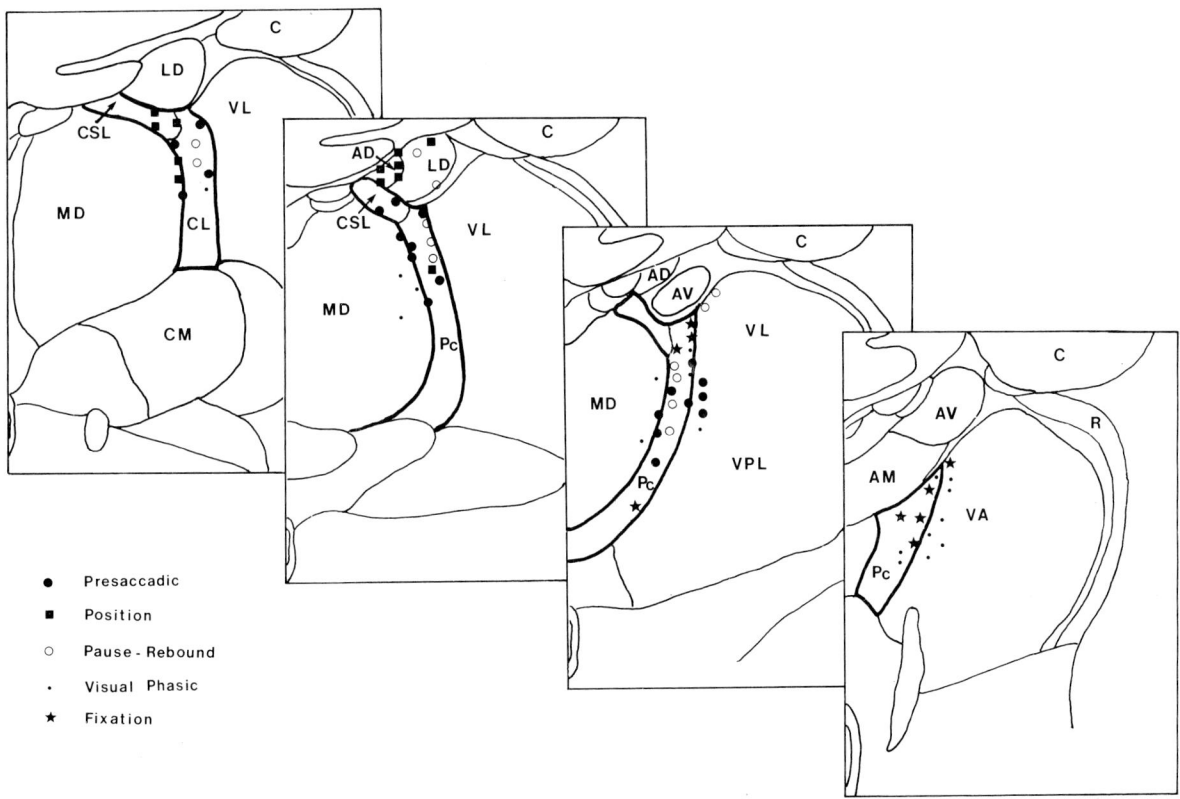

Fig. 5. Location of unit types on four successive coronal sections through central thalamus. VTEM units not represented because these were few and not clustered. Most rostral plane at right. IML outlined by thick line. Nuclei are: AD, anterior dorsalis; AM, anterior medialis; AV, anterior ventralis; C, caudate; CL, central lateralis; CM, centrum medianum; CSL, centralis superior lateralis; LD, lateralis dorsalis; MD, medialis dorsalis; Pc, paracentralis; R, reticularis; VA, ventralis anterior; VL, ventralis lateralis; VPL, ventralis posterolateralis.

Anatomical location

Fig. 5 shows the locations of unit types on four successive coronal sections through the central thalamus. The intralaminar territory is delineated by a thick outline. Each unit type is represented by a symbol, as shown in the legend. These maps summarize the detailed information on histologically identified sites of recording given in the original reports. Fig. 5 purports to illustrate the differences observed between unit types with respect to their relatively concentrated or widespread anatomical location from caudal (leftmost) to rostral planes of the thalamus; it does not provide means to compare the relative frequency of each cell type.

Discussion

If there is any common characteristic among the cell types described, it is that each one consistently signals, in its own way, one particular moment in the initiation of an eye movement: when a target appears, when the movement is going to start, when it starts, when it stops, where it goes, and whether or not the eyes will stay there. The key to understanding the role of the thalamic cell populations studied is that all these signals, individually observable in other structures, are here altogether emitted by neurons within a narrow territory. Obviously, it is not because they are all elaborated here. The intralaminar nuclei are not known to have the regular geometry of structures such as the superior colliculus, lateral geniculate nucleus, cerebellar or cerebral cortex, which seems required for the processing of information arriving in parallel on multiple input lines of common origin. If such information appears at the output of IML neurons, it ought to be assumed that it has been provided from elsewhere. The intralaminar nuclei are characterized by the convergence of afferents of many origins: mainly from the cerebellum (Thach and Jones, 1979), brain stem reticular formation (Büttner-Ennever and Henn, 1976), tectum (Benevento and Fallon, 1975) and pretectum (Benevento et al., 1977), but also from the vestibular nuclei (Kotchabhakdi et al., 1980a), ventral lateral geniculate nucleus (Kawamura et al., 1978) and perihypoglossal nucleus (Kotchabhakdi et al., 1980b). All these structures are implicated in gaze control. In addition, the intralaminar nuclei receive projections from many cortical areas such as frontal eye field and posterior parietal lobe (Graham et al., 1979; Leichnetz, 1980; Kaufman, 1982). Thus, although the contribution of each of these sources cannot easily be distinguished, there is no lack of possibilities to account for the discharge properties exibited by IML neurons.

On the other hand, IML neurons project to the striatum (Jones and Leavitt, 1974) and to several cortical areas, including frontal eye field (Barbas and Mesulam, 1981), inferior parietal lobule (Kasdon and Jacobson, 1978), anterior cingulate cortex (Vogt et al., 1979) and most visual areas (Kaufman, 1982). In a sense, their output connections are as multifarious as their inputs. Quantitatively, this output is not negligible since, according to a recent estimate (Brysch et al., 1984), the intralaminar nuclei contribute 10–20% of all corticothalamic projections, i.e., much more than would be expected given the small size of the IML region relative to the rest of the dorsal thalamus.

In short, anatomical data depict this central part of the thalamus as a node, i.e., a site of convergence and divergence, and physiological data indicate that it collects and distributes signals usable in gaze control. Such signals may not be needed if gaze control relies uniquely on prewired circuitry as, for instance, in a foveation apparatus like the one proposed by Schiller and Stryker (1972) for the superior colliculus. But, beyond purely reflexive mechanisms, we know that the gaze is involved in more complicated operations such as, for instance, selection, inspection, search, anticipation, and that, necessarily, the forebrain is responsible for making decisions. Characteristically, decision units have to be centralized, they must have access to information related to various kinds of contingencies and they must be able to call upon a variety of subroutines. Our claim is that the IML cell population seems ideally suited for such control functions.

Approaching the problem from the viewpoint of theoretical requirements, it seems first that a signal is needed to indicate the occurrence of external events. It is not sufficient that some receptors be impressed by a novel stimulus, the visual analyzers ought to be informed of a change, wherever it happens, in order to reappraise the whole scene. It may be the function of IML phasic visual neurons to initiate visual processing at such times. Second, a similar signal should also be emitted each time the gaze shifts to a new direction because new visual information then becomes available. Pause-rebound units, as the most reliable indicators of saccades among IML neurons, may be responsible for the stop-reset of visual processing after saccades (Schlag and Schlag-Rey, 1983b). Third, as long as the attention is retained on a target, there should be a hold-signal preventing any other input to gain access, for instance reflexively, to the gaze control. If it exists, such a signal would have the characteristics found in IML fixation units. Fourth, inasmuch as the gaze is directed by reading internal representations of the outside world, a signal of eye position would be required as a pointer of gaze direction on such maps. Very little is known as yet regarding these complicated operations, but the idea that retinal information is early combined with a signal of eye position is currently accepted (Robinson, 1975). Presumably, it is to the cerebral cortex that such a signal should be directed. IML eye-position units are presently the only known source satisfying theoretical requirements. Fifth, when a decision is finally made, a saccade is initiated and a signal is sent for this purpose. This may be the significance of the long-lead presaccadic units. Until recently, this view encountered serious difficulties because IML presaccadic units are active with spontaneous as well as visually triggered saccades, but nowhere in the cortex could spontaneous presaccadic activity be traced. Through where could this signal be relayed? Now we know that the dorsomedial cortex, at the rostral border of the supplementary motor area, contains units activated long before self-initiated saccades (Schlag and Schlag-Rey, 1984b).

As one will realize, these views are speculative, but we think they are sufficiently grounded in fact to serve as working hypotheses. As we mentioned earlier, they apply to a region of the central thalamus which is so particular in its organization that a generalization to other thalamic nuclei would not be warranted. However, another kind of generalization may be in order. If the intralaminar cell populations really operate as a controller, there is no reason to suppose that their role is limited to gaze. Other specific functions also require the coordinated analyses of past and present cues, presumably taking place in cortical networks working in parallel. One such function is speech, and it is interesting that stimulation effects were obtained in man in an area bounded by nuclei medialis dorsalis, ventralis lateralis, centrum medianum and medial pulvinar (Ojemann and Ward, 1971; Ojemann, 1975).

Summary

Stimulation, lesion and unit recording in cat initially disclosed that cells in the central — intralaminar — thalamus participate in the control of eye movements. Unit recording in monkey showed that different signals related to gaze shift and gaze fixation are emitted by neurons intermixed in intralaminar and juxtalaminar nuclei. Considering the multifarious connections of central thalamic cell populations, which give them access to practically all telencephalic structures involved in gaze mechanisms, it is proposed that these cell populations operate as a central controller.

Acknowledgments

We thank V. Pagano, S. Powell and H. King for their technical assistance at various stages of this study, and K. Zib for his help in analyzing the data. This research was supported by USPHS Grants NS04955 and EY02305.

References

Asanuma, H. and Hunsperger, R. W. (1975) Functional significance of projection from the cerebellar nuclei to the motor cortex in cat. Brain Res., 98: 73–92.

Barbas, H. and Mesulam, M.-M. (1981) Organization of afferent input to subdivisions of area 8 in the rhesus monkey. J. Comp. Neurol., 200: 407–431.

Benevento, L. A. and Fallon, J. H. (1975) The adcending projections of the superior colliculus in the rhesus monkey (*Macaca mulatta*). J. Comp. Neurol., 3: 339–362.

Benevento, L. A., Rezak, M. and Santos-Anderson, R. (1977) An autoradiographic study of the projections of the pretectum in the rhesus monkey (*Macaca mulatta*): evidence for sensorimotor links to the thalamus and oculomotor nuclei. Brain Res., 127: 197–218.

Brysch, I., Brysch, W., Creutzfeldt, O., Hayes, N. L. and Schlingensiepen, K.-H. (1984) The second, intralaminar thalamocortical projection system. Anat. Embryol., 169: 111–118.

Büttner-Ennever, J. A. and Henn, V. (1976) An autoradiographic study of the pathways from the pontine reticular formation involved in horizontal eye movements. Brain Res., 108: 155–164.

Goldberg, M. E. and Wurtz, R. H. (1972) Activity of superior colliculus in behaving monkey. II. Effect of attention on neuronal responses. J. Neurophysiol., 35: 560–574.

Graham, J. and Berman, N. (1981) Origins of the pretectal and tectal projections to the central lateral nucleus in the cat. Neurosci. Lett., 26: 209–214.

Graham, J., Lin, C.-S. and Kaas, J. H. (1979) Subcortical projections of six visual cortical areas in the owl monkey, *Aotus trivirgatus*. J. Comp. Neurol., 187: 557–580.

Jones, E. G. and Leavitt, R. Y. (1974) Retrograde axonal transport and the demonstration of non-specific projections to the cerebral cortex and striatum from thalamic intralaminar nuclei in the rat, cat, and monkey. J. Comp. Neurol., 154: 349–378.

Kasdon, D. and Jacobson, S. (1978) The thalamic afferents to the inferior parietal lobule of the rhesus monkey. J. Comp. Neurol., 177: 685–706.

Kaufman, E. F. S. (1982) Connections of the intralaminar nuclei of the thalamus in the cat. Ph. D. Thesis, University of Pennsylvania, p. 171.

Kawamura, S., Fukushima, N., Hattori, S. and Tashiro, T. (1978) A ventral lateral geniculate nucleus projection to the dorsal thalamus and the midbrain in the cat. Exp. Brain Res., 31: 95–106.

Kotchabhakdi, N., Rinvik, E., Wallberg, F. and Yingchareon, K. (1980a) The vestibulothalamic projections in the cat studied by retrograde axonal transport of horseradish peroxidase. Exp. Brain Res., 40: 405–418.

Kotchabhakdi, N., Rinvik, E., Yingchareon, Y. and Wallberg, F. (1980b) Afferent projections to the thalamus from the perihypoglossal nuclei. Brain Res., 187: 457–461.

Leichnetz, G. (1980) An anterogradely-labeled prefrontal cortico-oculomotor pathway in the monkey demonstrated with HRP gel and TMB neurochemistry. Brain Res., 198: 440–445.

Maldonado, H. M. and Schlag, J. (1984) Unit activity related to head and eye movements in central thalamus of cats. Exp. Neurol., 86: 359–378.

Merker, B. and Schlag, J. (1985) Role of intralaminar thalamus in gaze mechanisms: evidence from electrical stimulation and fiber-sparing lesions in cat. Exp. Brain Res., 59: 388–394.

Mountcastle, V. B., Lynch, J. C., Georgopoulos, A., Sakata, H. and Acuna, C. (1975) Posterior parietal association cortex of the monkey: command functions for the operations within extrapersonal space. J. Neurophysiol., 38: 871–908.

Ojemann, G. A. (1975) Language and the thalamus: Object naming and recall during and after thalamic stimulation. Brain Lang., 2: 101–120.

Ojemann, G. A. and Ward, A. A. Jr. (1971) Speech representation in ventrolateral thalamus. Brain, 94: 669–680.

Orem, J., Schlag-Rey, M. and Schlag, J. (1973) Unilateral visual neglect and thalamic lesions in the cat. Exp. Neurol., 40: 784–797.

Robinson, D. A. (1975) Oculomotor control signals. In G. Lennerstrand and P. Bach-y-Rita (Eds.), Basic Mechanisms of Ocular Motility and their Clinical Implications, Pergamon Press, Oxford, pp. 337–374.

Scheibel, M. E. and Scheibel, A. B. (1967) Structural organization of nonspecific thalamic nuclei and their projection toward cortex. Brain Res., 6: 60–94.

Schiller, P. H. and Stryker, M. (1972) Single-unit recording and stimulation in superior colliculus of the alert rhesus monkey. J. Neurophysiol., 35: 915–924.

Schlag, J. and Schlag-Rey, M. (1971) Induction of oculomotor responses from thalamic internal medullary lamina in the cat. Exp. Neurol., 33: 498–508.

Schlag, J. and Schlag-Rey, M. (1982) Functional significance of visually triggered discharges in eye movement related neurons. In C. Woody (Ed.), Conditioning, Representation of Involved Neural Function, Plenum Press, New York, pp. 375–387.

Schlag, J. and Schlag-Rey, M. (1983a) Interfacing visual input to oculomotor command for directing the gaze on target. In A. Hein and M. Jeannerod (Eds.), Spatially Oriented Behavior, Springer-Verlag, Berlin, pp. 87–103.

Schlag, J. and Schlag-Rey, M. (1983b) Thalamic unit firing upon refixation may be responsible for plasticity in visual cortex. Exp. Brain Res., 50: 146–148.

Schlag, J. and Schlag-Rey, M. (1984a) Visuomotor functions of central thalamus in monkey. II. Unit activity related to visual events, targeting, and fixation. J. Neurophysiol., 51: 1175–1195.

Schlag, J. and Schlag-Rey, M. (1984b) Visuo-motor units in frontal dorsomedial cortex of monkey. Neurosci. Abstr., 10: 989.

Schlag, J., Lehtinen, I. and Schlag-Rey, M. (1974) Neuronal activity before and during eye movements in thalamic internal medullary lamina of the cat. J. Neurophysiol., 37: 982–995.

Schlag-Rey, M. and Schlag, J. (1977) Visual and presaccadic neuronal activity in thalamic internal medullary lamina of cat: A study of targeting. J. Neurophysiol., 40: 156–173.

Schlag-Rey, M. and Schlag, J. (1984) Visuomotor functions of central thalamus in monkey. I. Unit activity related to spontaneous eye movements. J. Neurophysiol., 51: 1149–1174.

Scollo-Lavizzari, G. and Akert, K. (1963) Cortical area 8 and its thalamic projection in *Macaca mulatta*. J. Comp. Neurol., 121: 259–270.

Thatch, W. T. and Jones, E. G. (1979) The cerebellar dentatothalamic connection: terminal field, lamellae, rods and somatotopy. Brain Res., 169: 168–172.

Vogt, B. A., Rosene, D. L. and Pandya, D. N. (1979) Thalamic and cortical afferents differentiate anterior from posterior cingulate cortex in the monkey. Science, 204: 205–207.

Watson, R. T. and Heilman, K. M. (1979) Thalamic neglect. Neurology, 29: 690–694.

Watson, R. T., Miller, B. D. and Heilman, K. M. (1978) Nonsensory neglect. Ann. Neurol., 3: 505–508.

Discussion

P. L. Strick

Research Service, V.A. Medical Center, Department of Neurosurgery and Physiology, SUNY-Upstate Medical Center, Syracuse, NY 13210, U.S.A.

The discussion following the presentations by Fetz and Fischer centered on the physiological properties of corticomotoneuronal (CM) cells identified in Dr. Fetz's studies. One aspect of the discussion focused on a comparison between CM cells and oculomotor neurons. It appears that an important difference between these two types of neurons is that CM cells receive considerable peripheral afferent input. Thus, the response of CM cells in any behavioral task is potentially the combination of centrally generated signals and feedback from the movement. This feature of the organization of CM cells makes comparisons with oculomotor neurons difficult.

Another issue raised in discussion was whether Fetz saw any examples of cross-correlations between CM cells. Fetz had recorded simultaneously from two CM cells in only one instance. These cells did demonstrate a peak in the cross-correlogram (a tonic CM cell appeared to facilitate a phasic CM cell). However, this interaction may not have been due to direct connections between the two neurons.

Wiesendanger wondered why there was a disparity between the time of CM cell discharge and the onset of EMG activity during voluntary movement versus the time of CM cell discharge and the onset of post-spike facilitation. Fetz agreed that there is a disparity in the timing of these two events, but suggested that the early onset of discharge in CM cells led to subthreshold facilitation of EMG activity. This facilitation is evident in the testing of H-reflexes, which show clear facilitation prior to the onset of EMG activity.

Two issues were raised following Fischer's presentation. The first focused on the type of errors made in his randomly triggered task. Fischer noted that when humans guess incorrectly they initiate a saccade in the wrong direction. These saccades characteristically have slower reaction times and do not reach the proper target location. The next question was whether visual cortex lesions differentially affected the accuracy of the two types of saccade. Apparently, there was little difference; both types of saccade were equally inaccurate.

Following Goldberg's presentation there were several questions about the activity of frontal eye field (FEF) neurons in relation to eye and head movements. One issue discussed was whether the direction and amplitude of eye movements could be unequivocally encoded by discharge frequency in an ensemble of FEF neurons. Goldberg suggested that somewhat different populations of FEF neurons would be involved in generating different magnitude saccades. For example, a large saccade would be represented in 2 or 3 mm along the length of the arcuate sulcus. In contrast, a small saccade would be represented by a somewhat smaller and more medial population. In response to another question, Goldberg noted that he had not observed any correlation between the end of the burst from FEF neurons and the termination of a saccade. A final issue raised was whether the discharge in FEF neurons was encoding eye vector or gaze coordinates. Goldberg responded that he could not answer this question since in his experiments the animal's head was fixed.

The discussion following Wurtz's presentation further explored the role of the substantia nigra in the generation of saccadic eye movements. One issue raised was whether the nigra should be viewed as a motor structure which provides the superior colliculus with an input responsible for initiating saccades. Or, should the nigra be viewed as a priming structure which prepares the colliculus to evoke motor responses following an appropriate afferent input? Wurtz responded that for the cells he described, his working assumption is that the nigra provides a motor input to the colliculus, which is important for generating visually guided saccades. He noted, however, that there were other nigra neurons which were clearly 'sensory'. Another issue raised was whether the muscimol injections affected spontaneous saccades, as well as visually guided ones. Wurtz noted that muscimol injections did change the frequency of spontaneous saccades. However, the interpretation of this observation is not straightforward because the injections would alter not only the phasic input to the colliculus, but also the tonic inhibition.

The discussion which followed DeLong's presentation further explored whether movement parameters were encoded in the discharge of basal ganglia neuurons. One issue raised was whether the discharge of basal ganglia neurons had been examined during isometric contractions. DeLong responded that this issue had not been thoroughly examined, although Hepp-Reymond had observed some neurons in the basal ganglia which appeared to be well related to isometric gripping movements. Another question for DeLong was how his results compared with Evarts' observations on coding of movement parameters in the motor cortex. DeLong felt that there were striking differences between the behavioral paradigms employed in his and Evarts' experiments. Thus, he did not believe that meaningful comparisons could be made between the studies.

Schlag was asked whether the responses he observed could be explained by proprioceptive feedback from the moving eye. Schlag responded that proprioceptive feedback cannot explain the activity of "position" cells.

SECTION IV-B

Specialized Areas in Motor Control: Infratentorial

A comparison of disorders in saccades and in fast and accurate elbow flexions during cerebellar dysfunction

T. Vilis and J. Hore

Departments of Physiology and Ophthalmology, University of Western Ontario, London, Ontario, Canada N6A 5C1

Introduction

In keeping with the theme of this symposium, the goal of this paper is to attempt to define one common role of the cerebellum in the oculomotor and skeletal motor systems. In particular, two types of movements will be considered: saccadic movements of the eyes and voluntary movements of the arm, both directed to a visual target. The strategy adopted here is to compare the disorders observed during cerebellar dysfunction in these two types of movement. The disorders occurring in each phase of the movements will be compared. These are divided into disorders occurring during movement initiation, movement transit, movement termination and, finally, when attempting to hold stationary or fixate at the end of a movement. Comparison of the two types of movements illustrates clear differences in the disorders in each of the four phases. However, in spite of these differences a common function can still be ascribed to the cerebellum. The hypothesis put forward is that the role of the cerebellum in both saccades and fast arm movements is to calibrate or compute correctly an efference copy signal.

Movement initiation

The current view is that the cerebellum participates in the initiation of voluntary limb movements. This view stems from the observation of Holmes (1917) that the time to initiate limb movements (reaction time) is lengthened on the side affected by the cerebellar lesion. More recently, this has been confirmed in monkeys (Meyer-Lohmann et al., 1977; Lamarre et al., 1978; Trouche and Beaubaton, 1980). Moreover, it was found that both the onset of EMG activity and the onset of movement-related unit activity in the motor cortex was delayed with lesions of the lateral cerebellar nuclei (Meyer-Lohmann et al., 1977; Lamarre et al., 1978). These findings, coupled with the observation that unit activity in the lateral cerebellum on average preceded that of the motor cortex in the normal animal (Thach, 1975), led to the suggestion that the command to initiate movement travels through the lateral cerebellum to reach motor cortex (Meyer-Lohmann et al., 1977; Lamarre et al., 1978; Brooks and Thach, 1981).

In contrast to limb movements, we found no change in the reaction time of saccades with lesions of either the medial or lateral cerebellar nuclei in the monkey (Vilis and Hore, 1981). Thus, it appears from this evidence that the command to initiate saccades does not travel via the cerebellum.

These different effects on reaction time may be due to mechanical differences between the eyes and the limbs. The most prominent difference is the comparatively small inertia of the globe. The consequence of inertia in the limb is that the limb movement exerts a reactive force on the rest of the skeletal motor system. Thus, before a limb movement is initiated proper postural support must be provided (Woollacott et al., 1984). This suggests the possibility that in the initiation of limb movements the cerebellum is involved in precomputing the necessary postural support rather than in initiating the movement directly.

Movement transit

One major difference between limb movements and saccades during cerebellar dysfunction is that oscillations occur in the former but not in the latter. This disorder in limb movements has been variously described as astasia (Luciani, 1915), discontinuities (Brooks et al., 1973), irregularities or tremor (Holmes, 1917). To understand the origin of this disorder the properties of normal limb movements must first be examined.

Unlike saccades, the velocity of limb movements is under voluntary control. Thus, there are no characteristic velocity amplitude or duration amplitude relations by which a normal limb movement can be defined. However, like saccades, normal skilled arm movements exhibit a symmetry between their acceleration and deceleration phases (Flament et al., 1984a). Peak velocity is achieved at approximately the midpoint of a movement, with the preceding acceleration phase being approximately equal in magnitude and duration to the deceleration phase which follows. One purpose of symmetry may be to optimize the energy expenditure in a movement (Nelson, 1983).

It has been suggested that movements resulting from rapid unloading of isometric contractions are terminated by velocity-sensitive stretch reflexes (Ghez and Martin, 1982; Soechting et al., 1976). Our evidence suggests that this is not the case for braking of voluntary movements. This can be seen by comparing small and large amplitude movements, of the same peak velocity, that terminate at the same end position (Fig. 1). If velocity-sensitive stretch reflexes determined the deceleration of movements, then the deceleration phase of both should be equal. Instead, that of the small amplitude movement is larger. It appears that this larger deceleration is a consequence of the larger acceleration of the small amplitude movement, that is, a consequence of symmetry. This symmetry suggests that a central mechanism is involved in the generation of the phasic antagonist burst which matches the antagonist command to the preceding agonist command. This can be achieved either by preprogramming both commands together or by computing the antagonist command on the basis of the preceding agonist command through the use of efference copy. The latter is discussed further in the final section of the paper.

This symmetry also results in an inverse relationship between the velocity of movements of the same amplitude and the latency of onset of antagonist activity (Lestienne, 1979). Thus, in high-velocity movements the onset of antagonist activity is early in the movement while in low-velocity movements the onset occurs later (Fig. 2A and B, Control). This inverse relationship is disrupted during cerebellar dysfunction. Here the onset is early (approximately 50–80 mseconds) for both slow and fast movements (Fig. 2B, Cool). This inappropriate antagonist activity produces a deflection in the movement which in turn triggers one or more oscillations, the number of which depends on movement duration. The characteristics of these oscillations are similar to those of intention tremor observed after the application of a perturbation to a stationary limb (Vilis and Hore, 1977). The magnitude and

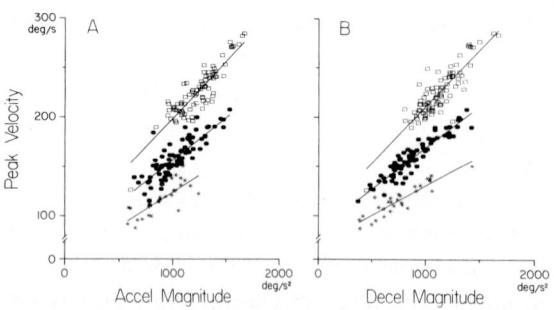

Fig. 1. Relationships between peak velocity and magnitude of acceleration (A) and magnitude of deceleration (B) in elbow flexions of the monkey. All movements were directed to the same final target position. The starting target position was varied by 60° (□), 35° (●) and 18° (*) relative to the final target position. The solid lines through the data points represent the regression lines. From Flament et al. (1984a).

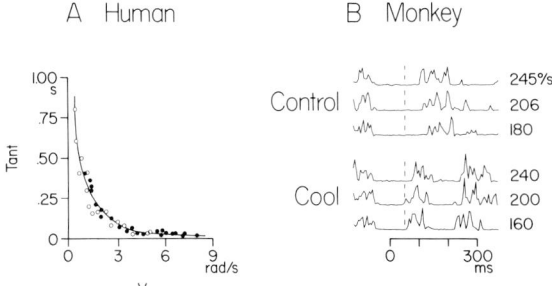

Fig. 2. Left side depicts the relationship between peak velocity (V) and onset of antagonist EMG activity (Tant) relative to start of movement in human elbow movements of similar amplitude. From Lestienne (1979). Right side compares onset of antagonist EMG activity in normal monkey flexions of three different velocities (Control) and those during reversible cooling lesions of the lateral cerebellar nuclei (Cool) synchronized to movement onset. The numbers beside each line indicate initial velocity. In all cases, the amplitudes of the movements were approximately the same.

prevalence of the early deflection is dependent on the load conditions imposed on the limb (Flament et al., 1984c). When a constant force is applied to the handle which loads the antagonist muscle, deflections become larger. In contrast, when inertia is added to the handle the deflections become smaller or are totally absent. The movements with no deflections are not normal in that the symmetry between the magnitude of the acceleration and deceleration becomes disrupted.

The probable cause of this early deflection in limb movements is a failure to suppress stretch reflexes adequately. This possibility is consistent with the short and relatively constant latency of antagonist onset in movements of different initial velocities during cerebellar dysfunction. Such a hypothesis is consistent with the absence of oscillations during saccades. Although the extraocular muscles are rich in receptors sensitive to muscle stretch and changes in tension, these receptors do not alter the firing frequency of the motor neurons when a load is imposed on the eye (Keller and Robinson, 1971). This difference may have evolved because unexpected load changes are not normally encountered by the eye.

Movement termination

The most striking disorder in saccadic eye movements with lesions of the cerebellum is saccadic dysmetria. In particular, the cerebellar vermis (Ritchie, 1976; Optican and Robinson, 1980) and the medial cerebellar nuclei (Vilis and Hore, 1981) appear to be implicated. The dysmetria is dependent on saccade direction, saccade magnitude and final eye position. As illustrated in Fig. 3, a lesion of the medial cerebellar nuclei in one monkey resulted in hypermetria when saccades were directed to the right, while saccades to the left were approximately normetric. In particular, all three studies noted a greater tendency for saccades to be hypermetric when they were directed towards the primary position than away from the primary position. The dysmetria was not equal in the two eyes (Fig. 3). The adducting eye produced smaller saccades than the abducting eye. This suggests that the cerebellum can exert a differential influence on the motor command to each eye.

The trajectory of these dysmetric saccades appeared to be normal. No attempt was made to correct for this dysmetria in the course of a saccade. Rather, one or more subsequent saccades were used to foveate the target properly. Because there is no voluntary control over a saccade's speed, a saccade of a particular magnitude has a fairly stereotyped velocity and duration. Thus, it is possible to ask whether dysmetric saccades maintain this relationship to this now incorrect amplitude. This question is important because, as we shall see in the concluding section, it provides a clue to the mechanism for saccadic dysmetria. The answer to this question is unfortunately inconsistent. For example, patients who had undergone partial cerebellar ablation (Ron and Nemet, 1977) demonstrated an increase in saccade duration when the eyes moved ipsilateral to the ablated side. However, cases involving atrophies or tumors suggest that a slowing of saccade velocity occurs only when the brainstem is also affected (Zee et al., 1976; Avanzini et al., 1979; Wennmo et al., 1983). Some animal cerebellar lesion studies (Aschoff and Cohen, 1971; Westheimer and

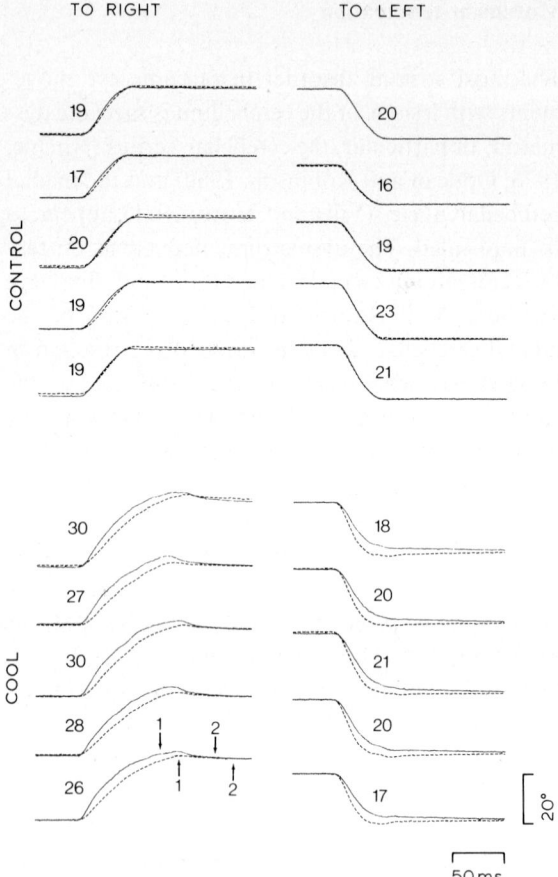

Fig. 3. Normal saccadic eye movements in the monkey and dysmetric saccades obtained during cooling of the left medial cerebellar nuclei to 10°C. Left column compares five successive normal saccades (top row, control) with five successive dysmetric saccades (Cool) for target displacements of 20° to the right, while the right column provides the same comparison for a 20° target displacement to the left. Solid line indicates the right eye and dashed line the left eye. Numbers beside each trace denote the saccade magnitude of the right eye in degrees. From Vilis et al. (1983).

Blair, 1973; Vilis and Hore, 1981) have reported no change in these saccade characteristics, while Ritchie (1976) observed abnormal saccade durations. A possible explanation of this discrepancy is the existence of post-saccadic drift in dysmetric saccades. This makes it difficult to determine when a saccade ends and drift begins, and in turn could result in various interpretations of saccade magnitude and saccade duration.

Dysmetria of the limbs is also a prominent feature during cooling of the lateral cerebellar nuclei in monkeys if dysmetria is defined as either an initial overshoot or undershoot of the target. Unlike saccades, which for a particular target displacement produce a consistent dysmetria, that in limb movements varies from trial to trial (Fig. 4). This variable limb dysmetria appears to be a consequence of the oscillations in the movement. However, in spite of these oscillations the affected limb eventually reaches the target and, if tremor persists, oscillates about the correct target position, whether or not visual feedback is provided (Flament et al., 1984b). If oscillations are abolished by adding inertia to the limb an initial hypermetria occurs, followed by a low-frequency temor about the target region. Thus, the subject's position sense of the affected limb is not impaired in cerebellar disorders. This was well demonstrated by Holmes (1917), who observed that patients could accurately point, with their unaffected limb and their eyes closed, to the position of the affected limb.

Disorders when holding or fixating

An obvious disorder in limbs at the end of a movement is a 3–4 Hz cerebellar intention tremor. We recently reported a number of characteristics of this tremor (Flament et al., 1984b). The phase of the tremor was synchronized by the termination, not the initiation, of the movement. The tremor was not driven by some visual error signal, since its characteristics were unchanged whether or not vision was present. Rather, the tremor, like the tremor that was initiated by a perturbation (Vilis and Hore, 1977), was dependent on the mechanical load imposed on the limb. Thus, if a spring-like force was added to the limb the frequency of the tremor increased. If an inertial load was added the frequency decreased. This behavior is consistent with the tremor being driven by unstable stretch reflexes.

Although various forms of oscillatory eye movements have been ascribed to cerebellar disorders (Dichgans and Jung, 1975; Hotson, 1982), only those related to saccade termination will be con-

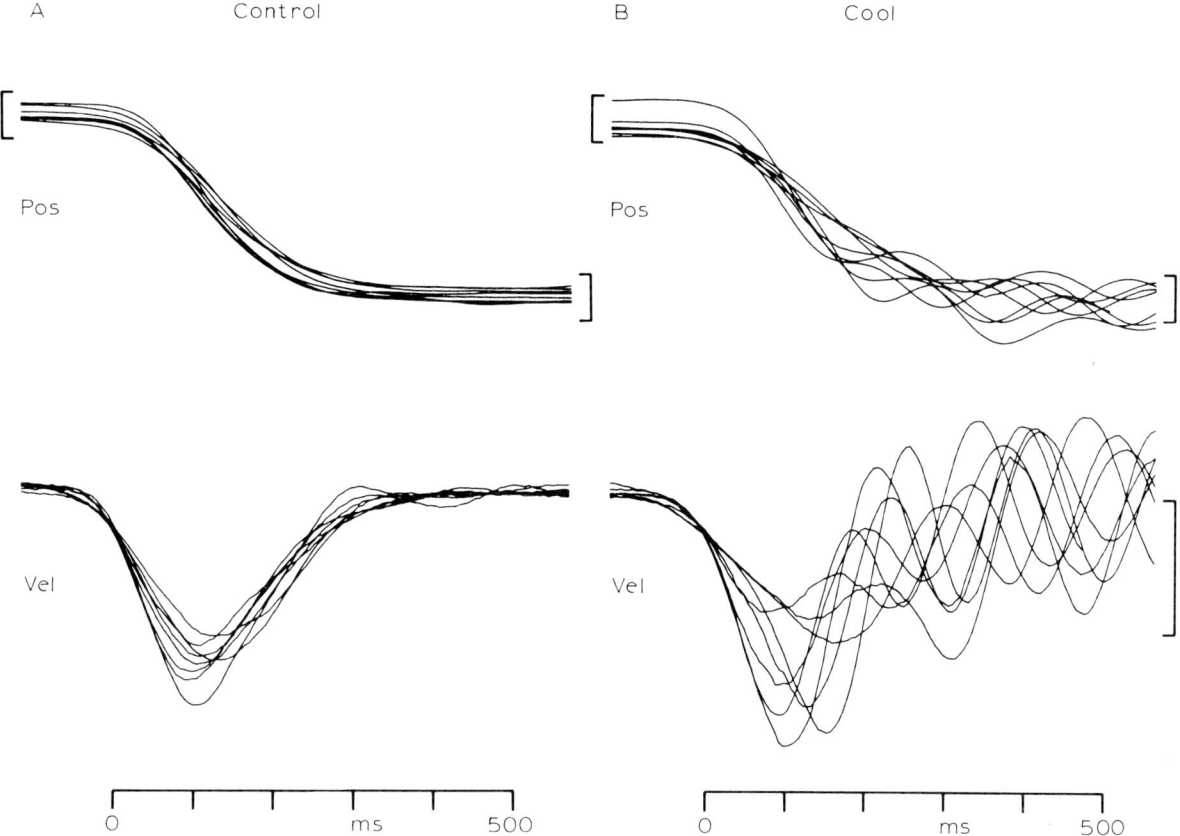

Fig. 4. A comparison of normal elbow flexion movement (A, Control) in the monkey and dysmetric movements (B, Cool) induced by cooling of the lateral and interposed cerebellar nuclei to 10°C. Top traces represent the superimposed positions (Pos) of eight movement trials while the bottom traces illustrate the corresponding velocity (Vel). Calibration bar is 12° for position and 200°/sec for velocity.

sidered here. These are ocular flutter, macrosaccadic oscillations, and gaze paretic nystagmus. The first, ocular flutter, while most closely resembling cerebellar intention tremor of the limb, is unlikely to have the same etiology. Rather, these oscillations appear to consist of a series of saccades without the usual intersaccadic interval and reflect an instability of the intrinsic brainstem saccade-generating circuits (Zee and Robinson, 1979). Macrosaccadic oscillations occur when saccades are hypermetric in both directions (Selhorst et al., 1976). In this situation any corrective saccade initiates a series of hypermetric saccades in alternating directions. The final type of oscillation occurs as a result of post-saccadic drift followed by corrective saccades (gaze paretic nystagmus).

One type of drift associated with saccades and cerebellar lesions is an exponentially decaying drift towards some position of rest, usually the primary position. This drift is usually associated with lesions of the flocculus (Zee et al., 1981). No dysmetria is observed in this case. In contrast, chronic lesions of the vermis result in dysmetria, with no post-saccadic drift (Ritchie, 1976; Optican and Robinson, 1980). These disorders can be interpreted in terms of the two commands that are thought to generate a saccade: a pulse which moves the eyes and a step which then holds the eyes in their new position. It has been proposed by Optican and Robinson (1980) that the vermis is responsible for adjusting the pulse to the correct amplitude. The flocculus then adjusts the step magnitude so that it correctly matches the amplitude of the pulse. This suggests that when in purely vermal lesions the pulse size becomes incorrect, the intact flocculus maintains the ability of adjusting the step in order to suppress post-saccadic drift. Consistent with this view is the observation that acute lesions of the medial cerebellar nuclei, produced by cooling, result in dysmetric saccades accompanied by post-saccadic drift (Vilis and Hore, 1981).

Discussion

In summary, the disorders in limb movements and saccades produced by lesions of the cerebellum appear to have more differences than similarities. Limb movement initiation is delayed during cerebellar dysfunction while that of saccades is not. Oscillations occur during limb movements but not during saccades. The oscillations in limb movements appear to be initiated by inappropriate stretch reflexes. Dysmetria can occur in limb movements as a consequence of the oscillations. However, the correct sense of target and limb position remains intact. Dysmetria occurs in saccades. Corrective saccades then follow after a refractory period. Termination of saccades is accompanied by post-saccadic drift while that of limb movements is followed by intention tremor. The latter is again attributed to inappropriate alternating stretch reflexes. Thus, the main differences in the disorders that occur in the execution and termination of saccades and limb movements may be due to the absence of stretch reflexes in the former and their presence in the latter.

In spite of these differences in the observed disorders, is there a common role for the cerebellum in the control of saccades and arm movements? There is considerable evidence that saccades are terminated by an efference copy signal. For example, the elimination of both visual feedback and extraocular muscle proprioception fails to disrupt saccade termination (Guthrie et al., 1983). According to the scheme proposed by Robinson (1981), burst neurons, located in the brainstem gaze centers, initiate the pulse or move command to the oculomotor neurons. A copy of this move command is directed to tonic neurons. The tonic neurons generate an internal estimate of eye position which serves two functions. First, it directs a step or hold command to the motor neurons which maintains eye position after saccade termination. Second, it is involved in the termination of the move command. According to Robinson's model, the activity of burst neurons is terminated when the error, the difference between target position in the orbit and the internal estimate of eye position, returns to zero. The internal estimate of eye position is predictive in that it precedes actual eye position. This predictive element is necessary because of the high speed and consequent short duration of saccades.

The experiments of Optican and Robinson (1980) clearly demonstrate that the cerebellum exerts a modulatory or calibrative role on this saccade-generating circuit. On the basis of microstimulation of the cerebellum, Keller et al. (1983) suggested that the cerebellum is involved in the creation of the internal eye position signal (efference copy). However, on the basis of computer simulations of the saccade-generating circuit (Optican, 1978) a change in the efference copy should produce a change in the velocity-duration relationships of dysmetric saccades. As mentioned previously, there is as yet no consensus as to whether this occurs.

As for arm movements, our previous studies on limb perturbations provided evidence for an efference copy mechanism for braking. In this situation we found that the role of the cerebellum was to generate an early antagonist response which prevented the return movement from overshooting the target (Vilis and Hore, 1980; Hore and Vilis, 1984). We proposed that an efference copy of the motor cortex agonist command is directed to the cerebellum, which in turn initiates the appropriate antagonist command (Fig. 5). This command is predictive in that it precedes the actual antagonist muscle stretch.

We now propose that the same mechanism could account for the symmetry observed in normal voluntarily generated limb movements. Here (Fig. 5), some internal movement command, rather than a

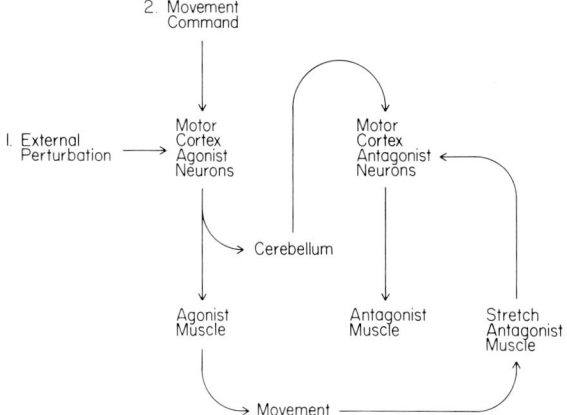

Fig. 5. A hypothetical efference copy mechanism by which the cerebellum could generate an appropriate antagonist command during normal elbow movements initiated either by an external perturbation (1) or by an internal movement command (2).

perturbation, activates motor cortex agonist neurons and generates the agonist command. The command to the antagonist muscle, as in the previous case, would be generated from motor cortex antagonist neurons on the basis of an efference copy computed by the cerebellum. Such a mechanism could ensure that the magnitude of the antagonist command was related to the magnitude of the previous agonist command. According to this scheme the mechanism for generating the antagonist activity that contributes to the braking of normal movements would be lost during cerebellar dysfunction. Instead, during cerebellar dysfunction antagonist activity would now be driven by stretch reflexes (spinal and transcortical). These abnormal stretch reflexes would then initiate oscillations in movements or, in movements with no oscillations, they would generate the antagonist activity at the end of the movement. This mechanism is consistent with the hypothesis proposed by Ito (1970). This stated that as motor learning occurs, an external feedback loop, in this case consisting of the pathway involving stretch of the antagonist muscle (Fig. 5), is gradually supplanted by an internal feedforward loop, in this case consisting of the efference copy signal generated by the cerebellum.

Why don't stretch reflexes disrupt normal movements? Von Holst and Mittelstaedt (1950) were faced with a similar problem. The question they asked is how a voluntary rotational movement is initiated by the common housefly, when such a movement should normally be impeded by a similar servomechanism, the optokinetic response. The conclusion they came to is that voluntary movements are normally accompanied by an efference copy signal whose function is to cancel precisely afferent feedback. It is important to note that afferent feedback is not turned off during the movement. Rather, the efference copy signal simply subtracts out the expected afferent feedback. If for some reason, such as an unexpected perturbation, the movement does not proceed as planned, the afferent feedback will differ from the efference copy signal and a corrective reflex response will be generated.

This hypothesis offers an explanation for the initial deflection that initiates oscillations in limb movements during cerebellar disorders. It may be that here the cerebellar disorder results in a failure of the efference signal and, in turn, a failure in the cancellation of afferent feedback and stretch reflexes. There are two possible modes whereby efference copy could cancel or regulate afferent feedback in normal limb movements. The first is similar to the classical Von Holst formulation. Here, the efference copy signal provided by the cerebellum would simply cancel afferent feedback (e.g., at the level of the spinal cord and motor cortex). In the second mode regulation would occur at the level of the muscle spindle. The gamma efferent discharge can be viewed as an efference copy in that it represents the expected movement trajectory (Granit et al., 1955; Matthews, 1981). This implies that alpha-gamma coactivation occurs not in a fixed ratio but in proportions depending on the prevailing load imposed on the muscles. As discussed by Matthews, if two identical movements are executed, one against no load and the other against a large load, the gamma drive, representing the expected movement trajectory, should be identical. However, the alpha drive in the loaded movement should be larger than that

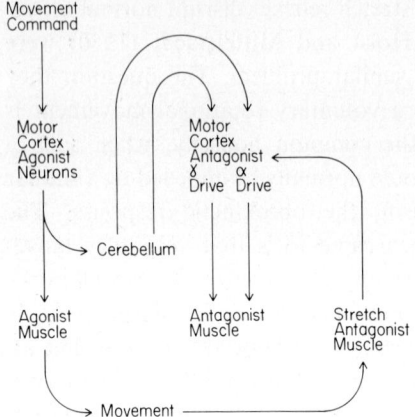

Fig. 6. A hypothetical efference copy mechanism by which the cerebellum could generate the appropriate alpha:gamma ratio for regulating stretch reflexes.

of the no-load case. Thus, the elimination of the reflex response from the stretched antagonist muscle in a normal movement would occur when the ratio of alpha and gamma drive is adjusted to reflect the prevailing mechanical load conditions. If, as suggested previously, the antagonist alpha command is computed by the cerebellum on the basis of the previous agonist command, the same should hold for the antagonist gamma drive (Fig. 6). Thus, in this formulation the inappropriate stretch reflex that occurs during cerebellar disorders represents a failure to adjust the alpha-gamma ratio to the prevailing load conditions. Here, the gamma drive no longer represents the correct efference copy of movement trajectory produced by the alpha drive. This is consistent with our observations, mentioned previously, that the magnitude of the initial deflections in disordered limb movements is dependent on the load conditions imposed on the limb.

In conclusion, in spite of differences observed in the disorders in saccades and limb movements during cerebellar dysfunction, a common role may be ascribed to the cerebellum, that of correctly computing or calibrating the efference copy signal. In saccades efference copy appears to have the single function of terminating the movement. In limb movements it may serve a dual role: cancelling stretch reflexes during movements and generating the antagonist command that terminates movements.

Summary

A comparison is made of the disorders that occur as a result of cerebellar dysfunction in saccadic eye movements and voluntary movements of the arm. One major difference in the observed disorders is the presence of oscillations (tremor) during and following arm movements but not saccades. These oscillations are ascribed to inappropriate stretch reflexes, both spinal and transcortical. It is proposed that under normal conditions the cerebellum has a common function in both arm movements and saccades: that of computing or calibrating an efference copy signal which serves to terminate both types of movements. In limb movements this cerebellar-dependent efference copy signal may serve an additional function of cancelling stretch reflexes.

References

Aschoff, J. C. and Cohen, B. (1971) Changes in saccadic eye movements produced by cerebellar cortical lesions. Exp. Neurol., 32: 123–133.

Avanzini, G., Girotti, F., Crenna, P. and Negri, S. (1979) Alterations of ocular motility in cerebellar pathology. An electro-oculographic study. Arch. Neurol., 36: 274–280.

Brooks, V. B. and Thach, W. T. (1981) Cerebellar control of posture and movement. In V. B. Brooks (Ed.), Handbook of Physiology. The Nervous System, Vol. II, Motor Control, Part 2, American Physiological Society, Bethesda, MD, pp. 877–946.

Brooks, V. B., Kozlovskaya, I. B., Atkin, A., Horvath, F. E. and Uno, M. (1973) Effects of cooling dentate nucleus on tracking-task performance in monkeys. J. Neurophysiol., 36: 974–995.

Dichgans, J. and Jung, R. (1975) Oculomotor abnormalities due to cerebellar lesions. In G. Lennerstrand and P. Bach-y-Rita (Eds.), Basic Mechanisms of Ocular Motility and their Clinical Implications, Pergamon Press, Oxford, pp. 281–298.

Flament, D., Hore, J. and Vilis, T. (1984a) Braking of fast and accurate elbow flexions in the monkey. J. Physiol., 349: 195–203.

Flament, D., Vilis, T. and Hore, J. (1984b) Dependence of cerebellar tremor on proprioceptive but not visual feedback. Exp. Neurol., 84: 314–325.

Flament, D., Vilis, T. and Hore, J. (1984c) Abnormal antagonist muscle activity occurs in elbow flexions during cerebellar dysfunction. Abst. Soc. Neurosci., 10: 905.

Ghez, C. and Martin, J. H. (1982) The control of rapid limb movement in the cat. III. Agonist-antagonist coupling. Exp. Brain Res., 45: 115–125.

Granit, R., Holmgren, B. and Merton, P. A. (1955) The two routes for excitation of muscle and their subservience to the cerebellum. J. Physiol. (Lond.), 130: 213–224.

Guthrie, B. L., Porter, J. D. and Sparks, D. L. (1983) Corollary discharge provides accurate eye position information to the oculomotor system. Science, 222: 1193–1195.

Holmes, G. (1917)The symptoms of acute cerebellar injuries due to gunshot injuries. Brain, 40: 461–535.

Hore, J. and Vilis, T. (1984) Loss of set in muscle responses to limb perturbations during cerebellar dysfunction. J. Neurophysiol., 51: 1137–1148.

Hotson, J. R. (1982) Cerebellar control of fixation eye movements. Neurology, 32: 31–36.

Ito, M. (1970) Neurophysiological aspects of the cerebellar motor control system. Int. J. Neurol., 7: 162–176.

Keller, E. L. and Robinson, D. A. (1971) Absence of a stretch reflex in extraocular muscles of the monkey. J. Neurophysiol., 34: 908–919.

Keller, E. L., Slakey, D. P. and Crandall, W. F. (1983) Microstimulation of the primate cerebellar vermis during saccadic eye movements. Brain Res., 288: 131–143.

Lamarre, Y., Bioulac, B. and Jacks, B. (1978) Activity of precentral neurones in conscious monkeys: effects of deafferentation and cerebellar ablation. J. Physiol. (Paris), 74: 253–264.

Lestienne, F. (1979) Effects of intertial load and velocity on the braking process of voluntary limb movements. Exp. Brain Res., 35: 407–418.

Luciani, L. (1915) Human Physiology, Muscular and Nervous System, Vol. 3, MacMillan, London.

Matthews, P. B. C. (1981) Muscle spindles: their messages and their fusimotor supply. In V. B. Brooks (Ed.), Handbook of Physiology. The Nervous System, Vol. II, Motor Control, Part 1, American Physiological Society, Bethesda, MD, pp. 189–228.

Meyer-Lohmann, J., Hore, J. and Brooks, V. B. (1977) Cerebellar participation in generation of prompt arm movements. J. Neurophysiol., 40: 1038–1050.

Nelson, W. L. (1983) Physical principles for economies of skilled movements. Biol. Cybern., 46: 135–147.

Optican, L. M. (1978) Cerebellar-dependent adaptive control of the saccadic eye movement system. Ph. D. Dissertation, The Johns Hopkins University.

Optican, L. M. and Robinson, D. A. (1980) Cerebellar-dependent adaptive control of the primate saccadic system. J. Neurophysiol. 44: 1058–1076.

Ritchie, L. (1976) Effects of cerebellar lesions in saccadic eye movements. J. Neurophysiol., 39: 1246–1256.

Robinson, D. A. (1981) Control of eye movements. In V. B. Brooks (Ed.), Handbook of Physiology. The Nervous System, Vol. II, Motor Control, Part 2, American Physiological Society, Bethesda, MD, pp. 1275–1320.

Ron, S. and Nemet, P. (1977) The cerebellum involvement in the generation of saccades. Doc. Ophthalmol., 43: 109–114.

Selhorst, J. B., Stark, L., Ochs, A. L. and Hoyt, W. F. (1976) Disorders in cerebellar ocular motor control. II. Macrosaccadic oscillation. An oculographic, control system and clinico-anatomical analysis. Brain, 99: 509–522.

Soechting, J. F., Ranish, N. A., Palminteri, R. and Terzuolo, C. A. (1976) Changes in a motor pattern following cerebellar and olivary lesions in the squirrel monkey. Brain Res., 105: 21–44.

Thach, W. T. (1975) Timing of activity in cerebellar dentate nucleus and cerebral motor cortex during prompt volitional movement. Brain Res., 88: 233–241.

Trouche, E. and Beaubaton, D. (1980) Initiation of a goal-directed movement in the monkey. Role of the cerebellar dentate nucleus. Exp. Brain Res., 40: 311–321.

Vilis, T. and Hore, J. (1977) Effects of changes in mechanical state of limb on cerebellar intention tremor. J. Neurophysiol., 40: 1214–1224.

Vilis, T. and Hore, J. (1980) Central neural mechanisms contributing to cerebellar tremor produced by limb perturbations. J. Neurophysiol., 43: 279–291.

Vilis, T. and Hore, J. (1981) Characteristics of saccadic dysmetria in monkeys during reversible lesions of medial cerebellar nuclei. J. Neurophysiol., 46: 828–838.

Vilis, T., Snow, R. and Hore, J. (1983) Cerebellar saccadic dysmetria is not equal in the two eyes. Exp. Brain Res., 51: 343–350.

Von Holst, E. and Mittelstaedt, H. (1950) Das Reafferenzprinzip. Wechselwirkung zwischen Zentralnervensystem und Peripherie. Naturwissenschaften, 37: 464–476.

Wennmo, C., Hindfelt, B. and Pyykkö, I. (1983) Eye movements in cerebellar and combined cerebellobrainstem diseases. Ann. Otol. Rhinol. Laryngol., 92: 165–171.

Westheimer, G. and Blair, S. M. (1973) Oculomotor defects in cerebellectomized monkeys. Invest. Ophthalmol., 12: 618–621.

Woollacott, M. H., Bonnet, M. and Yabe, K. (1984) Preparatory process for anticipatory postural adjustments — Modulation of leg muscles reflex pathways during preparation for arm movements in standing man. Exp. Brain Res., 55: 263–271.

Zee, D. S. and Robinson, D. A. (1979) A hypothetical explanation of saccadic oscillations. Ann. Neurol., 5: 405–414.

Zee, D. S., Optican, L. M., Cook, J. D., Robinson, D. A. and Engel, W. K. (1976) Slow saccades in spinocerebellar degeneration. Arch. Neurol., 33: 243–251.

Zee, D. S., Yamazaki, A., Butler, P. H. and Gücer, G. (1981) Effects of ablation of flocculus and paraflocculus on eye movements in primate. J. Neurophysiol., 46: 878–899.

Cerebellar relation to muscle spindles in hand tracking

W. T. Thach, M. H. Schieber, J. Mink, S. Kane and M. Horne

Departments of Anatomy and Neurobiology, Neurology and Neurosurgery, and The McDonnell Center for Study of Higher Brain Function, Washington University School of Medicine, St. Louis, MO 63110, U.S.A.

Introduction

The limb and the eye are similar in their capacity to move in planned trajectories. To do this, the central processes that control the two members must face similar problems in selecting the muscles, force, direction, position (and its time derivatives), and times of initiation and termination that are needed to program a trajectory. Yet the limb and the eye are very different in many respects, and the question is whether any of the differences creates special control problems unique to the one member. One such difference is the tendency of the limb to oscillate. The limb has much greater inertial mass, and external loads of infinite variety are routinely added to it. Its muscles are elastic, and lack viscous damping comparable to that provided by the tissues of the orbit. These purely mechanical factors determine that the limb will oscillate when perturbed or set in motion. The problem is compounded by the powerful stretch reflexes that regulate the limb but not the eye. Length-sensitive stretch reflexes with long conduction times sense and actively amplify the oscillation (Henatsch, 1967; Lippold, 1970; Nichols et al., 1978; Hagbarth and Young, 1979; Matthews, 1981). From an engineering point of view, the limb would be an extremely poorly designed system if there were not special routines for compensating the inherent mechanical and neural instability. Indeed, the problem is one that fascinated engineers at the very beginnings of thinking about feedback control. One reason Wiener named his landmark treatise on the subject "Cybernetics: Control and Communications in the Animal and the Machine" (Wiener, 1948) was the tremor of neurological disease states. He speculated freely that tremor might reflect the removal of a critical stabilizing component from an inherently unstable feedback (reflex) control system. By contrast, neurologists have traditionally adhered to the doctrine of Hughlings-Jackson, eloquently expressed by F. M. R. Walshe (1921, 1927) in specific reference to "cerebellar ataxy". His thesis was that it is illogical to define the normal function of a part of the brain as controlling the abnormalities that occur upon its removal. His analogy was that the removal of a tooth from a gear in an automobile drive train may cause noise and jarring, but that it is wrong to infer that the tooth was designed specifically to prevent noise and jarring. His specific admonition was that the cerebellum is not attached to the brain to prevent ataxia and tremor.

Until some recent work in our laboratory, we sided with Walshe's train of thought, preferring to think that the cerebellum took major executive roles in programming the direction, position, velocity, force and muscle selection parameters of movement trajectory (cf. Brooks and Thach, 1981). However, the outcome of the following experiments has caused us to question this opinion. The crucial finding was that in wrist trajectories made in opposite directions at different velocities and against different torque loads all cerebellar neurons recorded in dentate and interpositus discharged in a single pattern unrelated to any of these parameters. What the cerebellar neurons did relate to was the pattern of discharge in Ia spindle afferents, and physiological tremor.

Neuron recording during wrist ramp tracking in trained monkeys

Single unit discharge was recorded in the dentate and interposed cerebellar nuclei, motor cortex and C7 and C8 dorsal root ganglia during trained slow hold-ramp-hold tracking, rapid alternating movement, torque pulse perturbation, and action tremor of the monkey's wrist. The following is a summary of those experiments (Elble et al., 1984; Schieber and Thach, 1980a,b; Thach and Schieber, 1980).

57 dentate and 45 interposed neurons were found in two monkeys that discharged in relation to slow tracking movement. Nearly all neurons had a distinct bidirectional pattern of discharge consisting of an abrupt increase (or decrease) in firing frequency at or before the onset of movement that was variably maintained throughout the ramp and was independent of movement direction. None of the neurons showed a clear relationship to direction, position, velocity or load during the performance of this task. Nevertheless, these neurons usually discharged in relation to rapid alternation and (for interpositus) torque pulses in patterns that were directionally reciprocal. Some interpositus neurons showed a modulation related to tremor superimposed on the bidirectional discharge related to slow ramps.

29 neurons in motor cortex of one monkey discharged during slow hold-ramp-hold tracking in two patterns. Class I neurons (14/29) showed gradually changing, directionally reciprocal modulations of firing frequency for movements in opposite directions. These neurons were often related to torque load and/or to wrist position, but not to velocity. The discharge pattern was similar to the pattern of activity of forearm muscles. Class II neurons (15/29) showed an abrupt change in firing frequency that was bidirectional. They were often related to torque load and/or to velocity but not to position. Motor cortex neurons discharged in relation to rapid alternating movements, torque pulses and tremor in similar patterns that did not distinguish the two classes.

The cerebellum is known to control gamma motor neurons and to be controlled by muscle spindle afferents (cf. cited articles by Denny-Brown, Glaser, Gilman, and their colleagues; Eldred et al. 1953; Granit et al., 1955; Henatsch et al., 1964; Soechting et al., 1978; MacKay and Murphy, 1979). Having observed the bidirectional cerebellar discharge pattern that we could not relate either to trajectory parameters or to activity of alpha motor neurons (EMG), we devised a method for recording from spindle afferent neurons in the spinal dorsal root ganglia during trained movement. Our purpose was to see if they behaved as though related to the bidirectional cerebellar activity. Five units in dorsal root ganglia were identified by their non-cutaneous deep receptive field, tonic discharge at rest, response to brief taps and maintained pressure on the receptive field, driving by application of a tuning fork at 128/sec or subharmonic of 64/sec, pause during electrically stimulated local muscle twitch, reciprocal response to opposite torque pulses to the wrist, and reciprocal discharge to rapid alternating movements as muscle spindle afferents.

During ramps, their pattern of discharge was bidirectional and resembled the bidirectional discharge patterns of neurons in motor cortex (class II) and cerebellum. For some cells the bidirectional pattern varied slightly in relation to the direction and velocity of movement and the amount of torque load, but was not related to the large changes in wrist position (muscle length). Modulation in relation to tremor was superimposed on the bidirectional pattern related to ramps. The comparison of spindle afferent discharge with the concurrent EMG of the parent muscle suggested that spindles were driven by gamma fusimotor activity dissociated from that of alpha skeletomotor neurons.

Based on these results, we were led to entertain the idea that during slow hold-ramp-hold wrist tracking, two parallel motor systems operated in relative dissociation. The first system included class

I motor cortex neurons, spinal alpha skeletomotor neurons and extrafusal muscle. The elements of this system were active in a directionally reciprocal fashion; their activity was related to load and position but not to velocity. This system could have directly produced the wrist movement. The second system included all cerebellar dentate and interposed nuclear neurons, class II motor cortex neurons, spinal gamma fusimotor neurons, and muscle spindle afferents. This system could have maintained a constancy of spindle afferent sensitivity despite widely varying peripheral conditions, so as to monitor continuously and precisely small rapid movement irregularities such as tremor, as originally proposed by Kuffler et al. (1951).

Neural discharge related to stiffness, damping, and stretch reflexes

These results have led us to look for some quantitative measure of stability of the limb. Such a measure is necessary for comparison with the EMG and CNS neural activity that is putatively maintaining that stability or altering it as needed in response to change in external load on the limb. From the following work, it would appear that relatively simple measures of stiffness and damping of oscillations following a torque pulse may be adequate for this purpose (Kane et al., 1984).

The oscillatory behavior of a monkey's wrist was modeled as a classical spring-dashpot system, successfully quantitating the differences in damping and stiffness associated with tremor (r_2 values of 0.98 to 0.99+ for each task). Three rhesus monkeys were trained to insert their hands, with fingers extended, into a wedge-shaped manipulandum and to perform hold-ramp-hold movements by flexing and extending about the wrist while tracking a visual target. Trajectories at velocities of 28°/sec were performed in each direction through 70° of wrist arc with and against uniform torque loads (0.10 and 0.14 Nm). Each task was performed in blocks of ten trials, two of which included a 50-msecond loading or unloading torque pulse (0.77 and 0.11 Nm), one delivered during the hold 0.5 second before movement began, the other during the ramp after the monkey had moved 15° from the hold position. Position was measured by a potentiometer circuit, averaged for 6–10 trials, and stored in 6-msecond bins. Position data were chosen to begin after the torque pulse discontinuity and end 100–400 mseconds later, when either the oscillations died away or the monkey made a volitional, nonoscillatory movement. The damping coefficient g (1/sec) and natural frequency f_0 (Hz) were determined by fitting the position as a function of time to $\theta(t) = A\exp(-gt/2)\cos(wt+a)$ for the eight task conditions and averaging for holds and ramps:

	g-hold	g-ramp	f_0-hold	f_0-ramp
Monkey 1	76.8 ± 10.8	59.1 ± 7.9	10.2 ± 0.7	8.74 ± 0.39
Monkey 2	54.3 ± 7.4	64.6 ± 8.7	7.49 ± 0.17	9.17 ± 0.47
Monkey 3	20.8 ± 3.5	20.0 ± 3.6	7.37 ± 0.41	7.30 ± 0.34

Monkeys 1 and 2 had more damping than monkey 3 (paired t-test, $P < 0.01$) and had little physiological tremor. Monkey 3 had relatively poor damping (oscillating for periods up to 400 mseconds after perturbation), relatively more compliance (proportional to $f_0 - 2$), and a large-amplitude, 8–10 Hz tremor. In sum, stiffness (f_0) and damping (g) coefficients varied markedly across monkeys. High damping coefficients were accompanied by little physiological tremor. Nevertheless, each animal appeared to have a unique pattern of stiffness and damping when comparing holds and ramps, suggesting strategies of stability control were to some extent unique for each animal.

We then wondered whether the large differences in stiffness and damping between holds and ramps and especially across different monkeys were in turn correlated with (and produced by) differences in the stretch reflexes as measured by the EMG. We found that the monkey with the shortest latency reflex had the best damping and the least physiological tremor, and the monkey with the longest latency reflex had the least damping and the most tremor. These studies are summarized as follows (Mink et al., 1984).

In the three rhesus monkeys above, the hold and ramp-tracking tasks were performed in blocks of ten trials, two of which included a 50-msecond torque pulse that was delivered either during the initial hold or after the monkey had tracked the first 15° of trajectory (Kane et al., 1984). EMG activity was monitored while the monkey performed rapid alternating movements to ensure that the electrodes were not picking up activity of the antagonist muscles (Mink and Thach, 1983). Following torque pulse application, the monkey's wrist position exhibited a pattern of damped oscillation which was accompanied by periodic bursting in the EMG that continued for 100–300 mseconds after the end of the torque pulse. Three EMG patterns were seen in three monkeys: (1) agonist bursts with no phasic activity in the antagonists, (2) agonist bursts alternating with antagonist bursts, and (3) agonist and antagonist bursts occurring simultaneously. All three patterns were seen to some degree in each monkey, but one had a clear predominance of pattern 1, and another of pattern 3. The monkey with periodic bursting after torque pulse in the agonist without periodic bursting in the antagonist had the best damping of the oscillations after the torque pulse and the least amount of physiological tremor in holds and ramps. The monkey with periodic bursting after torque pulses simultaneously in both agonist and antagonist had the worst damping of the oscillations after the torque pulse and the largest amplitude, 8–10 Hz, physiological tremor in holds and ramps. The relationship between the EMG pattern and the degree of damping was seen within each monkey as well as between monkeys, e.g., when the monkey with the worst damping of oscillations used pattern 1, the degree of damping increased. The monkey with worst tremor and damping had a mean stretch reflex latency (perturbation to onset of EMG) of about 50 mseconds, while the monkey with the least tremor and the best damping (g value 5 times greater) had a mean latency of around 30 mseconds. These differences were significant at the $P = 0.0001$ level of significance. Our hypothesis is that these differences in stretch reflex latency may reflect a different bias in each monkey of the relative activities of type Ia and II stretch receptors and of gamma dynamic and gamma static neurons. The slower reflex would be produced by a predominance of type II and Ia (under gamma static control) receptors driven by absolute length changes: the muscles would tend to be elastic and the wrist would oscillate. The faster reflex would be produced by a predominance of type Ia receptors (under gamma dynamic control) driven by velocity/acceleration: the muscle would tend to be viscous and oscillations would be damped.

Finally, we wanted to know how Purkinje cells discharge during ramp tracking, oscillations produced by torque pulses, and tremor.

Purkinje cells had been shown to discharge in relation to anticipated torque pulse perturbations of the hand that require a prompt compensatory return to the initial position (Gilbert and Thach, 1977). The torque pulse amplitude had then been changed unexpectedly to a novel value. This made the previous response inappropriate, resulting in an undershoot or an overshoot of the initial position, depending on whether the torque pulse amplitude was larger or smaller than previously. As the monkey adapted the response over successive trials to an appropriate magnitude, the Purkinje cells behaved as though playing a role in the adaptation process. This consisted of a transient increase in the complex spike frequency, and a persistent decrease in simple spike frequency, both changes timelocked to the perturbation. An idea at the time was that the adaptation may have focussed on stretch reflexes — segmental, long loop, or both (cf. Vilis and Hore, 1977, 1980). The more recent observations cited below also suggest that Purkinje cell output may be focussed on the control of stretch reflexes, and that this may be an appropriate variable to manipulate experimentally in further tests of the cerebellar adaptive motor control theories.

Up to this point, we did not know how Purkinje cells might behave in the ramp-tracking task, our observations (Schieber and Thach, 1980a) having been confined to interposed and dentate nuclear cells. We also wanted to see how Purkinje cells responded to unexpected torque pulses, which threw the hand into oscillations and spoiled the trial, but which required no response (or adaptation) from the monkey. Therefore, the discharge of cerebellar Purkinje, cortical interneuronal, and deep nuclear cells was recorded as monkey 3 of the above studies performed hold-ramp-hold wrist tracking in flexor and extensor directions with and against maintained torque load (Thach et al., 1984). Wrist flexor and extensor EMG, position and force were monitored during all recordings. Loading and unloading torque pulses were applied on occasional trials during hold or ramp. This monkey had the marked 8–10/sec "physiological" tremor. After torque pulses, 3–5 beats of poorly damped oscillation of position and force occurred, accompanied by periodic EMG bursts simultaneously in agonist and antagonist (despite loading) muscles. During holds, discharge was poorly if at all related to position or load direction. During ramp movement, discharge at or before movement onset increased (most cells) or decreased (some cells) for the duration of movement, independent of direction or load. After torque pulses during holds and ramps, discharge increased or decreased, usually with periodic fluctuation related to wrist oscillation. Cells changing discharge in relation to ramp movement and torque pulse often underwent periodic changes in relation to tremor as well.

Complex spikes of Purkinje cells bore no strict time relation to torque pulse or oscillation, which stood in sharp contrast to their behavior in the previous experiment, when an adaptive response was required (Gilbert and Thach, 1977).

These results confirm the observations of Mano and Yamamoto (1980) that some Purkinje cells are bidirectional in slow pursuit tracking, and add that, under the conditions of our task performance, virtually all are. This is the pattern seen also in nearly all cerebellar nuclear cells and in primary muscle spindle afferents, and suggests that in this task Purkinje cells, like nuclear cells, have an important and possibly exclusive role in controlling stretch reflexes.

Discussion

Our specific objectives for the work now in progress address the following questions in an attempt to support causal relationships:

Are the parameters of wrist stiffness and damping, as measured after torque pulse perturbations of holds and ramp tracks, quantitatively related to tremor? Do these in turn relate quantitively to the length- and velocity- (and higher time-derivative) sensitivity of stretch reflexes? If so, by what route — segmental or transcortical? Are these in turn quantitatively related to the bidirectional discharge in these cerebellar neurons and spindle afferents? Are the stiffness, damping, and tremor of the limb, and the bidirectional discharge, length- and velocity-sensitivity of the stretch reflexes impaired critically and in parallel by cerebellar ablation? Does the compensation for inertial, viscous, and spring loads to maintain stability critically depend on the cerebellum?

If these studies are successful in supporting damping and load compensation mechanisms through cerebellar modulation of stretch reflexes, we should then be in a better position to examine further the hypothetical roles of Purkinje cells during natural adaptations of the behavior with which they are specifically concerned.

As to Walshe's warning against inferring abnormal function as the negative of the ablative deficit, one should point out the obvious, that the ablation does nevertheless negate the normal function, and that the defect is therefore the negative of the normal function. More than a question of semantics, it depends upon what one is willing to accept as normal function in the light of contemporary knowledge. In this case, the control of stability would be the normal function. While this concept owes much to control theory and to the increasing knowledge of limb mechanics and the stretch reflexes themselves (cf. especially MacKay and Murphy, 1979), clinical neurologists were among the first to question the categorical imperative of F. M. R. Walshe. Indeed, the results and interpretations we offer here seem to us quite in keeping with those of Denny-Brown (Denny-Brown and Gilman, 1965), of Glaser, Higgins and Partridge (Glaser and Higgins, 1966; Higgins and Glaser, 1964; Higgins et al., 1962), of Dow (Henatsch et al., 1964), of Gilman and his colleagues (Gilman et al., 1976; Gilman and Ebel, 1970; Gilman and McDonald, 1967; Van der Meulen and Gilman, 1965), and of Neilson and Lance (1978). One should also point out that the prevention of oscillation needn't be the only result of cerebellar control of stretch reflexes. The clinical signs judged empirically over the years to be the most successful in detecting cerebellar injury (cf. Holmes, 1939) consist not only of the unwanted oscillations in perturbed positions and smooth trajectories, but also of the inability to make rapid alternating movements — oscillations! We submit that the same controls that operate to adjust the spring and damping elements of stretch reflexes to prevent unwanted oscillation may also adjust them to produce wanted oscillation (cf. Thach, 1968; Hagbarth et al., 1975; E. G. Walshe, 1977). The use of reflexes at a segmental level may make possible an oscillation generator capable of higher resonant frequency than a generator forced to use exclusively long central conduction times in its loop. Finally, the cerebellar influence on the stretch reflex apparatus needn't be restricted to the control of oscillation. In the prompt ballistic movements triggered by an expected "go" signal, stretch reflex inputs could be used to bring alpha motor neurons to just under threshold firing level, freeing all the faster descending pathways to participate in the initiation of movement at the "go" signal (Thach, 1978). Such a presetting of the spindle afferents would also offset spindle unloading caused by movement onset. In both mechanisms, the cerebellar-spindle axis would be used to help initiate and maintain the fastest possible motor reponse. Thus, one may conceive of the same cerebellar-spindle mechanism being used in various different roles to damp oscillation in slow precise movements, to assist in producing oscillations of a desired high frequency, and to boost the speed of predictive ballistic movements.

How does this work on limb movements compare with that on eye movements? One might conclude that there are qualitative differences, since the eye has relatively little of this kind of instability, no stretch reflexes and rather primitive spindles. Cerebellar ablation has shown abnormalities in the fine adjustment of many different kinds of eye movements (Robinson, Section V), and the inference has been that each type is controlled separately. The cautionary warning these limb studies raise is whether each eye movement is indeed governed separately from all others, or whether all are affected through a differential control of a common neural element, such as the muscle spindle and the stretch reflexes.

Summary

Our reasons for believing that one normal function of the intact cerebellar dentate and interposed nuclei is the control of oscillation through adjustment of stretch reflexes are: 1, in precise ramp tracking, these cerebellar neurons do not relate to parameters of trajectory; 2, in precise ramp tracking, these cerebellar neurons do relate to spindle afferent discharge as though controlling it or being controlled by it, or both; 3, in precise ramp tracking, the one parameter of movement that these cerebellar neurons obviously monitor is tremor; 4, oscillation is itself a problem inherent in the design of the normal neuromusculoskeletal system; and 5, tremor is itself a normal phenomenon that may be kept within acceptable limits, but never prevented entirely.

References

Brooks, V. B. and Thach, W. T. (1981) Cerebellar control of posture and movement. In J. M. Brookhart, V. B. Mountcastle, and V. B. Brooks (Eds.), Handbook of Physiology, Section 1, The Nervous System, Vol. II, Motor Control, Part 2, American Physiological Society, Bethesda, MD, pp. 877–946.

Denny-Brown, D. and Gilman, S. (1965) Depression of gamma innervation by cerebellectomy. Trans. Am. Neurol. Assoc., 90: 96–101.

Elble, R. J., Schieber, M. H. and Thach, W. T. (1985) Activity of muscle spindles, motor cortex and cerebellar nuclei during

action tremor. Brain Res., 323: 330–334.
Eldred, E., Granit, R. and Merton, P. A. (1953) Supraspinal control of the muscle spindles and its significance. J. Physiol., 122: 498–523.
Gilbert, P. F. C. and Thach, W. T. (1977) Purkinje cell activity during motor learning. Brain Res., 128: 309–328.
Gilman, S. and Ebel, H. C. (1970) Fusimotor neuron responses to natural stimuli as a function of prestimulus fusimotor activity in decerebellate cats. Brain Res., 21: 367–384.
Gilman, S. and McDonald, W. I. (1967) Cerebellar facilitation of muscle spindle activity. J. Neurophysiol., 30: 1494–1512.
Gilman, S., Carr, D. and Hollenberg, J. (1976) Kinematic effects of deafferentiation and cerebellar ablation. Brain, 99: 311–330.
Glaser, G. H. and Higgins, D. C. (1966) Motor stability, stretch responses, and the cerebellum. In R. Granit (Ed.), Muscular Afferents and Motor Control. Proceedings of the Nobel Symp. I., Almquist & Wiksell, Stockholm, pp. 121–138.
Granit, R., Holmgren, B. and Merton, P. A. (1955) The two routes for excitation of muscles and their subservience to the cerebellum. J. Physiol., 130: 213–224.
Hagbarth, K.-E. and Young, R. R. (1979) Participation of the stretch reflex in human physiological tremor. Brain, 102: 509–580.
Hagbarth, K.-E., Wallin, G. and Lofstedt, L. (1975) Muscle spindle activity in man during voluntary fast alternating movements. J. Neurol. Neurosurg. Psych., 38: 625–635.
Henatsch, H. D. (1967) Instability of the proprioceptive length servo: its possible role in tremor phenomena. In M. D. Yahr and D. P. Purpura (Eds.), Neurophysiological Basis of Normal and Abnormal Motor Activities, Raven Press, New York, pp. 75–89.
Henatsch, H. D., Manni, E., Wilson, J. H. and Dow, R. S. (1964) Linked and independent responses of tonic alpha and gamma hind-limb motoneurons to deep cerebellar stimulation. J. Neurophysiol., 27: 172–192.
Higgins, D. C. and Glaser, G. H. (1964) Stretch responses during chronic cerebellar ablation. A study of reflex instability. J. Neurophysiol., 27: 49–62.
Higgins, D. C., Partridge, L. D. and Glaser, G. H. (1962) A transient cerebellar influence on stretch responses. J. Neurophysiol., 25: 684–692.
Holmes, G. (1939) The cerebellum of man. Brain, 62: 1–30.
Kane, S. A., Mink, J. W. and Thach, W. T. (1984) A mathematical analysis of movement (oscillation) following perturbation during hold-ramp-hold wrist movements in the monkey. Soc. Neurosci. Abstr., 10: 332.
Kuffler, S. W., Hunt, C. C. and Quilliam, J. P. (1951) Function of medulated small-nerve fibers in mammalian ventral roots: efferent muscle spindle innervation. J. Neurophysiol., 14: 29–54.
Lippold, O. C. J. (1970) Oscillation in the stretch reflex arc and the origin of the rhythmical 8–12 c/s component of physiological tremor. J. Physiol. (Lond.), 206: 359–382.

MacKay, W. A. and Murphy, J. T. (1979) Cerebellar modulation of reflex gain. Progr. Neurobiol., 13: 361–417.
Mano, N.-I. and Yamamoto, K.-I. (1980) Simple spike activity of cerebellar Purkinje cells related to visually guided wrist tracking movement in the monkey. J. Neurophysiol., 43: 713–728.
Matthews, P. B. C. (1981) Muscle spindles, their messages and their fusimotor supply. In J. M. Brookhart, V. B. Mountcastle and V. B. Brooks, (Eds.), Handbook of Physiology, Section 1: The Nervous System, Volume II, Motor control, Part 1, American Physiological Society, Bethesda, MD, pp. 189–228.
Mink, J. W. and Thach, W. T. (1983) Cocontraction of antagonist muscles during training of wrist movements in monkeys. Soc. Neurosci. Abstr., 9: 634.
Mink, J. W., Kane, S. A. and Thach, W. T. (1984) Agonist-antagonist muscle activity in oscillation after torque-pulse perturbation of the monkey's wrist. Soc. Neurosci. Abstr., 10: 332.
Neilson, P. D. and Lance, J. W. (1978) Reflex transmission characteristics during voluntary activity in normal man and patients with movement disorders. In J. E. Desmedt (Ed.), Cerebral Motor Control in Man: Long Loop Mechanisms, Progress in Clinical Neurophysiology, Vol. 4, Karger, Basel, pp. 263–299.
Nichols, T. R., Stein, R. B. and Bawa, P. (1978) Spinal reflexes as a basis for tremor in the premammillary cat. Can. J. Physiol. Pharmacol., 56: 375–383.
Schieber, M. H. and Thach, W. T. (1980a) Bidirectional neuronal discharge in cerebellar nuclei and motor cortex during slow hold-ramp-hold tracking. Soc. Neurosci. Abstr., 6: 762.
Schieber, M. H. and Thach, W. T. (1980b) Alpha-gamma dissociation during slow tracking movements of the monkey's wrist: preliminary evidence from spinal ganglion recording. Brain Res., 202: 213–216.
Soechting, J. F., Burton, J. E. and Onoda, N. (1978) Relationships between sensory input, motor output and unit activity in interpositus and red nuclei during intentional movement. Brain Res., 152: 65–79.
Thach, W. T. (1968) Discharge of Purkinje and cerebellar nuclear neurons during rapidly alternating arm movements in the monkey. J. Neurophysiol., 31: 785–797.
Thach, W. T. (1978) Correlation of neural discharge with pattern and force of muscular activity, joint position, and direction of intended next movement in motor cortex and cerebellum. J. Neurophysiol., 41: 654–676.
Thach, W. T. and Schieber, M. H. (1980) Bidirectional spindle afferent discharge during slow tracking movements: evidence for alpha-gamma dissociation. Soc. Neurosci. Abstr., 6: 762.
Thach, W. T., Mink, J. W. and Kane, S. A. (1984) Cerebellar Purkinje cells have bidirectional discharge during ramp tracking and phasic modulation during oscillation of the monkey's wrist. Soc. Neurosci. Abstr., 10: 333.
Van der Meulen, J. P. and Gilman, S. (1965) Recovery of muscle spindle activity in cats after cerebellar ablation. J. Neurophy-

siol., 28: 943–957.
Vilis, T. and Hore, J. (1977) Effects of changes in mechanical state of limb on cerebellar intention tremor. J. Neurophysiol., 43: 279–291.
Vilis, T. and Hore, J. (1980) Central neuronal mechanisms contributing to cerebellar tremor produced by limb perturbations. J. Neurophysiol., 43: 279–291.
Walshe, E. G. (1977) Persistense of stretch reflexes following cerebellar ablation, and a resonance theory of cerebellar function. In F. C. Rose (Ed.), Physiological Aspects of Clinical Neurology, Blackwell Scientific Publications, Oxford, pp. 215–224.
Walshe, F. M. R. (1921) On disorders of movement resulting from loss of postural tone, with special reference to cerebellar ataxy. Brain, 44: 539–556.
Walshe, F. M. R. (1927) Discussion on "The significance of the voluntary element in the genesis of cerebellar ataxy". Brain, 50: 377–385.
Wiener, N. (1948) Cybernetics: Control and Communications in the Animal and in the Machine, John Wiley, New York, pp. 113–136.

Cerebellar control of eye movements

U. Büttner, R. Boyle and G. Markert

Department of Neurology, University of Düsseldorf, Moorenstrasse 5, D-4000 Düsseldorf, F.R.G.

Introduction

In the oculomotor system, in contrast to the skeletalmotor system, functionally different types of movements with anatomically separate premotor structures can be distinguished (Henn et al., 1982). There are five different types of eye movements in higher mammals: 1. Fast eye movements, i.e., saccades and the fast phases of vestibular and optokinetic nystagmus. 2. The vestibulo-ocular reflex (VOR), which is used to stabilize the eyes in space during head movements. 3. Large moving visual fields which induce compensatory eye movements, called optokinetic nystagmus (OKN). 4. Smooth pursuit eye movements which occur during visual tracking of small moving objects. 5. Vergence movements are disconjugate eye movements which allow binocular fixation of nearby objects. The following article will restrict itself to the cerebellar control of slow, conjugate eye movements, i.e., the vestibulo-ocular reflex (VOR), optokinetic nystagmus (OKN), and smooth pursuit eye movements. The cerebellar control of fast eye movements (saccades) is considered in the contribution of Vilis and Hore (Section IV-B). Very little is known about cerebellar influences on vergence movements.

Most emphasis will be laid on single-unit studies in alert, behaving primates. As it will be shown, the understanding of the cerebellar control of slow, conjugate eye movements depends largely on the knowledge of vestibular nuclei activity during these eye movements. Therefore, the activity pattern of both vestibular nuclei neurons and Purkinje cells (the only output element of the cerebellum) will be presented. First, the different types of neurons in the vestibular nuclei and the cerebellum will be reviewed briefly.

Vestibular nuclei neurons

In relation to individual eye movements and responses to angular head acceleration several groups of neurons can be distinguished within the vestibular nuclei complex (Fuchs and Kimm, 1975; Buettner et al., 1978): (I) Vestibular only. Neurons respond to vestibular stimulation, but show no modulation with individual eye movements. (II) Vestibular plus saccade. Beside the vestibular response neurons burst or pause with saccades (Fig. 1A, 2). (III) Vestibular plus position. During spontaneous eye movements these neurons show activity changes related to eye position. Vestibular stimulation leads to additional, specific activity changes. (IV) Saccade plus position (burst-tonic). These neurons within the vestibular nuclei complex behave qualitatively like ocular motoneurons with a burst-tonic pattern during spontaneous eye movements. During vestibular stimulation no additional, specific activity changes occur (Fuchs and Kimm, 1975).

Cerebellar activity

In single unit studies in alert animals one distinguishes input elements (mossy fibers, granule cells), interneurons and output elements (Purkinje cells)

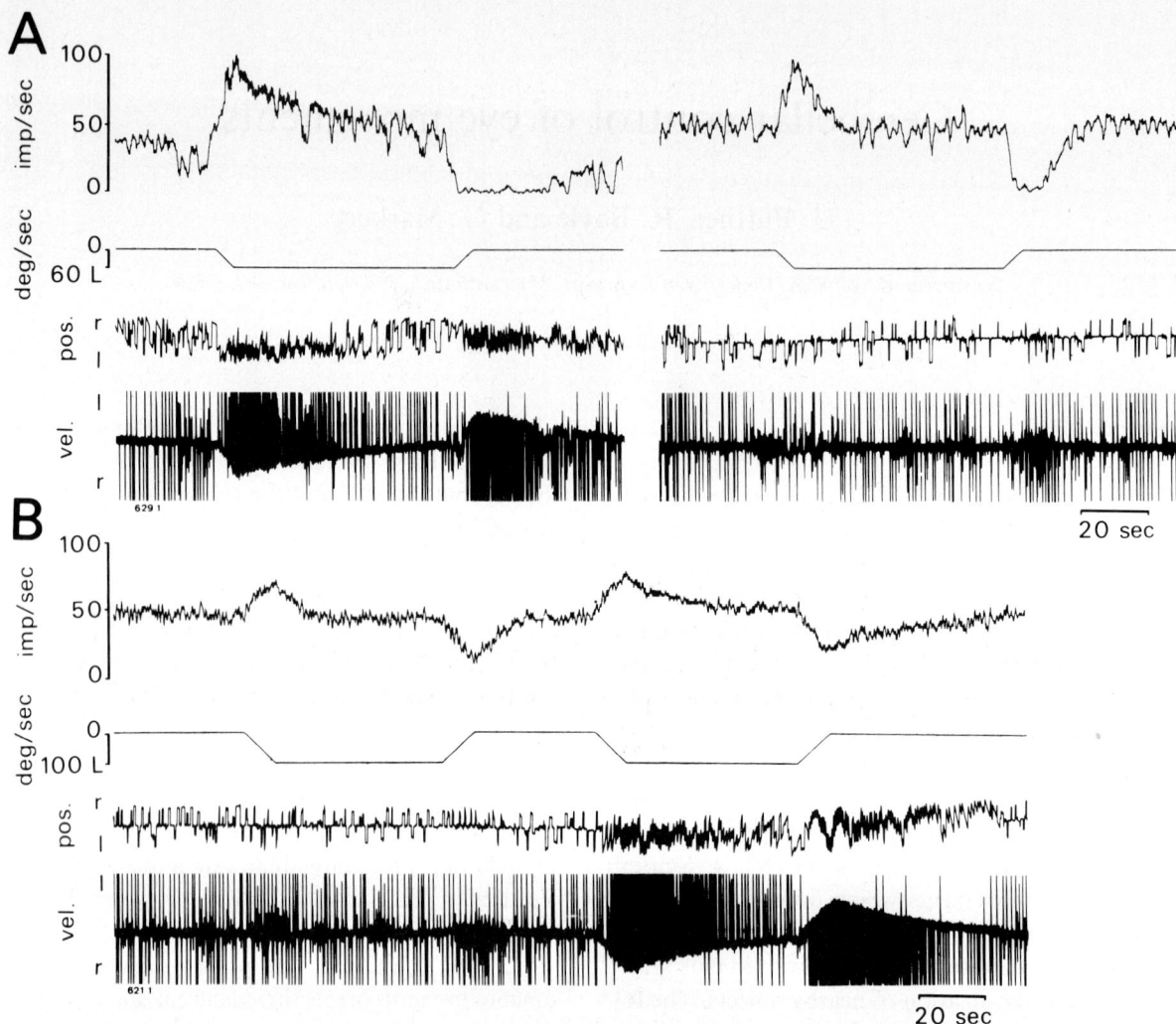

Fig. 1. Group II (A) and group I (B) vestibular nuclei neuron during vestibular nystagmus (A, first half of trace; B, second half of trace) and its suppression by fixating a small light spot attached to the turntable. Stimuli are velocity trapezoids in the dark. Traces, from above: neuronal activity (running average), stimulus velocity (acceleration and deceleration, 10°/sec²; constant velocity, 60°/sec (A) and 100°/sec (B)), horizontal eye position and eye velocity (first derivative of eye position). Velocity of saccades are arbitrarily cut off. During vestibular nystagmus neuronal activity decays in parallel with a long time constant of 15–25 seconds. During nystagmus suppression response amplitude is the same, but time constant of decay is considerably shorter. imp/sec, inpulses/sec. From Buettner and Büttner (1979).

(Lisberger and Fuchs, 1978; Miles et al., 1980; Waespe et al., 1981). In records from Purkinje cells, simple spikes (SS) and complex spikes (deriving from the climbing fiber input) can be distinguished. In the following accounts only the simple spike activity of Purkinje cells will be considered.

Most cerebellar studies in alert behaving primates have been performed in the flocculus. Here, Purkinje cells show some activity changes related to eye movements, but only about 20–40% of the population respond specifically during the eye movement paradigms described here (Lisberger and

Fuchs, 1978; Miles et al. 1980; Waespe and Henn, 1981). In the posterior vermis (lobule VI and VII) Purkinje cells related to smooth pursuit and those related to saccades have also been described (Kase et al., 1980; Suzuki et al., 1981).

Anatomy

The following cerebellar structures are considered to play some role in the control of slow, conjugate eye movements: the vestibulo-cerebellum consisting of the flocculus, paraflocculus, nodulus and uvula, and parts of the posterior vermis (lobulus VI and VII).

Recently, it has been shown in the monkey that the flocculus projects exclusively to the ipsilateral vestibular nuclei (Langer et al., 1985). Nodulus and uvula project to the vestibular nuclei, but apparently to different areas of the vestibular nuclei than those from the flocculus (Angaut and Brodal, 1967; Haines, 1977). Also, vermis lobule VI and — less intense — lobule VII send fibers to the ipsilateral vestibular nuclei (Haines, 1975).

The vestibulo-ocular reflex (VOR)

The VOR in the horizontal plane is usually investigated while the animal, with its head held stationary, is rotated about a vertical axis in complete darkness. The stimulus is applied sinusoidally (0.02–2 Hz) or as a velocity trapezoid (acceleration 10–80°/sec^2, constant velocity 10–180°/sec; Fig. 1). The VOR can be suppressed (VOR-supp.) by fixating a small light spot attached to the turntable, which moves simultaneously with the head.

During sinusoidal rotation (0.1–2 Hz) the vestibularly modulated neurons carry a signal related to eye velocity (Fig. 2A) (Fuchs and Kimm, 1975; Buettner et al., 1978). In response to a velocity trapezoid, vestibular nystagmus decays during constant velocity rotation with a time constant of 15–25 seconds (Fig. 1) (Waespe and Henn, 1977a; Buettner and Büttner, 1979), which is much longer than that found for primary afferent vestibular fibers (5–6 seconds, Fernandez and Goldberg, 1971;

Büttner and Waespe, 1981). These long time constants of the vestibular nystagmus are the result of a central "velocity storage" mechanism, which also reflects itself in similarly long decay time constants of activity of vestibular nuclei neurons (Fig. 1)

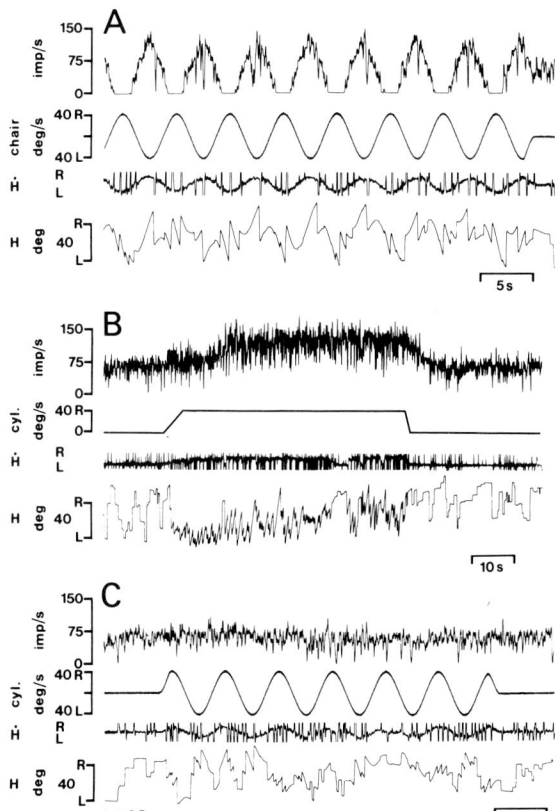

Fig. 2. Vestibular nuclei neuron during vestibular (A), constant velocity (B) and sinusoidal (C) optokinetic stimulation. Traces, from above: neuronal activity (running average), stimulus velocity, horizontal eye velocity, i.e., the first derivative of the horizontal eye position shown below. Stimulus frequency in A and C is 0.2 Hz, maximal stimulus velocity in A, B and C is 40°/sec. Neuronal activity pauses with saccades to the left (group II vestibular nuclei neuron). In A, the monkey is rotated about a vertical axis in the dark. Neuronal activity is in phase with turntable velocity to the left and silenced ("cut off") during rotation in the opposite direction. As for all vestibular nuclei neurons, the optokinetic stimulus has to move in the opposite direction, i.e., to the right, to elicit an increase in neuronal activity during constant velocity rotation B. Note the long time course for neuronal activity increase. In C, no modulation occurs during sinusoidal optokinetic stimulation.

(Buettner et al., 1978). During suppression of the VOR by visual fixation vestibular nuclei neurons are still modulated (Keller and Daniels, 1975; Buettner and Büttner, 1979). As Fig. 1 shows, the amplitude of the response is not, or only weakly, reduced by the fixation.

Thus, an oculomotor control signal similar but opposite in sign to the vestibular nuclei activity is necessary to cancel the vestibular activation and maintain fixation. This signal is thought to be provided by the flocculus (Lisberger and Fuchs, 1978; Miles et al., 1980; Büttner and Waespe, 1984). Here Purkinje cells can be found which are only weakly, if at all, modulated during VOR, but strongly modulated during VOR-supp. A sinusoidal stimulus under these conditions in the absence of reflex-induced eye movements results in activity changes in phase with head velocity; for most Purkinje cells activation occurs during VOR-supp. to the ipsilateral side. Thus, signals used for rapid changes in eye velocity, as during VOR-supp., are provided by the flocculus.

As described above, the "velocity storage" mechanism leads to time constants of vestibular nystagmus decay longer than predicted by vestibular nerve activity. Naive animals have time constants of 20–50 seconds, which decrease after repeated testing to values of 10–15 seconds. The decay of nystagmus can also be shortened by brief presentations of a stationary visual surround or by head tilting during postrotatory nystagmus (Waespe et al., 1985). These findings led to the postulation of a "dump" mechanism, which dynamically influences "velocity storage" (Raphan et al., 1981). Recently, it could be shown that this "dump" mechanism depends on the nodulus and uvula (Waespe et al., 1985). Lesions here leave the animals with the originally long time constants of 20–30 seconds, and the decay of vestibular nystagmus cannot be influenced by tilt or short visual surround presentation. Thus, all evidence suggests that in the normal animal the velocity storage is under influence of the nodulus and uvula. This "dump" mechanism is also active during VOR-supp. and its influence can be seen directly in the activity pattern of vestibular nuclei neurons. As mentioned earlier, the amplitude of the response is not altered during VOR-supp., but the time constant of decay is considerably shorter (5–9 seconds) and approaches that of the primary afferents (Buettner and Büttner, 1979). This reflects an inactivation of the "velocity storage" mechanism (Fig. 1).

Smooth pursuit eye movements

The same Purkinje cells in the flocculus, which are modulated during VOR-supp., are also activated during smooth pursuit eye movements (Lisberger and Fuchs, 1978; Miles et al., 1980; Büttner and Waespe, 1984). They encode eye velocity and activity increases for most neurons during smooth pursuit eye movements to the ipsilateral side (Fig. 4). Neurons are not activated by moving visual stimuli in the absence of eye movements (Büttner and Waespe, 1984). This led to the conclusion that Purkinje cells in the flocculus encode "gaze velocity" of eyes in space (Lisberger and Fuchs, 1978; Miles et al., 1980).

Another structure in the monkey cerebellum, where Purkinje cell activity related to smooth pursuit eye movements has been found, is the posterior vermis (lobulus VI and VII) (Suzuki et al., 1981). Purkinje cells in the vermis also encode eye velocity. In contrast to the flocculus, Purkinje cells in the vermis are in addition activated by moving visual stimuli. Since these neurons encode both (retinal slip and eye velocity), it was suggested that the activity of these Purkinje cells reflects target velocity (Suzuki et al., 1981).

In the vestibular nuclei group I and II neurons do not respond during smooth pursuit eye movements. Group III and IV neurons show a modulation, which is related to the position and weak eye velocity sensitivity seen in tonic and burst-tonic neurons (Keller and Daniels, 1975; Fuchs and Kimm, 1975).

Optokinetic nystagmus (OKN)

Whereas the VOR and smooth pursuit eye move-

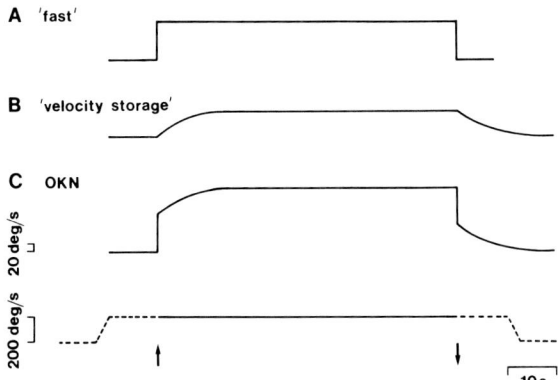

Fig. 3. Schematic drawing of the velocity profile for the "fast" (A) and "velocity storage" (B) component of OKN, and OKN slow-phase velocity (C) in response to sudden presentation and termination of a high, constant velocity optokinetic stimulus. Upward arrow indicates "light on" and downward arrow "light off". The "fast" component is characterized by rapid changes in eye velocity, whereas those of the "velocity storage" component are more gradual. Both components summate during high-velocity OKN. The nystagmus continuation after light-off is called optokinetic afternystagmus (OKAN).

vestibular nuclei neurons increase their activity direction-specifically up to nystagmus velocities of 40–60°/sec (Fig. 2B). Activity changes occur already at low nystagmus velocities. At higher nystagmus velocities (above 60°/sec) neurons tend to saturate. OKN in the opposite direction leads to a decrease in neuronal activity (Waespe and Henn, 1977a).

Only Purkinje cells in the flocculus, which are activated during VOR-supp. and smooth pursuit eye movements, respond during constant velocity optokinetic stimulation (Büttner and Waespe, 1984). The response pattern of Purkinje cells is complementary to that found for vestibular nuclei neurons. Purkinje cells do not respond if slow-phase nystagmus velocity is below 40–60°/sec (Fig. 4) (Waespe and Henn, 1981). It should be stressed that these are eye velocities which lead to a clear modulation of neuronal activity for the same neurons during smooth pursuit eye movements (Büttner and Waespe, 1984). However, at constant ny-

ments can be considered as a relatively uniform oculomotor response, it is now quite obvious that two components participate in the generation of slow phase of OKN (Ter Braak, 1936; Cohen et al., 1977; Büttner et al., 1983). One is called the "fast" or "direct" component, leads to rapid changes in slow-phase nystagmus velocity (Fig. 3A) and has been related to smooth pursuit mechanisms (Robinson, 1981). The other is called "velocity storage" or "indirect" component. It leads to more gradual eye velocity changes (Fig. 3B), and correlates with neuronal activity changes in the vestibular nuclei (Waespe and Henn, 1977a,b). The "velocity storage" mechanism is identical with the one mentioned previously in connection with vestibular nystagmus. It expresses itself most clearly during optokinetic afternystagmus (OKAN), i.e., the continuation of optokinetic nystagmus in the dark. It should be stressed that the terms "direct" and "indirect" refer to functional aspects of the response, not to anatomical connections.

With constant velocity optokinetic stimulation

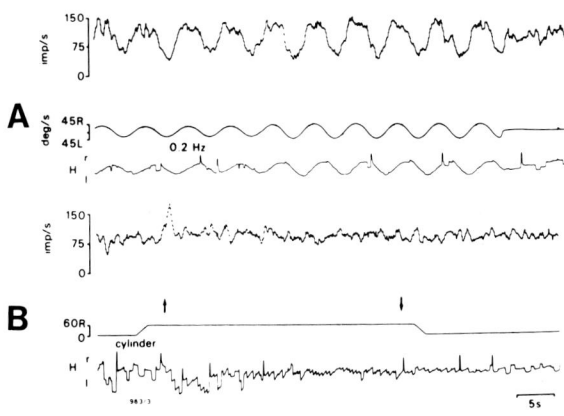

Fig. 4. Neuronal activity of a Purkinje cell in the primate flocculus during smooth pursuit eye movements (A) and constant velocity OKN (B). Traces, from above: neuronal activity (running average), stimulus velocity (light diode (A) and optokinetic cylinder (B)) and horizontal eye position (distorted by occasional blink artefacts). In A, neuronal activity is strongly modulated during smooth pursuit eye movements. Activity is in phase with stimulus velocity. In B, the animal is suddenly exposed to the optokinetic stimulus at "light on" (upward arrow). Beside a transient, short activity increase no activity changes occur during OKN, despite the fact that eye velocity is higher in B than in A. Nystagmus continues after "light off" (downward arrow) as OKAN (Büttner and Waespe, unpublished results).

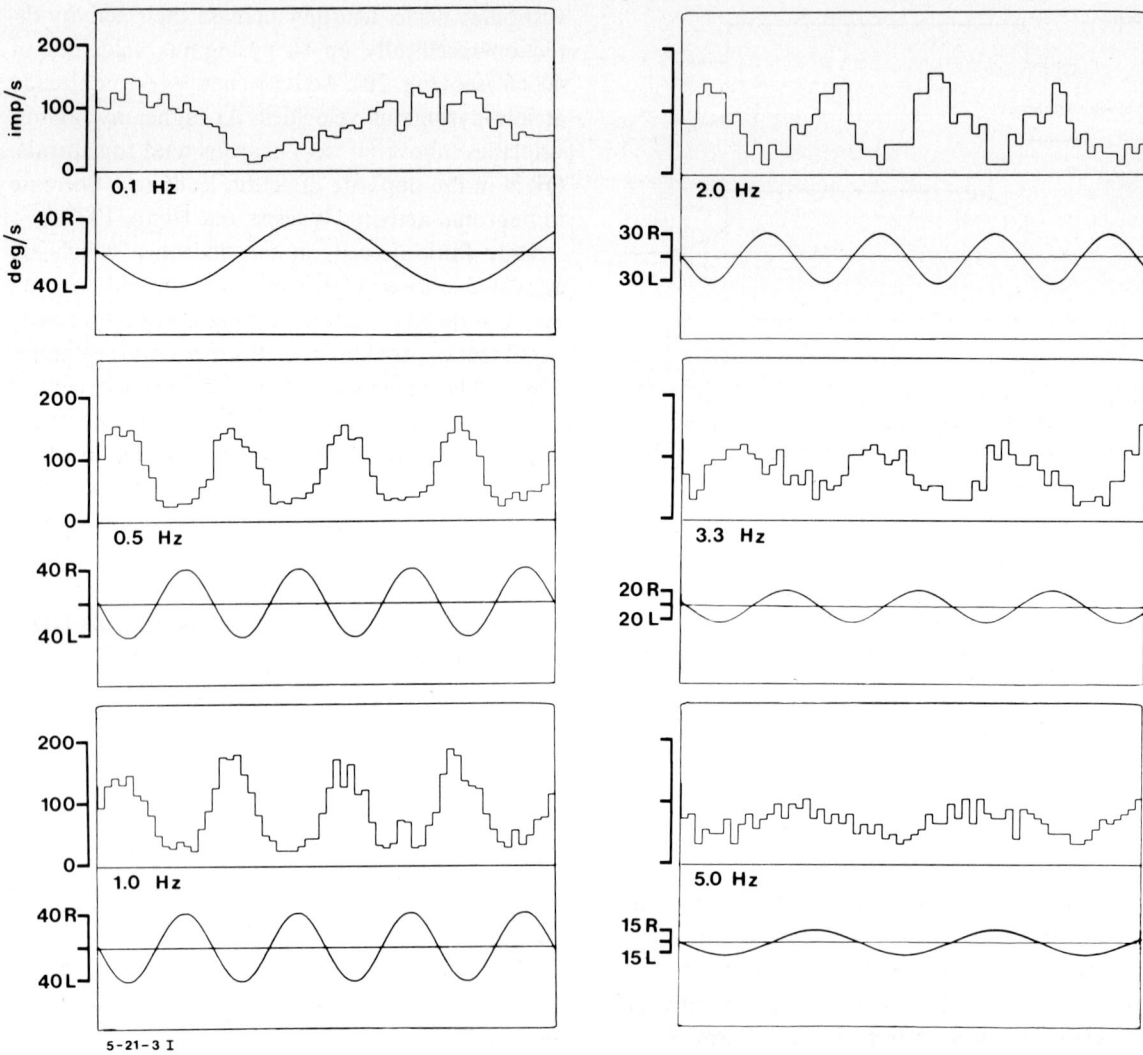

Fig. 5. Purkinje cell activity in the primate flocculus during sinusoidal optokinetic stimulation. The firing rate of this neuron, which was not modulated during VOR and constant velocity optokinetic stimulation of 40°/sec (not shown here), is clearly modulated at sinusoidal stimulation between 0.1 and 5 Hz.

stagmus velocities above 60°/sec Purkinje cells start to show an activity increase which is in parallel with further increases in nystagmus velocity.

If, instead of constant velocity, sinusoidal optokinetic stimulation (keeping the maximal stimulus velocity at 40°/sec or below) is applied, Purkinje cells show a clear modulation at frequencies above 0.05 Hz (Fig. 5). Activity changes follow stimulus frequencies above 3 Hz, in some instances up to 5 Hz (Boyle et al., 1984). At these high optokinetic stimulus frequencies compensatory eye movements still occur; however, with a low gain of about 0.3 (Paige, 1983; Boyle et al., 1985). Neuronal activity shows an increasing phase lag relative to stimulus velocity with higher frequencies (Fig. 5). However, basically neuronal activity stays in phase with eye velocity, which is similarly lagging stimulus velocity at higher frequencies (Boyle et al., 1985). At low frequencies of optokinetic stimulation (below 0.05 Hz) Purkinje cells are not, or only weakly, modulated.

Similar to the constant velocity responses, vestibular nuclei neurons and floccular Purkinje cells show a complementary response pattern during sinusoidal optokinetic stimulation. Thus, vestibular nuclei neurons respond with a high sensitivity (compared to the constant velocity response) at low frequencies (0.02 Hz). Sensitivity decreases with higher frequencies, responses are minimal at 0.1 Hz and absent at 0.2 Hz (Boyle et al., 1985) (Fig. 2).

Comments

The cerebellum and, in particular, the flocculus as part of the vestibulo-cerebellum play an important role in the control of slow, conjugate eye movements. This is also emphasized by lesion studies in man (Dichgans et al., 1978) and monkey (Zee et al., 1981), which demonstrate that smooth pursuit, VOR-supp. and OKN are severely affected. A comparison of single unit responses in the flocculus and the vestibular nuclei demonstrates a complementary action of neuronal activity in the generation of slow, conjugate eye movements (flocculus/vestibular-nuclei complementary hypothesis, Waespe and Henn, 1981).

Certain, generally more basic, functions, like the VOR and low constant-velocity OKN, can be attributed to the vestibular nuclei. In contrast, Purkinje cells in the flocculus are modulated when the oculomotor system, in order to minimize retinal slip, has to respond to visual stimuli with a response pattern that cannot be provided by the vestibular nuclei, as during smooth pursuit eye movements, VOR-supp., and high-frequency and high-constant velocity optokinetic stimuli. In some instances vestibular nuclei and flocculus act synergistically, as during high-velocity OKN, which leads to higher eye velocities than can be provided by each structure alone. In other situations, as during VOR-supp., the signals from the vestibular nuclei and the flocculus act antagonistically and the eyes remain stationary in the orbit.

	vestibular nuclei	flocculus	eye movements
VOR	↑	ø	contralateral
VOR-suppression	↑	↑	ø
OKN const. vel. below 60 deg/s	↓	ø	ipsilateral
OKN const. vel. above 60 deg/s	↓	↑	ipsilateral (high veloc.)
OKN-sinus below 0.1 Hz	↓	ø	ipsilateral
OKN-sinus above 0.1 Hz	ø	↑	ipsilateral
smooth pursuit	ø	↑	ipsilateral

Fig. 6. Complementary activity of a vestibular nuclei neuron and a Purkinje cell in the flocculus during different oculomotor paradigms. The responses to stimuli (vestibular, optokinetic and smooth pursuit) moving ipsilaterally to the recording side are shown qualitatively. This leads to activation (upward arrow) during the VOR for the vestibular nuclei neuron and during smooth pursuit eye movements for the Purkinje cell. Downward arrow: decrease in neuronal activity. ø: no changes. Direction and occurrence of slow eye movement component is shown on the right. Note the different pattern of activity in the vestibular nuclei neuron and the Purkinje cell during VOR suppression and high-velocity OKN.

The eye movements resulting from the various response patterns of floccular Purkinje cells and vestibular nuclei neurons can be explained if one assumes interaction at the single neuron level (Fig. 6). In both structures signals are encoded in relation to eye velocity. One major question is where does this interaction take place? Anatomical evidence clearly demonstrates that the flocculus projects exclusively to the vestibular nuclei complex (Langer et al., 1985). However, in behaving monkeys no direct effect of floccular activity changes has yet been seen in vestibular nuclei neurons (Fig. 1) (Keller and Daniels, 1975; Buettner and Büttner, 1979). The reason probably is that different functional groups of vestibular nuclei neurons exist. Most results described here were obtained from group I and II vestibular nuclei neurons, neurons without eye position sensitivity. Recently, it was shown that floccular Purkinje cells project to group III (vestibular + position) vestibular nuclei neurons (Lisberger and Pavelko, 1984). These neurons probably receive a disynaptic input from the vestibular nerve. Thus, functionally these group III neurons are situated between pure vestibular neurons (group I and II) and cculomotor nuclei neurons, but anatomically they lie within the vestibular nuclei complex, and may relay floccular activity to the oculomotor nuclei. The influence of nodulus and uvula on the vestibular nuclei takes place at a different level. As described above, nodulus and uvula regulate the dominant time constant of the "velocity storage" mechanism. The effect of this influence can already be demonstrated on group I and II vestibular nuclei neurons (Fig. 1). In accordance with this, nodulus and uvula project to different areas of the vestibular nuclei complex than does the flocculus (Angaut and Brodal, 1967; Haines, 1975). The precise role of the posterior vermis in the control of slow, conjugate eye movements has yet to be determined.

Generally, it is assumed that the cerebellum regulates and improves motor performance, for which the basic program is generated elsewhere. This concept certainly applies also for certain oculomotor functions, specifically saccades. Here, the paramedian pontine reticular formation (PPRF) in the brainstem is the immediate premotor structure for saccades (Büttner-Ennever, 1979; Henn et al., 1982). Cerebellar dysfunction leads to saccade impairment, but basically saccades can be performed (see Vilis and Hore, Section IV-B). In contrast, for smooth pursuit eye movements the flocculus itself could be considered as a premotor structure. Stimulation here leads to smooth pursuit eye movements (Lisberger and Pavelka, 1984). As described above, anatomical evidence suggests that the flocculus projects exclusively to the vestibular nuclei complex (Langer et al., 1985). Interaction between signals from the flocculus and from group I and II vestibular nuclei neurons takes place within the anatomical boundaries of the vestibular nuclei. Thus, with regard to smooth pursuit eye movements it seems possible that the flocculus plays a more basic role which is different from the general concept of the regulatory function of the cerebellum. However, several questions have to be answered before this hypothesis can be accepted. Particularly, further studies are necessary to elaborate the role of the brainstem in the generation of smooth pursuit eye movements. Eckmiller and Bauswein (Section V) recorded smooth pursuit-related activity in the vicinity of the abducens nucleus of the monkey. The functional role of this area, particularly in relation to the flocculus, needs further investigation. Furthermore, lesions in the flocculus do not abolish smooth pursuit eye movements completely (Zee et al., 1981), but total cerebellectomy does (Westheimer and Blair, 1974). Whether the remaining smooth pursuit eye movements after flocculectomy depend on the posterior vermis has to be further investigated.

Acknowledgements

The authors wish to thank Ms. B. Liebold and B. Pfreundner for typing the manuscript. This work was supported by Deutsche Forschungsgemeinschaft SFB 200, A2.

References

Angaut, P. and Brodal, A. (1967) The projection of the "vestibulo-cerebellum" onto the vestibular nuclei in the cat. Arch. Ital. Biol., 105: 411–479.

Boyle, R., Büttner, U. and Markert, G. (1984) Flocculus Purkinje cell response to high frequency and sudden high velocity optokinetic stimuli. Soc. Neurosci. Abstr., 10: 538.

Boyle, R., Büttner, U. and Markert, G. (1985) Vestibular nuclei activity and eye movements in the alert monkey during sinusoidal optokinetic stimulation. Exp. Brain Res., 57: 362–369.

Büttner-Ennever, J. A. (1979) Organization of reticular projections onto oculomotor neurons. In R. Granit and O. Pompeiano (Eds.), Reflex Control of Posture and Movement, Progress in Brain Research, Vol. 50, Elsevier, Amsterdam, pp. 619–630.

Büttner, U. and Waespe, W. (1981) Vestibular nerve activity in the alert monkey during vestibular and optokinetic nystagmus. Exp. Brain Res., 41: 310–315.

Büttner, U. and Waespe, W. (1984) Purkinje cell activity in the primate flocculus during optokinetic stimulation, smooth pursuit eye movements and VOR-suppression. Exp. Brain Res., 55: 97–104.

Büttner, U., Meienberg, O. and Schimmelpfennig, B. (1983) The effect of central retinal lesions on optokinetic nystagmus in the monkey. Exp. Brain Res., 52: 248–256.

Buettner, U. W. and Büttner, U. (1979) Vestibular nuclei activity in the alert monkey during suppression of vestibular and optokinetic nystagmus. Exp. Brain Res., 37: 581–593.

Buettner, U. W., Büttner, U. and Henn, V. (1978) Transfer characteristics of neurons in the vestibular nuclei of the alert monkey. J. Neurophysiol., 41: 1616–1628.

Cohen, B., Matsuo, V. and Raphan, T. (1977) Quantitative analysis of the velocity characteristics of optokinetic nystagmus and optokinetic after-nystagmus. J. Physiol., 270: 321–344.

Dichgans, J., Van Reutern, G. M. and Römmelt, U. (1978) Impaired suppression of vestibular nystagmus by fixation in cerebellar and non-cerebellar patients. Arch Psychiat. Nervenkr., 226: 183–199.

Fernandez, C. and Goldberg, J. M. (1971) Physiology of peripheral neurons innervating semicircular canals of the squirrel monkey. II. Response to sinusoidal stimulation and dynamics of peripheral vestibular system. J. Neurophysiol., 34: 661–675.

Fuchs, A. F. and Kimm, J. (1975) Unit activity in vestibular nucleus of the alert monkey during horizontal angular acceleration and eye movement. J. Neurophysiol., 38: 1140–1161.

Haines, D. E. (1975) Cerebellar corticovestibular fibers of the posterior lobe in a prosimian primate, the lesser bushbaby (*Galago senegalensis*). J. Comp. Neurol., 160: 363–398.

Haines, D. E. (1977) Cerebellar corticonuclear and corticovestibular fibers of the flocculonodular lobe in a prosimian primate (*Galago senegalensis*). J. Comp. Neurol., 174: 607–630.

Henn, V., Hepp, K. and Büttner-Ennever, J. A. (1982) The primate oculomotor system. II. Premotor system. Human Neurobiol., 1: 87–95.

Kase, M., Miller, D. C. and Noda, H. (1980) Discharges of Purkinje cells and mossy fibers in the cerebellar vermis of the monkey during saccadic eye movements and fixation. J. Physiol. London, 300: 539–555.

Keller, E. L. and Daniels, P. D. (1975) Oculomotor related interaction of vestibular and visual stimulation in vestibular nucleus cells in alert monkey. Exp. Neurol., 46: 187–198.

Langer, T., Fuchs, A. F., Chubb, M. C., Scudder, C. A. and Lisberger, S. G. (1985) Floccular efferents in the rhesus macaque as revealed by autoradiography and horseradish peroxidase. J. Comp. Neurol., 235: 26–37.

Lisberger, S. G. and Fuchs, A. F. (1978) Role of primate flocculus during rapid behavioral modification of vestibulo-ocular reflex. I. Purkinje cell activity during visually guided horizontal smooth-pursuit eye movements and passive head rotation. J. Neurophysiol., 41: 733–763.

Lisberger, S. G. and Pavelko, T. A. (1984) Functional properties of brainstem cells inhibited from the cerebellar flocculus in monkey. Soc. Neurosci. Abstr., 10: 988.

Miles, F. A., Fuller, J. H., Braitman, D. J. and Dow, B. M. (1980) Long-term adaptive changes in primate vestibuloocular reflex. III. Electrophysiological observations in flocculus of normal monkeys. J. Neurophysiol., 43: 1437–1476.

Paige, G. D. (1983) Vestibuloocular reflex and its interactions with visual following mechanisms in the squirrel monkey. I. Response characteristics in normal animals. J. Neurophysiol., 49: 134–151.

Raphan, T., Cohen, B. and Henn, V. (1981) Effects of gravity on rotatory nystagmus in monkeys. Ann. NY Acad. Sci., 374: 44–55.

Robinson, D. A. (1981) Control of eye movements. In V. B. Brooks (Ed.), Handbook of Physiology, Section 1: The Nervous System, Vol. II, Part 2, American Physiological Society, Bethesda, MD, pp. 1275–1320.

Suzuki, D. A., Noda, H. and Kase, M. (1981) Visual and pursuit eye movement-related activity in posterior vermis of monkey cerebellum. J. Neurophysiol., 46: 1120–1139.

Ter Braak, J. W. G. (1936) Untersuchungen über optokinetischen Nystagmus. Arch. Neerl. Physiol., 21: 309–376.

Waespe, W. and Henn, V. (1977a) Neuronal activity in the vestibular nuclei of the alert monkey during vestibular and optokinetic stimulation. Exp. Brain Res., 27: 523–538.

Waespe, W. and Henn, V. (1977b) Vestibular nuclei activity during optokinetic after-nystagmus (OKAN) in the alert monkey. Exp. Brain Res. 30: 323–330.

Waespe, W. and Henn, V. (1981) Visual-vestibular interaction in the flocculus of the alert monkey. II. Purkinje cell activity. Exp. Brain Res., 43: 349–360.

Waespe, W., Büttner, U. and Henn, V. (1981) Visual-vestibular interaction in the flocculus of the alert monkey, I. Input activity. Exp. Brain Res., 43: 337–348.

Waespe, W., Cohen, B. and Raphan, T. (1985) Dynamic modification of the vestibulo-ocular reflex by the nodulus and uvula. Science, 228: 199–202.

Westheimer, G. and Blair, S. M. (1974) Functional organization of primate oculomotor system revealed by cerebellectomy. Exp. Brain Res., 21: 463–472.

Zee, D. S., Yamazaki, A., Butler, P. H. and Gücer, G. (1981) Effects of ablation of flocculus and paraflocculus on eye movements in primates. J. Neurophysiol., 46: 878–899.

The functional organization of the primate superior colliculus: A motor perspective

David L. Sparks and Martha F. Jay

Department of Physiology and the Neurosciences Program, University of Alabama in Birmingham, University Station, Birmingham, AL 35294, U.S.A.

Introduction

The deeper layers of the superior colliculus (SC) are a site where visual, auditory and somatosensory signals converge and an area that contains neurons with motor properties (see Sparks and Mays, 1983; Schiller, 1984; Stein, 1984, for recent reviews). Based upon this observation, many investigators have suggested that the SC may be a brain region where signals from various sensory modalities are translated into common motor commands — commands for orienting the eyes, head and pinnae toward the source of significant or novel environmental stimuli. This chapter summarizes what is known about the motor signals found in the SC and, based upon this information, discusses the transformations of sensory signals that are required for a sensory/motor interface.

Results

Although electrical stimulation studies suggest that the SC may contain neurons related to movements of the eye, head, and external ears (Schaefer and Schneider, 1968; Syka and Radil-Weiss, 1971; Robinson, 1972; Schiller and Stryker, 1972; Harris, 1980; Roucoux et al., 1980; Stein and Clamann, 1981; McHaffie and Stein, 1982), only the signals involved in initiating saccadic eye movements have been studied in detail (Schiller and Koerner, 1971; Wurtz and Goldberg, 1972; Sparks et al., 1976).

One type of neuron found in the intermediate layers of the SC generates a high-frequency burst of spike activity that begins 18–20 mseconds before saccade onset (see Fig. 1). The activity of these neurons is tightly coupled to saccade onset, and in behavioral situations in which a visual target sometimes elicits a saccade and sometimes fails to do so, the probability of the high-frequency spike burst is almost perfectly correlated with the probability of saccade occurrence (Sparks, 1978). Collicular neurons discharge prior to saccades of a particular direction and amplitude, regardless of initial eye position (Schiller and Koerner, 1971; Wurtz and Goldberg, 1972, Sparks et al., 1976). Thus, their discharge is not related to moving the eye to a particular position in the orbit but to motor error, the change in eye position required to direct gaze to the target location. As illustrated in Fig. 1, each of these neurons has a movement field — i.e., each neuron discharges before a range of saccades that have particular directions and amplitudes (Wurtz and Goldberg, 1972; Sparks et al., 1976).

Neurons with motor properties are arranged topographically within the SC. In the monkey, this motor map has been described in detail using microstimulation methods (Robinson, 1972) and chronic single unit recording experiments have confirmed the basic features of the motor map (Schiller and Stryker, 1972; Wurtz and Goldberg, 1972; Sparks et al., 1976). Since each neuron fires before a range of saccades, it follows that a large popula-

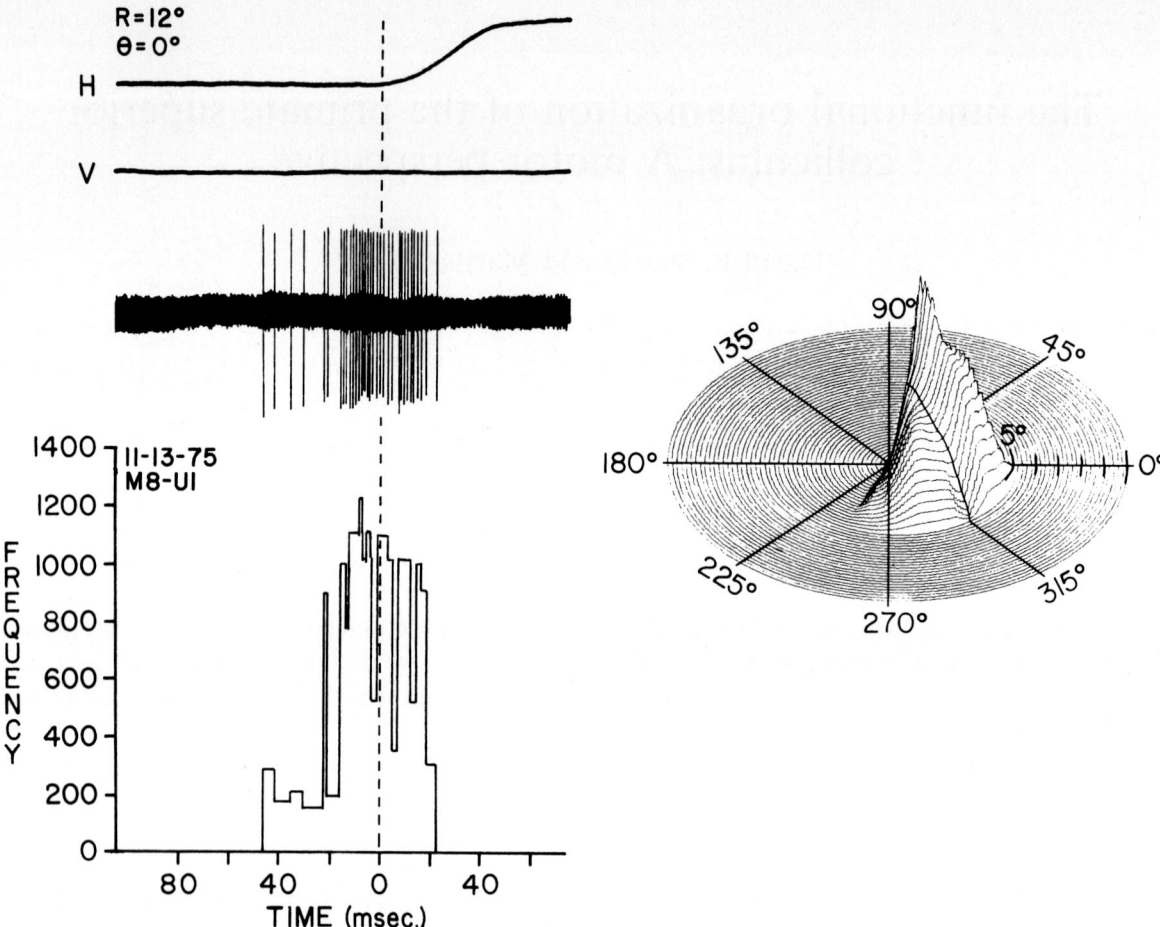

Fig. 1. Left. Discharge pattern recorded from a typical saccade-related burst neuron in the superior colliculus. H, Horizontal eye position; V, vertical eye position. Middle tracing: spike discharge. Bottom graph: instantaneous spike frequency as a function of time. The dotted line represents the onset of the eye movement. Right. Three-dimensional representation of the number of spikes as a function of the angle and amplitude of eye movements. The maximal burst (48 spikes) preceded small, right saccades with a downward component (1° in amplitude at an angle of 320°). Movements within the movement field but less than or greater than 1° in amplitude were preceded by a less vigorous response. Similarly, if the angle of movement deviated from 320°, fewer spikes were observed. Adapted from Sparks et al. (1976).

tion of collicular neurons will discharge before a particular saccade (McIlwain, 1975; Sparks et al., 1976). The population response is characterized by a temporal and spatial gradient of activity (Sparks and Mays, 1980). Neurons in the center of the population fire earlier and more vigorously than surrounding cells. Neurons on the fringe of the active population fire weakly and their activity may follow, rather than precede, saccade onset.

Although the vigor of discharge of a particular saccade-related burst cell varies for different movements within the movement field, information concerning saccade direction and amplitude is not contained within the discharge of a single cell (Sparks and Mays, 1980). As illustrated in Fig. 2, except for the maximal discharge which precedes saccades to the center of the movement field, the discharge of SC neurons is ambiguous with respect to saccade

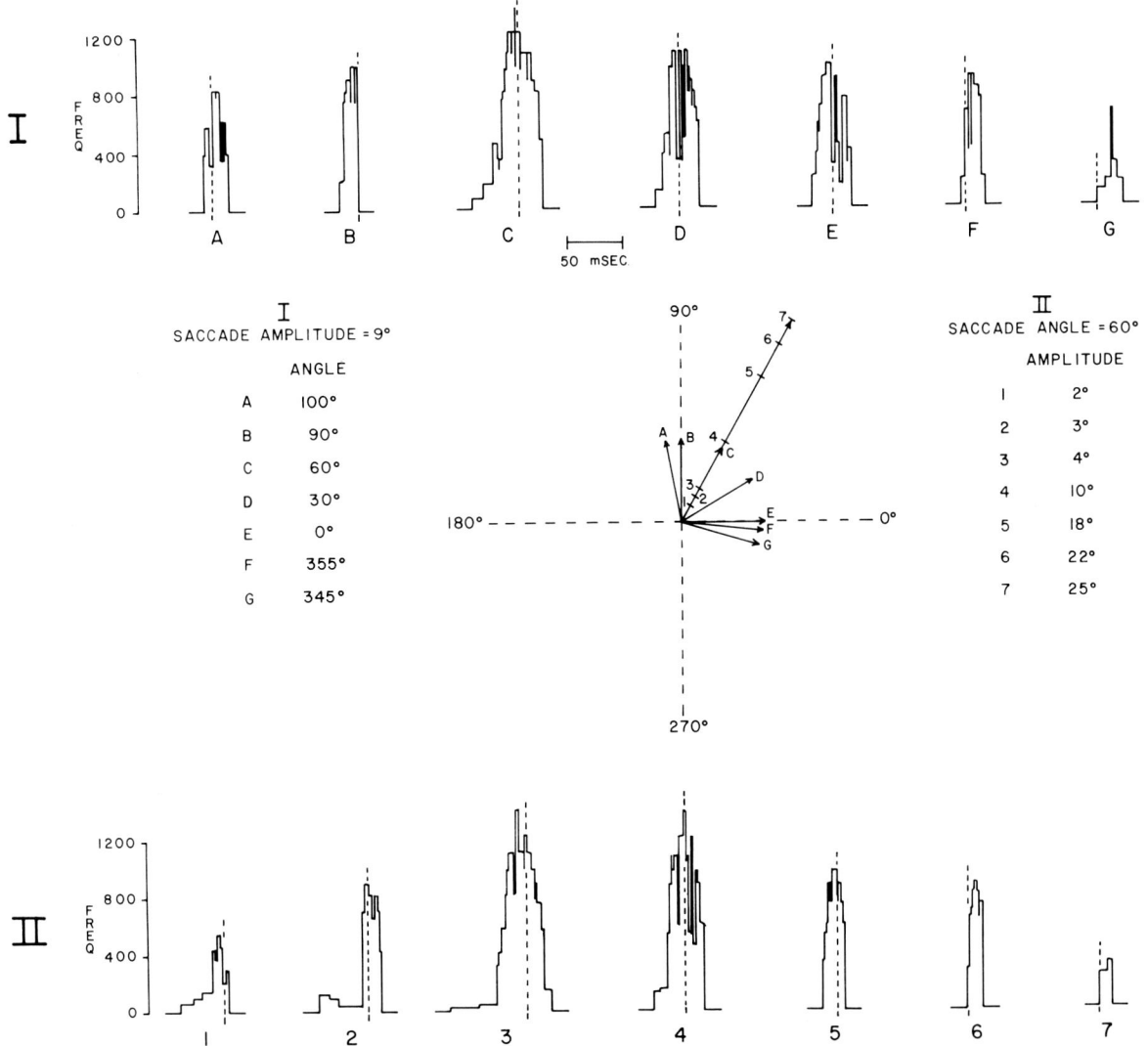

Fig. 2. Variations in the configuration and timing of the discharge of a typical saccade-related burst neuron. I. Instantaneous spike frequency records for seven saccades of the optimal amplitude (9°) but differing in direction. The dotted line represents saccade onset. II. Instantaneous spike frequency records for seven saccades of the optimal direction ($\theta = 60°$) but differing in amplitude. Note that for saccades on the fringe of the movement field, the neural discharge may follow, rather than precede saccade onset. Note, too, the similarity of the burst profile in B, F, 2 and 6, although these bursts preceded saccades with large differences in direction and amplitude. From Sparks and Mays (1980).

direction or amplitude. Identical discharges may precede many saccades having different directions and amplitudes (Sparks and Mays, 1980). Also, the discharge of different saccade-related burst units, some which discharge maximally to small saccades and some which discharge maximally to large saccades, is indistinguishable (Sparks and Mays, 1980). Thus, unlike the primary vestibular afferents, for example, which encode head velocity by firing rate, the SC does not generate specific rates of firing for different amounts of motor error.

In summary, two major conclusions can be

reached concerning the saccade-related motor signals found in the SC. First, the activity of collicular neurons encodes the desired change in eye position, not a movement to a particular orbital position. Secondly, saccade direction and amplitude are encoded anatomically. It is the location of the active neurons within the topographical map of movement fields, not their frequency of firing, that specifies the trajectory of a saccade.

What are the implications of these findings for the sensory/motor transformations that are thought to occur within the SC? First, since the collicular command specifies a change in eye position rather than a movement that directs gaze to a particular spatial location, sensory systems must provide a signal of the desired change in eye position, not just the location of a stimulus in head, body or retinal coordinates. Secondly, since it is the site of activity within the SC that encodes saccade direction and amplitude, sensory signals must be translated into a format compatible with this anatomical code — i.e., a particular subset of collicular neurons must be activated in order to produce a specific change in eye position. Consider, for example, the translation of an auditory signal into a command for a saccadic movement. The auditory system uses interaural differences in time, intensity and phase to localize targets in "head" coordinates. However, in order to compute the difference between the current direction of gaze and target position, the position of the eye in the orbit must also be known.

We have recently completed experiments conducted to test these hypotheses (Jay and Sparks, 1984). Monkeys were trained to look to both visual and auditory targets in a completely darkened room. A hoop, 6 feet in diameter, surrounded the monkey seated inside magnetic fields used to measure eye position. Rotation of the hoop by a computer-controlled stepping motor changed the elevation of the miniature speaker attached to the hoop. Another stepping motor controlled the azimuth of the target by moving the speaker around the hoop. A small light-emitting diode (LED) mounted at the center of the speaker permitted the presentation of visual or auditory stimuli. Also, three additional LEDs were used to control initial fixation. The center LED was placed directly in front of the monkey; the others were 24° to the left and right of center. On a typical trial, one of the three fixation lights was illuminated. If the animal looked to the fixation target and maintained fixation for a variable period, an eccentric stimulus (light or noise burst) was presented while the center fixation target remained illuminated. Reward was contingent upon maintaining fixation of the center target until, after a variable interval, it was extinguished, and then looking to the location of the eccentric auditory or visual stimulus. This delayed saccade task permitted unit activity linked to stimulus onset to be distinguished from activity coupled to saccade onset.

The goal of the experiment was to answer two basic questions. First, do neurons that discharge before saccades to visual targets also discharge before saccades to auditory targets? If they do, this indicates that auditory and visual signals have already been converted into the same coordinates and are sharing a motor circuit. If, however, some SC neurons burst before visually triggered saccades and other SC neurons burst before saccades to auditory targets, then separate motor circuits are being used, at least at the level of the SC. Secondly, are auditory signals reaching the SC in "head" or "motor error" coordinates? If auditory signals are organized in head coordinates, then in our experiments (in which the head was fixed) the response of acoustically responsive neurons should be independent of initial fixation position and depend entirely upon the azimuth and elevation of the speaker. However, if auditory signals have been translated into motor error coordinates, then the neural response to acoustic stimuli should depend upon both the position of the speaker in space and the position of the eyes in the orbit.

We found (Jay and Sparks, 1984) that SC neurons that burst prior to saccades to visual targets also burst before saccades to auditory targets. This indicates that, at or before reaching the level of the SC, auditory and visual signals have converged onto a common motor pathway for the generation of saccadic movements.

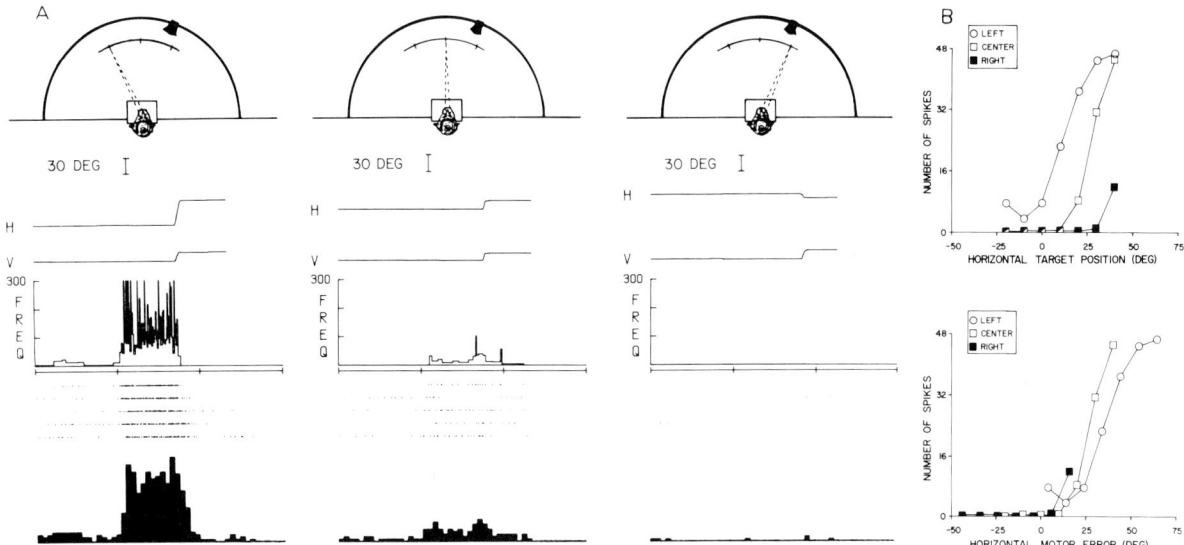

Fig. 3. The effects of eye position on the response of a single SC cell to an auditory stimulus. A. The speaker was placed 20° to the right and elevated 6° while the fixation position was varied between 24° left (left), center (center) and 24° right (right). The time base represents 3 seconds; target onset occurred at 1 second. Horizontal (up = right) and vertical (up = up) eye position traces are shown in the top row. Instantaneous firing rates are shown for single trials in the second row. Next, rasters displaying unit activity for five trials are illustrated. A cumulative histogram for these trials is displayed on the bottom row. B. A plot illustrating the shift in the position of the receptive field (top) when eye position was varied. The same data are aligned when plotted in motor error coordinates. From Jay and Sparks (1984).

The effects of varying eye position upon the response to auditory stimulation were tested in 121 cells, all but two of which were responsive to visual and auditory stimulation. Statistically significant ($P<0.05$) effects were obtained in 99 of the 121 SC cells tested. Typical data are illustrated in Fig. 3. For the trials shown, the speaker was positioned 20° to the right and 6° above the primary eye position. Presentation of the noise burst evoked a vigorous neural discharge when the monkey was looking at the left fixation target. When the monkey was viewing the center or right fixation lights, an identical noise burst presented in the same spatial location resulted in a response that was markedly attenuated or completely absent. The average number of spikes evoked by the noise burst is plotted as a function of the horizontal position of the speaker for the three different fixation positions in Fig. 1b (top). The receptive field of the neuron shifted with the position of the eyes in the orbit. Below, the average number of spikes is plotted as a function of horizontal motor error, the horizontal component of the movement required to look to the auditory targets. The data obtained while the monkey viewed the three fixation lights are closely aligned in this plot. Thus, the discharge of this neuron depended upon the movement required to look to the target, a factor that is a function of the position of the eyes in the orbit as well as the position of the target.

These findings suggest that a representation of motor error is formed by subtracting eye position from a head-centered representation of target location. Consequently, the map of auditory space found in the monkey SC is not static. With each movement of the eyes in the orbit, the population of neurons responsive to a stationary auditory stimulus changes to a new location within the SC — a location that represents the new motor error signal.

These results complement earlier experiments (Mays and Sparks, 1980; Sparks and Porter, 1983) in which we found that the discharge of visual neurons in the intermediate layers of the SC does not depend upon stimulation of a specific region of the retina. Using trials in which an intervening saccade changed the position of the eyes after a brief visual target had been extinguished, we discovered neurons (quasi-visual or QV cells) that were visually responsive but with discharge patterns that were best described as encoding motor error. If the eyes moved after a brief target had disappeared, the site of QV cell activity shifted to a location representing the trajectory of the eye movement required to look to the remembered position of the target.

Conclusions

In summary, results of several recent experiments can best be explained by assuming that the SC is organized in motor coordinates. Motor error is encoded anatomically; it is the site of activity within the colliculus, not discharge frequency, that specifies saccade direction and amplitude. This command format imposes constraints upon the configuration of signals that can initiate saccades and determines the required transformations of sensory signals. Inputs to the colliculus must specify (by activating a particular subset of collicular neurons) the desired change in eye position, not merely the location of the target in head, body or retinal coordinates. This requires dynamic maps of auditory and visual space. With each change in eye position, the site of acoustically and visually induced activity shifts to a location that specifies the eye movement required to direct gaze to the target location. In this manner, auditory and visual signals are translated into common motor error coordinates, are maintained in register with the static motor map, and converge onto a shared motor pathway for the generation of saccadic eye movements.

Acknowledgment

This research was supported by National Institutes of Health Grants R01EY01189 and P30EY03039.

References

Harris, L. R. (1980) The superior colliculus and movements of the head and eyes in cats. J. Physiol., 300: 367–391.

Jay, M. F. and Sparks, D. L. (1984) Auditory receptive fields in primate superior colliculus shift with changes in eye position. Nature, 309: 345–347.

Mays, L. E. and Sparks, D. L. (1980) Dissociation of visual and saccade-related responses in superior colliculus neurons. J. Neurophysiol., 43: 207–232.

McHaffie, J. G. and Stein, B. E. (1982) Eye movements evoked by electrical stimulation in the superior coliculus of rats and hamsters. Brain Res., 247: 243–253.

McIlwain, J. T. (1975) Visual receptive fields and their images in superior colliculus of the cat. J. Neurophysiol., 38: 219–230.

Robinson, D. A. (1972) Eye movements evoked by collicular stimulation in the alert monkey. Vision. Res., 12: 1795–1808.

Roucoux, A., Guitton, D. and Crommelinck, M. (1980) Stimulation of the superior colliculus in the alert cat. Exp. Brain Res., 39: 75–85.

Schaefer, K.-P. and Schneider, H. (1968) Reizversuche im Tectum Opticum des Kaninchens. Arch. Psychiat., 211: 118–137.

Schiller, P. H. (1984) The superior colliculus and visual function. In J. M. Brookhart, V. B. Mountcastle, I. Darian-Smith and S. R. Geiger (Eds.), Handbook of Physiology. Section 1: The Nervous System; Vol. III. Sensory Processes, Part 1, American Physiological Society, Bethesda, pp. 457–506.

Schiller, P. H. and Koerner, F. (1971) Discharge characteristics of single units in superior colliculus of the alert rhesus monkey. J. Neurophysiol., 34: 920–936.

Schiller, P. H. and Stryker, M. (1972) Single-unit recording and stimulation in superior colliculus of the alert rhesus monkey. J. Neurophysiol., 35: 915–924.

Sparks, D. L. (1978) Functional properties of neurons in the monkey superior colliculus: Coupling of neuronal activity and saccade onset. Brain Res., 156: 1–16.

Sparks, D. L. and Mays, L. E. (1980) Movement fields of saccade-related burst neurons in the monkey superior colliculus. Brain Res., 190: 39–50.

Sparks, D. L. and Mays, L. E. (1983) The role of the monkey superior colliculus in the spatial localization of saccade targets. In A. Hein and M. Jeannerod (Eds.), Spatially Oriented Behavior, Springer-Verlag, New York, pp. 63–86.

Sparks, D. L. and Porter, J. D. (1983) Spatial localization of saccade targets. II. Activity of superior colliculus neurons preceding compensatory saccades. J. Neurophysiol., 49: 64–74.

Sparks, D. L., Holland, R. and Guthrie, B. L. (1976) Size and distribution of movement fields in the monkey superior colliculus. Brain Res., 113: 21–34.

Stein, B. E. (1984) Development of the superior colliculus. Annu. Rev. Neurosci., 7: 95–125.

Stein, B. E. and Clamann, H. P. (1981) Control of pinna movements and sensorimotor register in cat superior colliculus.

Brain Behav. Evol., 19: 180–192.

Syka, J. and Radil-Weiss, T. (1971) Electrical stimulation of the tectum in freely moving cats. Brain Res., 28: 567–572.

Wurtz, R. H. and Goldberg, M. E. (1972) Activity of superior colliculus in behaving monkey. III. Cells discharging before eye movements. J. Neurophysiol., 35: 575–586.

Horizontal saccades and the central mesencephalic reticular formation

Bernard Cohen, David M. Waitzman, Jean A. Büttner-Ennever and Victor Matsuo

Department of Neurology, Mount Sinai School of Medicine of the City University of New York, New York, NY 10029, U.S.A.

Introduction

Brainstem mechanisms for rapid eye movements have been studied extensively, but it is still not clear how activity responsible for shifts in gaze is processed through the cerebrum and transmitted to the brainstem. It seems certain that the superior colliculus (SC) plays an important role in directing orientation of gaze. SC has the appropriate neural activity and requisite anatomic connections to sense peripheral targets and to initiate saccades and head movements in all directions (Schiller and Stryker, 1972; Wurtz and Goldberg, 1972a; Sparks, 1975; Sparks and Mays, 1980; for review, see Wurtz and Albano, 1980). However, destruction of SC has a relatively minor effect on the generation of saccades (Wurtz and Goldberg, 1972b), suggesting that other areas in the cerebrum may also participate in their production. In agreement with this, combined SC and frontal eye field lesions produce a more profound deficit in eye movements (Schiller et al., 1980).

Stimulation and lesion experiments originally suggested that portions of the mesencephalic reticular formation (MRF) might play an important role in producing horizontal eye movements (Szentágothai, 1943; Bender and Shanzer, 1964; Komatsuzaki et al., 1972). Stimulation induced contralateral deviation of the eyes in cat (Szentágothai, 1943) and monkey (Bender and Shanzer, 1964), while lesions of the MRF caused transient deficits in contralateral gaze (Bender and Shanzer, 1964; Komatsuzaki et al., 1972). As the MRF has now been shown to contain output fibers from the superior colliculus destined for the pontine reticular formation (Harting, 1977; Harting et al., 1980), the earlier stimulation results could have been due to activation of the tectal output. Moreover, electrolytic lesions would not differentiate between damage to the intrinsic neuronal mechanisms in the MRF and damage to fibers in passage. Therefore, we determined if neurons in the MRF were active in association with horizontal saccades. These results are summarized in this report. In addition, we will describe other facets of organization between the collicular output, the MRF and saccade-generating portions of the pontine reticular formation. The data indicate that the central MRF is an area that can contribute to production of saccades and gaze movements in the horizontal plane.

Region of the mesencephalic reticular formation related to horizontal saccades, central MRF

The area related to horizontal saccades in the monkey occupies only a restricted portion of the MRF. It lies within the region that is termed nucleus subcuneiformis in the human (Olszewski and Baxter, 1954), and nucleus cuneiformis in the cat (Edwards, 1975). We have referred to it as the central MRF (cMRF) to distinguish it from morphologically similar surrounding areas (Cohen and Büttner-Ennev-

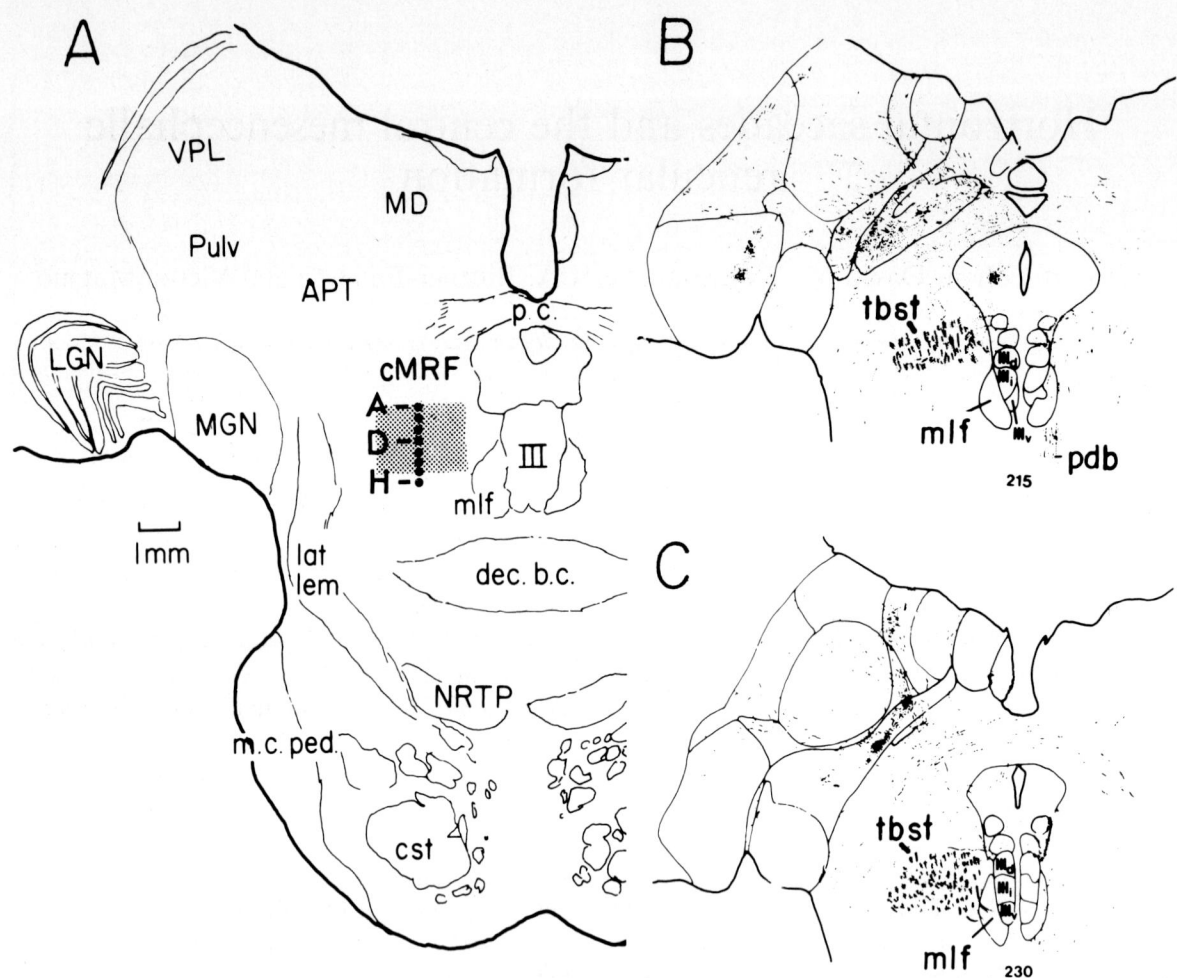

Fig. 1. A. Cross-hatched area shows the approximate region of the cMRF of the rhesus monkey. Cells recorded in this region had activity that was related to contralateral saccades, and electrical stimulation of this region elicited horizontal saccades. The dots show approximate sites of stimulation for the data in Fig. 4. They are separated by 0.25 mm. Locations A, D and H of that figure are marked. B, C. Sections adapted from Harting et al. (1980) showing location of tecto-bulbo-spinal tract (tbst) and predorsal bundle (pdb) in the rhesus monkey. The fibers in tbst and pdb have been darkened for emphasis. Note that tbst approximates the region defined as cMRF in A. From Cohen et al. (1985). APT, area pretectalis; cst, corticospinal tract; dec.b.c., decussation of the brachium conjunctivum; lat lem, lateral lemniscus; LGN, lateral geniculate nucleus; m.c.ped., middle cerebral peduncle; MD, medialis dorsalis; MGN, medial geniculate nucleus; mlf, median longitudinal fasciculus; NRTP, nucleus reticularis tegmenti pontis; Pulv, pulvinar; VPL, ventralis posterolateralis.

er, 1984). The approximate location of the cMRF in the rhesus monkey is shown in the cross-hatched region in Fig. 1A. It is approximately 2 mm wide, 1.5 mm deep and 3 mm in rostro-caudal extent. It lies lateral to the oculomotor nucleus and central gray matter and in its rostral portions is dorsolateral to the red nucleus, pars magnocellularis.

cMRF is lateral to the rostral iMLF, the interstitial nucleus of Cajal, and adjacent portions of the MRF that have been associated with vertical eye movement (Büttner-Ennever and Büttner, 1978). The rostro-caudal extent of cMRF corresponds roughly to the levels at which the interstitial nucleus of Cajal is found. As shown by Harting and colleagues

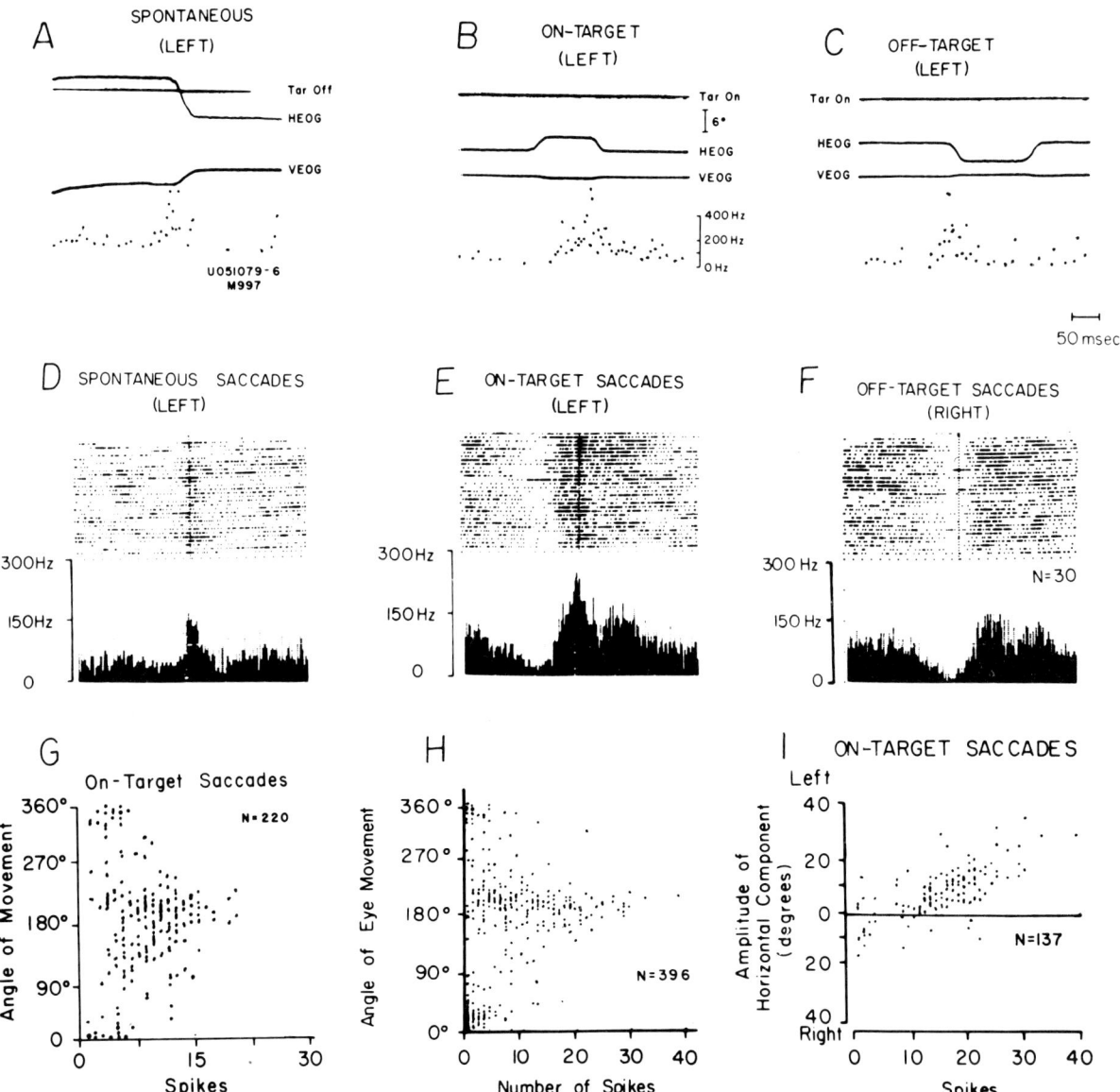

Fig. 2. A–F. Activity of a burst neuron recorded in the right cMRF with a high spontaneous firing rate (50–75 impulses/sec). A–C. Traces are from top to bottom, target on-off, horizontal and vertical EOG, and instantaneous frequency of firing. The calibrations for the EOGs and the firing frequencies are shown by the vertical bars in B. The time base is shown in C. D–F. Raster displays of firing associated with 30 consecutive spontaneous saccades (D), on-target saccades (E) and off-target saccades (F). The firing rates were aligned on saccade onset (vertical dotted lines). The dots under the raster displays occur each 32 mseconds. Below each raster is a histogram of the unit activity normalized for a peak frequency of 300 Hz. G. Number of spikes in the period from 32 mseconds before saccade onset to 4.8 mseconds before the movement ended (abscissa) associated with on-target eye movements in various directions for the neuron whose records are shown in A–F. The angle of eye movement is shown on the ordinate. 180° designates a movement to the left. H. Similar graph from another burst neuron, also recorded in the right cMRF, for on-target saccades. I. The horizontal component of on-target movements for the neuron of H is represented on the ordinate. Note the increasing number of spikes as the size of the horizontal component to the left increased. Adapted from Waitzman (1982).

(1977, 1980), the output fibers of the superior colliculus, destined for the pons and medulla via the dorsal tegmental decussation, course through cMRF (Fig. 1B, C). This must kept in mind when interpreting the effects of electrical stimulation in the normal animal that will be described below.

Activity of neurons in cMRF

To investigate whether cMRF subserves oculomotor function, single neurons were recorded extracellularly in the cMRF of several monkeys trained to fixate spots of light displayed at various locations on a TV screen (Waitzman and Cohen, 1979; Waitzman, 1982). When the target light dimmed, the monkeys were required to release a bar press within 500 mseconds to receive a water reward (Wurtz, 1969). Neurons were encountered in cMRF that had bursts of activity in association with contralateral spontaneous saccades as well as with saccades made to the visual target. A typical example is shown in Fig. 2A–F. Increases in activity began 30–100 mseconds before the onset of saccades and terminated in bursts of firing. Peak frequencies could be as high as 600–700 Hz and preceded saccades by 10–20 mseconds. Bursts often outlasted eye movements by 50–100 mseconds. Peak activity was greater in most neurons when the animal made saccades to the visual target (Fig. 2B, second saccade; Fig. 2E) than during spontaneous saccades (Fig. 2A, D) or saccades away from the target (Fig. 2C, first saccade). There was no overt visual response of the neurons, and many cells fired during saccades or quick phases of nystagmus in darkness. The neurons did not change their firing rates during pursuit movements, slow phases of nystagmus or vergence movements. Thus, cMRF activity was primarily related to the motor command for rapid conjugate eye movement. In addition, there was an important attentional component to the activity.

Firing of cMRF burst neurons was directional-specific, being related to contralateral horizontal eye movements. When there were more than seven to ten spikes in the burst, the associated eye movement had a contralateral horizontal component (Fig. 2G, H). There was no relationship to the vertical component of gaze. Despite the fact that the cells fired vigorously before and during contralateral saccades, the number of spikes in the portion of the burst just preceding the movement was not specifically related to the amplitude of the horizontal component. Therefore, the cMRF volley, if it produced saccades, must have done so in a manner similar to SC and frontal eye field neurons, namely, by acting as a trigger signal.

If the period of analysis was extended to include the time of the on-target saccade, the number of spikes in the burst increased in some cells as a function of the horizontal component of movement (Fig. 2I). Since neural activity was not specifically related to the size of the movement in the period before the onset of saccades (see above), activity responsible for the relationship of Fig. 2I must have occurred after the movement had been initiated. Results of stimulation have shown that the size of induced saccades is largely determined by the time the movement begins (see Fig. 3A, for example). Hence, activity that occurs after the onset of movement must serve another function. It might be used to help produce head movements during gaze shifts. Another possibility is that it could act as an efference copy signal, designating the horizontal component of saccades to structures that receive output from cMRF.

Many cMRF neurons had an irregular rate of background firing (Fig. 2A, D) that was enhanced when the animal was performing the behavioral task, i.e., when it was watching for dimming of the target light (Fig. 2B, C, E, F). The background activity was not associated with target or surround illumination or with eye position and appeared related to attention to the task. Similar background activity is not present in SC cells and frontal eye field neurons (Wurtz and Goldberg, 1972a; Sparks, 1975; Sparks and Mays, 1980; Goldberg and Bushnell, 1981).

cMRF burst neurons were not only excited during eye movements in the contralateral direction, but they were inhibited during ipsilateral saccades (Fig. 2B, first saccade; Fig. 2F). Pauses in firing

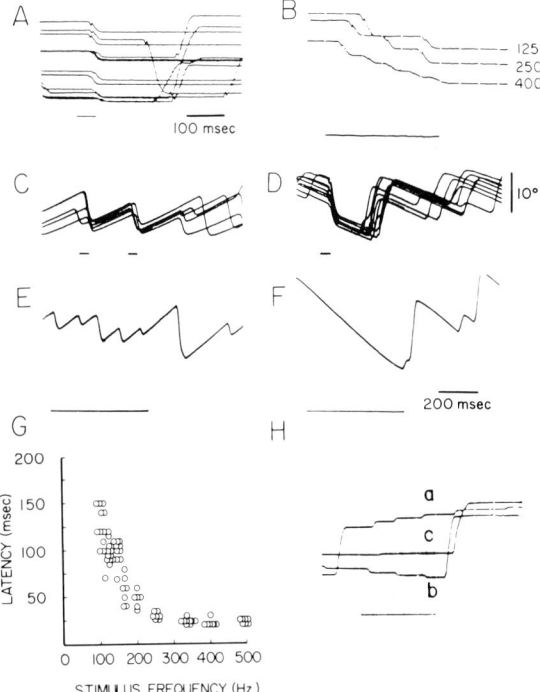

Fig. 3. Saccades induced by right cMRF stimulation. A. In dorsal cMRF short trains of pulses induced small saccades to the contralateral side in the alert animal. The movements were of approximately the same size regardless of the initial position of the eyes in the orbit. Each saccade was followed by a period of 100–200 mseconds when no further saccade tended to occur. B. Longer trains of pulses induced "staircase saccades" to the contralateral side, not slow eye movements. The latency was dependent on the frequency of stimulation which is designated by the numbers on the right. C, D. Stimulation of right cMRF during OKN with leftward (C) or rightward (D) quick phases elicited typical contralateral rapid eye movements. The velocity of the slow phases was not affected by the occurrence of the induced movements. E, F. Low-frequency cMRF stimulation (110 impulses/sec) during OKN facilitated (E) or inhibited (F) quick phase generation depending on whether the quick phases of OKN were to the contralateral (E) or ipsilateral (F) side. G. Plot of latency of induced saccades of the type shown in A (ordinate) against frequency of stimulation (abscissa). The pulse train contained 15 pulses and induced only a single saccade. H. Bilateral stimulation of cMRF. In a, the left cMRF was stimulated, causing movements to the right. In b, the right cMRF was stimulated, causing movements to the left. When both were activated simultaneously (c), the eyes did not move. From Cohen et al. (1985).

began 60–100 mseconds prior to the onset of movement and continued throughout the saccade. The reduction in firing was more profound and began earlier during ipsilateral saccades away from the target (Fig. 2B, first saccade) than during ipsilateral on-target (Fig. 2C, second saccade) or spontaneous eye movements. This indicates that the neuronal activity related to eye movements is reciprocal, with cMRF on both sides participating in the production of eye movements in either direction.

In summary, cMRF contains neurons whose activity is related to the horizontal component of saccades, particularly when they are made to targets of interest in the contralateral field. The latency of activity in cMRF neurons before the onset of eye movement is such that they could trigger saccades during shifts of gaze in the horizontal plane. cMRF neural activity could also signal the occurrence of the horizontal component of saccades to other parts of the nervous system.

Eye movements induced by stimulation of cMRF

In order to determine more about the processing of activity in cMRF neurons and possibly in tecto-bulbo-spinal fibers that pass through cMRF, the region was electrically stimulated in the alert monkey (Cohen et al., 1982, 1985). Saccadic eye movements were induced to the contralateral side at latencies of 18–35 mseconds (Fig. 3A). The characteristics of the induced horizontal movements were identical to those of spontaneously occurring saccades, suggesting that cMRF stimulation had excited natural pulse-generating mechanisms in the pontine reticular formation (PPRF). If stimuli were given during slow phases of optokinetic nystagmus (OKN), rapid eye movements were elicited, and the velocity of the slow phases was not affected (Fig. 3C, D). Smooth eye deviations were not produced in the alert animal, even by continuous cMRF stimulation (Fig. 3B). This is consistent with recordings from cMRF neurons that demonstrate a relationship to saccades, not to pursuit or vergence movements. It is a further indication that the function of cMRF neurons and/or pathways that lie within it is related to generation of rapid eye movements.

Experiments were done to establish the relationship between frequency of stimulation and the number of pulses necessary to trigger a movement. Similar to saccades induced from SC and the frontal eye fields (Robinson and Fuchs, 1969; Robinson, 1972), the frequency of stimulation was unrelated to the size of the induced movements, and their amplitude depended solely on the region of cMRF that was activated. When the stimulation frequency was lower, the latency to saccade onset was longer (Fig. 3B). The relationship between latency and stimulus frequency approximated the curve of a constant product (Fig. 3G), suggesting that saccades had been induced after a fixed number of pulses had been given. This would imply that the impulses elicited by the stimulating train had been integrated within the PPRF to trigger a saccade.

Cells or fibers in cMRF could also be shown to have a tonic effect on saccade generation. When cMRF was stimulated during OKN at impulse rates that were too low to elicit rapid eye movements, the frequency of quick phases was modulated according to the direction of the nystagmus: contralateral quick phases were faciliated (Fig. 3E) and ipsilateral quick phases were inhibited or suppressed (Fig. 3F). When the cMRF on both sides were stimulated simultaneously (Fig. 3Hc), the eyes were fixed in place, and no further movements occurred until the stimulus had ended. The absence of horizontal and vertical saccades during bilateral stimulation implies that saccade initiation had been inhibited in all directions.

Thus, activity in pathways and/or cells in cMRF was not only able to trigger saccades, but could also raise or lower the excitability of saccade-generating networks in the PPRF. Data on the suppressive effects of simultaneous bilateral stimulation on saccade initiation may be related to the increase in background activity of cMRF burst neurons that occurred while the animal was fixating during the attentional task (Fig. 2C, D, E, F). Such activity, which would occur bilaterally, might help inhibit the production of further saccades until a burst of activity from one side and a decrease in activity on the other caused the eyes to move to a new target.

Constant and variable amplitude saccades; topographic organization of activity related to constant amplitude saccades

Two types of saccades were elicited from cMRF, constant amplitude saccades and variable amplitude saccades. These are similar to the retinotopic movements and craniotopic movements described in studies of the superior colliculus (Guitton et al., 1980; Roucoux et al., 1980). From a given electrode location in dorsal cMRF the induced saccades tended to be of the same size, regardless of the initial position of the eye in the orbit. A typical example of retinotopic saccades is shown in Fig. 3A. A striking finding was that there was a topographic organization within cMRF for constant amplitude saccades of different sizes. Dorsally, small saccades were induced that were just at the limit of resolution of the EOG (Fig. 4A). (The approximate positions of the stimulus locations in Fig. 4A–H are shown by the dots in the cross-hatched region in Fig. 1A, with locations A, D and H being marked.) As the stimulating electrode was advanced in 0.25-mm increments, the constant amplitude saccades became progressively larger, increasing in size to about 10–15° over the next mm (Fig. 4B–D). The relationship between electrode position and size of induced movement was found in every animal that was stimulated, regardless of rostro-caudal or medial-lateral location of the electrode in cMRF. This suggests that cMRF neurons and/or fibers of passage from the SC are organized in a topographic fashion in the monkey, with cells and fibers responsible for horizontal components of movement of increasing size being layered in broad bands, one beneath another.

In ventral portions of cMRF, saccades were elicited whose sizes were dependent on eye position (variable amplitude saccades). The induced movements were larger when the eyes were on the ipsi-

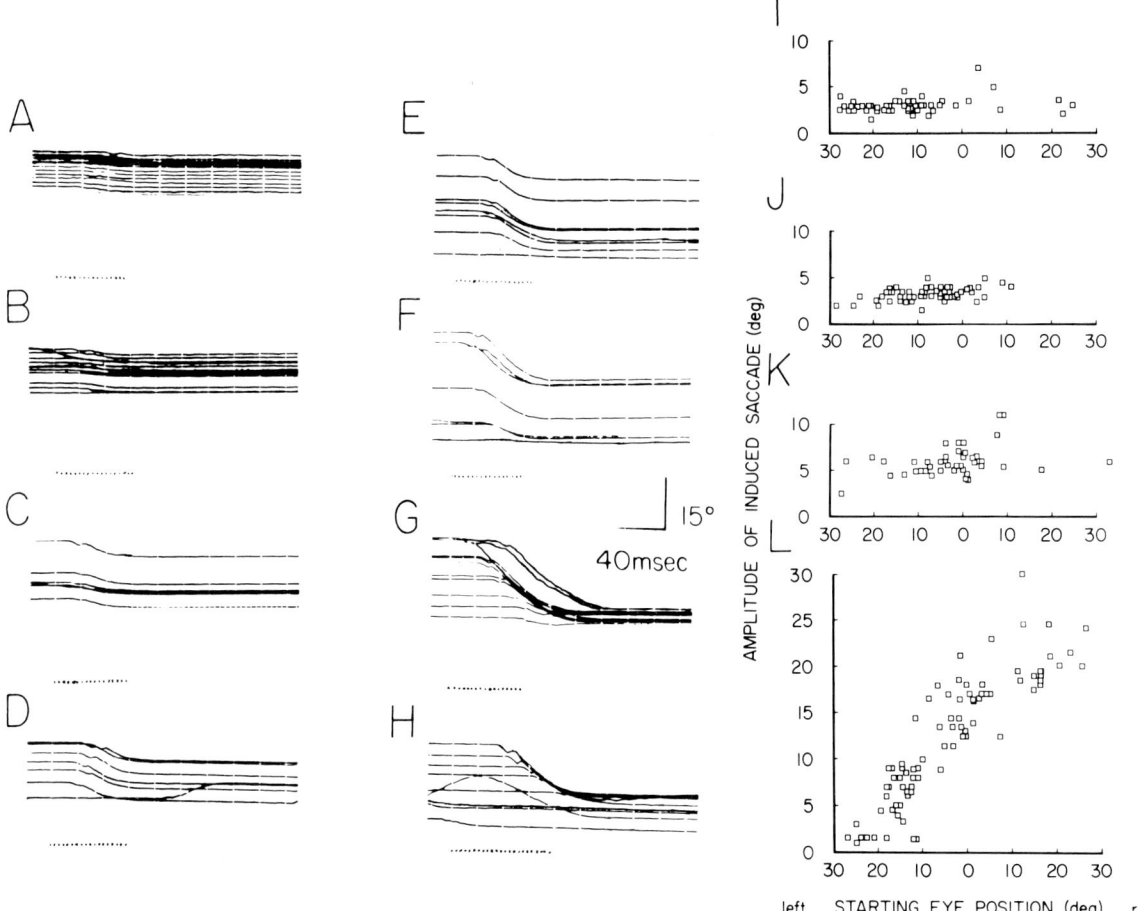

Fig. 4. A–H. Horizontal saccades induced by right cMRF stimulation at the approximate locations shown in Fig. 1A. The stimuli were given with the eyes in different initial positions. In each panel positions on the right (ipsilateral side) are at the top and positions on the left (contralateral side) are at the bottom. The sites of stimulation were each 0.25 mm apart from top (A) to bottom (H). I–L. Graphs of size of eye movement (ordinate) against initial position in the orbit (abscissa) for stimulation at different sites in another animal. I–K. Constant amplitude movements of increasing size were induced from sites in dorsal cMRF which were 0.25 mm apart. L. Variable amplitude movements were induced 0.5 mm below the site for K. From Cohen et al. (1985).

lateral side and smaller when the eyes were on the contralateral side (Fig. 4F–H). Consequently, when this region was stimulated, the eyes tended to move toward a sector of the contralateral field. The relationship between saccade size and initial eye position in another animal is shown in Fig. 4I–L. The stimulus locations for each graph were successively deeper in cMRF by 0.25 mm, except for L, which was 0.5 mm below the location for K. The slope of the relationship between saccade size and initial eye position was flat in the constant amplitude regions in dorsal cMRF (Fig. 4I–K) and positive in the variable amplitude region (Fig. 4L). Although "sector-directed" movements of the type shown in G and L have not been described before in the monkey, they have been found by stimulating posterior portions of SC in the cat (Guitton et al., 1980). If cMRF-induced movements are utilized in shifting gaze in the monkey, as in the cat (Roucoux et al., 1980), the larger variable amplitude move-

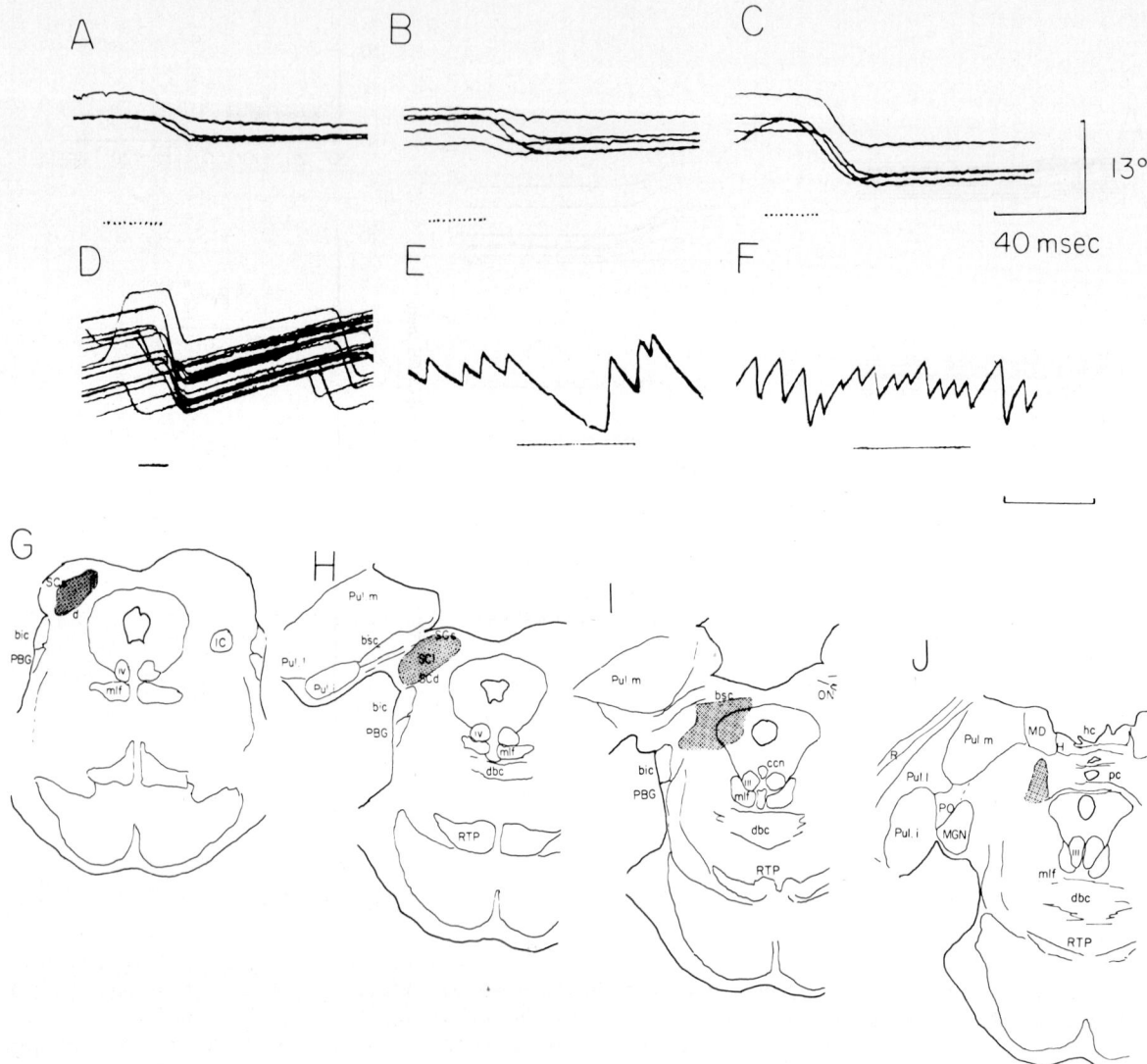

Fig. 5. Eye movements induced by right cMRF stimulation after cells in the intermediate and deep layers of the ipsilateral SC were destroyed by kainic acid. The region of cellular destruction is shown by the cross-hatched area in G–J. After the tectal output to cMRF had been largely removed, saccades of increasing size to the left were still induced by stimulating progressively deeper in the right cMRF (A–C). Pulse trains during OKN (D) caused typical leftward saccades, with a period following the saccades in which no movements tended to occur. Low-frequency stimulation caused quick phases to be suppressed (E) or facilitated (F), depending on whether the quick phases of OKN were ipsilateral (E) or contralateral (F) to the side of stimulation. bic, brachium of the inferior colliculus; bsc, brachium of the superior colliculus; dbc, decussation of the brachium conjunctivum; IC, inferior colliculus; hc, habenular commissure; PBC, parabigeminal nucleus; PC, posterior commissure; Pul i, m, l, intermediate, medial and lateral pulvinar; RTP, nucleus reticularis tegmenti pontis; SC d, i, s, deep, intermediate and superficial layers of SC; III, oculomotor nucleus; IV, trochlear nucleus.

ments may be accompanied by head movements. As the animals' heads were fixed in these experiments, however, this could not be determined.

Effects of SC lesions on cMRF stimulation

Since cMRF contains the output from SC to areas of the pons responsible for producing horizontal saccades, the question arose whether the results of stimulation were solely due to activation of tecto-bulbo-spinal fibers, or whether cMRF neurons were also capable of generating saccades. In one monkey the intermediate and deep layers of SC were lesioned on one side with kainic acid. These layers contain cells which give rise to the tectal output that reaches the contralateral pons, medulla and spinal cord (Kawamura et al., 1974; Harting, 1977; Grantyn and Grantyn, 1982; Edwards and Henkel, 1978; Edwards, 1980). The extent of the destruction is shown in Fig. 5G–J. There was extensive gliosis in the intermediate and deep layers of SC after lesion, and neurons were not seen in the cross-hatched regions.

After lesion characteristic saccades could still be induced by stimulating cMRF on the side of the injection, although initially the threshold was higher and the latency was longer. Saccades were elicited both with the eyes stationary (Fig. 5A–C) or in motion (Fig. 5D), and their amplitude increased as the electrode penetrated cMRF from dorsal to ventral (Fig. 5A–C). It was still possible to suppress or facilitate saccade generation by stimulation at low frequencies (Fig. 5E, F). Since few cells were present in the intermediate or deep layers of SC after lesion, it is unlikely that activation of their axons was responsible for the generation of eye movements. Other regions that are involved in production of saccades, such as the frontal eye fields, do not project to cMRF (Astruc, 1971; Kuenzle and Akert, 1977). It seems likely that activation of cells in cMRF was responsible for the saccades that were induced in the SC-lesioned animal, and that both cMRF cells and tecto-bulbo-spinal fibers lying in cMRF contributed to the result of stimulation observed in the normal animal.

Relationships between cMRF and SC

The orderly dorsal-ventral organization of bands of cells and fibers associated with horizontal saccadic components of different sizes in cMRF is reminiscent of the rostral-caudal topography for saccades found in SC (Robinson, 1972; Schiller and Stryker, 1972). A major difference is that cMRF is related only to horizontal eye movements whereas all movement directions are represented in the neurons of SC on the two sides. Tectal neurons project to the MRF in the cat (Grantyn and Grantyn, 1982), and the same is probably true in the monkey (Harting, 1977). Thus, it seemed possible that there might be a topographically organized connection from SC to cMRF.

This possibility was addressed in experiments in which regions of cMRF that were related to small or large eye movements were identified by electrical stimulation, and one of two retrograde tracer substances, horseradish peroxidase (HRP) or radioactive wheatgerm agglutinin (WGA), was placed at these sites. The advantage of having two independent injections in the same animal was that the location of the labelled cell groups could be compared more accurately.

The results from one such experiment are shown in Fig. 6. The eye movements induced by stimulation are shown in A and B, the sites of injection in C, and the location of the labelled cells in D. Cells labelled by both WGA and HRP were found in the intermediate and deep layers of SC and the adjacent central gray matter on the ipsilateral side. Injection of WGA into the dorsal cMRF (Fig. 6C, section 41), at a site where small saccades were induced (Fig. 6A), caused labelling of cells in the rostral intermediate layer of SC (Fig. 6D, dots, sections 28–32). Injection of HRP into the ventral cMRF (Fig. 6C, section 40), at a point where large saccades were elicited (Fig. 6B), caused labelling of cells in the caudal intermediate layer of SC (Fig. 6D, open circles, sections 22–28). The distribution of the labelled cells was different for the WGA and HRP injections. Findings were similar in two other animals (Cohen and Büttner-Ennever, 1984). We

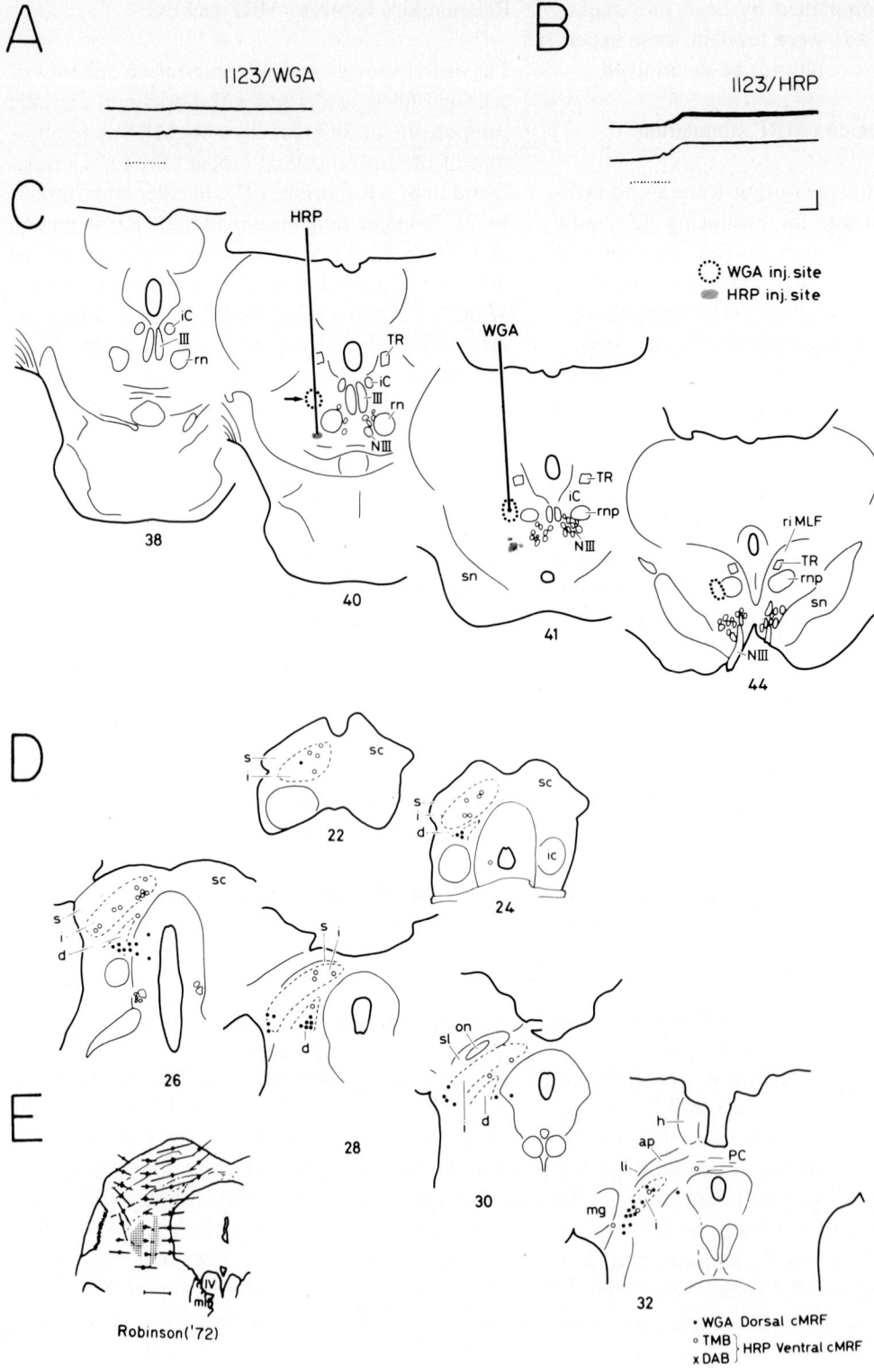

infer from these results that the intermediate layer of SC sends axonal projections to the horizontal eye movement region of MRF in a topographic fashion, with regions of SC and cMRF related to small or to large eye movements being interconnected. The same is probably true for cells related to eye movements with intermediate-sized horizontal components.

Although the data shown in Fig. 6 were from the cynomolgus monkey, there is a striking correspondence with data obtained from the rhesus monkey. Robinson (1972) electrically stimulated SC to determine which regions were associated with saccades of different sizes and directions. Results from the mid-colliculus, adapted from Fig. 3 of Robinson (1972), are shown in Fig. 6E. They can be compared to the data in Fig. 6D, sections 26 and 28. Electrical stimulation of the deepest layers of SC, just lateral to the central gray matter, elicited eye movements with a small horizontal component (surrounded by shaded area, Fig. 6E). This was where cells were located in our animals (Fig. 6D, dots, sections 26 and 28), that were labelled by injection in dorsal cMRF (Fig. 6C, section 41), where small saccades were elicited (Fig. 6A). Large eye movements were induced in the rhesus monkey by stimulation of the intermediate layers of SC at this level (Fig. 6E). As shown by the open circles in Fig. 6D, sections 26 and 28, the intermediate layer at this level projects to ventral cMRF (Fig. 6B, section 40), where larger saccades were elicited (Fig. 6B).

In several animals there was heavy labelling of cells in a region of the central gray matter after dorsal cMRF injections (Fig. 6D, dots, section 26). This region projects to the ipsilateral SC and MRF in both cat and monkey and receives projections from neurons in the contralateral intermediate layer of SC (Grofova et al., 1978; Mantyh, 1983). Thus, cells in this region of the central gray matter may also be related to oculomotor function.

These results suggest that activity related to the horizontal component of saccades is transmitted from SC to cMRF over size-ordered channels, where it encounters a similar neural organization. As shown by both the single neuron and stimulation studies, only the horizontal component of movement is represented in activity of cells and fibers in cMRF. The vertical component of movement from SC must be directed elsewhere.

cMRF not only receives projections from SC, but it also projects back onto the intermediate layer of SC (Edwards and DeOlmos, 1976). Thus, cMRF could provide SC with information about the occurrence of the horizontal component of saccade. Whether this projection is also topographically organized according to the size of eye movement remains to be determined. Alternatively, cMRF and SC may serve as parallel output pathways for the generation of contralateral horizontal saccades during gaze shifts. As suggested by the different characteristics of the unit activity in the two structures, cMRF and SC could supply different aspects of information about saccades from various brain regions, and/or excite different elements of the sac-

---

Fig. 6. Injection of cMRF with tracer substances, HRP and WGA (C), at locations where small (A) or large (B) saccades were induced caused cells in SC to be labelled (D). The time base and eye movement calibrations for A and B are shown by the horizontal and vertical bars under B. They are 20 mseconds and 12°, respectively. Cells in the rostral intermediate layer (dots, sections 28–32) were tagged by the dorsal cMRF injection (section 41). Those in the caudal intermediate layer (open circles, sections 22–28) were labelled by the ventral cMRF injection (section 40). Cells in the deep layer of SC and the adjacent central gray matter (dots, sections 24, 26 and 28) were also labelled by the dorsal cMRF injection. Adapted from Cohen and Büttner-Ennever (1984). E. Section redrawn from Fig. 3 of Robinson (1972). The arrows show the direction of saccades induced by SC stimulation in the alert rhesus monkey. All movements were to the contralateral side. The underlying bar shows 1 mm for the anatomic section and 25° for the induced eye movements. The region from which small eye movements were induced in the deep layers of SC is surrounded by cross-hatched marking to facilitate comparison with similar regions of sections 26 and 28. ap, area pretectalis; h, habenular; iC, interstitial nucleus of Cajal; li, nucleus limitans; mg, medial geniculate body; on, olivary nucleus; ri MLF, rostral interstitial nucleus of the MLF; rn, red nucleus pars magnocellularis; rnp, red nucleus pars parvocellularis; sc s, i, d, superficial, intermediate and deep layers of the SC; sn, substantia nigra.

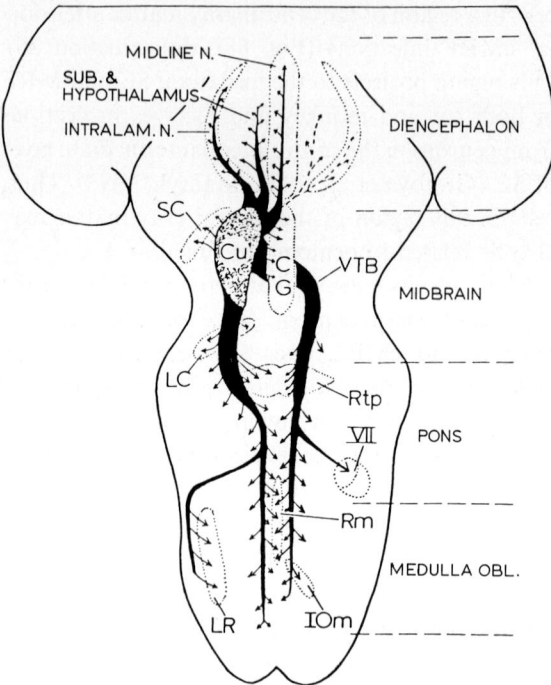

Fig. 7. Ascending and descending projections of nucleus cuneiformis in the cat, as determined with orthograde axonal transport of [^{3}H]leucine and [^{3}H]proline. CG, central gray; Cu, cuneate nucleus; IOm, medial accessory inferior olive; LC, locus coeruleus; LR, lateral reticular nucleus; Rm, raphe magnus; Rtp, nucleus reticularis tegmenti pontis; VII, facial nucleus; VTB, ventral tegmental bundle. From Edwards and DeOlmos (1976).

cade generating mechanism in the pons (Raybourn and Keller, 1977).

cMRF efferents

Relatively little is known about how activity is transmitted from cMRF to regions of the pons where saccadic eye movements are generated. Edwards (1975) originally showed that nucleus cuneiformis in the cat has heavy projections to the brainstem on both sides (Fig. 7). These projections descend ipsilaterally in the central tegmental tract to innervate a wide variety of structures, including NRTP, nucleus reticularis pontis oralis and caudalis, and the raphe nuclei in the medial pontine reticular formation. The contralateral output of the MRF joins that from SC and the two are "fused into a single massive fiber bundle" that decussates through the oculomotor rootlets just rostral to the oculomotor nucleus, before turning ventrally to descend in the predorsal bundle to the pontine and medullary tegmentum and the inferior olive (Fig. 7; Edwards, 1980).

Comparative studies of the projection from cMRF to the PPRF are currently in progress in the monkey (Büttner-Ennever, Pause and Cohen, unpublished data). Initial results (Cohen et al., 1981) indicate that cMRF has similar connections to regions of the pons and medulla, where burst and pause neurons are to be located (Keller, 1974; Raybourn and Keller, 1977). A complete description of these projections is beyond the scope of this paper, but it is clear that cMRF has the appropriate neural connections to participate in producing saccades. It also projects widely to areas of the forebrain that are known to have activity related to saccades.

Summary

(1) A region of the mesencephalic reticular formation, designated as the central MRF or cMRF, contains burst neurons whose activity is related to the horizontal component of contralateral saccadic eye movements, particularly when monkeys make saccades to targets of interest. There is a decrease in the firing rates of cMRF during ipsilateral saccades. Bursts have the appropriate latency before the onset of eye movement to contribute to the triggering of saccades.

(2) Stimulation studies in cMRF show that tectal efferent fibers and/or cMRF neurons can be activated to produce contralateral saccades. The size of the movements depends on the location of the stimulating electrode in cMRF, small movements being induced more dorsally and larger movements more ventrally. A continuum of movement sizes is induced in between. Constant amplitude or variable amplitude saccades made toward sectors of the contralateral field are induced by stimulation of different portions of cMRF. Contralateral saccades were also induced by cMRF stimulation after a

kainic acid lesion of the superior colliculus had largely eliminated cells in the region where the tectal efferent outflow originates.

(3) Retrograde axonal tracer studies show that there are projections from the intermediate and deep layers of SC to cMRF. These projections are organized in a topographic fashion, with areas related to small or to large eye movements being connected in the two structures. Anatomic data in the cat and preliminary results in the monkey indicate that cMRF projects to regions of the brainstem that are involved in control of horizontal gaze. Thus, a circumscribed region of the MRF contains neurons that could provide a parallel pathway to that from SC for the generation of the horizontal component of gaze.

Acknowledgements

Supported by NIH Research Grant EY 02296, Core Center Grant EY 01867, DFG Grant SFB 200/A3, and a grant from the Young Men's Philanthropic league

References

Astruc, J. (1971) Corticofugal connections of area B (frontal eye field) in *Macaca mulatta*. Brain Res., 33: 241–256.
Bender, M. B. and Shanzer, S. (1964) Oculomotor pathways defined by electric stimulation and lesion in the brainstem of monkeys. In M. B. Bender (Ed.), The Oculomotor System, Harper and Row, New York, pp. 81–140.
Büttner-Ennever, J. A. and Büttner, U. (1978) A cell group associated with vertical eye movements in the rostral mesencephalic reticular formation of the monkey. Brain Res., 151: 31–47.
Cohen, B. and Büttner-Ennever, J. A. (1984) Projections from the superior colliculus to a region of the central mesencephalic reticular formation (cMRF) associated with horizontal eye movements. Exp. Brain Res., 57: 167–176.
Cohen, B., Büttner-Ennever, J. A., Waitzman, D. and Bender, M. B. (1981) Anatomical connections of a portion of the dorsolateral mesencephalic reticular formation associated with horizontal saccadic eye movements. Soc. Neurosci. Abstr., 7: 132.
Cohen, B., Matsuo, V., Raphan, T., Waitzman, D. and Fradin, J. (1982) Horizontal saccades induced by stimulation of the mesencephalic reticular formation. In A. Roucoux and M. Crommelinck (Eds.), Physiological and Pathological Aspects of Eye Movements. Dr. W. Junk Publishers, The Hague, pp. 325–335.
Cohen, B., Matsuo, V., Fradin, J. and Raphan, T. (1985) Horizontal saccades induced by stimulation of the central mesencephalic reticular formation. Exp. Brain Res., 57: 605–616.
Edwards, S. B. (1975) Autoradiographic studies of the projections of the midbrain reticular formation: Descending projections of nucleus cuneiformis. J. Comp. Neurol., 161: 341–358.
Edwards, S. B. (1980) The deep cell layers of the superior colliculus: Their reticular characteristics and structural organization. In A. Hobson and M. Brazier (Eds.), The Reticular Formation Revisited, Raven Press, New York, pp. 193–209.
Edwards, S. B. and DeOlmos, J. C. (1976) Autoradiographic studies of the projections of the midbrain reticular formation: Ascending projections of the superior colliculus in the cat. J. Comp. Neurol., 173: 23–40.
Edwards, S. B. and Henkel, C. K. (1978) Superior colliculus connections with the extraocular motor nuclei in the cat. J. Comp. Neurol., 179: 451–468.
Goldberg, M. E. and Bushnell, M. C. (1981) Behavioral enhancement of visual responses in monkey cerebral cortex. II. Modulation in frontal eye fields specifically related to saccades. J. Neurophysiol., 46: 773–787.
Grantyn, A. and Grantyn, R. (1982) Axonal pattern and sites of termination of cat superior colliculus neurons projecting in the tecto-bulbar-spinal tract. Exp. Brain Res., 46: 243–250.
Grofova, I., Ottersen, O. P. and Rinvik, E. (1978) Mesencephalic and diencephalic afferents to the superior colliculus and periaqueductal gray substance demonstrated by retrograde axonal transport of horseradish peroxidase in the cat. Brain Res., 146: 205–220.
Guitton, D., Crommelinck, M. and Roucoux, A. (1980) Stimulation of superior colliculus in the alert cat. I. Eye movements and neck EMG evoked when the head is restrained. Exp. Brain Res., 39: 63–73.
Harting, J. K. (1977) Descending pathways from the superior colliculus: An autoradiographic analysis in the rhesus monkey (*Macaca mulatta*). J. Comp. Neurol., 173: 583–612.
Harting, J. M., Huerta, M. F., Frankfurter, A. J., Strominger, N. L. and Royce, G. J. (1980) Ascending pathways from the monkey superior colliculus: An autoradiographic analysis. J. Comp. Neurol., 192: 853–882.
Kawamura, K., Brodal, A. and Hoddevik, G. (1974) The projection of the superior colliculus onto the reticular formation of the brainstem. An experimental anatomical study in the cat. Exp. Brain Res., 19: 1–19.
Keller, E. L. (1974) Participation of medial pontine reticular formation in eye movement generation in monkey. J. Neurophysiol., 37: 316–322.
Komatsuzaki, A., Alpert, J., Harris, H. E. and Cohen, B. (1972) Effect of mesencephalic reticular formation lesions on optokinetic nystagmus. Exp. Neurol., 34: 522–534.
Kuenzle, H. and Akert, K. (1977) Efferent connections of cortical Area B (frontal eye field) in *Macaca fascicularis*. A rein-

vestigation using the autoradiographic technique. J. Comp. Neurol., 173: 147–164.

Mantyh, P. W. (1983) Connections of midbrain periaqueductal gray in the monkey. I. Descending efferent projections. J. Neurophysiol., 49: 567–581.

Olszewski, J. and Baxter, D. (1954) Cytoarchitecture of the Human Brain Stem. Karger, Basel, pp. 1–199.

Raybourn, M. S. and Keller, E. L. (1977) Colliculoreticular organization in primate oculomotor system. J. Neurophysiol., 40: 861–878.

Robinson, D. A. (1972) Eye movements evoked by collicular stimulation in the alert monkey. Vision Res., 12: 1795–1808.

Robinson, D. A. and Fuchs, A. F. (1969) Eye movements evoked by stimulation of frontal eye fields. J. Neurophysiol., 32: 637–648.

Roucoux, A., Guitton, D. and Crommelinck, M. (1980) Stimulation of the superior colliculus in the alert cat. II. Eye and head movements evoked when the head is unrestrained. Exp. Brain Res., 39: 75–85.

Schiller, P. H. and Stryker, M. (1972) Single unit recordings and stimulation in superior colliculus of the alert rhesus monkey. J. Neurophysiol., 35: 915–924.

Schiller, P. H., True, S. D. and Conway, J. L. (1980) Deficits in eye movements following frontal eye field and superior colliculus ablations. J. Neurophysiol., 44: 1175–1189.

Sparks, D. L. (1975) Response properties of eye movement-related neurons in the monkey superior colliculus. Brain Res. 90: 147–152.

Sparks, D. L. and Mays, L. E. (1980) Movement fields of saccade-related burst neurons in the monkey superior colliculus. Brain Res., 33: 241–256.

Szentágothai, J. (1943) Die zentrale Innervation der Augenbewegungen. Arch. Psychiatr. Nervenkr., 116: 721–760.

Waitzman, D. (1982) Burst neurons in the mesencephalic reticular formation (MRF) associated with saccadic eye movements. Ph. D. Thesis, City University of New York.

Waitzman, D. and Cohen, B. (1979) Unit activity in the mesencephalic reticular formation (MRF) associated with saccades and positions of fixation during a visual attention task. Neurosci. Abstr., 5: 389.

Wurtz, R. H. (1969) Visual receptive fields of striate cortex neurons in awake monkeys. J. Neurophysiol., 32: 727–742.

Wurtz, R. H. and Albano, J. E. (1980) Visual-motor function of the primate superior colliculus. Annu. Rev. Neurosci., 3: 189–226.

Wurtz, R. H. and Goldberg, M. E. (1972a) Activity of superior colliculus in behaving monkey. III. Cells discharging before eye movements. J. Neurophysiol., 35: 575–586.

Wurtz, R. H. and Goldberg, M. E. (1972b) Activity of superior colliculus in behaving monkey. IV. Effects of lesions on eye movements. J. Neurophysiol., 35: 587–596.

Brainstem neurons are peculiar for oculomotor organization

Robert Baker

Department of Physiology, New York University Medical Center, 550 First Avenue, New York, NY 10016, U.S.A.

Introduction

The purpose of this paper is to comment generally on the structural and functional aspects of neurons and neural circuits in the oculomotor system, including some comparisons to the skeletal motor system. Although I conclude that little can be learned from the latter attempt, the last part of this presentation describes what I consider a reasonably important convergent similarity between the two motor systems — namely, the necessity to have "selectively adapted for" a neuronal feature which dictates the sequence of motor unit recruitment. Since this view implies order in the sense of "orderly recruitment of neurons", it also must include "orderly graduation of firing frequency" underlying the development of muscle force. The discussion is centered around applicability of the 20-year-old size principle of Henneman et al. (1965a, b), even though Enoka and Stuart (1984) recently have pointed out this concept's provocative nature, including their opinion that the results have been largely inconclusive in assessing exactly "What size related mechanism(s) produces orderly recruitment?" and the accompanying hypothesis "To which group of motor units does the size principle, if applicable, operate for specific motor performances?" (cf. Burke et al., 1982; Kernell and Zwaagstra, 1981; Ulfhake and Kellerth, 1982). Although herein I offer no new insight or resolution to these two important questions, I conclude that in the mammalian oculomotor system, as in the skeletal motor, a size principle is applicable to organization of extraocular motor nuclei. Thus, I propose that as a significant evolutionary convergent adaptation underlying CNS organization, the above two questions deserve further study in sensory-motor systems.

Quite possibly a more compelling, even fundamental, reason for emphasizing the role of "size" is its applicability to a population of internuclear neurons that directly contact other oculomotoneurons (Figs. 1 and 2). There are few comparable studies of spinal cord interneurons (any non-motoneuron), but they should be contemplated because the findings concerning internuclear neurons demonstrate that the size principle is not a "unique feature" for translating neural encoding only to mechanical operation of the ocular (or skeletal) motor plant. Size is significant for neural to neural translation. Furthermore, if these particular internuclear neurons are "new" — in the sense of being "specific" — to the mammalian CNS then they illustrate selective adaptation for neural circuitry capable of more precise, symmetrical motor control (in this particular case, conjugate movement of the two eyes). Arguing that idea is beyond the scope of this paper; however, it introduces use of phylogenetic evaluation, vis-a-vis comparative neuroscience, as an important tool for understanding the successful integration of structural and functional properties in the brain (Cambell and Hodos, 1970; Hodos, 1970; Bullock, 1983). Therefore, the second and larger topic of this paper is to address the issue

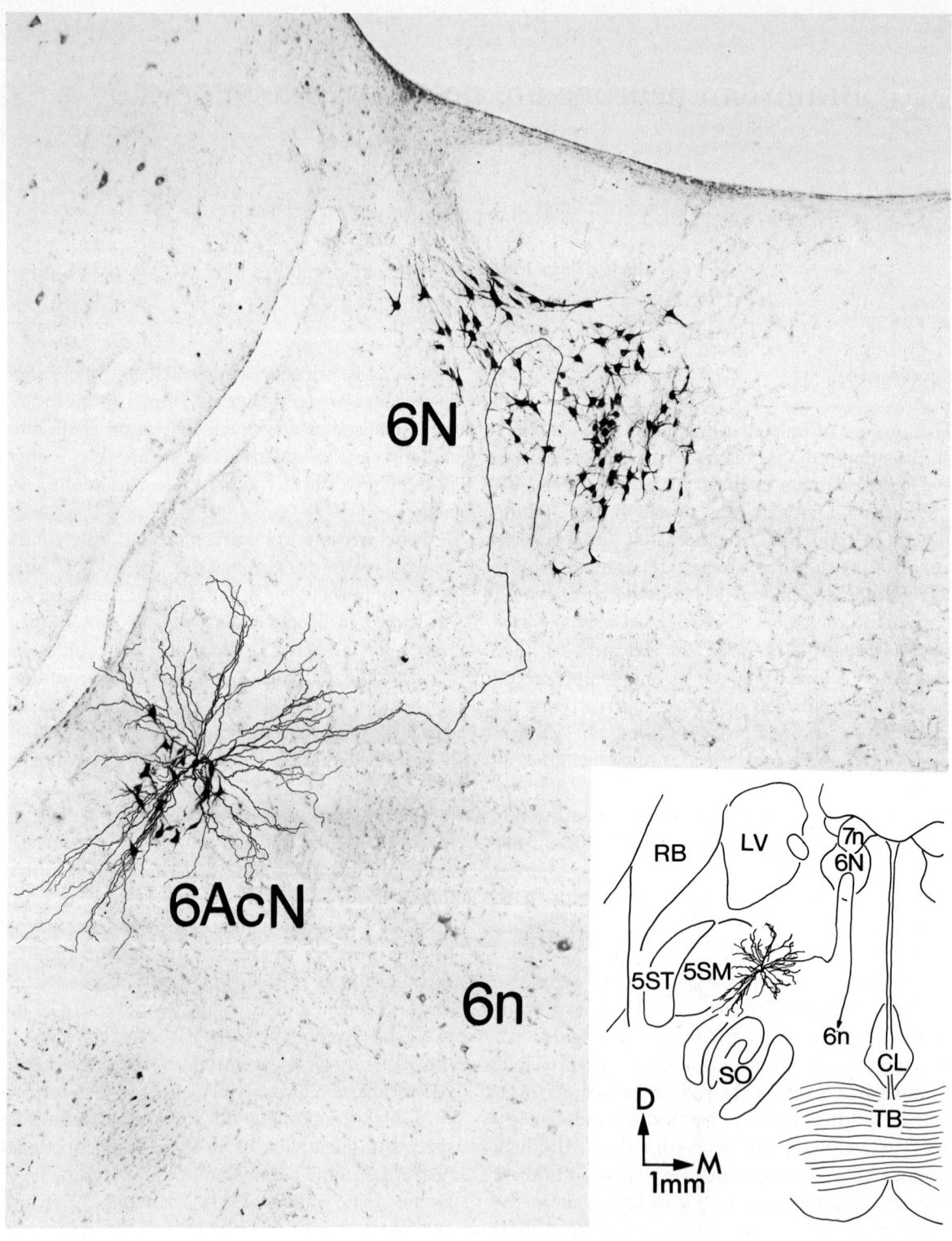

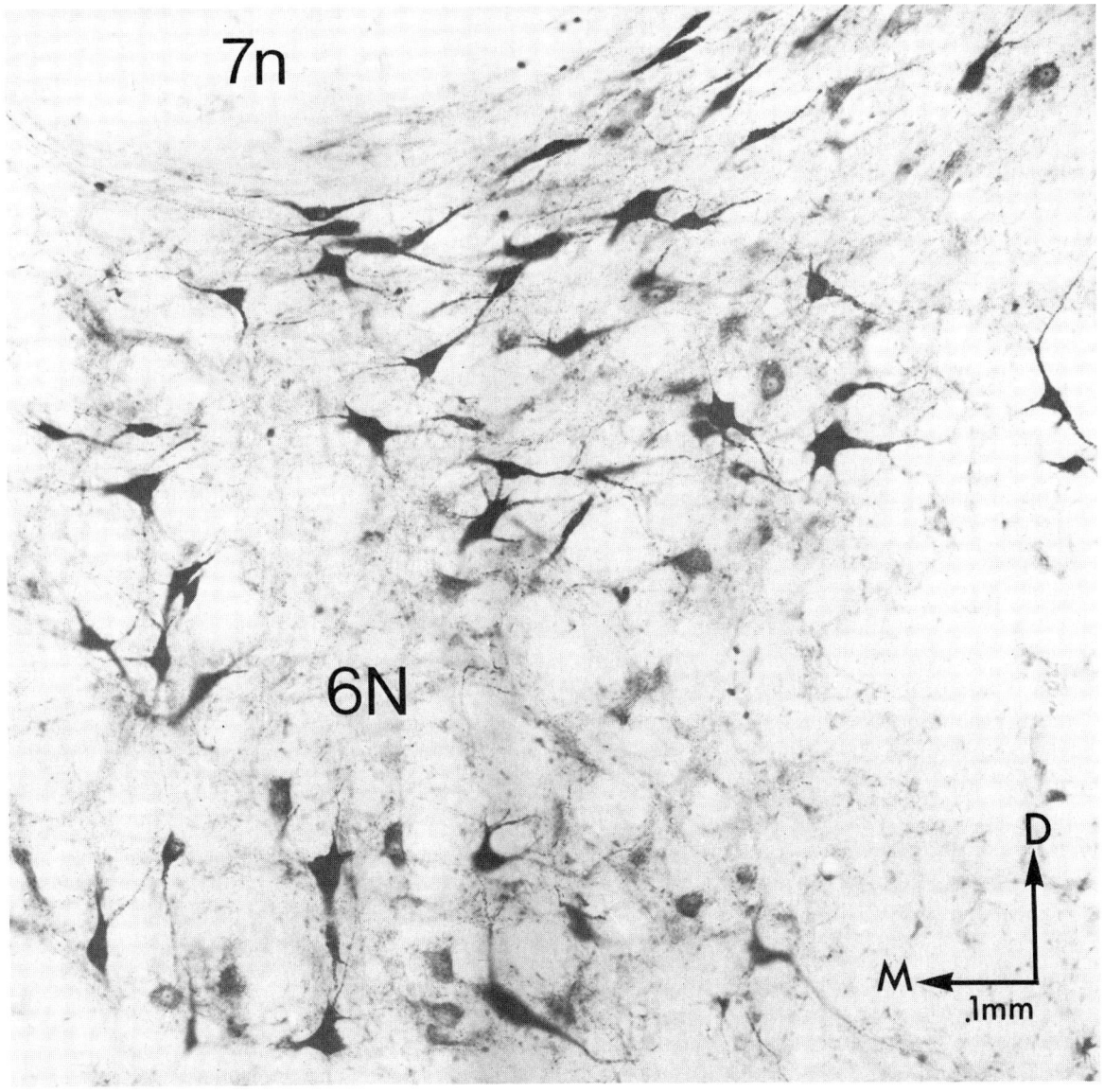

Fig. 2. Distribution of internuclear neurons in the cat abducens nucleus illustrated by retrograde labelling following HRP injection in the medial rectus subdivision of the oculomotor complex. Note the variation in cell size and intermingling dendritic trees of the abducens motoneurons and internuclear neurons. Abbreviations as in Fig. 1 legend. (cf. Spencer and Sterling, 1977).

Fig. 1. Microphotograph and schematic illustration of the abducens and accessory abducens nucleus in the cat. The motoneurons were retrogradely labelled following injection of HRP into the lateral rectus and retractor bulbi muscle. A reconstruction of an intracellularly injected accessory abducens motoneuron (6AcN) was photographically superimposed on the microphotograph. Nomenclature and size are indicated on the inset on the lower right. Note the relationship between the two nuclei (6N and 6AcN), extension of the 6AcN dendritic tree and trajectory of the 6AcN axon. Dorsal (D) and medial (M) directions are indicated. Abbreviations are: 7n, genu; 6n, VIth nerve; 6N, abducens nucleus; 6AcN, accessory abducens nucleus; LV, lateral vestibular nucleus; RB, restiform body; SO, superior olive; CL, claustrum; TB, trapezoid body; 5SM and 5ST, trigeminal spinal nucleus and tract. (see also Spencer et al., 1981).

of "peculiarity", in the sense of morphological uniqueness, at the single cell and circuit level in mammalian extraocular organization. Realizing at the outset that a little phylogenetic history would be helpful, if not essential, for understanding my conclusions, it is presented, but with apology for its brevity. An appropriately scaled account will be undertaken.

Phylogeny of the extraocular motor system

Eye muscles appear in the most antecedent vertebrates, save the pre-chordate Amphioxus, which lacks eye balls. Surprisingly, they appear in essentially the same form as in man. It can be argued that for all practical purposes the number of muscles and their motor nerve innervation (notably not the pattern) exhibit the same relationships in mammals as they do in the very earliest fish (Neal, 1918). Except for the appearance in amphibians of a retractor bulbi muscle that persists up through mammals, comparative embryology seems to justify the assertion that eye muscles are remnants of the lateral trunk muscles which in the ancestors of vertebrates extended in an unbroken series throughout the entire length of the body (Gilbert, 1947). By contrast, a remarkable scenario of cell migration(s) has been observed in the movement of central oculomotor-related nuclei throughout phylogeny that in fact has been paralleled, if not prompted by, extensive elaboration of the vestibular and visual sensory systems. These events appear to have exerted strong neurobiotaxic pressures, as first envisioned by Ariens-Kappers (1910) (see also Addens, 1933), upon the final disposition of central nuclei as well as structural characteristics of individual cells. The important question now is: To what extent can the above phylogenetic processes be visualized and interpreted in the extraocular system by use of contemporary experimental techniques?

The evolutionary sequence

Throughout phylogeny two consistent selection processes are described in the sense of producing adaptive radiation (Hodos, 1970; Northcutt, 1983). First, neurons of similar form and function have become arranged into compact aggregates termed "nuclei" and this anatomical differentiation can be viewed as a means of "specialization". Motoneurons innervating extraocular muscle illustrate, may even epitomize, this principle and the phylogenetic realization of internuclear neurons with their subsequent migration into, and distribution throughout, the mammalian abducens nucleus provides a perfect ontogenetic model to investigate such adaptive radiation. Recent study of this "newly derived" state by my colleagues is described in detail later.

By contrast, there is a simultaneous de-differentiation process, sometimes called "degeneration" or "regression", occurring in evolution. The phenomenon may be reflected at the whole brain level, as exemplified best by amphibians, or restricted to individual structures that become less important for successful radiations of the species (Ebbesson, 1980; Bullock, 1984). Particular neural systems are then lost. In principle, the accessory abducens nucleus is a particularly good example of degeneration. Its phylogenetic timetable is particularly relevant because the disappearance of this nucleus is most evident in a single order of mammals, namely primates. Paradoxically, and of course for the wrong reason, the accessory abducens nucleus has been of little fascination for oculomotor research; however, it has provided a major substrate for the study of mammalian CNS plasticity (McCormick and Thompson, 1984).

Adaptive radiation and contemporary research

Not so strangely, most work in the oculomotor system has focussed on studying adaptive specializations in neurons and neural circuitry that underlie acquisition of sophisticated mammalian motor behaviors such as smooth pursuit and saccades up to, and including, whole new motor systems that move the eyelid and external ear. Indeed, all may be equally fascinating, but I would point out that their neural substrates are not equivalent in respect to "amenity of" experimental attack. For example, it might be more rewarding to explore the superior colliculus in respect to ear rather than eye orientation. Earlier, that structure had already solved the sensorimotor transformation for eye movement (clearly we have not). After considering the discussion by Northcutt (1983) and Vanegas (1983) on the evolution of cell populations and lamination in the optic tectum only of typical fish, it is difficult to believe that any phylogenetic solution for a new behavior could be simpler. It probably won't. Yet there is reason to believe that synaptic organization related to "new" neural circuitry is likely to be more direct. And that means accessible.

One tenent to which neurobiology now seems largely to subscribe is that augmentation (in the sense of acquisition) of new pathways is not achieved by inserting new neurons in sequence between existing neuronal populations. Functionally, this means that nuclei or their neuronal operations may not be viewed "simplistically" as relays without addition of new information. The increasing diversity of signal observed in vertebrate (largely mammalian) vestibular neurons and the structural specialization(s) accompanying their new behavioral roles substantiate the above viewpoint, but evolution of these neurons needs further elaboration from the angle of their presumed common ancestry. The issue is to recognize homologous cell populations among different vertebrates.

In the skeletal system development of limbs in terrestrial vertebrates is one of the most important factors in evolution of "new centers" for motor control and coordination in the telencephalon and cerebellum (Petras, 1969; Bullock, 1984). Herein lies an important contrast between the extraocular and skeletal systems. Phylogenetically older motor centers were sufficient for mass movements of axial muscles, but they did not provide for the precision required by terrestrial animals with extremities. In fish, fins were largely used as directional rudders, with propulsion through the water produced by rhythmical movement of the trunk and tail. By contrast, the extraocular system present in fish was already well designed for both rotation and translation of the globe (Easter, 1971). It can be argued that the oculomotor system reached a higher level of specialized adaptation earlier than the skeletal motor. Yet, to what extent can one accept such sketchy phylogenetic arguments in that direction? They remain unconvincing, given that it is virtually impossible to decide whether any adaptive radiation at the level of extant neuronal circuitry is really a successful — or unsuccessful — experiment of nature because of the existing diversity in species (Northcutt, 1983; Bullock, 1984).

Another, even larger, consideration looming on the horizon has been pointed out by Pellionisz and Llinas (1981). It is the concept of "overcompleteness" (in the sense of overdetermined) that likely is extensively developed in mammalian sensory-motor systems. At its simplest level, this may be envisioned as a signal distributed so subtly that its causality cannot be assessed. That feature alone (i.e., without its sequelae) argues against the success of any contemporary approach based on usual experimental techniques even to broach acceptable (i.e., convincing) teleological solutions. This author finds it alarming, if not amusing, that the majority of work, especially that in the area of sensory-motor control, seems to focus on mammals — notably, the newly evolved primate variety. Generally, it is argued that we can understand the mammalian brain through interpretation of its neurobiology manifested as a singular endpoint onto itself. I believe that assumption to be seriously flawed, given my estimation of so-called progress over the last cycle.

The thesis of my above stated philosophical position would argue that it is not possible really to comprehend how a motor system, such as the oculomotor, works until insight is gained into the range of its operation in representative classes of vertebrates. General cellular mechanisms and fundamental principles may not be found more quickly in any other fashion (see Bullock, 1984). Essential for establishing structure-function relationships in either the oculomotor or the skeletal motor system is a thoughtful careful comparison of diverse animal species and stages of their development. For example, could one argue the relative advantages of visual or locomotor systems in a particular species or class? Both systems de-differentiate, that is, become degenerate, under a variety of environmental influences — and they do so with some long-term success, as aquatic forms, especially mammals, exemplify (Ebbesson, 1980). Without elaborating on this general point, evidence is already available that some motor systems widely differ in circuit organization in various classes, orders and even families. As described later, this is also true for oculomotor organization with regard to eye movement.

Homology, homoplasy and convergence

Given the fundamental debates over the different evolutionary scenarios that have been plausibly proposed for the oculomotor system alone, it is difficult to envision how information from this system could be re-directed to an understanding of the skeletal motor system. This point is particularly relevant in light of the difficulty in distinguishing between homoplasy (resemblances not due to inheritances from common ancestry) and homology (those from common ancestry with or without resemblance in form or function) (Smith, 1967; Cambell and Hodos, 1970). This task is especially problematic since homology has been used with both phylogenetic and structural definitions. If embryonic origin cannot be easily established in a well characterized system, then distinguishing homoplasy from homology is a useless, if not impossible, task in the brain (Northcutt, 1983). Excluding motoneurons, the status for most circuitry in the oculomotor system is indeterminate, solely because of inadequate knowledge concerning phenotypic expression of genetically similar, or independent, ancestry.

The skeletal motor system presents a good example in this regard. It has been argued that the "so-called" convergent development of the cortico-spinal motoneuronal system shows evolution of major groups to have proceeded by radiation and not in a so-called ladder-like sequential sequence (Petras, 1969). Is organization of the cortico-ocular motoneuronal system the same? This issue hasn't been addressed at all, let alone from the above vantage point of species comparison. By contrast, based on the straightforward gross dissection of muscle origin and insertion in the orbit of numerous vertebrate species, Isomura (1981) has concluded that evidence points to the evolutionary process proceeding by radiation rather than a so-called ladder-like sequence. If this observation holds for the very periphery of the motor plant itself, then what can one conclude about organization of the CNS? Without reviewing any evidence here, more support can be found for radiation in the oculomotor system, but with convergent evolutionary development in function. The remaining part of the chapter presents examples to support this conclusion.

Oculomotor motoneurons and nuclei

A particularly interesting phylogenetically homologous neuron found in all vertebrates is the oculomotoneuron itself. There are many dissimilarities between these neurons and skeletal motoneurons innervating the appendages. For example, one large difference is in absolute soma-dendritic size, but not in the absence of axon collaterals, as has been classically held. Recently, axon collaterals were found on particular types of mammalian extraocular motoneurons but not in all species of mammals, and not at all in non-mammals (Evinger et al., 1982). All cat, but no rabbit, medial rectus motoneurons have axon collaterals. Neither species have collaterals on abducens motoneurons, but both do on some superior rectus motoneurons. This particular illustration points to a specific adaptive radiation for axon collaterals. Isn't it likely dependent upon acquisition of a new behavior (presently unknown)? Indeed, if so, it might well be an example of convergent radiation not proceeding in ladder-like sequence, as believed for the cortico-motoneuronal projection.

Distribution of the oculomotoneuronal collateralization may be used to illustrate that the functional nature of the modification, even though presently not specified, is not at all the same as in the skeletal motor system. Since the local axon collaterals terminate on neurons whose axons leave the oculomotor nucleus, they cannot provide recurrent motoneuronal inhibition. This difference, therefore, may be a demonstration of a non-convergent evolutionary development. Finally, it is worth noting that the very presence of selective collateralization in diverse mammalian classes, particularly in motoneurons that arise from the same analage within one species (Gilbert, 1947; and unpublished results), emphasizes the extent of genomic specificity available for expression of a particular neuronal property.

Internuclear neurons of the abducens nucleus

This second example illustrates both positive and negative attributes of convergent evolution. The population of non-motoneurons associated with the abducens nucleus are specifically adapted for relaying conjugate gaze signals to medial rectus motoneurons (Baker and Highstein, 1975; Delgado-Garcia et al., 1977). They are argued to be essential for conjugate horizontal movement of both eyes in lateral- and frontal-eyed mammals (Baker and McCrea, 1979). This particular system seems to be a specialization that might be relatively, if not entirely, new to the mammal. The extent of its functional variation, in terms of information or morphological variation, remains to be rigorously assessed across species by my colleagues. For instance, it is not known whether precursor (recognizable antecedent) neurons exist in any fish, amphibian or reptile. For certain, there are putative candidates that lie in the vicinity of, but not in, the abducens nucleus of some species. Existing evidence suggests that, before frontalization and fovealization with the intent of true stereopsis, horizontal movement of the eyes did not develop with close adherence to the principle of "shared conjoint circuitry" purely for purposes of conjugate movements. This viewpoint would argue that there was little adaptive pressure (advantage) to move both eyes in a parallel, symmetric, simultaneous fashion. This author believes that neuronal circuits have evolved separately with the expressed intent of moving each eye independently, and then, secondarily, maybe together. Nevertheless, independent of eye position in the head, phylogenetic pressures placed more emphasis (in the sense of survival) upon conjugate movement of the eyes in order fully to utilize binocular overlap in respect to object position and movement in the visual surround. Yet it does not imply that members of two classes quite disparate upon the evolutionary scale, such as the lateral-eyed fish and rabbit, are at all comparable vis-a-vis individual neurons or eye movement circuitry. I believe that the above conclusion is almost certain, given what is already known about their respective CNS organization, but it is still largely ignored due to the outward similarity in the behavioral descriptions of how the eyes move in response to visual ("world") or vestibular ("self movement") stimuli.

Nonetheless, it is clear that all mammals examined have definable populations of internuclear neurons but their disposition is quite disparate according to species. In some lateral-eyed animals, such as the rat, guinea pig and mouse, putative internuclear neurons lie rostral to the abducens nucleus. They are not interdigitated or, if you like, they have not migrated to "interdigitate with" the abducens motoneurons to the extent described in the frontal-eyed cat and monkey. What is the most successful specialization? Wouldn't a distribution of internuclear neurons overlapping the population of motoneurons facilitate a more economic, and equal, distribution of any afferent oculomotor signals to the abducens nucleus? The answer is probably yes. But the abducens nucleus certainly didn't start out with that principle in mind. In fact, the teleost abducens nucleus itself appeared in two separate structural parts (Fig. 3), each with a different functional role (Gestrin and Sterling, 1977). Motoneurons in the rostral part were largely related to maintaining eye position and those in the caudal part to actual movement of the eye. In the amphibian, Dieringer and Precht (1983) found evidence for a separation of function along the above lines in identified motoneurons, but in a species where the abducens nucleus has become a contiguous popu-

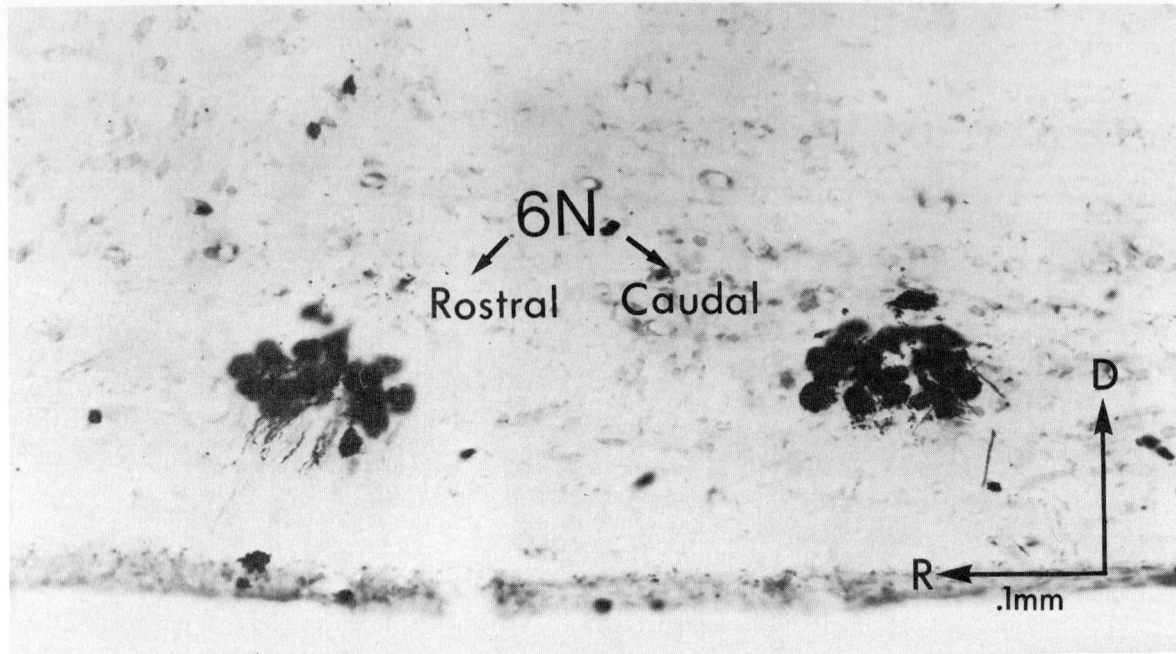

Fig. 3. The abducens nucleus in saggital section through the ventral part of the medulla in the catfish, *Icatalurus punctatus*. The rostral and caudal subdivisions are indicated. Motoneurons were retrogradely labelled with injection of HRP into the lateral rectus muscle.

lation of cells. These findings show that a specific oculomotor afferent system can distribute its "characteristic" signal to a "particular" target. In addition, some motoneurons in both the above species exhibited both signals. This observation showed that very early in phylogeny motoneurons had already begun to combine the static (tonic) and dynamic (phasic) signals. As shown for the three cell types in Fig. 4, neuronal size, and even shape, is not a given structural feature that determines (i.e., is dependent on) eventual function. Thus, the oculomotor system of antecedent species originally evolved with quite different operating principles than that found in the mammal. The overwhelming majority, if not all, mammalian oculomotoneurons exhibit all aspects of any signal (i.e., static and dynamic) that have been envisioned as synaptic input to the motor nuclei. In another dimension, I would argue that this adaptive specialization is a natural sequelae of what might be anticipated in a motor system that operates over a wide dynamic frequency range, and generally amplitude, with spatial accuracy and precision. More importantly, the above motoneurons manifest the requisite measure of "overcompleteness" that should be represented in the mammalian brain. This rationalization is of consequence when expanded to consider questions of adaptation and plasticity.

Adequacy of the above proposition has been critically assessed at a structural and functional level for internuclear neurons in the cat abducens nucleus by my colleagues during the past decade. These still largely unpublished data substantiate a view that the internuclear neuron population can be considered what I would call a "highly specialized nuclei" that has nearly reached optimum differentiation. Fundamental in this regard is its association with the known behavior of ensuring conjugate gaze. But at the same time, I would like to express with equal weight the opinion that the internuclear neuron adaptation is still largely incomplete in the sense of adequacy. Roughly speaking,

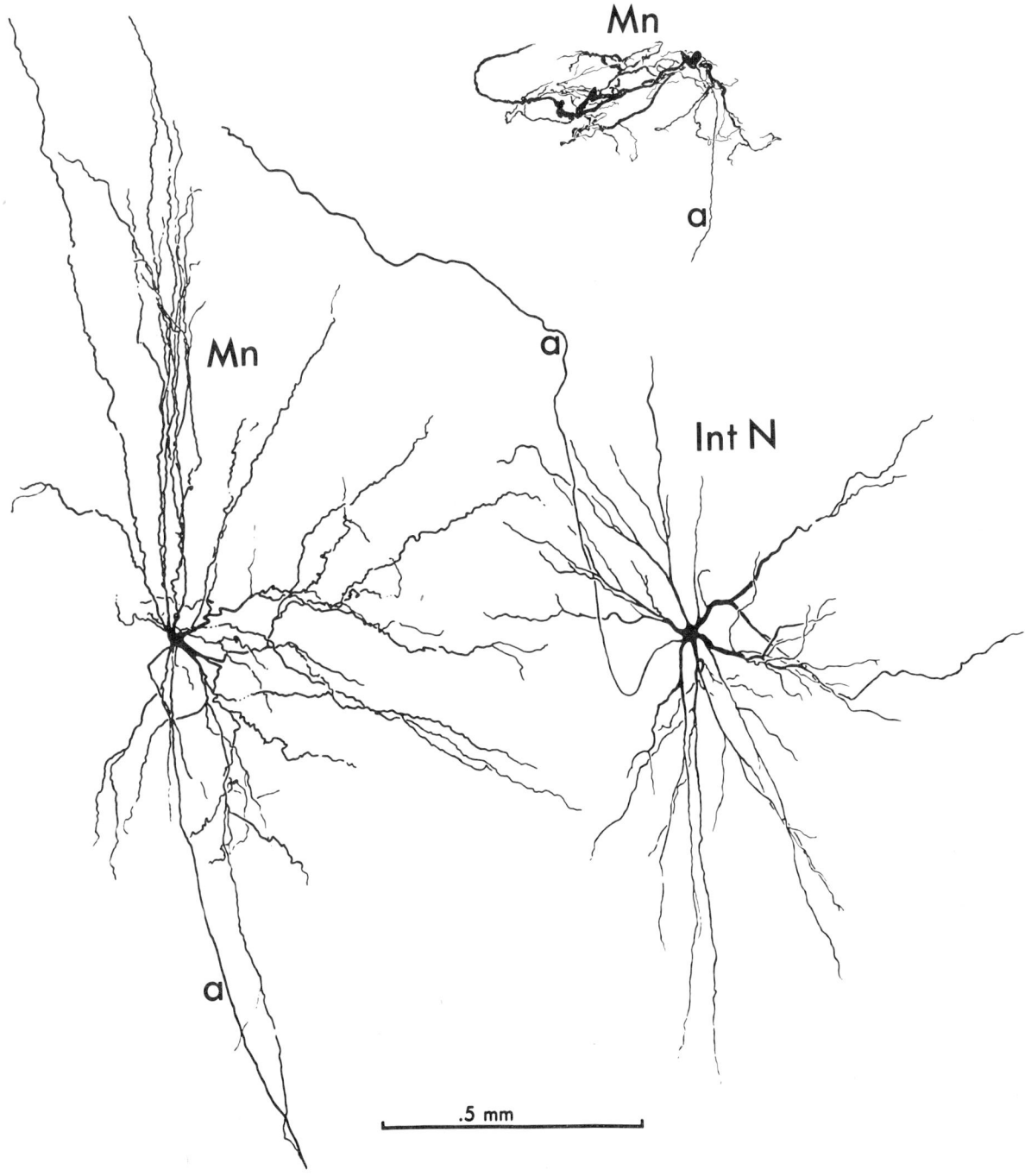

Fig. 4. Graphic reconstruction of oculomotor neurons following intracellular injection of HRP. The lower two neurons represent a typical cat abducens motoneuron (Mn) (on left) and internuclear neuron (Int N) (on right). The motoneuron on the upper right is from the flounder, *Pseudopleuronectes americanus*. Axons (a) are indicated. (cf. Highstein et al., 1982).

about 10% of the tested human population does not deploy this machinery in a fashion well enough to maintain binocular vision. Without delving into details regarding interocular alignment, critical periods, etc., and the role these neurons might play in those phenomena, I would maintain that the adaptive specialization is still an on-going phylogenetic experiment. The perfect "neuronal solution" to conjugate gaze is yet to be achieved. This hypothesis can continue to be examined, even though the most desirable experimental species for its test is not within the foreseeable future. The point is that I believe a thorough approach to the phylogenetic development of internuclear neurons offers high probability for a contemporary answer. The bottom line again is the reminder that the best study in the primate will only be as good as comparable work in other species permits.

The accessory abducens nucleus

In the oculomotor system, the phylogenetic story surrounding specialization of the accessory abducens nucleus and its subsequent de-differentiation serves perfectly to illustrate both structural and functional principles during evolution. The accessory abducens nucleus was best described in birds, where we (Spencer et al., 1981), as did Terni (1922a), concluded that it reached nearly the pinnacle of evolutionary development (Terni, 1922b). This highly specialized group of cells first seems to have appeared in the transition of aquatic to terrestrial environment by the amphibians (Fig. 5 legend; Addens, 1933). Structurally, the accessory abducens motoneurons (like internuclear neurons) probably derive their cellular origin from anlage of the abducens nucleus (Gilbert 1947; Isomura 1981). These motoneurons successfully migrated

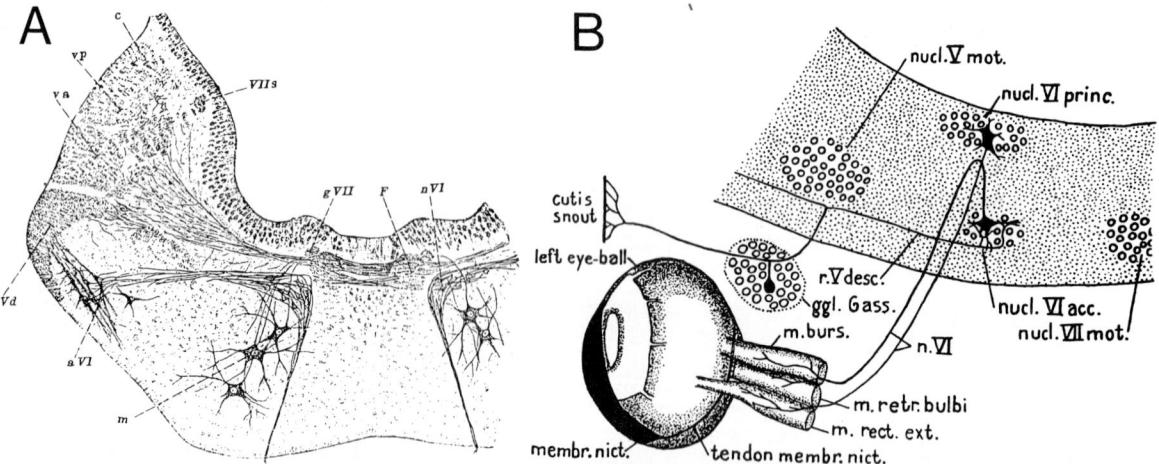

Fig. 5. A diagram showing the anatomical substrate and functional role of the accessory abducens nucleus as first described by Terni (1922a, b) in the reptile, *Gongylus ocellatus*. The coronal section in A is a direct reproduction of Fig. 5 from Terni (1922a). The original Italian legend is below. The diagram in B is my reproduction of Addens' Fig. 4 (1933) which he had modified from a figure on p. 308 of Terni (1922b) entitled "Schema che illustra la base anatomica del reflesso trigemino-abducente in *Gongylus ocellatus* Wagl.". My modified figure legend follows in B. (A. Sezione trasversa dell'oblongata di un embrione di *Gongylus o*. allo stadio 4. Coloraz. met. Cajal, Ingr. 240 × circa. c, radice cocleare; va, vp, radice vestibolare anteriore e posteriore; VII s, radice sensitiva del faciale; Vs, radice discendente del trigemino; aVI, nucleo accessorio dell'abducente; m, nucleo magnicellulare disseminato; gVII, porzione ascendente della radice del faciale; F, fascicolo longit. mediale; nVI, nucleo principale dell'abducente.) (From Terni, 1922a.) B. This diagram illustrates the anatomical basis and presumed functional operation of the trigemino-accessory abducens reflex according to Terni (1922b). The nictitating membrane covers about half the cornea in this species. The tendon is shown to pass medial to the lateral rectus (m. rect. ext.) and extend through the bursalis muscle (m. burs.) near its insertion on the sclera. Note that the accessory abducens nucleus (nucl. VI acc.) is shown to innervate both the retractor bulbi (m. retr. bulbi.) and the bursalis muscle. The remarkable coronal section in A provides an accurate topographical relationship of other central nuclei to the acessory abducens. The scheme in B is equally well conceived except for the direct synaptic relationship between trigeminal afferents (ggl. Gass.) and acessory abducens.

laterally toward the sensory trigeminal nucleus, from which they receive their major source of afferent input. As expected, the accessory abducens nucleus performs the specific reflex function of eye retraction subsequent to stimulation of cornea and permits reflex elevation of the nictitating membrane in most species. As a protective mechanism, evolution of the accessory abducens nucleus, in many ways, parallels that of the levator palpebrae and orbicularis motoneurons that innervate musculature associated with development of a true eyelid (Evinger et al., 1984). The latter mechanical innovation provided an adequate form of protection without a nictitating membrane. One could surmise that the success of the eyelid, and its peculiar CNS neuronal circuitry, as a specific adaptation closely "mimicking" eye retraction with elevation of the nictitating membrane became a large, but not exclusive, reason why the accessory abducens nucleus is no longer with us today.

Although not yet thoroughly tested, it will likely be found that the accessory abducens nucleus and its innervation of the retractor bulbi muscle is not the only means of producing eye retraction. Clearly, it was never part of the antecedent neuronal solution to translational eye movement because the accessory abducens does not appear in any of the diverse species of fish where eye retraction, including the so-called "stretching" response (as named by Easter, 1971), is indeed a significant aspect of the oculomotor repertoire. This situation is also true for elasmobranchs, who have a kind of nictitating membrane and "retraction-like" response (Bell and Satchell, 1963). In all vertebrate species so far tested, co-contraction of extraocular muscles, largely the recti, produce transient as well as maintained translational movement of the eye. Nonetheless, the argument appears valid that the accessory abducens nucleus specifically evolved for the behavior of reflex translational movement of the eye. Delgado-Garcia, Evinger and I (unpublished results) have tested this hypothesis in the alert cat, and unequivocally conclude that accessory abducens motoneuronal activity is related to both reflex and volitional retraction, but never to rotational eye movement.

In one sense, that role appears logical. It removes a time-sharing component of translation from the presumed main role of rotation for the extraocular muscles. In this regard, recent studies by Evinger et al. (1984) of cat brainstem neurons suggest there may be separate reflex circuitry associated with translational, as distinguished from rotational, eye movement. An intriguing species-related question is what this disassociation implies for trigeminal (and other) brainstem reflex pathways establishing synaptic connections with motoneurons that now move the eye in all directions. This could be the reason why evidence indicates that neuronal circuitry producing lid movement may also be distinct from oculomotor circuitry (Evinger, unpublished results). In summary, these points all illustrate that parallel evolutionary processes can produce highly specialized brainstem circuitry independently (i.e., non-convergent).

Finally, in spite of the well-developed accessory abducens nucleus within the class of mammalia as typified in the lateral-eyed rabbit and frontal-eyed cat, it apparently has de-differentiated in primates (Spencer et al., 1981). There are a few ventrally located motoneurons below the main accessory abducens nucleus, and only a vestige of the retractor bulbi muscle in the presumed homologous accessory lateral rectus muscle. Yet, the latter muscle, itself, has now largely become a horizontal eye mover for rotation, rather than one purely deployed for translational movement of the eyeball. However, the eye in the primate retracts significantly during lid movement associated with blinking. And in this particular species, as in fish, retraction is accomplished through activity of the original set of extraocular muscles (Evinger et al., 1984). Would it not be of relevance to understand what successful adaptive pressures were exerted on a presumably adequate reflex mechanism, such as the accessory abducens, to result in its degeneration? Was it the successful frontalization of the eyes with an extensive protective bony encapsulation? Or was it the need for the precision and speed of a lid system with separate CNS circuitry? Possibly, it was something as simple as the ability to place a finger in, or a hand in front of, the eye. Without excluding any form of phenomenological causality, all existing features in the primate oculomotor system attest to the tremendous importance of the visual system, but one, or more, led to the demise of the accessory abducens. There should be little concern as it survived more than 300 million years. Moreover, it could re-emerge at any time.

Uniqueness of brainstem neurons in oculomotor function

There is little doubt that the composition of central brainstem circuitry related to generating any particular oculomotor function must be very specific for that behavior. From the viewpoint of translational eye movement, the abducens nucleus, the accessory abducens nucleus, levator palpebrae and orbicularis motoneurons illustrate final common motor pathways extending from "older" to "newer" neurons. Each must have acquired appropriate, but quite unique, sets of "newer" and "older" neuronal patterns underlying eye retraction and movement. Take, for instance, the abducens nucleus of a particular species. Can a particular structural or functional emphasis be placed upon one vestibular, reticular or prepositus neuron, all of which terminate in common in the nucleus, but also individually select many other brainstem areas for extensive collateral distribution (Baker et al., 1981; Baker and Spencer, 1981)? For instance, in a particular species the vestibular — prepositus — cerebellar circuitry producing horizontal eye movement represents an intertwined sequential and parallel pathway specifically adapted to implement only that particular behavior. In a general sense it is quite certain that the neuronal ensemble consisting of all those basic properties related to that one solution will be quite peculiar to each species. Yet current study of the normal physiology, and especially adaptive behavior, of oculomotor function largely ignores this basic structure caveat. Fortunately, and on the positive side, the vestibular system turns out to be a particularly fruitful place to engage the above hypothesis. On the other hand, and unfortunately, most mammalian neurons and their pathways are simply too formidable to consider at the present moment.

Why vestibular neurons?

Signal diversity on vestibular neurons, in the context of information, has been evident from the first single cell study. Table 2 of Lisberger and Miles (1978), showing 22 functionally defined types in one part of the vestibular nucleus, can best be used to indicate that all combinations of activity are possible. Coupled with a large amount of recent work in the vestibulo-oculomotor field, these findings illustrate that nearly all the usual position and velocity signals that can be correlated with eye movement are present to varying degrees (cf. Chubb et al., 1984). One can envision a scenario that argues for successive adaptive convergences of "newer" signals at the level of individual vestibular neurons so that advantage may be taken of a particular vestibular neuron's "given" (in the sense of "endowed") synaptic space on oculomotoneurons. This proposition is in no way a simple alternative to the "competition hypotheses" as advanced in the visual system. The extraocular motor system needed to adapt specifically in response to a quite different set of physiological and structural requirements in order to retain and successfully deploy newer eye movements. Apparently, in so doing it capitalized on adaptive specialization at the level of the vestibular nucleus. The experimental focus of these arguments is very much in the process of development and needs further elaboration before fuller presentation (cf. Graf and Baker, 1983; Simpson et al., 1981). However, in common, the studies are evaluating the concept that even for homologous neurons (either phylogenetic or structural), signal information is specific for a particular vestibular neuron in a particular species. And then, when necessary, new (not in the sense of phylogenetic origin) neurons appear to assume other functional roles. As such, the primate vestibular nucleus is tantamount to Pandora's box for an experimentalist with imagination.

On the structural side it is clear that from the outset in the most antecedent vertebrates that vestibular neurons arborized widely to other targets related to the larger purpose of gaze. Given the specialization of the visual system and the presumably newly developed phylogenetic capacity for eye movements such as pursuit and saccades, together with head and body movements, then how are homologous vestibular neurons different? Assuredly, they will be both functionally and morphologically unique as adaptive specializations in a particular species! They could not be "replacement parts" for other vestibular neurons in any other "closely related" animal. I conclude that a given vestibular (or for that matter prepositus) neuron, and associated circuitry, appears necessary, sufficient and appropriate for the oculomotor system of a particular species but no other. It certainly goes without elaboration that the skeletal motor system is excluded. I would equally stress my earlier conclusion that there will be general principles in each of the motor systems, but they indeed will probably follow understanding of the details, not precede.

Applicability of the size principle

The one particular neuronal feature between oculomotor and skeletal motor systems exhibiting convergent homoplasy is what I referred to earlier as applicability of the size principle. The following observations are based on both structural and functional arguments that necessitate an appreciation of a large background of work that cannot be provided here. In short, the activity of antidromically identified abducens motoneurons and internuclear neurons have been analyzed in alert cats during spontaneous, visual and vestibular induced eye movement (Delgado-Garcia et al., 1977). Numerical proportionality constants were obtained that could be correlated with both the position and velocity profiles of eye movement. Such measurements permitted an indirect assessment of a size principle rule contending that hierarchical organization of neurons within a pool is based on size alone, with rank order functionally defined in terms of excitability (Henneman et al., 1965a, b). When the quantitative data were reduced to a single line for comparison, it illustrated a significant relationship between eye position threshold for which a motoneuron and an internuclear neuron began to fire and the slope of their rate position regression lines. It also indicated a consistent relationship between position sensitivity and conduction velocity. Since threshold and conduction velocity were also co-correlated, it permitted the conclusion that both recruitment and frequency potentiation in the cat abducens nucleus are largely dependent on morphological uniqueness intrinsic to cell size (Cullheim, 1978). The size principle was shown not to be a rigid absolute criterion because the values of velocity sensitivity varied significantly for individual neurons, depending on whether they were computed during fast (including saccades) or slow phases of vestibular nystagmus. This was expected because separate sources of presynaptic afferents are known to be involved and, therefore, the differences reflect unique arborization patterns onto target motoneurons (Baker and Spencer, 1981). Nonetheless, these velocity values were correlated, but less well, with conduction velocity and position sensitivity. This led to the conclusion that both motoneurons and internuclear neuron properties during recruitment and frequency potentiation are dependent upon the distribution of neuronal properties throughout the pool as well as the pattern of synaptic effects from separate afferent systems. In addition, the interdigitated population of motoneurons and internuclear neurons in the abducens nucleus co-varied in other ways, such as their extent of static hysteresis, the influence of alertness and position-dependent non-linearities. The conclusion followed that independent of whether the latter features were innate to cellular architecture they were not a function of target, i.e., muscle fibers or neurons. Given the phylogenetic uniqueness of the internuclear neuron population for the mammal, it is a rather convincing demonstration of a general cellular principle that seems to develop independent of a phylogenetic timetable. Can it not be interpreted as a strong evolutionarily convergent adaptive pressure in CNS organization?

As far as general principles and fundamental information are concerned, the above conclusion is in good agreement with findings of motoneuronal organization in the spinal cord (not excluding the vestibular system), and thus it can be considered as a "principle in common" for oculomotor and skeletal motor systems. The particular caveats of any such arguments are related to the specific behaviors each of the circuits are involved with in real life. Nonetheless, my final conclusion is unaltered. General principles will only arise in retrospect to the understanding of particular neurons and their role in circuits underlying identified behavior. As such, they cannot be used as the pretext for understanding the neuronal composition of newly acquired behaviors. Moreover, the evolutionary history of particular mammalian nuclei have been shaped by such diverse selective pressures that it is unlikely we will discern the phylogenetic path easily and without error, but the endeavor is essential.

References

Addens, J. L. (1933) The motor nuclei and roots of the cranial and first spinal nerves of vertebrates. Part I. Introduction. Cyclostomes. Z. Anat. Entwicklungsgesch., 101: 307–410.

Ariens Kappers, C. V. (1910) The migration of the motor cells of the bulbar trigeminus, abducens and facialis in the series of vertebrates, and the differences in the course of their root fibres. Verh. Akad. Amsterdam, 16: 1–195.

Baker, R. and Highstein, S. M. (1975) Physiological identification of interneurons and motoneurons in the abducens nucleus. Brain Res., 91: 292–298.

Baker, R. and McCrea, R. A. (1979) The para-abducens nucleus. In H. Asanuma and V. Wilson (Eds.), Integration of the Nervous System, Igakaku Shoin Ltd., New York, pp. 97–122.

Baker, R. and Spencer, R. (1981) Synthesis of horizontal conjugate eye movement signals in the abducens nucleus. Jpn. J. EEG EMG Suppl., 31: 49–59.

Baker, R., Evinger, C. and McCrea, R. A. (1981) Some thoughts about the three neurons in the vestibulo-ocular reflex. Ann. NY Acad. Sci., 374: 171–181.

Bell, J. P. and Satchell, G. H. (1963) An undescribed unilateral ocular reflex in the dogfish *Squalus acanthias* L. Austr. J. Exp. Biol., 41: 221–234.

Bullock, T. H. (1983) Why study fish brains? Some aims of comparative neurology today. In R. E. Davis and R. G. Northcutt (Eds.), Fish Neurobiology and Behavior, Vol. 2, University of Michigan Press, Ann Arbor, pp. 361–368.

Bullock, T. H. (1984) Comparative neuroscience holds promise for quiet revolutions. Science, 225: 473–478.

Burke, R. E., Dum, R. P., Fleshman, J. W., Glenn, L. L., Lev-Tov, A., O'Donovan, M. J. and Pinter, M. J. (1982) An HRP study of the relation between cell size and motor unit type in cat ankle extensor motoneurons. J. Comp. Neurol., 209: 17–28.

Cambell, C. B. G. and Hodos, W. (1970) The concept of homology and the evolution of the nervous system. Brain, Behav. Evol., 3: 353–367.

Chubb, M. C., Fuchs, A. F. and Scudder, C. A. (1984) Neuron activity in monkey vestibular nuclei during vertical vestibular stimulation and eye movement. J. Neurophysiol., 52: 724–742.

Cullheim, S. (1978) Relations between cell body size, axon diameter and axon conduction velocity in the cat sciatica α-motoneurons stained with HRP. Neurosci. Lett., 8: 17–20.

Delgado-Garcia, J., Baker, R. and Highstein, S. M. (1977) The activity of internuclear neurons identified in the abducens nucleus of the alert cat. In R. Baker and A. Berthoz (Eds.), Control of Gaze by Brainstem Neurons: Developments in Neuroscience, Vol. I, Elsevier/North Holland, New York, pp. 291–301.

Dieringer, N. and Precht, W. (1983) Fibre types in the extraocular muscles of the frog. Neurosci. Lett. Suppl., 14: S92.

Easter, S. S. (1971) Spontaneous eye movements in restrained goldfish. Vision Res., 11: 333–342.

Ebbesson, S. O. E. (1980) The parcellation theory and its relation to interspecific variability in brain organization, evolutionary and ontogenetic development and neuronal plasticity. Cell Tissue Res., 213: 179–212.

Enoka, R. M. and Stuart, D. G. (1984) Henneman's size principle: current issues. Trends Neurosci., 7: 226–228.

Evinger, C., Spencer, R. and Baker, R. (1982) Comparison of oculomotor motoneuron axon collaterals in mammals. In G. Lennerstrand, D. Zee and E. Keller (Eds.), Functional Basis of Ocular Motility Disorders, Pergamon Press, New York, pp. 531–534.

Evinger, C., Shaw, M. D., Peck, C. K., Manning, K. A. and Baker, R. (1984) Blinking and associated eye movements in humans, guinea-pigs and rabbits. J. Neurophysiol., 52: 323–339.

Gestrin, P. and Sterling, P. (1977) Anatomy and physiology of goldfish oculomotor system. II. Firing patterns of neurons in abducens nucleus and surrounding medulla and their relationship to eye movements. J. Neurophysiol., 40: 573–588.

Gilbert, P. W. (1947) The origin and development of the extrinsic ocular muscles in the domestic cat. J. Morphol., 81: 151–193.

Graf, W. and Baker, R. (1983) Adaptive changes of the vestibulo-ocular reflex in flatfish are achieved by reorganization of central nervous pathways. Science, 221: 777–779.

Henneman, E., Somjen, G. and Carpenter, D. O. (1965a) Functional significance of cell size in spinal motoneurons. J. Neurophysiol., 28: 789–792.

Henneman, E., Somjen, G. and Carpenter, D. O. (1965b) Excitability and inhibitability of motoneurons of different size. J. Neurophysiol., 28: 599–620.

Highstein, S. M., Karabelas, A., Baker, R. and McCrea, R. A. (1982) Comparison of the morphology of physiologically identified abducens motor and internuclear neurons in the cat: A light microscopic study employing the intracellular injection of horseradish peroxidase. J. Comp. Neurol., 208: 369–387.

Hodos, W. (1970) Evolutionary interpretation of neural and behavioral studies of living vertebrates. In F. O. Schmitt (Ed.), The Neurosciences Second Study Program, Rockefeller University Press., New York, pp. 26–39.

Isomura, G. (1981) Comparative anatomy of the extrinsic ocular muscles in vertebrates. Anat. Anz. Jena., 150: 498–515.

Kernell, D. and Zwaagstra, B. (1981) Input conductance, axonal conduction velocity and cell size among hindlimb motoneurons of the cat. Brain Res., 206: 311–326.

Lisberger, S. G. and Miles, F. A. (1978) Role of primate medial vestibular nucleus in long-term adaptive plasticity of vestibuloocular reflex. J. Neurophysiol., 41: 733–763.

McCormick, D. A. and Thompson, R. F. (1984) Cerebellum: Essential involvement in the classically conditioned eyelid response. Science, 223: 296–299.

Neal, H. V. (1918) The history of the eye muscles. J. Morphol., 30: 433–453.

Northcutt, R. G. (1983) Evolution of the optic tectum in ray-finned fishes. In R. E. Davis and R. G. Northcutt (Eds.), Fish Neurobiology and Behavior, Vol. 2, University of Michigan Press, Ann Arbor. pp. 1–42.

Pellionisz, A. and Llinas, R. (1980) Tensorial approach to the geometry of brain function: Cerebellar coordination via a metric tensor. Neuroscience, 5: 1125–1136.

Petras, J. M. (1969) Some efferent connections of the motor and somatosensory cortex of simian primates and felid, canid and procyonid carnivores. Ann. NY Acad. Sci., 167: 469–505.

Simpson, J. I., Graf, W. and Leonard, C. (1981) The coordinate system of visual climbing fibers to the flocculus. In A. F. Fuchs and W. Becker (Eds.), Progress in Oculomotor Reearch, Elsevier/North-Holland, Amsterdam, pp. 475–484.

Smith, H. M. (1967) Biological similarities and homologies. Syst. Zool., 16: 101–102.

Spencer, R. F. and Sterling, G. P. (1977) An electron microscope study of motoneurons and interneurons in the cat abducens nucleus identified by retrograde intra-axonal transport of HRP. J. Comp. Neurol., 176: 65–85.

Spencer, R. F., Baker, R. and McCrea, R. A. (1981) Morphological and physiological organization of the accessory abducens nucleus in the cat and primate. In A. F. Fuchs and W. Becker (Eds.), Progress in Oculomotor Research, Elsevier/North-Holland, Amsterdam, pp. 271–279.

Terni, T. (1922a) Richerche sul nervo abducente e in special modo intorno as significato del suo nucleo accessorio d'origine. Folia Neurobiol., 12: 277–327.

Terni, T. (1922b) Il sostrato anatomico del riflesso di chiusura dell membrana nittitante nei Sauropsidi. Arch. Fisiol., 20: 305–311.

Ulfhake, B. and Kellerth, J.-O. (1982) Does alpha motoneuron size correlate with motor unit type in the cat triceps. Brain Res., 251: 201–209.

Vanegas, H. (1983) Organization and physiology of the teleostean optic tectum. In R. E. Davis and R. G. Northcutt (Eds.), Fish Neurobiology and Behavior, Vol. 2, University of Michigan Press, Ann Arbor, pp. 43–90.

Spinal programs for locomotion

Gerald E. Loeb

Laboratory of Neural Control, IRP, National Institute of Neurological and Communicative Disorders and Stroke, National Institutes of Health, 9000 Rockville Pike, Bethesda, MD 20205, U.S.A.

Introduction

In comparing the current level of knowledge regarding the function and control of the oculomotor system with that for the skeletomotor system, one is immediately struck by a disparity. Oculomotor research is characterized by accurate quantitative methods, well-defined performance criteria, mathematical models of control and feedback regulation, and a highly evolved theoretical basis in engineering control systems. Skeletomotor research has been and continues to be plagued by phenomenological description, intractable, unstable and inappropriate models, and an allied field of robotic engineering whose greatest contribution continues to be proofs of the impossibility of trajectory planning in real time (Loeb, 1983).

Of course, it might be argued that the skeletomotor system is simply a more complicated embodiment of the principles underlying oculomotor control, and that the state of knowledge simply lags behind for that reason. However, I shall argue that the oculomotor system represents an almost singular exception to the more general function and control of striate muscles. Rather than offering a cleaner crucible in which to concoct and test general theories of motor control, it has provided a protected niche for the preservation of a seductive oversimplification inherited from the study of isolated muscles. Muscle physiology research continues to be artificially constrained by the undeniable observation that activated muscles contract. If the muscle is attached to an initially stationary but movable object, then the object moves when the muscle contracts, providing a class of phenomena for measurement by the muscle physiologist. However, the primary process within the muscle that is modulated by changes in the neurally controlled state of activation is not length or even tendon strain. Rather, it is a complex, statistically distributed set of forces in the cross-bridges, which are highly dependent on the direction and magnitude of cross-bridge motion.

It is only in circumstances such as the eyeball and ear pinna that muscles find themselves controlling the unopposed motion of virtually massless, inelastic objects in a frictionless, low-viscosity medium. Under such circumstances, muscles are well described and easily replaced by simple actuator mechanisms of the sort commonly employed in conventional electromechanical engineering. However, in more typical skeletomotor configurations, the addition of large inertial effects, gravity and other external loads, and elastic storage represent not mere complexities, but rather compel the motor system to adapt entirely different modes of operation. In such systems, one frequently encounters muscles with highly specialized internal architectures to improve performance under such kinematically diverse conditions as active shortening, active lengthening, and isometric force generation. The torques and length changes of a given muscle acting across one joint may depend on the position of the joint and possibly of other joints spanned by multiarticular muscles. Such actuators are a far cry from the simple torque motors of robotic systems, so it is not surprising that mechanical engineering has had little to offer in the way of biologically relevant computational models or control theories.

In studying the function of any single muscle in such a dynamic system, the muscle should not be considered directly as a cause of the observed motion; rather, it is better considered as a generator of an "impulse" added to the system. Impulse is the kinetic contribution to momentum given by the product of force and time. The impulse is the resultant of the interaction of the activated crossbridge sites (bearing calcium and ATP but not necessarily attached) with the motion that is largely imparted to the muscle by the inertia of limb segments and the action of other forces external to the muscle, including other muscles. As we shall see, there is evidence that both the anatomical architecture and the neurophysiological control circuitry for the muscles of locomotion are highly dependent on the particular kinematic conditions under which each muscle is called upon to provide this impulse. If there are any single, unifying principles of motor control, they must be expressed in terms that transcend the concerns local to any such specialized structure as the extraocular muscles, which deal with only one kinematic condition.

The locomotor program in the cat hindlimb

The phenomenology of terrestrial locomotion has been thoroughly studied in many species having two, four or six legs used in a variety of gait patterns. There has been special interest in the cat hindlimb during walking and trotting because of the ease with which these gaits are elicited in various intact and reduced preparations, and the wealth of data available on the anatomical and physiological properties of the myoskeletal and neural systems as they have been studied in this species in isolation over the past century (for reviews, see Grillner, 1975; Wetzel and Stuart, 1976). The cat hindlimb model is a fortuitous choice, because it appears to represent a highly evolved and thus presumably optimized structure for the efficient generation of sustained locomotion needed for predatory hunting. This is not to say that such locomotion is the sole activity of the hindlimb or that it has been entirely optimized with efficiency as the only goal. Rather this suggests the likelihood that the highly organized and largely invariant structures to be found in the cat hindlimb derive from real function rather than evolutionary accident and that this function is likely to be expressed during locomotion. While much of the general structure of the cat hindlimb is undoubtedly inherited from other, perhaps very different ancestors, the specifics have come to embody a great wealth of constructive and instructive improvements resulting from the interplay of random mutations with their consequences in situations with various probabilities of occurrence (for discussion, see Partridge, 1982).

A fairly complete phenomenology of cat locomotion has been available in the literature for some time (see Table I), but it has been only superficially analyzed biomechanically. Data collection methods external to the animal (cinephotography and force plates) have permitted analysis of the stability of the quadrupedal patterns and extraction of joint angles and some muscle lengths. The availability of reasonably reliable EMG signals spurred the observation that at least some muscles tended to become active when operating near their optimal lengths, as determined during tetanic electrical stimulation of single muscles in acute preparations (Stephens, 1975). However, even more important than the length/tension properties of muscle are the velocity/tension properties (see Joyce et al., 1969). These have large, nonlinear effects on force output, energetic efficiency, and on the generation of proprioceptive signals from muscle spindles. Only a few muscles having suitable tendon structures have been monitored by surgically implanted force transducers (Walmsley et al., 1978; O'Donovan et al., 1982; Abraham and Loeb, 1985), and there has been no quantitative analysis of muscle velocity in any of the kinesiological studies. A further weakness is the absence of a thorough analysis of the free-body forces operating in this complex open-

TABLE I

Phenomenology of cat locomotion

Quadrupedal locomotion studies	Classical references
Myoskeletal anatomy	Crouch (1969)
Gait patterns and stride lengths	Hildebrand (1966) Arshavsky et al. (1965) Stuart et al. (1973)
Step cycle phase times	Goslow et al. (1973) Miller et al. (1975a,b)
Ground forces	Manter (1938)
Joint angles	Engberg and Lundberg (1969) Goslow et al. (1973)
Muscle lengths	Goslow et al. (1973)
EMG phasing	Engberg and Lundberg (1969) Tokuriki (1973a,b)
Length/tension correlate	Stephens et al. (1975) (incomplete)
Muscle forces	incomplete — see text
Muscle velocity	not available
Velocity/tension correlate	not available
Joint torques and segmental momentum	not available

linked segmental structure, a difficult but tractable problem of inverse dynamic analysis which has been addressed in humans.

Thus, for most hindlimb muscles, it is not possible to state the kinematic conditions under which they generate their output impulses, whether or not these kinematic conditions are homogeneous, or (for multiarticular muscles) how they arise from the complex motion of multiple limb segments. Conversely, it is thus not possible to state which muscles perform their roles by actively shortening, which serve as nearly isometric stiffeners, and which constitute highly elastic force conveyors. As we shall see (and as one might have guessed), these different functional roles are accompanied by substantial and specific specializations at a variety of levels ranging from muscle fiber architecture to the generation and reflexive use of proprioceptive feedback.

Fig. 1 shows a summary of the actions of the major muscle groups in the cat hindlimb at various points in the walking step cycle (phases from Phillipson, 1905). It is derived from many different experimental sources and from biomechanical modeling techniques still under development in a collaborative project with Professor William Levine of the Electrical Engineering Department of the University of Maryland (Loeb et al., 1983; Marks et al., 1984). The stick figure sequence at the bottom represents every second field of a 60 field per second videotaped walking sequence, with joint positions determined by a combination of skin markers and trigonometric equations based on post-mortem measurement of limb segments. In each figure at the top, the location of each of eleven major muscle groups is shown by a fine line if the muscles are inactive (or nearly so) and by a spindle-shaped thickening if the muscles are generating substantial amounts of active force (relative to the peak for each muscle in the step cycle as measured by EMG and, in some cases, tendon strain gauges). Each active muscle is depicted with one or two arrows signifying the length changes imparted to the muscle by the motion at the one or two joints crossed by the muscle. Arrows pointing distally (from proximal origin to distal insertion) indicate lengthening motion while arrows pointing proximally indicate shortening motion. When there are two arrows, the more proximal indicates the sign of the motion imparted by the more proximal joint crossed. Arrows pointing towards or away from each other thus indicate that the active tension in the muscle is causing an acceleration of the motion at one joint with a deceleration of the motion at another joint. The net length change experienced by the muscle depends on the relative magnitude of the effects of motion at each joint, and is not shown here. Also not shown and still in progress is a quantitative reconciliation of the various active muscle torques acting across each joint with the net joint torques obtained from inverse dynamic analysis of the observed limb motion and measured ground forces.

One of the most striking general findings is the scarcity of muscles in which the active mechanical action is an unambiguous shortening (all arrows

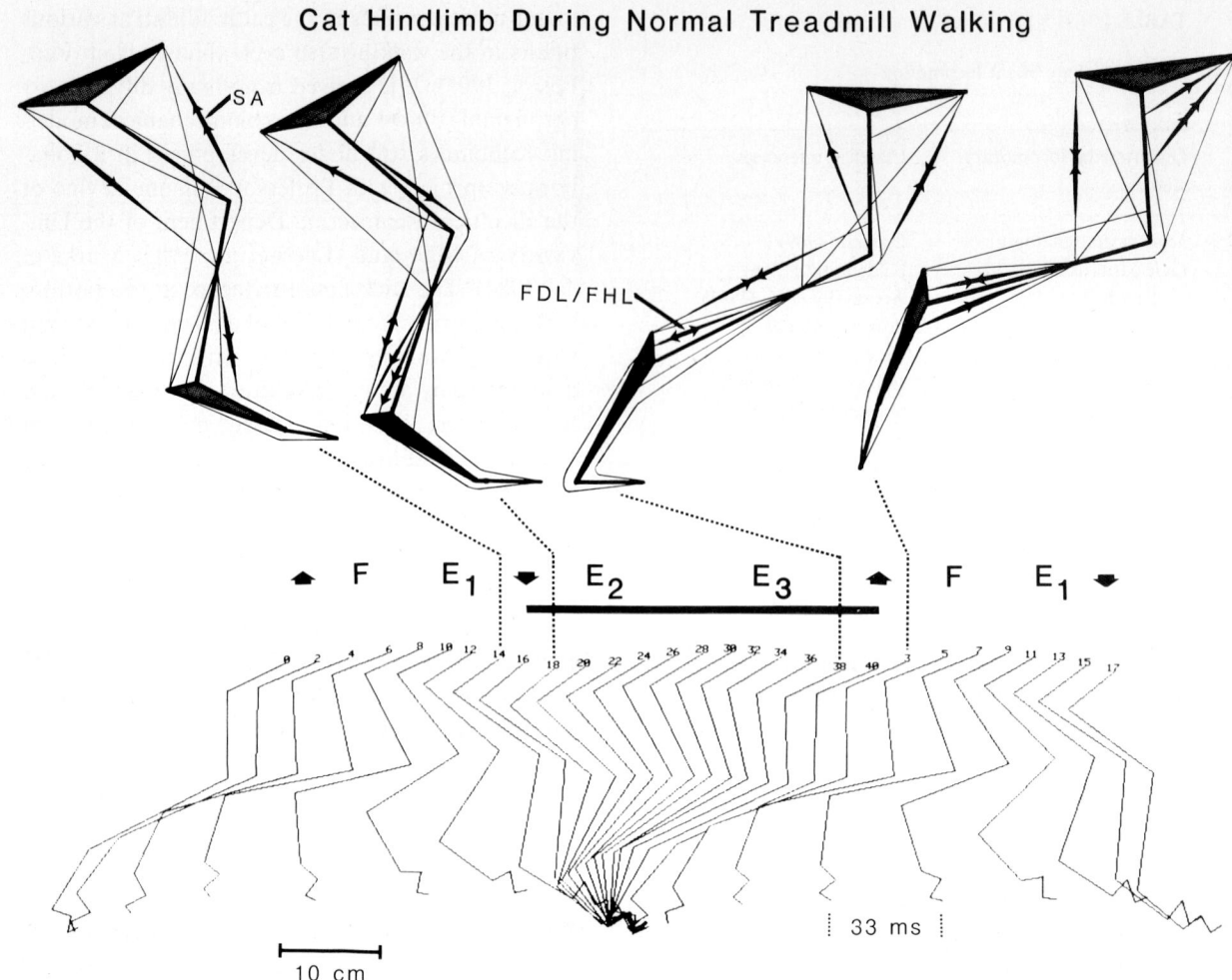

Fig. 1. Stick figure sequence at bottom taken from videotape stills of cat walking, showing corresponding phases from Phillipson (1905) step cycle (flexion, F; first extension during swing, E_1; yield during early stance, E_2; and push-off at late stance, E_3). Arrows indicate footlift (up) and footfall (down); heavy line indicates period of foot contact with treadmill surface. Four stick figures at top taken from the points indicated by the dotted lines, showing approximate anatomical course of eleven major muscle groups as fine lines (inactive) or spindle-shaped thickened lines (generating active force output) with arrows as described in text. SA, sartorius pars anterior muscle; FDL/FHL, anatomically synergistic pair of flexor digitorum and hallucis longus muscles.

pointing proximally). This simple, classical notion of a muscle at work arises only in some of the lightly loaded flexors during swing phase (far left and far right diagrams) and in the pure hip extensors during stance (E_2 and E_3, middle two diagrams). Some of the flexion motions at the knee and toes are generated by muscles that pass excessive flexion momentum at a proximal joint (hip and ankle, respec-

tively) to the more distal joint by becoming stiffly elastic. Most of the early stance phase muscle activity is concerned with limiting the yielding under the load of the body weight. At the end of the stance phase, the highly extended position of the joints places the monoarticular knee and ankle extensors at a disadvantageous length for tension generation, so much of the final push-off is generated by biarticular muscles, with compensatory stretching at one of their joints. This provides the fringe benefit of decelerating the hyperextending angular momentum (particularly in the thigh and shank), making the ensuing flexion task less difficult.

From the foregoing description, it should be clear that the contribution of any single muscle to the locomotor behavior is not evident from a simple gross anatomical description of the actions of the muscle at the joint(s) it crosses. Even less obvious is the identity of the muscles which are in some way "synergistic" and the nature of the proprioceptive information which such muscles might need to exchange for their coordinated control. Such functional dilemmas may well underlie at least some of the dismaying complexity evident in the interneuronal projections among motor nuclei (Jankowska and McCrea, 1983; Harrison et al., 1983). However, some interesting patterns of muscle recruitment have emerged that begin to suggest that the central pattern generators may use kinematics as at least one organizing principle.

Existence of task groups of motoneurons in anterior sartorius

The anterior sartorius (SA) muscle originates on the anterior iliac crest (most rostral extreme of the pelvis) and inserts on the patella, permitting it to act as a flexor of the hip joint and an extensor of the knee. The diagrams indicate that it is active in the swing phase (E_1, first diagram) and again in the late stance phase (E_3, third diagram). The swing phase active tension assists in the motion of both hip and knee in ways that add constructively, resulting in high-speed shortening (1–3 muscle rest lengths per second, depending on gait speed). The stance phase activity occurs when the hip and knee motion are out of phase. In fact, the lengthening contributed by the extending hip outweighs the shortening occurring at the extending knee, causing a net active lengthening. Recordings during unrestrained walking from single alpha motoneurons projecting to this muscle (made using floating microelectrodes chronically implanted in the ventral roots) dem-onstrate that two entirely independently recruited groups of motoneurons are responsible for these two periods of EMG recruitment (Hoffer et al., 1980, 1982). More detailed studies of the recruitment patterns within the muscle and of the microanatomical organization of the spinal motor nucleus suggest that the segregation is purely functional rather than spatial (Pratt et al., 1984; Loeb et al., 1984). We have just begun a search for selective interneuronal projections from the central pattern generator and from the various proprioceptors, which connectivity might be expected to underlie such a functional specialization.

"Reciprocal" use of the long digit flexors

The flexor hallucis longus (FHL) and the flexor digitorum longus (FDL) muscles in the cat both originate on the tibia, pass around pulleys on the extensor side of the ankle joint, and insert on a common tendon distributed to all four distal phalanges (claws) (Goslow et al., 1972). The second through fourth diagrams in Fig. 1 (top) indicate apparently continuous periods of activity for this pair of anatomical synergists, but in fact stance phase activity occurs predominantly in flexor hallucis longus, while a brief EMG burst at the beginning of flexion occurs only in flexor digitorum longus (O'Donovan et al., 1982). The multiarticular path of the tendons causes both muscles to be rapidly lengthened during stance phase. The active flexor hallucis longus, a pinnate muscle, is thus an efficient generator of propulsive forces throughout the stance phase (lengthening muscles generate higher forces with lower ATP turnover than isometric or shortening muscles). The recruitment of flexor digitorum longus coincides with the unloaded flexion of the toes in the early swing phase, suggesting that it might be actively shortening, much like the other flexors. However, it is also a pinnate muscle (Sacks and Roy, 1982), which would exacerbate the inherent inefficiency of active shortening. A close examination of the force and length data from implanted transducers indicates that the stretch applied via the dorsiflexing ankle effectively reverses the shortening from the toe motion, resulting in more nearly isometric function (Abraham and Loeb, 1985; also seen in records of O'Donovan et al., 1982). Interestingly, the pulley radius for the two muscles at the ankle is substantially different (3 mm for flexor digitorum longus and 5 mm for flexor hallucis longus; Rindos and Loeb, unpublished data), presumably representing some optimization of the ratio of effective lever arms across the joints for each of the two kinematically different tasks.

Specialized fusimotor programming of the muscle spindles

As sensors of muscle length, muscle spindle afferents contribute kinesthetic information that almost certainly contributes to the coordinated regulation of muscle recruitment. However, the activity of these afferents is complexly and nonlinearly determined by length, velocity, and activity in intrafusal muscle fibers controlled by several kinds of gamma and beta motoneurons (Lennerstrand and Thoden, 1968; Hulliger et al., 1977). Theories suggesting that there are stereotyped rules for the use of the fusimotor system (e.g., alpha-gamma coactivation) have not taken into account these diverse effects on afferent sensitivity. In particular, the optimization of stretch sensitivity in a lengthening muscle (usually via gamma dynamic motoneurons) is incompatible with the generation of any activity at all in rapidly or even modestly shortening spindles. Conversely, the gamma static motoneuron influence needed to preserve afferent activity during shortening causes afferent discharge that is high and poorly sensitive to fluctuations in velocity in lengthening muscle. Thus, it should not be surprising that the patterns of recruitment of the various types of intrafusal regulatory motoneurons appear to be highly dependent on the normal kinematic function of the muscle (for review, see Loeb, 1984). However, this has resulted in some consternation among those who would hope to find single, unifying rules for the control of all muscles.

Conclusions

Skeletal muscles must contend with inertial loads and external forces, factors that do not exist in oculomotor control. These factors have resulted in complex, multiarticular specializations of muscles and tendons that allow them to operate in modes (e.g., spring-like) that do not occur in the extraocular muscles. These added factors represent not simply complications of underlying, uniform principles of muscle function and motor control, but rather force the neuromuscular systems into one or more modes of operation having no analogs in oculomotor control (see Loeb, 1985). It is likely that within single skeletal systems such as the cat hindlimb and even within some single muscles such as the anterior sartorius, the need arises for multiple, independent, and fundamentally different control schemes. It will be the task of the next few years to identify the number and roles of different control schemes arising in striate muscles throughout the body. Once such an understanding has been obtained, it may be fruitful to look again for underlying, unifying themes in motor control.

One analogy that seems to express the nature of this search is that of a novice computer programmer examining the codes of a large number of different compilers to figure out what they are. The structure evident in the code itself will depend almost entirely on the particular language being compiled and the machine language of the computer on which it will run. However, they are all compilers, with certain metastructural similarities deeply embedded in their disparate architectures. The similarities will be apparent only to someone with a broad, intimate knowledge of many different languages and computers, and a clear notion of the high level role of the compiler.

The identification of candidate unifying principles in motor control may be more imminent than one might assume. One approach is to look for performance criteria that might be optimized. At least some of the structure of any system will be dictated by attempts to optimize specifications such as speed or accuracy, albeit within other constraints. We have proposed that the major function of the fusimotor system in all muscles may be the optimization of the rate of information transmitted by the spindle afferents for the kinematic conditions anticipated during the normal function of the muscle (Loeb and Marks, 1986). Others have proposed that the temporal and spatial patterns of muscle performance during maximal height jumping may be attributed to motor programs optimized for such an experimentally specified criterion (Zajac et al., 1981). The common thread in these suggestions is that sensorimotor systems may be free to adapt control strategies that are in some way optimal for the task at hand rather than being constrained to a limited repertoire of simple, restricted patterns of recruitment. Such performance-based unifying notions seem a priori more encouraging than historical attempts to generalize from single, specific experimental findings.

Summary

A comparison of the control problems inherent in the biomechanics of the oculomotor versus skeletomotor systems reveals that the skeletal musculature must generally cope with much more diverse kinematic problems, including inertia, elasticity, and external loads. Because of the highly nonlinear properties of muscle, such factors can be expected to require very different and highly specialized structural and functional architectures in both the muscles and their neuronal control circuits. Studies of the cat hindlimb muscles during locomotion have revealed patterns of motoneuron and spindle afferent activity that appear to be segregated based on the kinematics of muscle function (e.g., active lengthening vs. active shortening). It is suggested that these "task groups" of the motor apparatus may represent optimization strategies for the performance and control of kinematically well-defined, frequently recurring motor tasks.

References

Abraham, L. D. and Loeb, G. E. (1985) The distal hindlimb musculature of the cat: Patterns of normal use. Exp. Brain Res., 58: 580–593.

Arshavsky, Y. I., Kots, Y. M., Orlovsky, G. N., Rodionov, I. M. and Shik, M. L. (1965) Investigation of the biomechanics of running by the dog. Biophysics, 10: 737–746.

Crouch, J. E. (1969) Text-Atlas of Cat Anatomy, Lea & Febiger, Philadelphia.

Engberg, I. and Lundberg, A. (1969) An electromyographic analysis of muscular activity in the hindlimb of the cat during unrestrained locomotion. Acta Physiol. Scand., 75: 614–630.

Goslow, G. E., Jr., Stauffer, E. K., Nemeth, W. C. and Stuart, D. G. (1972) Digit flexor muscles in the cat: Their action and motor units. J. Morphol., 137: 335–352.

Goslow, G. E., Jr., Reinking, R. M. and Stuart, D. G. (1973) The cat step cycle: Hind limb joint angles and muscle lengths during unrestrained locomotion. J. Morphol., 141: 1–42.

Grillner, S. (1975) Locomotion in vertebrates: Central mechanisms and reflex interactions. Physiol. Rev., 55: 247–304.

Harrison, P. J., Jankowska, E. and Johannisson, T. (1983) Shared reflex pathways of group I afferents of different cat hind-limb muscles. J. Physiol., 338: 113–127.

Hildebrand, M. (1966) Analysis of the symmetrical gaits of tetrapods. Folia Biotheoretica, 11: 9–22.

Hoffer, J. A., Loeb, G. E., O'Donovan, M. J. and Pratt, C. A. (1980) Unitary activity patterns during walking confirm the existence of two functionally distinct classes of sartorius motoneurones in cats. J. Physiol. (Lond.), 308: 20P.

Hoffer, J. A., Sugano, N., Marks, W. G. and Loeb, G. E. (1982) Cat sartorius: Three functionally distinct motoneuron pools supply a single muscle. Soc. Neurosci. Abst., 8: 272.6.

Hulliger, M., Matthews, P. B. C. and Noth, J. (1977) Static and dynamic fusimotor action on the response of Ia fibres to low frequency sinusoidal stretching of widely ranging amplitude. J. Physiol. (Lond.), 267: 811–838.

Jankowska, E. and McCrea, D. A. (1983) Shared reflex pathways from Ib tendon organ afferents and Ia muscle spindle afferents in the cat. J. Physiol. (Lond.), 338: 99–111.

Joyce, G. S., Rack, P. M. H. and Westbury, D. R. (1969) Mechanical properties of cat soleus muscle during controlled lengthening and shortening movements. J. Physiol. (Lond.), 204: 461–474.

Lennerstrand, G. and Thoden, U. (1968) Muscle spindle responses to concomitant variations in length and in fusimotor activation. Acta Physiol. Scand., 74: 153–165.

Loeb, G. E. (1983) Finding common ground between robotics and physiology. Trends Neurosci., 6: 203–204.

Loeb, G. E. (1984) The control and responses of mammalian muscle spindles during normally executed motor tasks. Exer. Sport Sci. Rev., 12: 157–204.

Loeb, G. E. (1985) Motoneuron task groups — coping with kinematic heterogeneity. J. Exp. Biol., 115: 137–146.

Loeb, G. E. and Marks, W. B. (1986) Optimal control principles for sensory transducers. In Proceedings of the International Symposium: The Muscle Spindle, MacMillan Ltd., London, in press.

Loeb, G. E., Marks, W. B., Rindos, A. J., O'Malley, M., Chapelier, J. P. and Levine, W. S. (1983) The kinematics and task group organization of bifunctional muscles during locomotion. Soc. Neurosci. Abst., 9: 107.16.

Loeb, G. E., Pratt, C. A. and Marks, W. B. (1984) Segregation of normal and reflex activity in the cat sartorius muscle. Soc. Neurosci. Abst., 10: 183.5.

Manter, J. T. (1938) The dynamics of quadrupedal walking. J. Exp. Biol., 15: 522–540.

Marks, W. B., Loeb, G. E., Levine, W. S., Chapelier, J. P. and Roberts, W. M. (1984) The work of the cat hindlimb muscles during locomotion. Soc. Neurosci. Abst., 10: 183.1.

Miller, S., Van der Burg, J. and Van der Meche, F. G. A. (1975a) Coordination of movements of the hindlimbs and forelimbs in different forms of locomotion in normal and decerebrate cats. Brain Res., 91: 217–237.

Miller, S., Van der Burg, J. and Van der Meche, F. G. A. (1975b) Locomotion in the cat: Basic programmes of movement. Brain Res., 91: 239–253.

O'Donovan, M. J., Pinter, M. J., Dum, R. P. and Burke, R. E. (1982) The actions of FDL and FHL muscles in intact cats: Functional dissociation between anatomical synergists. J. Neurophysiol., 47: 1126–1143.

Partridge, L. D. (1982) The good enough calculi of evolving control systems: evolution is not engineering. Am. J. Physiol., 242: R173–R177.

Phillipson, M. (1905) L'autonomie et la centralisation dans le systeme nerveux des animaux. Trav. Lab. Physiol. Inst. Solvay (Bruxelle), 7: 1–208.

Pratt, C. A., Yee, W. J., Chanaud, C. M. and Loeb, G. E. (1984) Organization of the cat sartorius motoneuron pool. Soc. Neurosci. Abst., 10: 183.4.

Sacks, R. and Roy, R. R. (1982) Architecture of the hind limb muscles of the cat: Functional significance. J. Morphol., 173: 185–195.

Stephens, J. A., Reinking, R. M. and Stuart, D. G. (1975) The motor units of cat medial gastrocnemius: Electrical and mechanical properties as a function of muscle length. J. Morphol., 146: 495–512.

Stuart, D. G., Withey, T. P., Wetzel, M. C. and Goslow, G. E., Jr. (1973) Time constraints for inter-limb co-ordination in the cat during unrestrained locomotion. In R. B. Stein, K. G. Pearson, R. S. Smith and J. B. Redford (Eds.), Control of Posture and Locomotion, Plenum Press, New York, pp. 537–560.

Tokuriki, M. (1973a) Electromyographic and joint-mechanical studies in quadrupedal locomotion. I. Walk. Jpn. J. Vet. Sci., 35: 433–446.

Tokuriki, M. (1973b) Electromyographic and joint-mechanical studies in quadrupedal locomotion. II. Trot. Jpn. J. Vet. Sci., 35: 525–533.

Walmsley, B., Hodgson, J. A. and Burke, R. E. (1978) Forces produced by medial gastrocnemius and soleus muscles during locomotion in freely moving cats. J. Neurophysiol., 41: 1203–1216.

Wetzel, M. C. and Stuart, D. G. (1976) Ensemble characteristics of cat locomotion and its neural control. Prog. Neurobiol., 7: 1–98.

Zajac, F. E., Zomlefer, M. R. and Levine, W. S. (1981) Hindlimb muscular activity, kinetics, and kinematics of cats jumping to their maximum achievable height. J. Exp. Biol., 91: 73–86.

Discussion

J. Dichgans

Neurologische Klinik der Universität, Liebermeisterstrasse 18–20, D-7400 Tübingen, F.R.G.

Comparison of the effects of cerebellar lesions on visually elicited eye saccades and elbow flexions (Vilis and Hore)

This paper elicited a number of comments and a very heated discussion, mainly because of its theoretical interpretation of the results. Thach doubted that the absence of oscillations of arm movement in intact animals as opposed to monkeys after cooling of the cerebellar dentate nucleus is really due to suppression of fusimotor activity in the antagonist, resulting in spindle unloading and consequent cancelling of the stretch reflex. He discussed the possibility that stretch reflexes are preserved but a velocity-sensitive component is added. This becomes active earlier in the phase of stretch and applies a viscous damping which terminates oscillations in the course of the stretch. He wondered why it should be necessary to cancel the stretch reflex entirely, since stretch reflexes are a rather complicated mixture of these sensitivities. Matthews felt that it would be a pity if the general ideas on efference copy and stretch reflex cancellation became too closely tied to the idea that gamma-discharge to muscle spindles of antagonists is shut off. He reported that all recordings in conscious animals show that when a muscle is stretched the spindles fire rather rapidly, even when the fusimotor bias is removed.

Strick addressed the authors' ideas about symmetry of acceleration and deceleration of elbow flexion and commented on some of the differences between arm and eye movements. In particular, one of the things that the arm can do and the eye cannot is to make step tracking movements at different speeds. The ability to vary the speed of an arm movement must in some way involve the ability to make movements asymmetrically and to control the antagonist brake. Strick mentioned some of his work, showing that one can in fact dissociate agonist and antagonist activity. If a subject is told to make a very accurate movement, a well-defined antagonist burst is observed. But if the subject is allowed to be inaccurate or to bang against a mechanical stop, there is no antagonist burst, even if the activity of the agonist is approximately the same. The other circumstance in which a dissociation of agonist and antagonist activity may be observed is when the subject is asked to move at different speeds. A large-amplitude movement executed very slowly and a small movement made very quickly may result in approximately the same agonist activity, but what differentiates the two movements is the antagonist activity. A small movement made very quickly will have a large antagonist burst braking it, whereas a large movement made slowly will have a delayed and smaller antagonist brake.

Hultborn felt that the authors had neglected the reciprocal inhibition in the spinal cord. It is known that there are parallel connections to alpha-motoneurons and Ia-inhibitory interneurons. He referred to the paper presented by Fetz that demonstrated disynaptic inhibition evoked from corticospinal cells. It remains to be determined how strictly these parallel lines to alpha-motoneurons and reciprocal inhibitory interneurons function, and to what extent they can be dissociated.

Hore conceded a role for parallel connections. He restated his opinion, however, that any command to the spinal cord for the antagonist has to be based on knowledge of the expected trajectory of the movement. Under different loading conditions the agonist may change but the trajectory of the movement is basically the same. So one cannot move an antagonist, purely based on the agonist. A structure like the cerebellum must calculate the difference between the different loading conditions, so that the signal generated to control the antagonist muscle can be dissociated from the activity of the agonist. How, and at what level, this signal operates, the fusimotor system or the spinal cord, is not clear.

Eccles contended that, as based on the present knowledge about the cerebral cortex and the cerebellum and all their connectivity including feedback loops, the concept of efference copy was useless.

Hore defended his concept by referring to earlier studies in which his group was able to demonstrate that after cerebellar cooling monkeys were no longer able to generate an early antagonist response to torque-pulse perturbations of arm movements. Normally this response was generated at a latency of 60 mseconds. After cerebellar cooling it was abolished. Only in response to stretching of the antagonist muscle could one see antagonist-related activity either at the level of the motor cortex or in EMG activity. It was assumed that the early response was elicited via an efference copy mechanism sending a collateral signal to the cerebellum, which then precalculated the earlier response of the antagonist. He felt that their work on torque pulses also made sense of Evarts' findings on the reflex versus intended response. He also referred to the work of Strick indicating that neurons of the dentate nucleus are related to this kind of activity.

Relation of cerebellar and spindle afferent unit activity to parameters of movement stability (Thach et al.)

Strick mentioned earlier studies by Thach in which he showed marked differences between the nucleus interpositus and the dentate nucleus, in terms of the timing of their neuronal activity related to movement. He asked whether there were similar differences between the two nuclei in the study presented. Thach replied that the interpositus nucleus carried the tremor signal alone. Differences in timing were not investigated. It is hypothesized that the interpositus signal monitors spindle discharge, whereas the dentate nucleus may cause the discharge of gamma-motoneurons but is not in the peripheral feed back loop.

Cerebellar control of slow eye movements (Büttner et al.)

Hepp invited comments on the role of the vermal region of the cerebellum in smooth pursuit and optokinetic eye movements.

Büttner mentioned the work of Zee, who found that even if both flocculi were ablated there was still some pursuit gain left. He speculated that possibly the paraflocculus or the vermis play an additional role, and reported that the signals recorded so far in the vermis are more closely related to target velocity. To him, this indicates that these responses at least carry some sensory component. Büttner felt that in the context of all the information available, even if it is not only the flocculus, it is still safe to assume that pursuit is processed entirely by the cerebellum.

Precht reported on his own experiments in rats, in which a floccular lesion considerably reduced the response of the eyes to sinusoidal optokinetic stimulation. If he added a vermal lesion, the previously maintained residual response disappeared almost completely. Thus, at least in the rat, the vermis takes part in the response. It was asked whether the vestibular nucleus obtains a direct output signal from smooth pursuit units of the flocculus. Büttner said that at the present time this question could not be answered.

Eckmiller restated the question, asking whether the proper premotor signal for smooth eye movements, i.e., an eye velocity signal, is generated in the flocculus. Probably, Purkinje cells mix their input, as indicated by Miles et al., who showed that the granular layer input elements of the flocculus know a surprising amount of what the Purkinje cells know. To find out whether the flocculus generates a smooth pursuit command internally or just mixes it, Eckmiller proposed to use stimuli that suddenly disappear for brief intermittent periods of time, so that the system has to generate the ongoing smooth pursuit input to the ocular motor nuclei for short intervals.

Cohen asked about the possible function of the cerebellar flocculus in animals that have neither much ocular pursuit nor a rapid response to optokinetic stimuli, e.g., the rabbit.

Büttner responded that even in the rabbit and the rat optokinetic nystagmus (OKN) has a direct component that comes via the cerebellum, despite the fact that one cannot elicit pursuit in these afoveate animals. He mentioned his own work in the monkey, in which he demonstrated that even with a large central and parafoveal scotoma due to a retinal lesion, he could still obtain a direct response.

The role of the primate superior colliculus in sensory motor integration (Sparks and Jay)

Grüsser mentioned studies in which he measured horizontal and vertical auditory saccades in man. He found that with an eccentricity below 40°, auditory saccades were always too large. His conclusion was that the spatial map representing auditory direction and amplitude must be much less precise than the visual map.

Sparks responded by stating that the auditory receptive fields in the colliculus are much larger than the visual ones. However, under his experimental conditions the accuracy of the final position of aurally elicited and visually elicited eye movements was roughly comparable, although the way the animal reached the final position was different. Usually more than one saccade was executed to the auditory target. The primary saccade was frequently grossly inaccurate, and a second saccade compensated for this inaccuracy. There was no tendency to overshoot.

Henn wondered about the similarities and differences in the organization of movement fields in the superior colliculus and the frontal eye fields.

Sparks pointed to the similarities. The movement fields are symmetrical for direction and asymmetrical for amplitude. There is also a quasi-logarithmic amplitude relationship.

Goldberg referred to the work of Wurtz and added that the amplitude-log normal relationship probably also holds for the transformation from striate cortex to the frontal eye field. He asked whether the cells investigated by Sparks, like those recorded by Wurtz and Hikosaka, in the upper part of the intermediate layers of the superior colliculus, were also sensory in that they did not discharge before spontaneous eye movements in the dark.

Sparks replied that his cells were sensory by several criteria, but not purely sensory, since their activity depended on the starting position of the eye and the movement required. Consequently, he assumes that there is a dynamic visual map that changes the response characteristics of the cell along with the change in eye position.

The central mesencephalic reticular formation and the oculomotor decussation (Cohen et al.)

Wurtz tried to characterize the similarities and differences between cells in the central mesencephalic reticular formation and the cells in the intermediate layer of the colliculus. He pointed out that in the upper part of the intermediate layer colliculus cells give a clean burst with low background activity, and these cells are not similar to the ones observed by Cohen, but deeper in the intermediate layer there are cells that look very similar. After it was made clear that cells in the central mesencephalic reticular formation lead saccades anywhere between 30 and 100 mseconds, Wurtz found them to be within the range of the deeper colliculus cells. Wurtz then invited a comment from J. Büttner-Ennever, who stated that there are projections from the deeper part of the intermediate layer of the colliculus to the central mesencephalic reticular formation. Wurtz asked whether the cells recorded by Cohen discharge before all kinds of eye movements, including spontaneous eye movements in the dark and visually elicited eye movements. Cohen confirmed this and added that the cells respond even before quick phases of optokinetic afternystagmus, but in the latter case the lead time tended to be shorter and the peak frequency lower. Cohen pointed out that the projection from the colliculus to the central mesencephalic reticular formation is probably weaker than that coming back from the central mesencephalic reticular formation to the colliculus. He considered the possibility that this latter pathway conveys information to the colliculus about the horizontal component of the spontaneous eye movements in the dark and vestibular nystagmus.

Precht mentioned earlier work by Szenthagothai who described a similar area in the cat, just lateral to the midline, which he claimed was mediating cortically induced eye movements. He felt that this was the connecting area from the frontal eye field to the oculomotor brain stem areas, with independent access not necessarily going through superior colliculus. Precht asked whether there is evidence for that direct connection.

Cohen responded by saying that it does not appear that there is a direct pathway from either area 8 or the parietal cortex.

Goldberg noted the fact that the central mesencephalic reticular formation shares a number of common target regions with the frontal eye field, such as the nucleus reticularis tegmenti pontis and the superior colliculus.

Brainstem neurons and oculomotor organization (Baker)

This discussion centered mainly on the claim that the size principle is applicable to the organization of both eye and limb movements.

Loeb had doubts about the similarities in recruitment of motor neurons in the oculomotor and skeletomotor systems. Baker mentioned that in the oculomotor complex synaptic density on motoneurons is carefully contrived so as to generate the reported size recruitment. He felt that as far as the skeletomotor system is concerned this is still quite controversial. Work from Burke's laboratory suggests to Loeb that at least for the Ia-projection there are rather simple notions about the projection density to the motor neuronal pool which could account for a great deal of the size principle effects. Only limited specified location and density of synapses on the dentritic tree are required for a functional size principle. Contrary to Baker, he also felt that in respect to the skeletomotor system recruitment of strength is not mainly a matter of recruitment of new motor units, but also of an increase in frequency of previously recruited units. Kernell pointed out that the average resistivity of small and large motoneurons in the spinal cord is different, and that this produces, with a sort of random distribution of synapses, a preferential recruitment of the small ones. He interpreted the data of Grantyn and Grantyn as suggesting that this difference does not exist for oculomotor neurons they investigated.

Eckmiller asked where the axon collaterals demonstrated by Baker in many oculomotor units project to, since Renshaw cells do not exist in the oculomotor complex. Baker replied that these collaterals terminate on internuclear neurons, which in turn project to the abducens nucleus, but he did not know exactly what signals are on them. Büttner asked how the internuclear neurons and abducens motor neurons behave during vergence movements. Baker responded that 10–15% of the internuclear neurons in the cat (25% in the monkey) have a small vergence signal. However, the vergence signal is small in comparison to the conjugate gaze signal, in terms of position and velocity sensitivity curves, and can be in both directions.

Precht mentioned that in the frog there are slowly contracting muscle fibres that are innervated by slowly conducting motor units. The slowly conducting motor units in the abducens nucleus code eye position, whereas the fast motoneurons that presumably go to twitch fibres have no eye position signal. Instead, they code retinal slip or head velocity. Thus, in the frog there is a rather sharp specialization of motoneurons within a nucleus that is generally considered to be homogenous.

Baker found this to be consistent with the flatfish and toadfish, and noted that this is different from the mammal.

SECTION V

Functional Organisation of Movements

Time control of hand movements

H.-J. Freund

Neurologische Klinik der Universität Düsseldorf, Moorenstrasse 5, D-4000 Düsseldorf, F.R.G.

Introduction

The time control of self-initiated voluntary limb movements is more difficult to assess than that in the oculomotor system, where saccadic and pursuit eye movements are regarded as products of two independent control systems. The different velocities of the two types of eye movement depend on vestibular and visual inputs as well as on movement amplitude. In contrast to these different types of eye movements, velocity control in the skeletal motor system is continuous, so that limb muscles can produce movements resembling the pursuit or saccadic type of eye movements. In spite of this continuum of possible performances, it is a widely held view that in the skeletal motor system ballistic and ramp movements represent different categories. Ballistic movements have been defined as being too short to allow sensory feedback to alter their execution. Therefore, one could compare ballistic with saccadic and ramp with pursuit movements. Such a comparison would be based on their different velocities and on the different role of sensory information for the motor performance.

A difficulty in a comparative analysis of time control in the two systems lies in their different accessibility to examination. Eye movements can be examined in response to visual and vestibular inputs and described in terms of input-output relationships. In reflex studies this is also possible for limb movements. However, the wide range of input variables and of possible performances of limb movements makes it difficult to explore the control strategies relevant for their performance.

Rapid isometric contractions

Freund and Büdingen (1978) studied the fastest possible self-paced isometric contractions because their velocity control is not subject to voluntary modification with respect to further increase. They represent the simplest motor performance not complicated by mechanical factors or the demands of sensory control. This allows the examination of the extent to which the limitation of speed is due to the motor program, the neural code or the contractile apparatus. These experiments showed for the isometric contractions that for a given muscle and subject the time to peak of the fastest voluntary contractions was approximately the same no matter how large the amplitude. This was achieved by a linear increase in the rate of rise of tension with force. In this respect the fastest possible voluntary contractions showed the same properties as those seen in muscle twitches elicited by single electric shocks applied to the muscle nerve. The times to peak of the fastest voluntary contractions were only slightly longer than those of the electrical twitch contractions (Miller et al., 1981).

Comparing different muscles showed a linear relationship between the amplitude-independent times to peak and the percentage of type I fibres of the muscle examined (Hefter et al., 1983). This correlation was shown for both electrical and voluntary contractions. The linear relation between force and rate of rise of tension constituting the basis for the amplitude-independent contraction times is therefore due to neuromuscular properties. Such a type of organization provides the simplest operational mechanism for the time control of synergistic movements: the synergistic muscles engaged in a motor act such as catching a ball can all start their contractions at the same time, irrespective of their relative force contributions.

Isotonic movements and sensory control

Isotonic movements show an increase of the time to peak with increasing amplitude. The slope of this increase depends on the mass to be moved: the increase in time can be manipulated by adding loads to the moving parts. The difference between isotonic movements and isometric contractions simply reflects Newtonian mechanics because the calculation of movement time requires 2-fold integration of acceleration.

A further factor augmenting movement or contraction times is sensory guidance. If the fastest voluntary contractions or movements are examined under target conditions requiring sensory guidance the situation is different. According to Fitts' law (1954), the duration of the fastest possible movements increases with the ratio of target size to amplitude of movement. The finer the adjustment required, the slower the movement.

Serial movements

If one considers repetitive movements instead of single movements and examines how fast they can be performed, the results are usually described in terms of frequency of movement reversals per second. As a psychological standard this is called motility. Such rapid repetitive movements are employed in a variety of everyday or artistic activities, such as stroking, typing, writing, pencil-shading or playing a musical instrument. The first measurements of the highest possible motility scores during key pressing lay between 8–9.3/sec (Ream, 1922). It is astonishing that despite a revived interest in motor physiology, psychology, psychophysics and motor control theory very little is known about this capacity. For musical instruments the fastest finger movements during the vibrato are performed at rates between 5–7.1/sec (Schlapp, 1973). For the piano Adams (1976) quotes an anecdote by Lashley (1951) that a pianist can move the fingers at a rate of 16/sec. The highest motility scores in musical performance seem to lie somewhere in the range between 5.5–16/sec. Nothing quantitative is known about interindividual differences and the effects of training.

We have recently conducted a systematic study of the highest motility scores that can be achieved by normal subjects for a few simple alternating movements and isometric contractions (Hefter, H., Hoemburg, V. and Freund, H.-J., unpublished data). The goal of this investigation was not only to find the highest motility scores for the different conditions tested, but also the mechanisms limiting the performance. The subjects were asked to perform an alternating finger movement starting from a slow alternating extension-flexion movement executed with the extended forefinger, and then to execute this movement at successively faster rates until the fastest possible performance was reached. The second instruction was to keep the amplitude of the movement as large as possible. Fig. 1 shows a typical amplitude-frequency relationship obtained from a normal subject. The full amplitude can only be maintained up to a rate of ≈2 Hz and

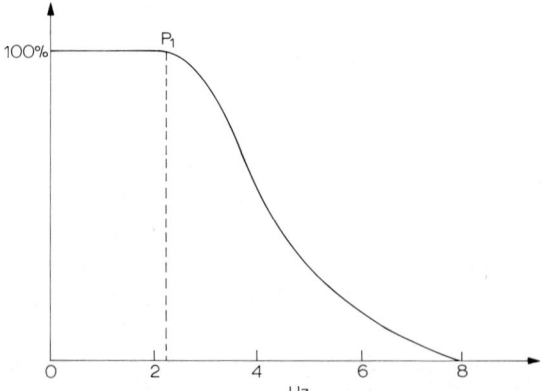

Fig. 1. Amplitude-frequency relationship of serial finger movements. Amplitude (ordinate) was measured by goniometer while the subject successively increased the rate of alternating movements trying to keep the amplitude maximal. Amplitude decreases at frequencies higher than 2 Hz (P_1).

then declines on to the highest frequency, at around 8 Hz. The decrease of amplitude with increasing frequencies was mainly the consequence of mechanical damping by means of subtraction of counteractive forces generated by the antagonistic muscles. When a similar paradigm was examined for an isometric condition, where the forefinger was fixed to a ring and the produced strength recorded by a strain gauge, a similar curve was obtained. As long as small masses have to be moved, the difference between the isotonic and isometric condition is small. This changes for larger masses, but also for different muscle groups. The turning point (P_1) of the frequency-amplitude relationship, from which onwards the amplitude decreases, is different for different muscle groups and subjects. The same is true for the maximum frequency that can be produced. As in the case of the fastest single contractions, the major determinant is the fibre-type composition of the muscles involved.

Due to their small amplitudes the fastest possible alternating movements performed voluntarily have a tremulous character. The highest possible motility scores are closely related to the peak frequency of isometric force tremor and for body parts with a small mass, such as the fingers, also to the rate of position tremor. The similarity between the fastest voluntary and involuntary movements has already been noted in a study in which the vibrato produced by a violinist had a similar frequency to that of the violinist's finger tremor (Schlapp, 1973). It is further illustrated by the fact that the decrease in tremor rate in pathological conditions is associated with a corresponding decrease in motility scores (Hefter et al., 1983).

The EMG during rapid alternating movements shows an antagonistic pattern similar to that in tremor records. At slower repetition rates (below P_1) a different EMG pattern can be observed. It is the typical triphasic pattern seen in rapid single movements. This triphasic pattern reflects the biomechanical demands of moving parts, and therefore is less pronounced or absent during small-amplitude finger movements or isometric contractions. If the triphasic pattern is employed at repetition rates below P_1, the subject follows a strategy of a succession of single rapid movements with a ramp--plateau type of pattern. If the subject wants to produce a smoother sinusoidal movement at the same rate, the alternating pattern will be employed instead. Therefore, at rates slower than P_1 the subject can choose between the single move strategy associated with the triphasic burst pattern and the alternating mode, depending on the intended action. Above P_1 it is no longer possible to employ the first strategy. The decrease in amplitude demonstrates that this is due to the damping properties of the moved parts. The movement initiated by the activity of the agonistic muscles does not reach full amplitude because the antagonist activity starts too early, so that the movement in the opposite direction commences before the maximum is reached. For this reason the activation of the antagonist as a breaking mechanism is not necessary. For finger and, similarly, for hand movements the range between P_1 and maximum frequency lies between 2 and 6–12 Hz. This is the range of restrained capacity of movement performance where full amplitude movements cannot be produced.

The isochrony principle

A large number of automized everyday performances of the hand and fingers are characterized by rapid, repetitive small-amplitude movements. These movements are usually performed at frequencies higher than P_1, so that they already fall into the range of reduced amplitudes. Their temporal organization follows a similar principle to that described for the fastest voluntary isometric contractions: the time of performance is approximately constant. This had already been noticed by Katz (1948) and was recently found to apply for a wide range of manual performances. Variation of the size of letters by a factor of 5 did not change their execution time (Katz, 1948). Enoka (1983) observed that the duration of the first component of a weightlifting movement did not vary with amplitude. The tangential velocity of a pen's tip was found to be closely related to the total linear extent

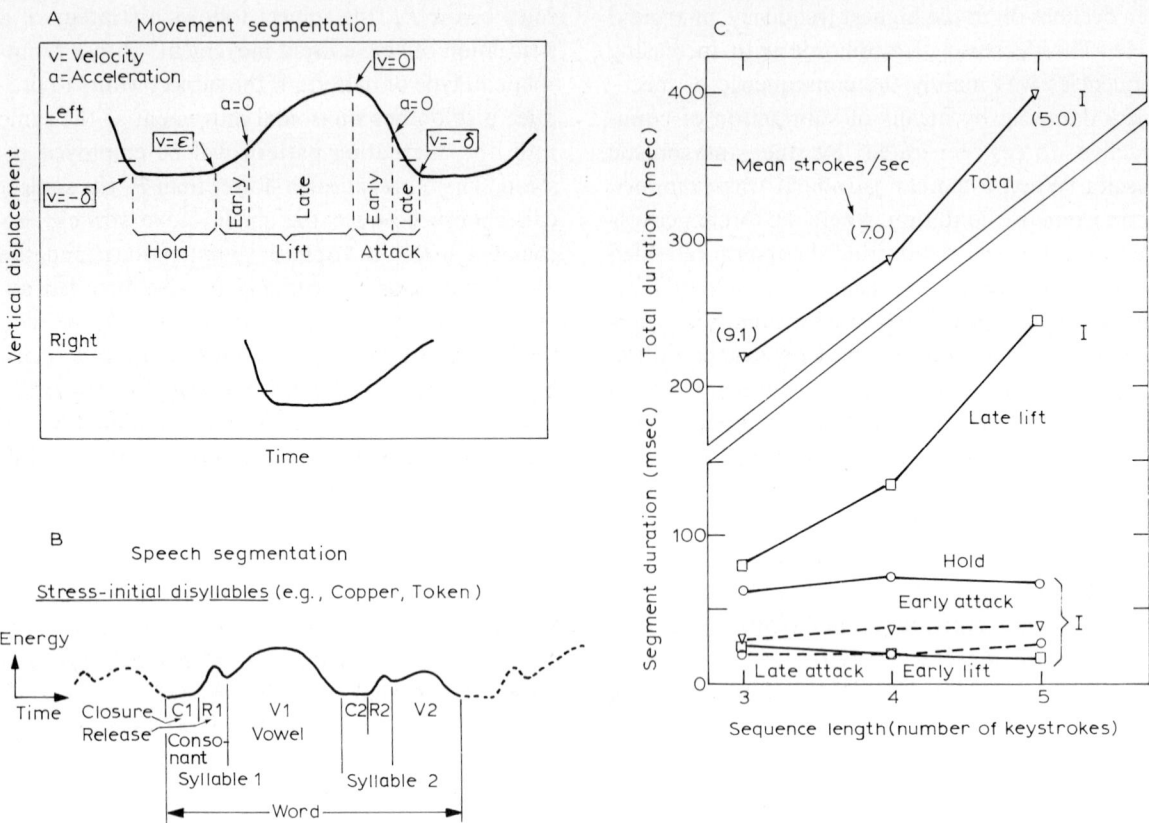

Fig. 2. Segmentation (A) of a finger trajectory during rapid typing and (B) of speech for a two-syllable word. The influence of sequence length on the duration of each segment of the finger movement is shown in C. Only the late lift phase showed major variation with sequence length. For the two-syllable word only the final, second vowel was length dependent. From Sternberg et al. (1984).

of the trajectory, keeping the execution time independent of movement size, even for complex trajectories (Viviani and Terzuolo, 1980). This relationship was found to apply to the linear extent of one cycle of movement as well as to the whole performance. These observations led Viviani and Terzuolo (1980) to formulate isochrony as a general principle in movement control. Similar observations have been made on the basis of experiments on the control of rapid action sequences in speech and typing (Sternberg et al., 1984). For typing they constructed a finger-trajectory apparatus and segmented the finger trajectory as illustrated in Fig. 2. The examination of the influence of sequence length on finger movement showed that the late lift segment was the only one revealing any substantial effect of sequence length. This was interpreted as reflecting that the control system must gain access to the next subprogram before the attack, fitting in with the idea of a retrieval process that is temporally discrete. A comparable segmentation of two-syllable spoken words into six segments also showed that all these time segments remained unaltered when the number of words was varied between two and five. Only the final, second vowel of the second syllable was length dependent. Sternberg et al. (1984) regarded this as evidence for the advanced planning of whole sequences. Their model employs an action unit containing several actions that are executed as part of the same unit, thus supporting the hypothesis of hierarchical control in the execution of two classes of rapid-action sequences. These experiments revealed that this type of time control operates at a fairly general level.

Eye-hand interaction

Although the interaction between eye and hand has been of some importance for human development it is astonishing how little is known about this issue. With respect to the temporal characteristics of eye movements, it is known that the eye will follow moving targets by means of smooth pursuit eye movements up to frequencies around 1 Hz. Further increase in frequency is associated with an increasing number of sacadic eye movements, until the ocular tracking stops completely at frequencies exceeding 2 Hz (Von Noorden and Mackensen, 1962; Mather and Putchat, 1983; Leist et al., 1986). This does not change significantly if active movements of the own hand or finger are pursued instead of an external object, although the accuracy of the tracking may improve (Mather and Putchat, 1983). The fastest hand or finger movements that can be produced lie in the range between 6–12 Hz. Hand and finger movements faster than 2 Hz are frequently employed in everyday activities. Since the eye will not pursue objects moving at frequencies above 2 Hz, these rapid hand and finger movements will not be followed by the eyes. As known from the high velocities that can be employed by the oculomotor system this limitation is not due to the motor side. This is illustrated by the ability to perform sinusoidal eye movements up to frequencies around 6–8 Hz, when the vestibulo-ocular reflex is brought into play by shaking the head as fast as possible while fixating the finger (Atkin and Bender, 1968). Leist et al. (1986) have explained the inability of the eyes to track at frequencies exceeding 2 Hz by the failure to see the target at faster frequencies even when a combination of saccades and smooth movements is used. Calculating the time spent in eye movement at 2 Hz and assuming that 20° saccades have durations between 50–60 mseconds, then 4 saccades/sec need 200–250 mseconds. This leaves less than 200 mseconds for each period of fixation, which is too short for visual perception because of the visual blanking by post-saccadic suppression. Therefore, Leist et al. arrived at the conclusion that the limitation of oculomotor tracking to frequencies below 2 Hz is visual rather than motor in nature.

Plotting the amplitude-frequency relationship for the eye movements in the same way as shown for the hand performance in Fig. 1 reveals that the larger part of the frequency range of human hand movements cannot be controlled by the eye (Fig. 3). Therefore, fast moving target and hand movements cannot be foveated. What the eye can do instead is a 'Ganzfeld-Kontrolle' (whole field control). In the context of this chapter I would like to call this control mode 'range control'. As obvious from everyday experience, the range of pencil-shading or handwriting, activities commonly executed at rates faster than 2 Hz, can be controlled well with fixed gaze, so that one can write within a demarcated area. These considerations are approximate and only valid for smooth regular movements. Grossly irregular movements may be different, because they contain a spectrum of different frequencies.

Another modality which is of major significance for the control of hand movements is somatosensory information gained from the hand. The hand is a somatosensory sense organ used for object manipulation. Tactual scanning has been compared

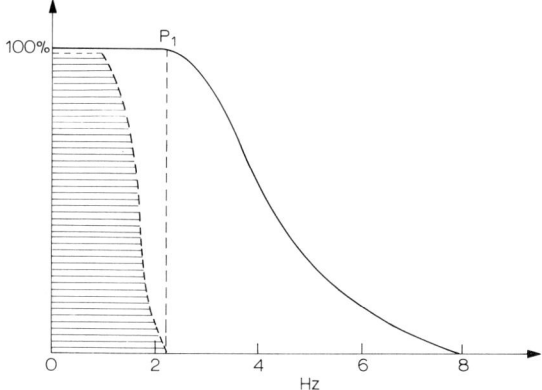

Fig. 3. Amplitude-frequency relationship of serial finger movements as shown in Fig. 1 (solid line) and of eye movements (dashed line), measured while the subject was trying to watch his moving finger.

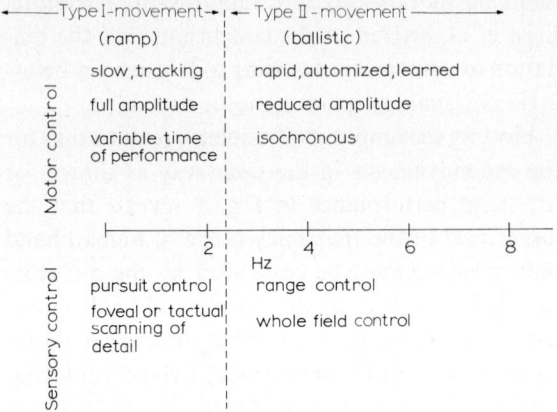

Fig. 4. Schematic illustration of the major differences between slow and rapid hand movements.

with visual scanning (Gibson, 1962), and it was assumed that the scanning procedures are closely similar for the eye and hand, as there is a high precision in cross-modal matching between the visual and somatosensory modalities. The speed of the exploratory movements of the hand is, to my knowledge, not known quantitatively. Watching the action of hand and fingers during tactile prehension and exploration of objects gives the impression that such movements are slow rather than fast. Therefore, it may be tentatively suggested that the sensory guidance of hand and finger movements, no matter whether visual, somatosensory, or both, will be restricted to the range of slower movements.

Conclusions

Two modes of eye-hand interaction

The analysis of the temporal characteristics of hand movements shows a continuum of possible performances between very slow and brisk. On the basis of the evidence discussed so far, I would like to propose a model of sensory motor interaction which is based on the temporal characteristics of eye and hand movements. This model is schematically represented in Fig. 4 and consists of two classes of hand movements:

1. Type I movements: slower movements; if repetitive, below 1–2 Hz. These movements can be executed under sensory guidance based on pursuit, foveal control or on tactual scanning.
2. Type II movements: rapid single or serial movements; if repetitive, commonly performed at rates above 2 Hz. They include many skilled and learned movements. The time of their individual performance is independent of amplitude for the usual operational range. This provides the basis for a stable relationship between the spatial and temporal code addressing fixed times to the formation of distinct trajectories or action units. This may be an important determinant for motor learning. These movements can be sensory controlled but the type of sensory control is a range control rather than a fine, foveal pursuit control mode, as employed in the sensory guided movements.

The eye also employs two modes of operation when interacting with the hand: 1. Smooth pursuit eye movements used for the sensory guidance of the slower hand movements. 2. Range control — with the eyes watching the range of performance — for the fast, learned, skilled hand movements.

This concept provides a new quantitative and qualitative basis for the old idea of separating ballistic movements from ramp movements. Ballistic movements have been regarded as movements that are terminated before sensory feedback can come into action, and therefore were referred to as single rather than repetitive movements. The term ballistic was frequently under attack because of its vague definition with respect to its temporal limits and to the continuous transition from ballistic to ramp movements.

A distinction between the two types of hand movement as shown in Fig. 4 is based on different mechanisms and operational strategies and can be applied to single as well as repetitive, serial movements. In contrast to the concept of ballistic movements, type II movements frequently are performed under sensory control, but this is a whole field, a range control rather than a pursuit foveation of detail. This type of sensory control can set the border conditions and control them. Therefore, the performance of learned movements may or may not be subject to sensory range control. What is impossible is foveation or precise tactual scanning.

The two types of hand movement have both different sensory control modes and different motor capacities. Although the latter are not as different as in the oculomotor system, the slower, type I movements belong to that range of motor control that allows full amplitude performance, employment of triphasic or alternating EMG patterns in antagonistic muscles, and the generation of motor patterns is variable in time. In contrast, the type II movements cannot reach full amplitude, cannot be generated as a sequence of single movements with triphasic patterns and their execution time is amplitude independent, allowing for invariant timing in the production of motor patterns.

There is not yet enough information about the actual extent of the frequency range to which isochrony applies. The examples given so far were all rapid performances. The relation between isochrony and motor learning and their frequent association with fast motor acts remains the subject of future research. Why is it so difficult, or sometimes impossible, to reproduce the typical features of one of the best learned movements, one's own signature, at very low speed? On the other hand, a pianist can play a learned musical sequence at slow as well as at high speed.

With respect to nomenclature, the term 'ballistic' seems difficult to adapt for rapid serial movements such as writing. Since 'saccadic' would not be suitable for a fast limb movement, the most adequate terms would possibly be those reflecting their different functional role, such as sensory guided slower and intrinsically patterned faster movements. Since no single term defines the sets of properties shown in Fig. 4 unambiguously, the designation of the functional categories as type I and type II movements may be the clearest one.

As compared with the smooth pursuit and the saccadic eye movements, there are more differences than similarities. The engagement of smooth pursuit or type I movements in sensory guidance of eye or hand is similar. However, almost everything else is different, including their functional context. Moving the eye back to a new fixation point has nothing to do with the rapid production of learned motor patterns. This differs as soon as the interaction between eye and hand comes into play. Then, the perceptive and executive aspects show astonishing mutually adaptive control modes underlying the type of sensory-motor organization illustrated in Fig. 4. Not only sensory control — pursuit or range — is different but also the characteristics of the movement as listed in this figure. A closer understanding of the mechanisms underlying the matching of certain temporal demands for perception and motor control is an intriguing problem for future research.

References

Adams, J. A. (1976) Issues for a closed-loop theory of motor learning. In G. E. Stelmach (Ed.), Motor Control: Issues and Trends, Academic Press, New York, pp. 525–533.

Atkin, A. and Bender, M. B. (1968) Ocular stabilization during oscillatory head movements. Vestibular system dysfunction and the relation between head and eye velocities. Arch. Neurol. (Chic.), 19: 559–566.

Enoka, R. M. (1983) Muscular control of a learned movement: the speed control system hypothesis. Exp. Brain Res., 51: 135–145.

Fitts, P. M. (1954) The information capacity of the human motor system in controlling the amplitude of movement. J. Exp. Psychol., 47: 381–391.

Freund, H.-J. and Büdingen, H.-J. (1978) The relationship between speed and amplitude of the fastest voluntary contractions of human arm muscles. Exp. Brain Res., 31: 1–12.

Gibson, J. J. (1962) Observations on active touch. Psychol. Rev., 69: 477–491.

Hefter, H., Reiners, K. and Freund, H.-J. (1983) Mechanisms underlying the limitation of speed and amplitude of rapid movements. Neurosci. Lett. Suppl., 14: S158.

Katz, D. (1948) Gestaltpsychologie, Schwabe, Basel, pp. 124–129.

Lashley, K. S. (1951) The problem of serial order in behavior. In L. A. Jeffress (Ed.), Cerebral Mechanisms in Behavior, Wiley, New York, pp. 112–136.

Leist, A., Freund, H.-J. and Cohen, B. (1986) Comparative characteristics of eye and head tracking in humans, submitted for publication.

Mather, J. A. and Putchat, C. (1983) Parallel ocular and manual tracking responses to a continuously moving visual target. J. Motor Behav., 15: 29–38.

Miller, R. G., Mirka, A. and Maxfield, M. (1981) Rate of tension development in isometric contractions of a human hand muscle. Exp. Neurol., 73: 267–285.

Ream, M. J. (1922) The tapping test — a measure of motility. Iowa Stud. Psychol., 8: 293–319.

Schlapp, M. (1973) Observations on a voluntary tremor — violinist's vibrato. Q. J. Exp. Physiol., 58: 357–368.

Sternberg, S., Knoll, R. L., Monsell, S. and Wright, C. E. (1984) Control of rapid action sequences in speech and typing. Bell Laboratories Technical Communication, pp. 1–20.

Viviani, P. and Terzuolo, C. (1980) Space-time invariance in learned motor skills. In G. E. Stelmach and J. Requin (Eds.), Tutorials in Motor Behavior, Elsevier/North-Holland, Amsterdam, pp. 525–533.

Von Noorden, G. K. and Mackensen, G. (1962) Pursuit movements of normal and amblyopic eyes. I. Physiology of pursuit movements. Am. J. Ophthalmol., 53: 325–336.

Reflex control of hand muscles

J. Noth and H.-H. Friedemann

Department of Neurology and Clinical Neurophysiology, Alfried Krupp Hospital, 4300 Essen, F.R.G.

Introduction

The skilled motor functions of the primate's hand depend not only on the action of the pyramidal tract (Tower, 1940; Lawrence and Kuypers, 1968) but also on continuous somatosensory input from receptors of the hand (Marsden et al., 1984).

The fact that impulses from skin receptors and proprioceptors of the hand are transmitted via oligosynaptic pathways to separate clusters of cells within area 4 of the motor cortex (Lemon, 1981; Strick and Preston, 1982) indicates a distinct functional link between the peripheral input and the cortical output. This is in line with Phillips' (1969) idea that a transcortical reflex loop plays a functional role in, at least, distal arm muscles of the primate.

Nevertheless, precise knowledge about the mode by which hand muscles are controlled by peripheral inputs is missing. Neither is it known which part is played by the spinal stretch reflex, which has not been abandoned completely even in intrinsic hand muscles (Stanley, 1978; Buller et al., 1980; Noth et al., 1983), nor is it agreed whether the proposed transcortical reflex acts in a "servo-like" or a "triggered" fashion (Tatton and Bawa, 1979; Chan and Kearney, 1982).

We decided to use a quantitative approach to study the balance in gain between the spinal stretch reflex and the "long-latency" reflex. Sinusoidal analysis was chosen, because this technique provides estimates of gain and loop time of a feed-back system in operation (Rosenthal et al., 1970; Rack, 1981). In the oculomotor system, sinusoidal analysis has been successfully applied to study the transfer function of various reflexes (cf. Büttner et al., section IV-B), which made it possible to describe some of the investigated subsystems in mathematical terms (Robinson, section V). It will be shown that in the skeletomotor system sinusoidal analysis can also provide data which may be used as a first building block of a quantitative description of the reflex control of hand muscles. To this end, the frequency response of the flexing force of the index finger to an imposed sinusoidal movement was analysed and plotted as a Nyquist diagram. The typical "epsilon-shaped" curve was best fitted by a model with two reflex arcs of different loop times. This supports the concept that, in addition to the short-latency spinal stretch reflex, a reflex route with a considerably longer latency participates in the control of finger muscles.

Methods

The present study consists of an experimental part, in which the force response of the voluntarily flexed index finger in response to imposed sinusoidal movements is analysed. Some aspects of the present work have been published previously (Noth et al., 1984), and therefore only essentials of the method will be given here. The second part deals with a simple model involving conduction delays, which is able to describe some characteristics of the experimentally obtained force responses.

Sinusoidal analysis

20 normal subjects without previous history of neurological disorders participated in the study. The principles of the stretching device and the motor paradigm are shown in Fig. 1A. The subject pressed the terminal phalanx of the index finger against a lever, exerting a steady voluntary torque of 20% maximal. The low-pass filtered force was displayed on an oscilloscope for visual control. The electromagnetic stretcher produced sinusoidal movements of the lever of 1° peak to peak. Stiffness of the stretching device was high enough to exclude distortions of the imposed length changes. A sequence of frequencies between 3 and 16 Hz was tested (Fig. 2A). This was done in a continuous run of either increasing or decreasing frequency. 15 cycles were applied at each test frequency, but only the last 10 cycles were digitized, thus allowing for biomechanical and neuronal adaptation after each frequency step. After each "active" frequency run, the subject was asked to relax his index finger and another "passive" run with the finger taped to the lever was carried out to correct for the mass of lever and finger. The length and torque signals were digitized on-line and averaged ($n = 10$ cycles). After subtraction of the "passive" torque cycle averages, least-square sinusoids were fitted to the corrected cycle averages at each frequency. The data were plotted as Nyquist stiffness diagrams (Fig. 1), in

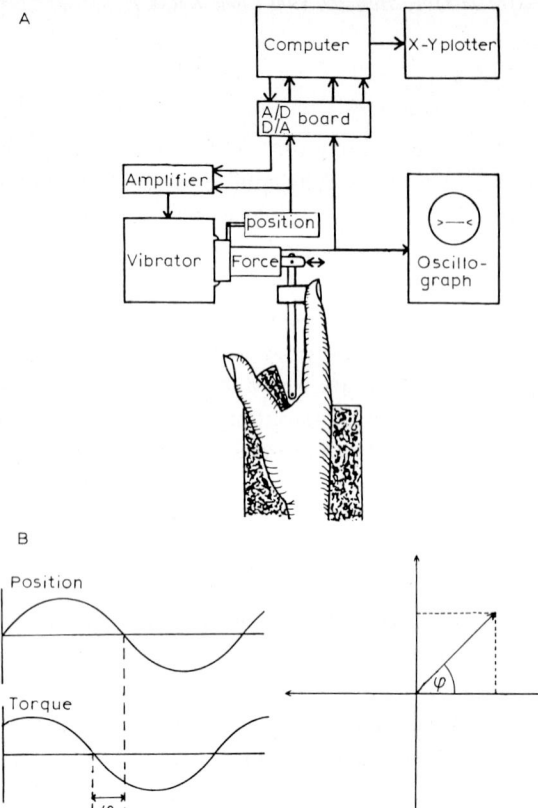

Fig. 1. Stretching device (A) and construction of Nyquist stiffness diagram (B). The modulated flexing force of the sinusoidally displaced index finger was measured by a force transducer connected between lever and vibrator. Correction for inertia and friction of the lever and for inertia of the finger was achieved by subtracting a "passive run" (relaxed index finger taped to the lever) from the "active run" (see text for details). Least-square sinusoids were fitted to the digitized length and force signals (averaged over ten cycles) for each test frequency (B) and displayed as a Nyquist diagram. Each frequency point (cf. Fig. 2A) represents a vector characterized by the phase shift between position and torque (φ) and the amplitude of the force modulation. In the following figures force signals are calibrated in terms of stiffness (Nm/rad).

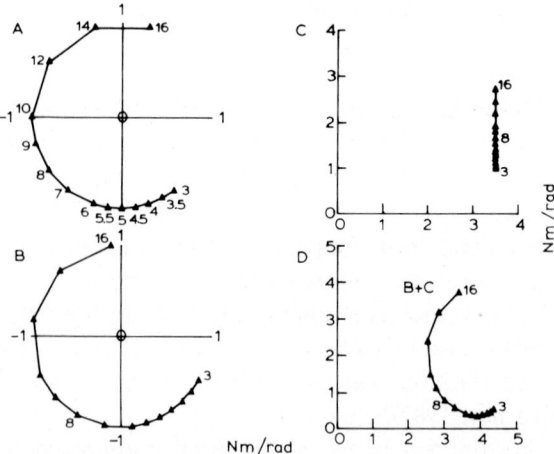

Fig. 2. Constructed vector diagrams. A. Flat frequency response of gain (1) and constant delay (50 mseconds) of torque over position. B. As A, but with additional frequency-independent phase advance (25°) of torque. C. Non-reflex stiffness of flexed index finger, taken from Noth et al. (1984). D. Vector addition of B and C, resulting in a "C"-shaped vector path.

which each dot represents a stiffness vector calculated for a particular frequency. The modulus of the vector is determined by the ratio of torque to position amplitude (stiffness), and the angle φ by the phase shift between position and torque cycle averages. The vector paths of Figs. 3 and 4A are averages of a number of individual frequency runs carried out with the same hand. A period of 2 minutes was given for rest between test runs.

Model

The vector path of a feedback system in which the force output is proportional to the length input and delayed by a constant time lag has been described by Rack (1981). It is a cycle around the origin, as exemplified in Fig. 2A for a constant time lag of 50 mseconds between length input and force output. For a description of the human stretch reflex, this model is, of course, an oversimplification, because the various subsystems involved have distinct transfer functions (Stein and Oğuztöreli, 1976), which, in the case of the human finger, are not all known. On the other hand, Rack (1981) has demonstrated that when the transfer functions of muscle spindles (Poppele and Bowman, 1970) and skeletal muscles (Mannard and Stein, 1973) are included in the model of Fig. 2A, the cycle is almost perfectly preserved. It seems that the velocity sensitivity of muscle spindle endings partially compensates for the low-pass filter properties of the skeletal muscle, resulting in a nearly flat over-all frequency response. In fact, experiments on the stretch reflex of cat triceps surae muscle support this assumption (Rosenthal et al., 1970). As the aim of the present study was to model some principle characteristics of the experimentally obtained transfer function, the assumption of a flat frequency response of reflex gain was therefore thought to be justified. Another implication of the experiments of Rosenthal et al. (1970) was considered in our model. These authors showed that in the cat, where the conduction delay in the peripheral nerves may be neglected, the reflex force leads the length change by 20–25°. The phase lag due to the muscles and the phase lead of the muscle spindles do not balance exactly. Although it is not clear whether this assumption is also valid for the human hand muscles, the vector path B in Fig. 2 is based on a linear over-all transfer function with an additional phase lead of 25°, which causes a counter-clockwise shift of the vector path A in Fig. 2.

It has been demonstrated that even after correction for the passive finger properties the vector path is not determined solely by reflex forces (Brown et al., 1982a; Noth et al., 1984). This is due to the visco-elastic properties of the muscles involved (Rack, 1966). This component of the total stiffness was estimated by applying an ischaemic conduction block (Noth et al., 1984). The resulting frequency response is that of the visco-elastic properties and can be described by a straight line parallel to the ordinate (Fig. 2C). This means that for small length changes the response is dominated by Newtonian friction. The geometrical addition of vector paths B and C in Fig. 2 results in a "C"-shaped vector path (D) which resembles those obtained experimentally on the thumb interphalangeal joint (Brown et al., 1982a) and on the index finger (Noth et al., 1984).

Results

The general shape of the Nyquist stiffness diagram has been delineated by Brown et al. (1982a) for the thumb and by Noth et al. (1984) for the index finger. The shape resembles a "C", but in many subjects it is better described as an "ε", with an inward notch at about 8 Hz. This notch may be only a slight indentation in the vector path, as seen in Fig. 3A, but in most subjects it was quite pronounced (Fig. 3B). It was always directed toward the centre of the vector path at a frequency between 7 and 9 Hz in the 20 normal subjects studied. The notch was highly reproducible for each individual subject. The consistency of the notch is best documented when vector diagrams from a number of individual runs of a subject are averaged as in Fig. 3B. Inconsistency of the notch frequency would attenuate the indentation, but this does not happen.

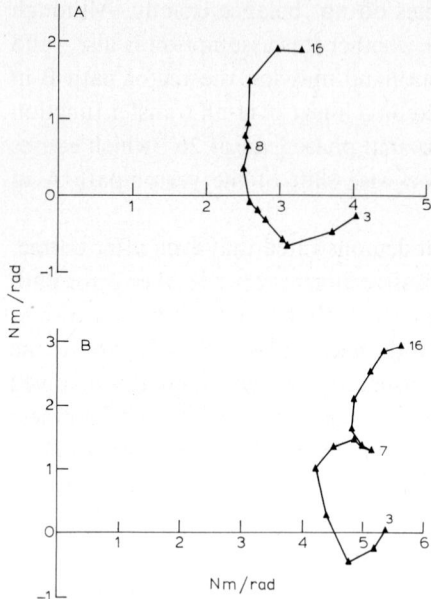

Fig. 3. Nyquist stiffness diagrams for index finger of two normal subjects. A. Average of four runs. B. Average of six runs. Note the uneven distribution of frequency points along the vector path, as in Fig. 2A.

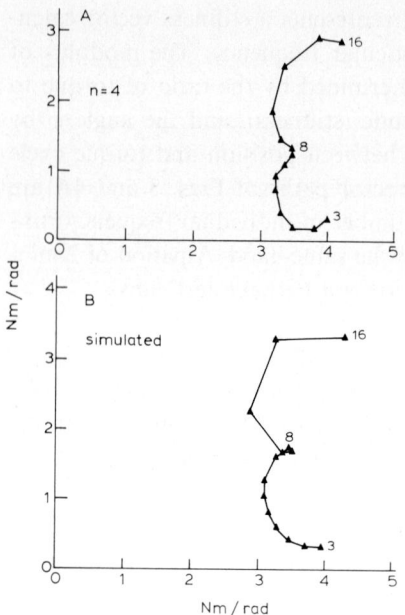

Fig. 4. Comparison between experimental Nyquist diagram (A) and simulated diagram (B). A. Averaged stiffness diagram of four normal subjects. B. Vector summation of non-reflex visco-elastic stiffness (Fig. 2C); short-latency reflex pathway: delay, 60 mseconds; long-latency reflex pathway: delay, 120 mseconds. Gain for both reflexes 0.5, with a frequency-independent phase advance of 45°. Frequency points in A and B identical, as in Fig. 2A. Further explanation in text.

Even in the grand average of three subjects with similar notch frequencies, a sharp indentation at 8 Hz was preserved (Fig. 4A).

Such an inward indentation can easily be simulated with the model outlined in Methods if the operation of two reflex pathways with different conduction delays is assumed (Fig. 4B). The best fit with the experimental vector path was obtained when the delay between both reflex arcs was around 60 mseconds, but even considerable variations in the choice of the variable parameters (gain and delay in both reflex arcs, phase advance of the torque) did not abolish the notch. Changes in these parameters only affected the final outline of the vector path, i.e., the depth of the indentation and the frequency at which it occurred.

Discussion

In confirmation of previous work the general shape of the Nyquist stiffness diagram of the flexing force of the index finger is "C"-shaped, and thus best explained by the action of a reflex force fed back to the muscle with an appreciable time lag (Rack, 1981). However, closer inspection of the stiffness diagram disclosed an inward indentation at stretching frequencies around 8 Hz, which manifests itself in the majority of the subjects studies (cf. also Noth et al., 1984). Outward displacements of the vector path, as occasionally observed by Brown et al. (1982b) at the thumb interphalangeal joint, were never detected in the present study.

It is unlikely that the inward notch was due to phase locking of α-motoneurones to the stretch cycle. As discussed by Brown et al. (1982b), phase locking should enhance the gain in the stretch reflex and thus should rather cause an outward displacement, in analogy to the increase in muscle spindle sensitivity during phase locking (Goodwin et al., 1975).

Which other mechanisms can account for the observed inward indentation of the vector path? Non-linearities of the stretching device can be excluded, since no displacements around 8 Hz were detected when the passive finger (no voluntary force exerted) was moved or when ischaemic conduction block was induced by a cuff on the upper arm, which interrupted the reflex transmission (Noth et al., 1984). Furthermore, the degree of indentation varied considerably between subjects (cf. Fig. 3), which does not favour an electro-mechanical origin of the indentation. Rack (1981) calculated vector diagrams for various combinations of mechanical loads and reflex transfer functions, but never obtained a vector path with an inward indentation. One restraint in his analysis was the consideration of only one reflex arc contributing to the force modulation. If two reflex arcs with different loop times are considered in his model, inward displacements around 8 Hz are readily encountered, as demonstrated in Fig. 4. It could be argued that the various non-linearities involved in length-force transmission impede any conclusion drawn from the similarities between the experimental stiffness diagram and the model. Such non-linearities have been analysed only recently at the human ankle joint during imposed sinusoidal movements (Evans et al., 1983; Rack et al., 1983). In spite of considerable non-linearities which were detected in the electromyogram of the stretched calf muscles, the vector path itself was a smooth "C", with no sign of inward or outward displacements. The study of Rack et al. (1983) also disclosed how important it is to take into account the compliance of the tendon in a quantitative description of reflex forces. In our motor paradigm, quite different muscle groups participate in the generation of the flexing force: the first dorsal interosseus muscle with a short tendon, and the flexor digitorum superficialis and profundus muscles with long tendons (Long et al., 1970). Although frequency-dependent distribution of the imposed length changes to these muscles should be considered as a reason for the inward indentation, the fact that inward indentations were also readily encountered (Brown et al., 1982b) at the thumb interphalangeal joint, where only one flexing muscle is involved, renders this possibility unlikely.

Long-latency reflex pathway

Our data suggest that a reflex pathway with a transmission time considerably longer than the spinal reflex delay contributes to the force of the hand muscles. This assumption is in line with numerous recent publications in which the electromyographic responses of human muscle to imposed stretches were investigated. The advantage of the method described here is that it circumvents the risk of grouped muscle spindle volleys being responsible for grouped EMG responses (Hagbarth et al., 1981), as brisk muscle stretches are prevented by the sinusoidal stretching.

In the modelled vector path of Fig. 4, the best fit to the experimental curve was achieved when the long-latency reflex had a loop time which was 60 mseconds longer than the spinal reflex delay. This is much more than the value which would result from the difference in spinal loop times between the intrinsic and extrinsic hand muscles which participate in the finger flexion (Long et al., 1970). This difference is also much longer than the time difference between the spinal stretch reflex and the presumed secondary muscle spindle effect on the electromyographic stretch response, which amounts to only 15 mseconds in the long flexor pollicis muscle (Matthews, 1984, and section II). Even the M_2 response (according to Lee and Tatton, 1975), which in hand muscles follows the M_1 response by about 20–25 mseconds (Marsden et al., 1978; Noth et al., 1985), can hardly account for such a large difference in reflex delays. Thus, a reflex pathway with an even longer transmission time must be considered.

Implications for reflex stability

The resonant frequency of such a "long-loop" reflex would be about 4 Hz, as this is the frequency point closest to the origin (Fig. 3). A detailed analysis of the tremor of the human thumb revealed in fact a low-frequency tremor at 3.5–6 Hz, which for several reasons was attributed to the action of reflex force (Brown et al., 1982c). Spontaneous low-frequency tremor at 4–6 Hz was also observed for the human wrist (Stiles, 1976) and the elevated middle finger (Gottlieb and Lippold, 1983). The implications of multiple reflex pathways for the stability of neuromuscular systems have been discussed by Oğuztöreli and Stein (1976), and for hand muscles the demand for high stability is especially great. The cooperation of the spinal stretch reflex and a long-loop reflex would certainly improve the stability in the feed-back system, but it seems unlikely that this is the only function of the long-loop reflex.

The data presented here give no hint as to which central pathways are involved, but preliminary results obtained in patients with cerebellar lesions show that the low-frequency part of the stiffness diagram is greatly enlarged in these patients (Friedemann et al., 1983). Therefore, the assumption that the cerebellum is involved in the gain control of the proposed long-loop reflex pathway in hand muscles may serve as a working hypothesis to be rejected or supported by further work.

Conclusions

Sinusoidal movements imposed on the voluntarily flexed index finger produce force modulations which can be expressed as a Nyquist stiffness diagram. In confirmation of previous work, this diagram is "C"-shaped, but in most subjects a reproducible inward notch appears at 7–9 Hz. A simple explanation for this notch is that two reflex pathways with quite different transmission times are acting. One possible functional role of such a multiple feed-back system is the improvement of stability. The timing of the long-latency reflex force would support the build-up of tremor at around 4 Hz. Such low-frequency tremor can occasionally develop in normal subjects and is seen frequently in patients with motor disorders. Thus, enhanced gain in long-loop reflex(es) may be the reason for pathological tremor at low frequencies.

Acknowledgements

We are grateful to Drs. S. Cleveland and A. Thilmann for critical reading of the manuscript and for valuable comments. The work was supported by grants of the Deutsche Forschungsgemeinschaft, SFB 200.

References

Brown, T. I. H., Rack, P. M. H. and Ross, H. F. (1982a) Forces generated at the thumb interphalangeal joint during imposed sinusoidal movements. J. Physiol., 332: 69–85.

Brown, T. I. H., Rack, P. M. H. and Ross, H. F. (1982b) A range of different stretch reflex responses in the human thumb. J. Physiol., 332: 101–112.

Brown, T. I. H., Rack, P. M. H. and Ross, H. F. (1982c) Different types of tremor in the human thumb. J. Physiol., 332: 113–123.

Buller, N. P., Garnett, R. and Stephens, J. A. (1980) The reflex responses of single motor units in human hand muscles following muscle afferent stimulation. J. Physiol., 303: 337–349.

Chan, C. W. Y. and Kearney, R. E. (1982) Is the functional stretch response servo controlled or preprogrammed? Electroenceph. Clin. Neurophysiol., 53: 310–324.

Evans, C. M., Fellows, S. J., Rack, P. M. H., Ross, H. F. and Walters, D. K. W. (1983) Response of the normal human ankle joint to imposed sinusoidal movements. J. Physiol., 344: 483–502.

Friedemann, H.-H., Diener, H. C., Matthews, H. R. and Noth, J. (1983) Enhanced long-latency reflexes in patients with lesions of the cerebellar hemispheres. Electroenceph. Clin. Neurophysiol., 56: 81.

Goodwin, G. M., Hulliger, M. and Matthews, P. B. C. (1975) The effects of fusimotor stimulation during small amplitude stretching on the frequency-response of the primary ending of the mammalian muscle spindle. J. Physiol., 253: 175–206.

Gottlieb, S. and Lippold, O. C. J. (1983) The 4–6 Hz tremor during sustained contraction in normal human subjects. J. Physiol., 336: 499–509.

Hagbarth, K.-E., Hägglund, J. V., Wallin, E. U. and Young, R. R. (1981) Grouped spindle and electromyographic responses to abrupt wrist extension movements in man. J. Physiol., 312: 81–96.

Lawrence, D. G. and Kuypers, H. G. J. M. (1968) The functional organization of the motor system in the monkey. I. The effects of bilateral pyramidal lesions. Brain, 91: 1–14.

Lee, R. G. and Tatton, W. G. (1975) Motor responses to sudden limb displacements in primates with specific CNS lesions and in human patients with motor system disorders. Can. J. Neurol. Sci., 2: 285–293.

Lemon, R. N. (1981) Functional properties of monkey motor

cortex neurones receiving afferent input from the hand and fingers. J. Physiol., 311: 497–519.

Long, C., Conrad, P. W., Hall, E. A. and Furler, S. L. (1970) Intrinsic-extrinsic muscle control of the hand in power grip and precision handling. J. Bone Joint Surg., 52: 853–867.

Mannard, A. and Stein, R. B. (1973) Determination of the frequency response of isometric soleus muscle in the cat using random nerve stimulation. J. Physiol., 229: 275–296.

Marsden, C. D., Merton, P. A., Morton, H. B., Adam, J. E. R. and Hallett, M. (1978) Automatic and voluntary responses to muscle stretch in man. In J. E. Desmedt (Ed.), Cerebral Motor Control in Man: Long Loop Mechanisms, Progress in Clinical Neurophysiology, Vol. 4, Karger, Basel, pp. 167–177.

Marsden, C. D., Rothwell, J. C. and Day, R. L. (1984) The use of peripheral feedback in the control of movement. Trends Neurosci., 7: 253–257.

Matthews, P. B. C. (1984) Evidence from the use of vibration that the human long-latency stretch reflex depends upon spindle secondary afferents. J. Physiol., 348: 383–415.

Noth, J., Friedemann, H.-H., Podoll, K. and Lange, H. W. (1983) Absence of long latency reflexes to imposed finger displacements in patients with Huntington's disease. Neurosci. Lett., 35: 97–100.

Noth, J., Matthews, H. R. and Friedemann, H.-H. (1984) Long latency reflex force of human finger muscles in response to imposed sinusoidal movements. Exp. Brain Res., 55: 317–324.

Noth, J., Podoll, K. and Friedemann, H.-H. (1985) Long-loop reflexes in small hand muscles studied in normal subjects and in patients with Huntington's disease. Brain, 108: 65–80.

Oğuztöreli, M. N. and Stein, R. B. (1976) The effects of multiple reflex pathways on the oscillations in neuromuscular systems. J. Math. Biol., 3: 87–101.

Phillips, C. G. (1969) Motor apparatus of the baboon's hand. Proc. R. Soc. (B), 173: 141–174.

Poppele, R. E. and Bowman, R. J. (1970) Quantitative description of linear behavior of mammalian muscle spindles. J. Neurophysiol., 33: 59–72.

Rack, P. M. H. (1966) The behavior of a mammalian muscle during sinusoidal stretching. J. Physiol., 183: 1–14.

Rack, P. M. H. (1981) Limitations of somatosensory feedback in control of posture and movement. In V. B. Brooks (Ed.), Motor Control, Handbook of Physiology, Section 1: The Nervous System, Vol. II, Waverly Press, Baltimore, pp. 229–256.

Rack, P. M. H., Ross, H. F., Thilmann, A. F. and Walters, D. K. W. (1983) Reflex responses at the human ankle: the importance of tendon compliance. J. Physiol., 344: 503–524.

Rosenthal, N. P., McKean, T. A., Roberts, W. J. and Terzuolo, C. A. (1970) Frequency analysis of stretch reflex and its main subsystems in triceps surae muscles of the cat. J. Neurophysiol., 33: 713–749.

Stanley, E. F. (1978) Reflexes evoked in human thenar muscles during voluntary activity and their conduction pathways. J. Neurol. Neurosurg. Psychiat., 41: 1016–1023.

Stein, R. B. and Oğuztöreli, M. N. (1976) Tremor and other oscillations in neuromuscular systems. Biol. Cybernet., 22: 147–157.

Stiles, R. N. (1976) Frequency and displacement amplitude relations for normal hand tremor. J. Appl. Physiol., 40: 44–54.

Strick, P. L. and Preston, J. B. (1982) Two representations of the hand in area 4 of a primate. II. Somatosensory input organization. J. Neurophysiol., 48: 150–159.

Tatton, W. G. and Bawa, P. (1979) Input-output properties of motor unit responses in muscles stretched by imposed displacements of the monkey wrist. Exp. Brain Res., 37: 439–457.

Tower, S. S. (1940) Pyramidal lesions in the monkey. Brain, 63: 36–90.

Pathophysiology of rapid eye movement generation in the primate

V. Henn[1] and K. Hepp[2]

[1]*Neurology Department, University Hospital, CH-8091 Zürich and* [2]*Physics Department, Swiss Federal Institute of Technology, CH-8093 Zürich, Switzerland*

Introduction

The oculomotor system is unique in its repertoire of movements: rapid, slow, and vergent eye movements are controlled separately. Rapid eye movements include saccades and fast phases of vestibular or optokinetic nystagmus. The generator of rapid eye movements can be localized in the brainstem. In disease it can be affected independently, leaving slow movements intact.

Dynamics of rapid eye movements

Rapid eye movements are too fast to allow for external feedback via the visual system. They usually exhibit a stereotypical trajectory of maximal velocity for a given amplitude. The trajectories approximate straight lines even for oblique saccades. The velocity profile is almost symmetrical, with no oscillation between acceleration and deceleration. Their dynamics have been described by Robinson (1964), and aspects of muscular mechanisms by Collins et al. (1975). Under normal conditions unexpected external forces do not act on the globe. Such external perturbations would have to be corrected by a second saccade, which as a rule follows only after a refractory period. However, internal, system-inherent perturbations occur very often. During a blink, saccades are slowed down markedly, which is already reflected in lower discharge rates in brainstem burst neurons. In a similar way, saccades are often slowed down in periods of reduced alertness (Henn et al., 1984a). In order to reach the target position under such conditions (Becker et al., 1981), internal feedback loops are needed.

At various times, rapid eye movements have been called ballistic. This is a term borrowed from the art of warfare, where it describes the path of a bullet with maximum initial acceleration and the following trajectory exclusively determined by passive forces. Instead of giving up such a misleading term, it had been redefined as rapid and preprogrammed. It seems that even this definition is too narrow, since movements induced by the vestibular system are also preprogrammed, and during rapid head turning can reach velocities higher than those of small saccades.

In comparison, movement patterns in the skeletomuscular system differ in that usually a stabilization of posture is needed before the execution of the movement; there is no refractory period at the end of movement; external loads can differ over a very wide range; extremities are not mechanically overdamped; therefore, to initiate and to stop rapid movements of the extremities neuronal pulse patterns must be different from those which move the eyes.

Loss of rapid eye movements after lesions

Clinical experience shows that the generation of rapid eye movements can selectively affect movements in the vertical or horizontal direction (Bender and Shanzer, 1964). The area for horizontal rapid eye movement generation has been localized as the paramedian pontine reticular formation (PPRF) (Fig. 1) (Cohen et al., 1968); and the area for vertical movement generation as the rostral interstitial nucleus of the medial longitudinal fasciculus (rostral iMLF) (Büttner et al., 1977; Büttner-Ennever and Büttner, 1978). As many movements occur in oblique directions needing coordination, this requires coordination by a common central input. In this sense the scheme proposed in Fig. 2 has proven useful (Henn et al., 1982a,b). In a very simplified way it proposes three spatially separate channels for the generation of rapid eye movements: one channel for the parametric determination of horizontal movement components; a second for vertical movement components; and a third channel affecting timing and coordination of movement. This scheme is supported by the results of single neuron recordings and lesion experiments. Recent lesion experiments have been done chemically by the local injection of kainic acid, which destroys cells but leaves fibers mostly unaffected (Henn et al., 1984b).

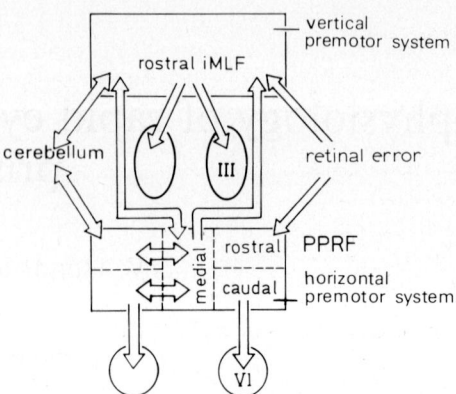

Fig. 2. Scheme of rapid eye movement generation. The medial PPRF gates and synchronizes eye movements in the horizontal and vertical directions. Temporal parameters of horizontal eye movements are elaborated in several steps in the rostral and caudal PPRF; determination of vertical movement parameters is achieved in the rostral iMLF. III, oculomotor complex; VI, abducens nucleus.

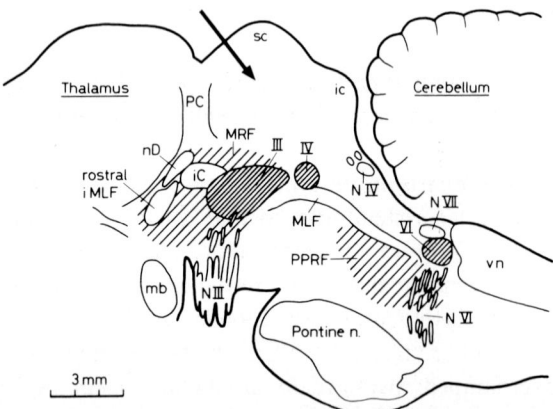

Fig. 1. Parasagittal section through the brainstem of a rhesus monkey. The third, fourth and sixth nuclei are heavily shaded. The PPRF and the rostral iMLF are immediate premotor areas for generation of horizontal and vertical rapid eye movements. iC, interstitial nucleus of Cajal; mb, mammillary body; nD, nucleus of Darkschewitsch; PC, posterior commissure; MRF, mesencephalic reticular formation; MLF, medial longitudinal fasciculus; sc and ic, superior and inferior colliculi, respectively; vn, vestibular nuclei. Arrow indicates vertical stereotaxic plane. From Henn et al. (1982a).

A unilateral PPRF lesion leads to a loss of all rapid eye movements to the ipsilateral side (Fig. 3); a bilateral lesion of the rostral PPRF results in the loss of all horizontal eye movements; a unilateral lesion of the rostral iMLF shows no effect, while a bilateral lesion leads to the loss of all vertical movements (Fig. 4); and a bilateral lesion of the medial and caudal PPRF leads to a severe disruption of eye movement in all directions. In all lesions the velocity-to-position integrator and the generators for slow eye movement programs remained intact.

These lesion experiments show that one can abolish movements in the direction of one coordinate in a Cartesian system. It has to be stressed that this is the result of the inactivation of a large number of units with different on-directions. If electrical stimulation and lesions suggest an organization strictly in Cartesian coordinates, then this is the result of the pooled activity of neurons, which when taken individually display a more complex spatial coding pattern (Hepp and Henn, 1983a). This is of importance when considering the interface to the visual input or motoneuron output, as neither of these systems use coding in a global Cartesian frame.

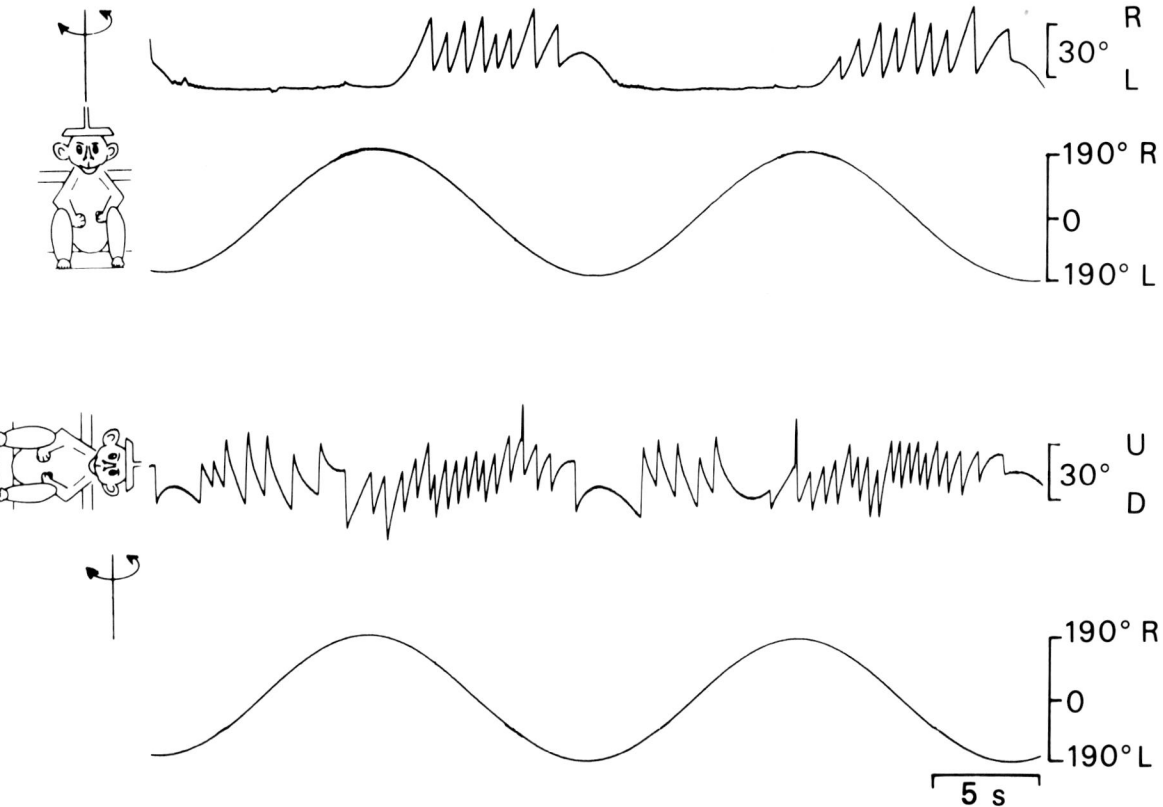

Fig. 3. Vestibular nystagmus in a monkey with a right-sided PPRF-lesion. The monkey was rotated over slightly more than a half-circle (190°) to the right and left with a sinusoidal velocity profile. During rightward rotation the eyes deviate fully to the left, as the monkey is unable to generate any rapid movements to the right. During leftward rotation the eyes make compensatory movements well across the midline into the right half-field, with normal quick phases to the left. Below, vertical nystagmus which is normal in both directions. From Henn et al. (1982b).

In comparison, no equivalent exists in the skeletal muscular system. A paresis can affect preferentially distal or proximal muscles, but not one type of movement in one geometrical plane, leaving movements in an orthogonal plane unaffected. Also, the strict separation between rapid and slow movements is not encountered.

Neuronal activity in the PPRF and rostral iMLF

Single-cell recordings in the alert monkey also suggest that there are subdivisions of the PPRF with specialized functions. Neuron populations, although not strictly separated, show an unequal distribution. Neurons in the rostral PPRF are mostly of the long-lead burst type. Their activity rises to the respective maximal level about 20 mseconds prior to the movement. In the caudal PPRF medium-lead burst neurons predominate, the activity of which precedes saccades by 4–12 mseconds. The on- and offset of their activity is sharp. Therefore, the number of spikes in a burst is unambiguously defined and shows a close correlation to the eye displacement component in the respective on-direction. For neurons in the caudal PPRF it is horizontal, whereas the equivalent class with vertical on-directions is found in the rostral iMLF. Electrophysiological investigations in the cat show that medium-lead burst neurons consist of two classes, excitatory or inhibitory, and project monosyn-

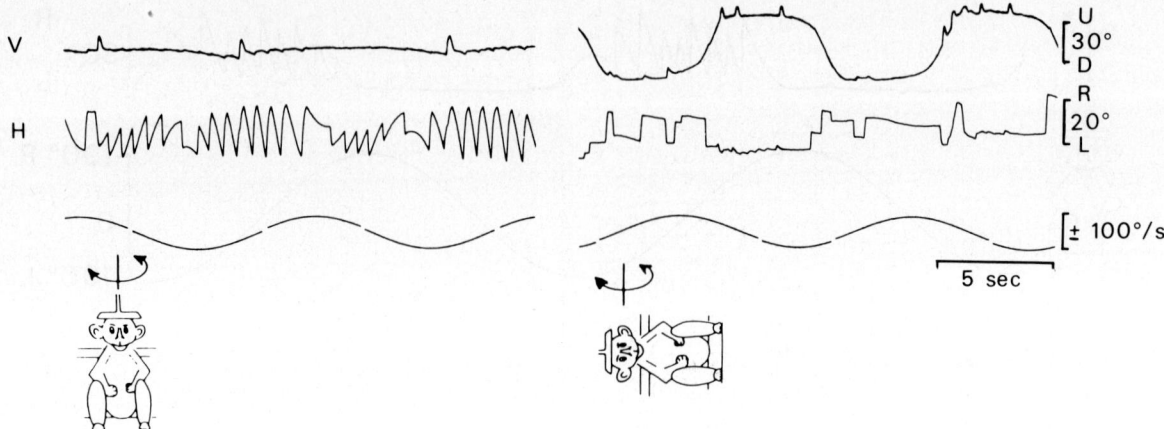

Fig. 4. Vestibular nystagmus in a monkey with a bilateral lesion of the rostral iMLF. All rapid eye movements in the vertical plane are lost. The blips on the vertical eye position trace indicate blinks which are preserved. Rapid eye movements in the horizontal direction are unaffected, as in nystagmus (left) or as spontaneous saccades (right).

aptically to motoneurons (for a review, see Shimazu, 1983).

In the medial PPRF pause neurons predominate (Keller, 1980). They discharge regularly at 150–200 Hz and pause for rapid eye movements in all directions approximately for the time of activity of medium-lead burst neurons.

These findings suggest the following simplified scheme of rapid eye movement generation: there are three channels for the generation of rapid eye movements, one in the PPRF for the horizontal component, and another one in the rostral iMLF for the vertical component. Part of the synchronization of both components during oblique saccades is effected by a third channel, a common input which times the sharp onset and termination of saccades. It is realized by pause neurons which act as inhibitory gates for the central input to the pulse generator.

Spatio-temporal recoding for visually evoked saccades

The visual system uses spatial maps for the location of a target. With different magnification factors the retinal topography is projected in different visual areas, of which the frontal eye field (FEF) and superior colliculus (SC) constitute an interface with the motor system. Their combined lesion severely disrupts the execution of visually evoked saccades (Schiller et al., 1980); low-amplitude stimulation elicits saccades; single unit activity can precede visually elicited saccades (SC: Schiller and Stryker, 1972; review: Wurtz and Albano, 1980; FEF: Goldberg and Bushnell, 1981); both areas directly project to brainstem oculomotor areas (FEF: Leichnetz, 1981; Schnyder et al., 1985; SC: Harting, 1977). Neurons in both structures are characterized as having movement fields in the sense that a neuron fires maximally for a movement of a particular amplitude and direction. If the amplitude is smaller or larger or in a different direction, unit activity is less. Examples and a more detailed description of neurons with movement fields in the SC are discussed by Sparks and Jay (Section IV-B) and for the FEF by Goldberg and Bruce (Section IV-A). With such an organization, the direction and amplitude of a saccade is determined by the spatial distribution of active neurons in a motor error map. Motoneurons, however, need a neuronal input which is organized differently. Instead of a spatial, they use a temporal code. The direction of movement is determined by the set of neurons activated for the different muscles, and the amplitude by how long neurons are active. For a lateral movement, for example, abducens and medial rectus motoneurons are activated in the monkey during 30 mseconds for a 10° saccade and during 50 mseconds for a 30° saccade. For horizontal rapid eye movements this spatio-temporal recoding is effected in the PPRF (Hepp and Henn, 1983a).

Long-lead burst neurons in the rostral PPRF are mostly spatially organized in movement fields similar to neurons in the FEF or SC, but they have not been shown to be topographically arranged in a map. An example is given in Fig. 5. The vectorial long-lead burst neuron in Fig. 5A has a small movement field, the center of which is about 12° left and slightly upward relative to the fovea. The directed

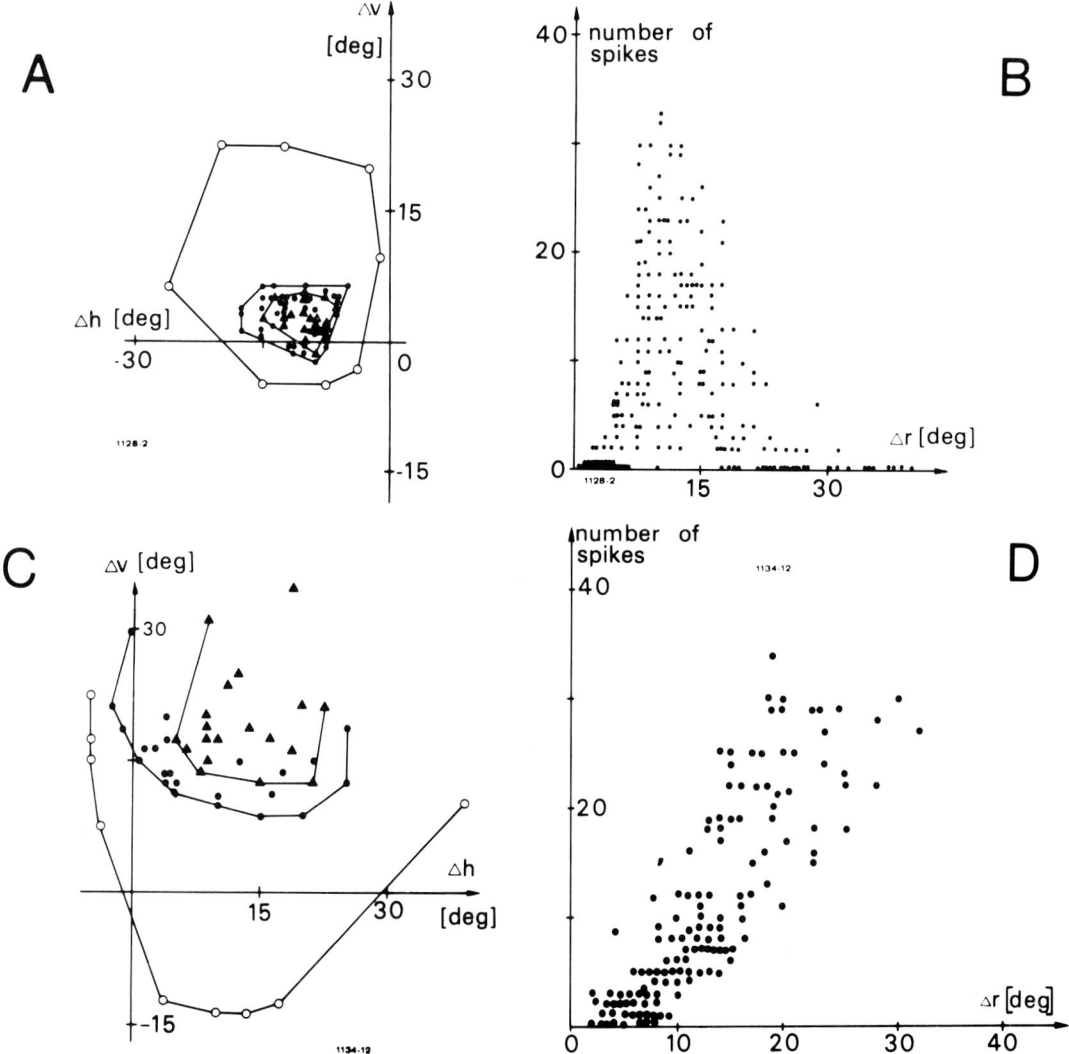

Fig. 5. Two long-lead burst neurons recorded from the PPRF. In A and C the eye displacement in a vertical (ordinate) and horizontal (abscissa) direction is plotted. The two innermost lines encircle all movements which occur together with bursts of more than 75 (triangles) or 50% (dots) of maximum number of spikes observed in the respective neurons. The outermost line (circles) defines the region of movement inside of which at least two high-frequency spikes had been observed. The neuron in A has a small movement field. In B, the number of spikes is plotted against amplitude of movement within a cone of 60° around its average on-direction left and up. One sees a peak for movements of about 12°. In C, a neuron with a much larger movement field open to the periphery. The diagram (D) shows that the number of spikes versus amplitude in a given direction increases monotonically. Therefore, this neuron already provides a temporal encoding of saccades in the right-upward direction. From Hepp and Henn (1983b).

long-lead burst neuron in Fig. 5C has a much larger field, with a center in the direction 20° to the right and up. Usually, a boundary to the periphery cannot be determined. These two examples are typical. With increasing distance from the fovea the size of movement fields increases. Movement fields are not circular: there is a steeper gradient of activity towards the fovea, while towards the periphery gradients are less steep. In these respects, neurons are similar to those in the FEF or SC. They are different in that the burst shape and maximal activity already show some relation to the onset, peak velocity and termination of the resulting saccade, which already contribute elements of a temporal code. The locations of movement fields of long-lead burst neurons in the rostral PPRF are distributed over the whole ipsilateral half-field. Recent investigations of neurons in the SC and PPRF under identical conditions show that the distinction between spatial and temporal code in neuron populations might not be as sharp (unpublished observations). Rather, there seems to be a gradual shift to a temporal code which is already visible in some SC neurons.

Neurons located more caudally in the PPRF increasingly show elements of a temporal code. Their on-directions shift towards horizontal, on-latencies decrease and reach a value between 5 and 12 msec-

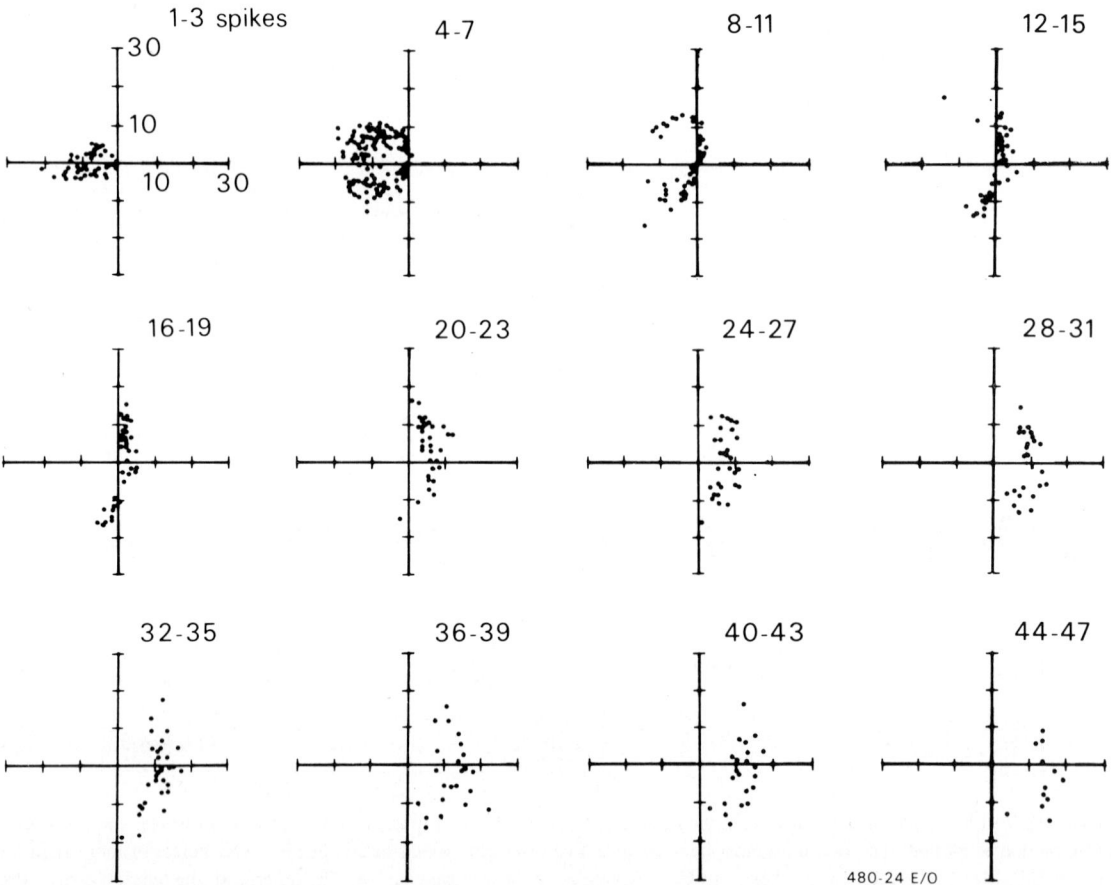

Fig. 6. Medium-lead burst neuron from the PPRF. The number of spikes per burst were counted and separated into bins. For each bin the horizontal and vertical displacement is plotted. For example, the bin of 16–19 spikes shows that most eye movements go to the right, but a few go down and to the left. If these data points were approximated by a line, one obtains an iso-burst curve indicating all possible eye displacements for a burst of a given strength. Only for the bins with more than 24 spikes, have all movements a rightward component.

onds which defines medium-lead burst neurons. For generating eye movements in the vertical plane the rostral iMLF is similar to the caudal PPRF, with medium-lead burst neurons displaying vertical on-directions. Fig. 6 gives an example of one PPRF medium-lead burst neuron and Fig. 7 shows representative iso-burst curves from a family of medium-lead burst neurons all recorded from the rostral iMLF of one monkey. One can see the still complex spatial organization of the single neuron, although their averaged on-directions would yield straight vertical on-directions. This might explain why lesions lead to deficits in one Cartesian plane.

For saccades in oblique directions, horizontal and vertical movement components have a similar time course. The initial signal is an activation of long-lead burst neurons located in the appropriate region on the motor map. The exact location on the motor map determines the strength of synaptic connection to medium-lead burst neurons with a horizontal or vertical on-direction. This connection might be direct, or through intermediate cells. As this information is transmitted synchronously to medium-lead burst neurons, their onset and duration of activation should be similar. This ensures that horizontal and vertical movement components have a similar time course independent of how large the vector components are in Cartesian coordinates. These considerations, derived from observations of motoneuron behavior (Henn and Cohen, 1973) and discharge patterns of burst neurons in the PPRF (Hepp and Henn, 1983a), have recently been modelled (Van Gisbergen et al., 1985). Computer simulation based on such a two-dimensional model could better predict oculomotor behavior than models which treated the horizontal and vertical systems separately.

In comparison, such clearly defined sensorimotor interfaces as the FEF or SC with spatially coded motor maps have not been found in the skeletal motor system. However, the logical problem of such a transformation will remain the same, independent of whether such postulated maps are arranged topographically in a laminar structure or in virtual space.

Eye movement and its parametric adjustment

There had been much controversy whether saccades are coded in fovea-centered coordinates which move the eyes relative to a prior position, or in head-centered absolute coordinates. Numerous experiments show that we can make saccades to remembered targets in the dark in head-centered coordinates. This suggests that such positional information is available, probably at a cortical level. Along the main brainstem pathways from the visual system one finds fovea-centered coordinates which are translated into a motor-error (Sparks and Porter, 1983). However, eye position has to enter at some level to adjust for non-linearities of firing pattern in neurons (thresholds, saturation) or of the oculomotor plant (asymmetry of orbital anatomy). Eye position signals, i.e., a head-centered code, are found in neurons near the output of the PPRF. The cerebellum seems to play a prominent role in com-

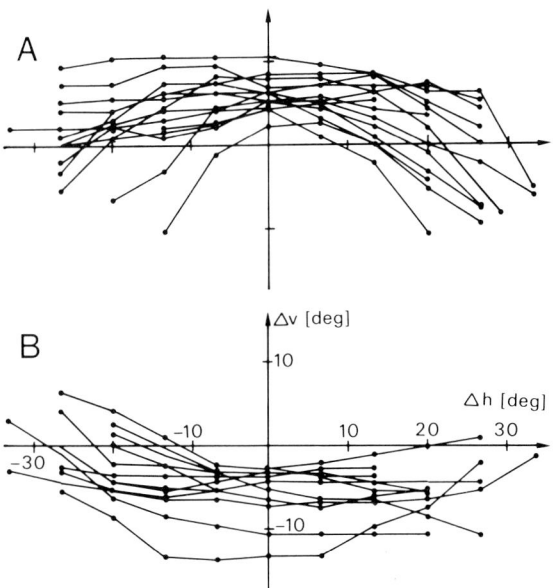

Fig. 7. Single representative iso-burst curves from medium-lead burst neurons recorded in the rostral iMLF from one monkey. Note the complex firing pattern of single units, although the average on-direction in A would be straight up, and in B straight down.

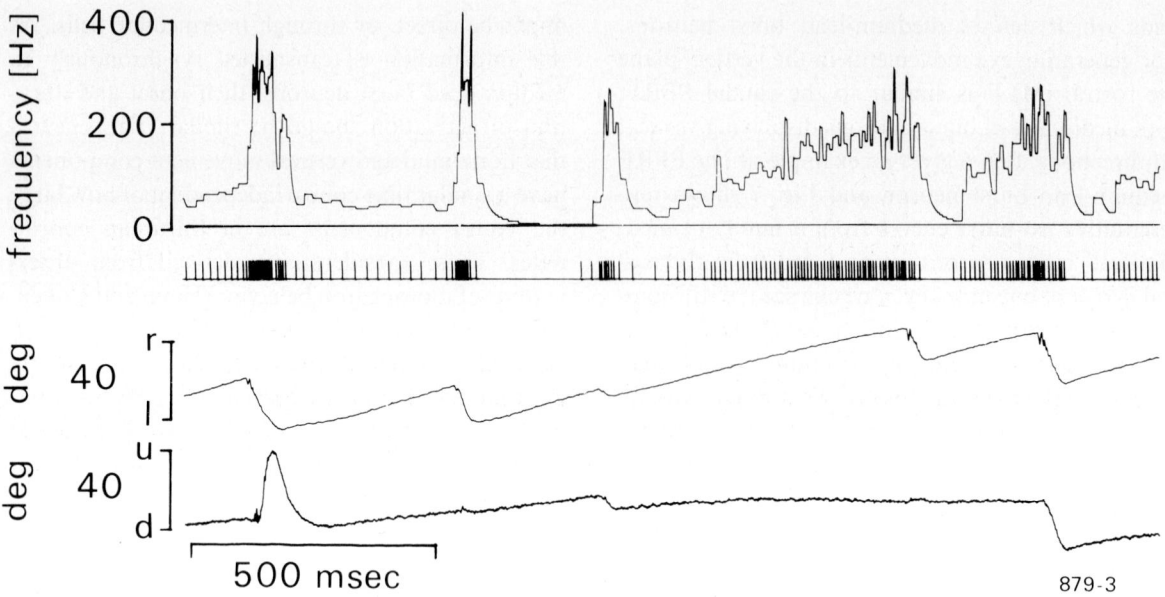

Fig. 8. Neuron recorded in the cerebellar nuclei. From above, instantaneous spike frequency, blips indicating occurrence of single spikes, horizontal and vertical eye position. During centrifugal rapid movements, unit activity increased, during centripetal movements into the same direction and of similar amplitude, unit activity decreased.

bining these codes and to perform corrections as necessary (Ritchie, 1976; Optican and Robinson, 1980; Hepp et al., 1982). An example of a neuron recorded from the cerebellar nuclei is given in Fig. 8. The neuron fires differently for saccades of similar size and direction, depending on whether the rapid movement is in a centripetal or centrifugal direction. The orbital mechanics are different for such movements, for which a correction signal is necessary. Further examples are discussed by Vilis and Hore (Section IV-B), who demonstrated that cooling of the cerebellar nuclei leads to a misalignment of the trajectories of the two eyes.

Oculomotor and skeletal motor systems

Movements for the extremities and eye movements have in common that muscles are activated to direct the limbs or the eyes to a particular target. For the limb the force required can vary over wide ranges and external perturbations are compensated using peripheral and central loops. For the eyes, any external perturbations of the movement are not compensated by a stretch reflex (Keller and Robinson, 1971).

The oculomotor system is highly specialized and rigid in the execution of its motor programs. The parametric elaboration of how motoneurons have to be innervated has been delegated to brainstem circuits. The main function of the FEF seems to be that it selects a visual target, remembered or present, and determines its time of occurrence. As the determination of the spatial location of a visual target seems to be also performed in the SC, a lesion of either structure alone leads to a prolonged processing time, but not to a paresis. A paresis only occurs with brainstem lesions, with the peculiarity that it can occur in one plane or even in one direction only, leaving the orthogonal plane unaffected.

Summary

Rapid eye movements are generated in two interconnected structures in the brainstem, the PPRF for horizontal movements, and the rostral iMLF for vertical movements. Their main input comes from the FEF and SC, and the output goes to extraocular motoneurons. Single unit recordings revealed several classes of neurons which could constitute the logical elements in establishing a link between FEF and SC, in which saccades are coded as a vector in spatial coordinates, to motoneurons which use a temporal code. This interpretation receives support from lesion studies in which the loss of well-defined classes of neurons leads to permanent deficits of movements.

Acknowledgement

The authors' laboratory is supported by the Swiss National Foundation for Scientific Research, grants 3.718-80 and 3.593-84.

References

Becker, W., King, W. M., Fuchs, A. F., Jürgens, R., Johanson, G. and Kornhuber, H. H. (1981) Accuracy of goal-directed saccades and mechanisms of error correction. In A. L. Fuchs and W. Becker (Eds.), Progress in Oculomotor Research, Elsevier/North-Holland, New York, pp. 29–37.

Bender, M. B. and Shanzer, S. (1964) Oculomotor pathways defined by electric stimulation and lesions in the brainstem of the monkey. In M. B. Bender (Ed.), The Oculomotor System, Harper and Row, New York, pp. 81–140.

Büttner, U., Büttner-Ennever, J. A. and Henn, V. (1977) Vertical eye movement related activity in the rostral mesencephalic reticular formation of the alert monkey. Brain Res., 130: 239–252.

Büttner-Ennever, J. A. and Büttner, U. (1978) A cell group associated with vertical eye movements in the rostral reticular formation of the monkey. Brain Res., 151: 31–47.

Cohen, B., Komatsuzaki, A. and Bender, M. B. (1968) Electrooculographic syndrome in monkeys after pontine reticular formation lesions. Arch. Neurol., 18: 78–92.

Collins, C. C., O'Meara, D. and Scott, A. B. (1975) Muscle tension during unrestrained human eye movements. J. Physiol. (Lond.), 245: 351–369.

Goldberg, M. E. and Bushnell, M. C. (1981) Behavioral enhancement of visual responses in monkey cerebral cortex. II. Modulation in frontal eye fields specifically related to saccades. J. Neurophysiol., 46: 773–787.

Harting, J. K. (1977) Descending pathways from the superior colliculus: an autoradiographic analysis in the rhesus monkey (*Macaca mulatta*). J. Comp. Neurol., 173: 583–612.

Henn, V. and Cohen, B. (1973) Quantitative analysis of activity in eye muscle motoneurons during saccadic eye movements and positions of fixation. J. Neurophysiol., 36: 115–126.

Henn, V., Büttner-Ennever, J. A. and Hepp, K. (1982a) The primate oculomotor system. I. Motoneurons — a synthesis of anatomical, physiological, and clinical data. Human Neurobiol., 1: 77–85.

Henn, V., Hepp, K. and Büttner-Ennever, J. A. (1982b) The primate oculomotor system. II. Premotor system — a synthesis of anatomical, physiological, and clinical data. Human Neurobiol. 1: 87–95.

Henn, V., Baloh, R. W. and Hepp, K. (1984a) The sleep-wake transition in the oculomotor system. Exp. Brain Res., 54: 166–176.

Henn, V., Lang, W., Hepp, K. and Reisine, H. (1984b) Experimental gaze palsies in monkeys and their relation to human pathology. Brain, 107: 619–636.

Hepp, K., Henn, V. and Jaeger, J. (1982) Eye movement-related neurons in the cerebellar nuclei of the alert monkey. Exp. Brain. Res. 45: 253–261.

Hepp, K. and Henn, V. (1983a) Spatio-temporal recoding of rapid eye movement signals in the monkey paramedian pontine reticular formation. Exp. Brain Res., 52: 105–120.

Hepp, K. and Henn, V. (1983b) Neurodynamics of the oculomotor system: space-time recoding and a non-equilibrium phase transition. In E. Basar, H. Flohr, H. Haken and A. J. Mandell (Eds.), Synergetics of the Brain, Springer, New York, pp. 139–154.

Keller, E. L. (1980) Oculomotor specificity within subdivisions of the brain stem reticular formation. In J. A. Hobson and M. A. B. Brazier (Eds.), The Reticular Formation Revisited, Raven Press, New York, pp. 227–240.

Keller, E. L. and Robinson, D. A. (1971) Absence of a stretch reflex in extraocular muscles of the monkey. J. Neurophysiol. 34: 908–919.

Leichnetz, G. R. (1981) The prefrontal cortico-oculomotor trajectories in the monkey. J. Neurol. Sci., 49: 387–396.

Optican, L. M. and Robinson, D. A. (1980) Cerebellar-dependent adaptive control of primate saccadic system. J. Neurophysiol., 44: 1058–1076.

Ritchie, L. (1976) Effects of cerebellar lesions on saccadic eye movements. J. Neurophysiol., 39: 1246–1256.

Robinson, D. A. (1964) The mechanics of human saccadic eye movement. J. Physiol. (Lond.), 174: 245–264.

Schiller, P. H. and Stryker, M. P. (1972) Single-unit recording and stimulation in superior colliculus of the alert Rhesus monkey. J. Neurophysiol., 35: 915–924.

Schiller, P., True, S. D. and Conway, J. L. (1980) Deficits in eye movements following frontal eye-field and superior colliculus ablations. J. Neurophysiol., 44: 1175–1189.

Schnyder, H., Reisine, H., Hepp, K. and Henn, V. (1985) Frontal eye field projection to the paramedian pontine reticular formation traced with wheat germ agglutinin in the monkey. Brain Res, 329: 151–160.

Shimazu, H. (1983) Neuronal organization of the premotor system controlling horizontal conjugate eye movements and vestibular nystagmus. In J. E. Desmedt (Ed.), Motor Control

Mechanisms in Health and Disease, Raven Press, New York, pp. 565–588.

Sparks, D. L. and Porter, J. D. (1983) The spatial localization of saccade targets. II. Activity of superior colliculus neurons preceding compensatory saccades. J. Neurophysiol., 49: 64–74.

Van Gisbergen, J. A. M., Van Opstal, A. J. and Schoemakers, J. J. M. (1985) Experimental test of two models for the generation of oblique saccades. Exp. Brain Res., 57: 321–336.

Wurtz, R. H. and Albano, J. E. (1980) Visual-motor function of the primate superior colliculus. Annu. Rev. Neurosci., 3: 189–226.

Smooth pursuit eye movements

R. Eckmiller and E. Bauswein

Division of Biocybernetics, Department of Biophysics, University of Düsseldorf, D-4000 Düsseldorf, F.R.G.

Introduction

Fixation of a visual target requires an initial aiming movement of the eye to center the target projection on the fovea, and a subsequent stabilization process. The precision of this centering and stabilization process can be described by the size of the residual position error or eccentricity, r, of the target projection relative to the foveal center. If either the target or the head, or both, move, smooth pursuit eye movements serve to continuously maintain vision of the target as occurs during fixation. Again, the position error r indicates how well maintenance of vision is achieved.

Smooth pursuit eye movements incorporate at least three well-known types of eye movements: (1) Foveal pursuit, with the goal of keeping the visual projection of a small moving target continuously on the center of the fovea, as first described by Dodge (1903). (2) Schau-nystagmus (look nystagmus), as described by Ter Braak (1936). In this case the subject deliberately "fixates" an object as part of the visual world which is moving relative to the unaccelerated head. (3) Compensatory eye movements, which are known as vestibulo-ocular reflex (VOR) in the light. They manifest the attempt to "fixate" a stationary target while the head performs rotatory or translatory movements. The largest contribution to the neural control of these compensatory eye movements is presumably of pure vestibular origin and can be estimated as the vestibulo-ocular reflex in the dark.

Various types of special pursuit eye movement can only be induced under certain laboratory conditions. They range from pursuit of an imagined swinging pendulum in the dark, via pursuit of a perceptually completed contour that was extrapolated from peripheral retinal information (Steinbach, 1976), to Sigma-pursuit movements on the basis of a stroboscopically illuminated stationary stimulus pattern (Behrens and Grüsser, 1978). Other types of smooth eye movement, although occurring involuntarily as a result of visual or vestibular stimulation, can hardly be called pursuit movements, since they are insufficient to maintain clear vision of moving objects. An example is Stier-Nystagmus (Ter Braak, 1936), which leaves vision rather blurred due to considerable retinal slip movements. Some types of smooth eye movements, such as the vestibulo-ocular reflex in the dark or the optokinetic afternystagmus, do not serve vision at all.

There is no reason to assume that all of the types of pursuit eye movements mentioned above, let alone smooth eye movements, are controlled by identical neural mechanisms.

The scope of this paper will be confined to a discussion of foveal pursuit during purely visual and combined visual-vestibular stimulus paradigms.

Foveal pursuit eye movements require well-defined stimulus conditions, in particular with regard to the following parameters: (1) Adaptation level: the pursuing eye should be adapted to a luminance in the upper part of the mesopic range (10^{-3}–5 cd/m^2; Le Grand, 1972) or in the photopic range (above 5 cd/m^2) in order to keep the foveal part of the retina in its physiological range of operation. During dark adaptation (luminance below 10^{-3} cd/m²) the fovea is functionally blind. The crucial dependence of foveal pursuit versus extrafoveal pursuit performance on the adaptation level has been well documented (Wheeless et al., 1967; Winterson and Steinman, 1978). Those many behavioral pursuit experiments which have been carried out during dark adaptation do not allow conclusions concerning foveal pursuit and the importance of position error minimization to be drawn. (2) Target size: The target should be small, to reduce the probability that the line of gaze switches between various parts of the target contour, but large enough to assure good visibility throughout the macula; a good size is about 1-10 minutes of arc in diameter. (3) Contrast: A moderate contrast between target and a homogeneous background assures that the subject actually sees the target with its color and contours rather than being blinded by it. At 1 cd/m² background luminance the contrast threshold, $\Delta L/L$, for small targets (diameter below 0.5°) ranges from about 10^{-2} to 1. (4) Target movement: A continuous movement time course of the target between about 10° left and right of center allows the experimenter to study not only the initiation of foveal pursuit but also its maintenance over several minutes, if the stimulus velocity and acceleration ranges are sufficiently small to allow the pursuit system, with its considerable time delay, to react to unpredicted changes of the target trajectory. In contrast, step-ramp time courses and triangular time courses, both of which imply very high acceleration values at each turning point, restrict the analysis to the initiation of foveal pursuit, since pursuit necessarily becomes interrupted soon after its initiation.

Contribution of cerebellum and brain stem to the control of foveal pursuit

The pursuit system is highly dependent on an intact cerebellum (particularly flocculus, paraflocculus and vermis), as revealed by numerous clinical observations as well as by lesion studies (Westheimer and Blair, 1974; Zee et al., 1981) and single unit studies in primates (Kase et al., 1979; Lisberger and Fuchs, 1978; Miles et al., 1980; Noda and Suzuki, 1979; Suzuki et al., 1981). However, extensive neonatal cerebellar ablations can be compensated as long as the cerebellar nuclei have been spared from the lesion (Eckmiller and Westheimer, 1983; Eckmiller et al., 1984). The flocculus received special attention since many of its Purkinje cells exhibit the dynamic activity pattern of gaze velocity neurons, in that they are modulated in phase with eye velocity during smooth pursuit (with head stationary) but in phase with head velocity during VOR suppression. Little or no modulation occurs during the VOR (light) paradigm. However, a qualitatively similar activity pattern has been found in presumed mossy fibers in the granular layer (Miles et al., 1980) and even in identified mossy fibers (Noda, personal communication). These findings support the hypothesis that the flocculus monitors and perhaps modifies, rather than generates, the neural control signal for pursuit eye velocity. Several recent neuroanatomical studies in rats (Blanks et al., 1983) and monkeys (Langer and Kaneko, 1984) demonstrated by retrograde transport of horseradish peroxidase (HRP) that a substantial number of afferent neurons to the flocculus are located just rostral and dorsal to the abducens nucleus (see also Results).

In the brain stem there are several classes of presumed pre-motor neurons which are specifically active during pursuit eye movements but exhibit only a low correlation, if any, with saccades or fixation. Two recent reports (Chubb and Fuchs, 1982; Tomlinson and Robinson, 1984) described pursuit-related neurons in the Y group of the vestibular nuclear complex whose activity was modulated in phase with upward eye velocity. Their dynamic properties resembled those of gaze velocity neurons in the flocculus. However, neurons with comparable dynamic properties for downward, left- or rightward pursuit movements have not been found in the vestibular nuclear complex, which is thought to be the main target for Purkinje cells from the flocculus.

Just ventral to the VIth nerve nucleus a class of velocity-sensitive pursuit neurons was found by the author (Eckmiller and Mackeben, 1980). The neural activity of these pursuit neurons was correlated with horizontal eye velocity in the direction ipsilateral to the recording site during the smooth pursuit paradigm, but showed little or no modulation in phase with head velocity during VOR (light). The following results present a detailed analysis of the dynamic activity pattern of these pursuit neurons and of another class of pursuit-related neurons (eye velocity neurons) in the vicinity of the VIth nerve nuclei during the three standard stimulation paradigms: smooth pursuit, VOR (light), and VOR suppression in the trained Java monkey.

Methods

This study is based on data from three monkeys (*Macaca fascicularis*) ranging from 2.5 to 4 kg in body weight. The monkeys had been trained (for details of training and recording procedures, see Eckmiller and Mackeben, 1978) to pursue a visual target (8 minutes of arc in diameter; target luminance: 1.9 cd/m^2) against a homogeneous background (1 cd/m^2) under three conditions: (a) Smooth pursuit: foveal pursuit eye movements during sinusoidal target movement (10° amplitude at frequencies between 0.3 and 1.3 Hz); (b) VOR (light): pursuit of a stationary target during head rotation (chair rotation about the vertical axis) with the same amplitude and frequency range as in (a); and (c) VOR suppression: fixation of the target which moved with the sinusoidally rotating chair.

While under barbiturate anesthesia, the monkeys were implanted with a headgear for the rigid attachment of the head to the upper portion of the primate chair, and a lucite chamber over a trephine hole in the vertex of the skull. During implantation, the headgear position was calibrated to assure that the stereotaxic horizontal plane of the head was kept exactly perpendicular to the gravity vector in the primate chair.

Eye movements were measured in two monkeys with implanted Ag/AgCl electrodes and in one monkey with an infrared oculometer (Bouis, Karlsruhe, see Bach et al., 1983).

The precise location of recording sites in the vicinity of the VIth nerve nuclei was reconstructed from stereotaxic coordinates of electrode tracks perpendicular to the horizontal plane and histologically verified by means of small electrolytic lesions. Histology was performed on serial sections of the Celloidin-embedded brain following perfusion under deep barbiturate anesthesia.

Results*

Pursuit neurons

Single unit activity of 41 pursuit neurons, which were located either ventral to the VIth nerve nucleus, as previously described (Eckmiller and Mackeben, 1980), or at the dorsal rim of the VIth nerve nucleus was analyzed at various frequencies during the three paradigms already described (see Methods).

Typical recordings of a pursuit neuron are displayed in Fig. 1 during both visual (smooth pursuit), and visual plus vestibular (VOR (light), VOR suppression) stimulation at 0.7 Hz. This neuron, D21-476, was recorded just ventral to the left VIth nerve nucleus and demonstrates our general finding that pursuit neurons are modulated about in phase with eye velocity ipsilateral to the recording site during smooth pursuit. During VOR (light) the peak-to-peak modulation of the impulse rate clearly is reduced. In fact, many other pursuit neurons showed no modulation at all during this paradigm. This reduced modulation typically occurred about in phase with contralateral eye velocity (ipsilateral head velocity). During VOR suppression, which is often less than perfectly achieved, the impulse rate modulation is clearly larger than during smooth pursuit; however, it is about in phase with head velocity ipsilateral to the recording site.

The frequency dependence of both peak-to-peak

---

* Preliminary results have already been reported (Eckmiller and Bauswein, 1984).

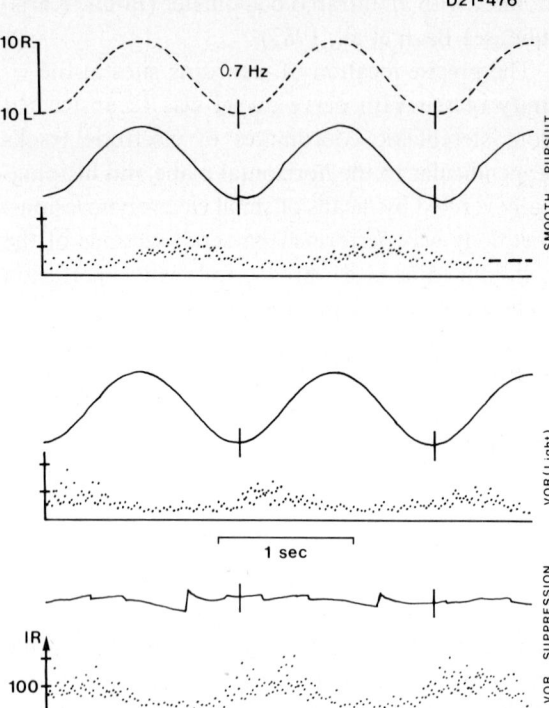

Fig. 1. Three recording episodes of a pursuit neuron located ventral to the left VIth nerve nucleus. Top trace (broken line): movement time course of the target in the horizontal plane between 10° right (10R) and 10° left (10L) at a distance of 1.5 m during smooth pursuit at 0.7 Hz; the same time course refers to chair rotation about the vertical axis (10R and 10L reversed) during VOR (light) and VOR suppression. Continuous traces above the IR(*t*) diagrams give horizontal eye movement of the left eye measured as EOG. Diagrams with dotted values: instantaneous impulse rate IR(*t*) in impulses per second for the three paradigms.

modulation and phase re. velocity for four pursuit neurons is plotted in Fig. 2. Two of them (D21-476 (see Fig. 1) and D21-831) were located ventral to the left VIth nerve nucleus whereas the other two neurons were located at the dorsal rim of the right VIth nerve nucleus.

The left diagram in Fig. 2 gives linear regression lines of peak-to-peak modulation of the impulse rate, indicating that the modulation typically was larger during VOR suppression than during smooth pursuit at a given frequency. The pair of phase plots in Fig. 2 indicates the dramatic phase shift (of about 180°) from ipsilateral eye velocity during smooth pursuit to ipsilateral head velocity during VOR suppression. Each data point is the average of five measurement values at different movement cycles. Please note the wide range of phase values for individual pursuit neurons between about 30° lead and 30° lag relative to velocity.

Only some of the pursuit neurons exhibited a measurable modulation during the VOR (light) paradigm, as indicated in both diagrams by the open symbols for two neurons (D21-476 and D21-831).

Eye velocity neurons

This newly identified class of pre-motor neurons has a dynamic activity pattern quite different from that of pursuit neurons. These differences are not necessarily significant during smooth pursuit but they become very clear during the VOR (light) and VOR suppression paradigms. Single unit activity of 34 eye velocity neurons located dorsal to the VIth nerve nucleus was analyzed at various frequencies during the three stimulus paradigms.

A typical recording of an eye velocity neuron is shown in Fig. 3. This neuron, D30-650, was located at the dorsal border of the right VIth nerve nucleus as histologically verified by means of a small electrolytic lesion at the recording site. The two upper sets of traces in Fig. 3 exemplify our general finding that eye velocity neurons were modulated in phase with eye velocity with similar modulation depth and in the same direction during both smooth pursuit and VOR (light). As a rule no measurable modulation was found during episodes of VOR suppression (not shown here). At variance with pursuit neurons, some eye velocity neurons were modulated in phase with eye velocity ipsilateral to the recording site (ipsilateral eye velocity) whereas others were modulated in phase with contralateral eye velocity. The bottom set of traces, recorded during a very unattentive smooth pursuit episode at 0.2 Hz, indicates very little eye position sensitivity during the 20° saccade to the left. The impulse rate is clearly increased during the episode of sloppy pursuit for the last third of this recording. Note, however, the

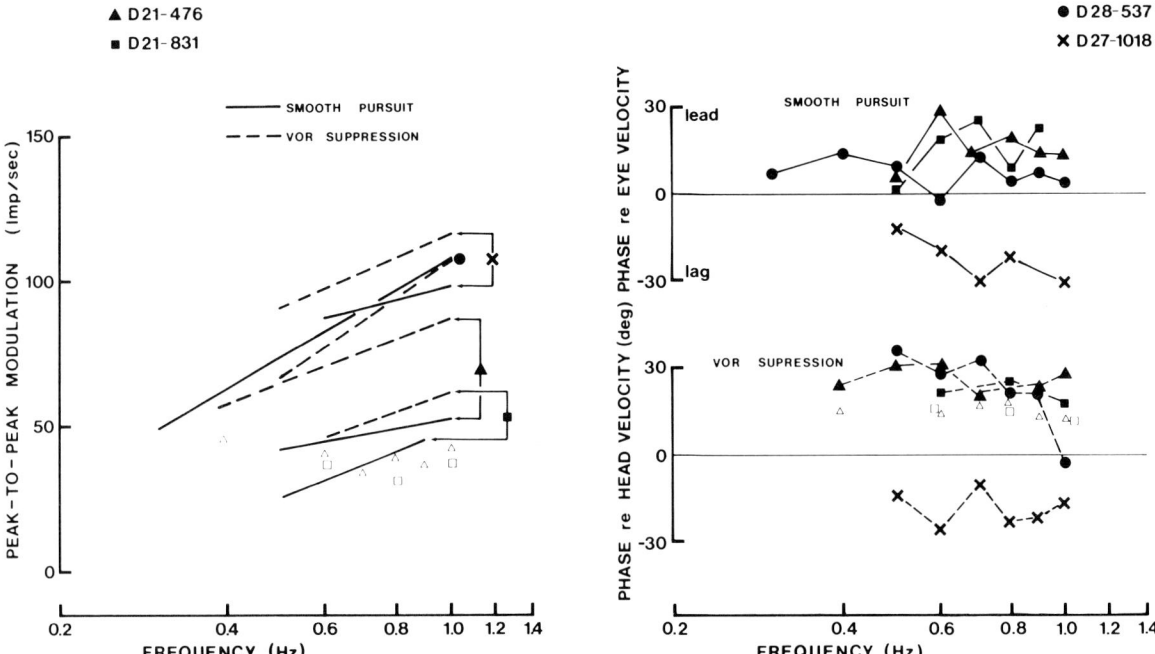

Fig. 2. Modulation and phase re. velocity of pursuit neurons as a function of stimulus frequency. The left diagram gives pairs of linear regression lines (continuous for smooth pursuit and interrupted for VOR suppression). Measurement values and regression lines of four pursuit neurons are distinguished by different symbols (triangle, square, circle, cross). The open symbols (triangle, square) in both diagrams indicate that these two pursuit neurons were also modulated during VOR (light).

brief impulse rate bursts for saccades to the left.

For four eye velocity neurons peak-to-peak modulation as well as phase re. eye velocity as a function of stimulus movement frequency are plotted in Fig. 4. With locations at the dorsal border of one of the VIth nerve nuclei, two of these neurons (D26-1755 and D26-1858) showed a modulation in phase with ipsilateral eye velocity whereas the other two neurons (D30-650 (see Fig. 3) and D32-382) were modulated in phase with contralateral eye velocity.

The modulation vs. frequency diagram indicates only small differences between the linear regression lines for smooth pursuit as compared with VOR (light). The two phase vs. frequency diagrams on the right half of Fig. 4 demonstrate that the phase values are rather close to eye velocity and show only little frequency dependence during both paradigms.

Fig. 5 summarizes the dynamic characteristics of a typical pursuit neuron and eye velocity neuron as compared with a typical second order vestibular neuron and an oculomotor motoneuron, for all three stimulus paradigms.

During smooth pursuit in the left section, the time courses of the target θ_t and of the left eye θ_e are nicely superimposed, while head position (θ_h) is constant. Accordingly, both the pursuit neuron and the eye velocity neuron are about in phase with eye velocity to the left. As a result of a postulated neural integrator, the impulse rate of the left lateral rectus motoneuron leads eye position to the left by about 20–30° at 0.7 Hz (Eckmiller and Mackeben, 1978), just enough to account for the mechanical lag of the orbit plant. During VOR (light) in the middle section, the modulation of the pursuit neuron is considerably reduced or even absent, whereas a strong modulation of the vestibular neuron occurs. As a result (according to our hypothesis), both the eye velocity neuron and the motoneuron show virtually the same modulation as during smooth pursuit. The neural events during VOR suppression

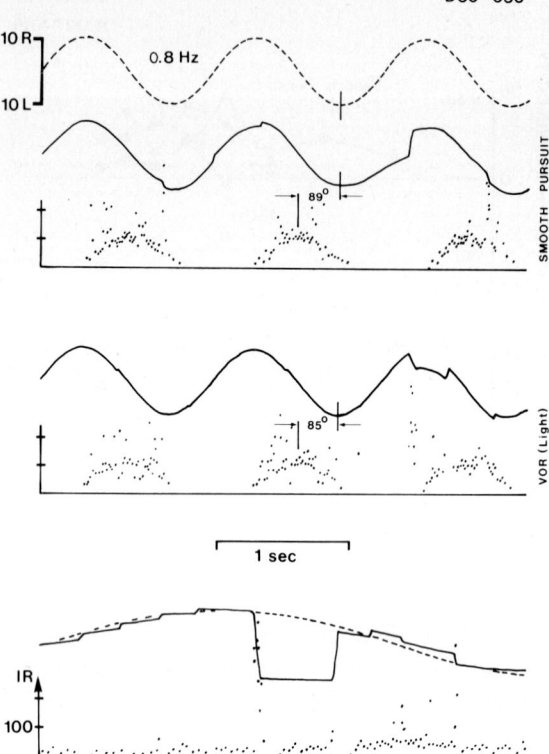

Fig. 3. Three recording episodes of an eye velocity neuron with a histologically verified location at the dorsal border of the right VIth nerve nucleus. Top trace (broken line): movement time course of the small target between 10° right (10R) and 10° left (10L) during smooth pursuit at 0.8 Hz, or chair position (10R and 10L reversed) during VOR (light). Diagrams with dotted values: instantaneous impulse rate, IR(t), in impulses per second. Continuous traces above the IR(t) diagrams: corresponding horizontal eye movement of the right eye measured with infrared oculometer. The lower recording belongs to an inattentive episode of smooth pursuit at 0.2 Hz (broken line gives target movement).

are summarized in the right section of Fig. 5. The data are compatible with the hypothesis that the pursuit neuron neutralizes the big vestibular modulation by generating an equivalent signal about 180° out of phase. According to this hypothesis, as indicated by the scheme in Fig. 5, the eye velocity neuron summates the activity of both the pursuit neuron and the vestibular neuron and feeds into the neural integration stage.

Discussion

Our findings demonstrate for the first time the existence of two classes of pre-motor neurons in the immediate vicinity of the VIth nerve nuclei which could serve to supply the oculomotor motoneurons with the necessary eye velocity signal for the control of pursuit eye movements. According to our hypothesis, the activity of pursuit neurons, which is quite similar to that of gaze velocity neurons at the input and output of the flocculus (see Introduction), assures foveal pursuit during the various paradigms with or without additional vestibular stimulation. Both neurophysiological and histological studies (see Introduction) are compatible with the hypothesis that pursuit neurons also project to the ipsilateral flocculus. Eye velocity neurons, which have not been described in the flocculus or elsewhere in the cerebellum, are the best candidates available to represent the eye velocity signal as input for the neural integration stage. This eye velocity signal possibly represents the algebraic sum of the two competing velocity signals from vestibular neurons and pursuit neurons (Fig. 5).

Comparison between oculomotor and skeletomotor pursuit systems

Various skeletomotor systems, e.g., for head or arm movements, successfully solve complex pursuit (or tracking) tasks. For example, the moving target to be pursued by the hand can be a visual object (even without visual feedback of the hand position), a sound source in the dark, or a moving tactile stimulus. Despite the existence of numerous important differences between oculomotor and skeletomotor systems, such as load compensation, multi-joint movements, or varying participation of a given muscle as co-agonist or antagonist (Freund, 1983), there probably exist many similarities in the neural strategies involved in pursuit of a moving object.

In principle, any given pursuit task requires the monitoring of the trajectory of the moving aim in space by means of one or several sense organs, and the generation of the appropriate neural control

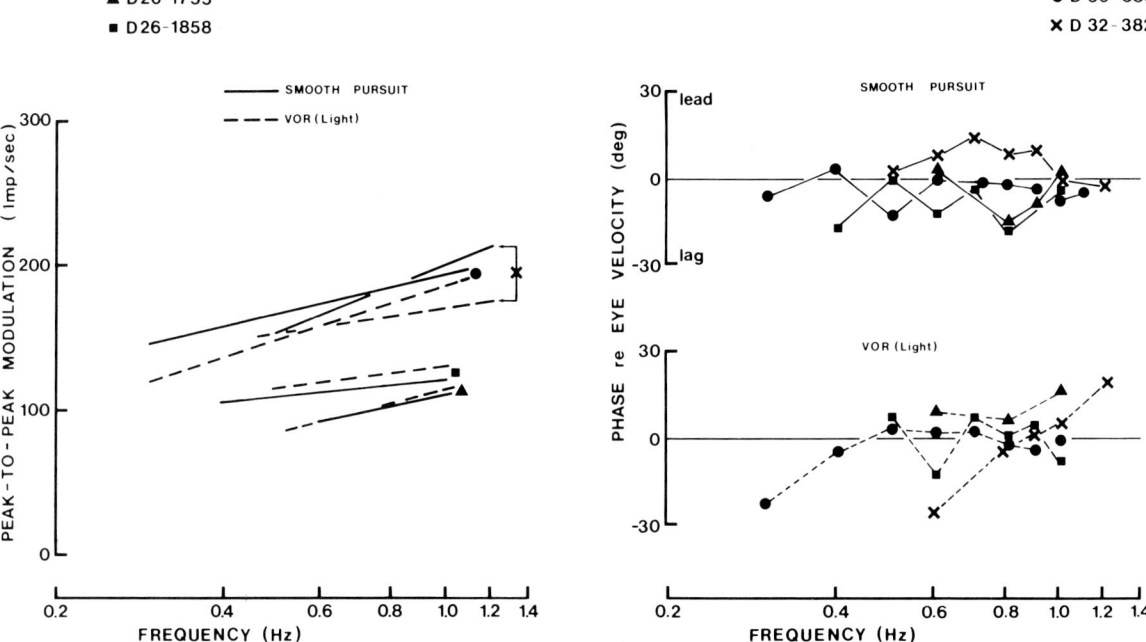

Fig. 4. Modulation and phase re. eye velocity of eye velocity neurons as a function of stimulus frequency. The left diagram gives pairs of linear regression lines (continuous for smooth pursuit and interrupted for VOR (light)). Measurement values and regression lines of four eye velocity neurons are distinguished by different symbols (triangle, square, circle, cross).

signals for the desired pursuit (eye, head or limb) movement. The goal of any pursuit system is to match (or at least approximate) the trajectory of the moved eye, head or limb with that of the moving target.

A general scheme for the foveal pursuit system has been proposed recently (Eckmiller, 1983) which may also partially apply to certain skeletomotor systems. Its main components are arranged into a sequence of three stages for: (1) spatio-temporal translation (STT), (2) motor-program generation (MPG) and (3) neural integration. The concept of STT for the control of movements was put forward initially to assign a functional role to the unique architecture of the cerebellar cortex (Braitenberg and Atwood, 1958) and was elaborated further and applied to the control of both eye and arm movements (Kornhuber, 1971; Robinson, 1973). The necessary task of STT is to turn the spatial coordinate values of the target position into a neural signal in the temporal domain so as to assure the appropriate pursuit movement.

In higher vertebrates many movements are controlled by internally generated motor programs which do not necessarily require, but can be guided and up-dated by, sensory information (Miles and Evarts, 1979; Tatton and Bruce, 1981). Very little is known about the neural realization of these different MPGs which generate time courses of neural activity to control voluntary or especially pursuit movements. Foveal pursuit probably requires a pair of MPGs in order to generate eye velocity signals to the left and right, respectively (Eckmiller, 1983). We assume that the activity of pursuit neurons represents the output signal of these MPGs. It is noteworthy in this context that trained monkeys (similar to humans) perform smooth post-pursuit eye movements for more than 1 second (Eckmiller and Mackeben, 1978) after sudden target disappearance during foveal pursuit. Pursuit neurons

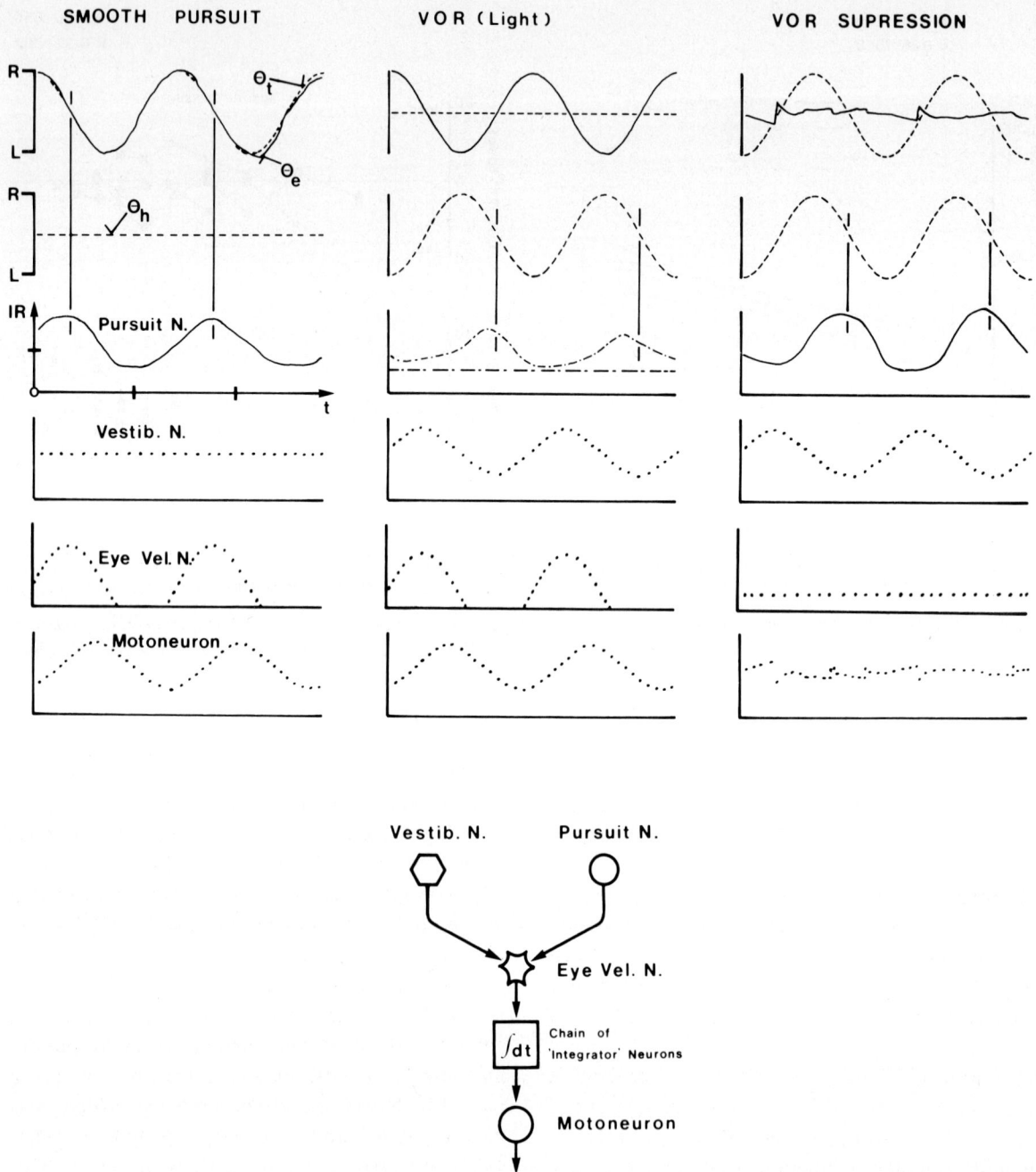

Fig. 5. Summary scheme of the dynamic properties of typical pursuit neurons and eye velocity neurons during the stimulus paradigms: smooth pursuit, VOR (light) and VOR suppression. Traces, from top to bottom: target position, θ_t, and eye position, θ_e; head position, θ_h; impulse rate of pursuit neuron: note that during VOR (light) some pursuit neurons show no modulation (straight line) whereas others are slightly modulated with ipsilateral head velocity; impulse rate of vestibular neuron as part of the vestibulo-ocular reflex; impulse rate of eye velocity neuron; impulse rate of oculomotor motoneuron. The wiring diagram below the summary scheme indicates a hypothesis of possible connections between vestibular neuron, pursuit neuron, eye velocity neuron, and a neural integrator.

continue being modulated with eye velocity during these post-pursuit episodes (Eckmiller and Mackeben, 1980) which resemble the most recent pursuit time course.

The basic arrangement that an internally generated (MPG) eye velocity signal gets transformed by means of a neural integrator into the required eye position signal (with an additional eye velocity component) at the motoneuronal level is well established for the various oculomotor subsystems, but remains doubtful for skeletomotor systems. Interestingly, however, the first evidence and possible explanations for the existence of neural integration came from the work of various skeletomotor physiologists (Ranson and Hinsey, 1930, with further references to Forbes and Sherrington), which led to the formulation of their "theory of reverberating circuits" before Lorente de Nó (1933) and much later Robinson (1971) applied the concept of a neural integrator to the oculomotor system.

In principle, a movement (of eye or limb) from an initial position in space P_1 to a desired position P_2 can be encoded in the CNS by means of a neural movement signal (MS) or a position signal (PS). MS is a velocity time course $\dot{P}(t)$ for a given time interval between t_1 and t_2 which will theoretically lead to the desired position change from P_1 to P_2 as a result of neural integration.

$$P_2 = P_1 + \int_{t_1}^{t_2} \dot{P}(t)\, dt$$

This encoding principle would have several advantages: (a) the tonic neural position signal to hold the new position P_2 is generated simply by integration. (b) MS can be a rather simple signal with a small information content. MS is almost independent of the absolute initial or final position values, because it encodes only the relative position change P_2-P_1. This feature makes it particularly easy to encode a movement (e.g., a foveating saccade) without the need to consider the absolute position of the reference coordinate system (e.g., eye and head location in space).

In contrast, the use of a neural position signal PS for encoding the desired position P_2 would demand an enormous amount of processing in order to keep track of the coordinates in the various coordinate systems which move relative to each other (e.g., head relative to trunk). In effect, PS only defines "where to move to" without specifying "how to get there". However, such a system could do without a neural integrator.

Further studies on skeletomotor control systems will show whether or not, and if so how, movements can be generated without neural integration close to the motoneurons. There is a good chance, however, that the oculomotor system in this regard will serve as a model for many skeletomotor systems.

Summary

Smooth pursuit eye movements serve continuously to maintain vision of a target (as during fixation) while either the target, and/or the head are in motion. The goal of the foveal pursuit system (in the mesopic or photopic range) in primates is to minimize the position error of the target projection relative to the foveal center.

Two classes of pursuit-related neurons (pursuit neurons and eye velocity neurons) were studied in three Java monkeys which had been trained to pursue a small visual target during three standard stimulus paradigms: (a) smooth pursuit, (b) VOR (light), and (c) VOR suppression.

Pursuit neurons (located ventral to, and occasionally also at the dorsal border of, the VIth nerve nuclei) were modulated about in phase with eye velocity ipsilateral to the recording site only during paradigm (a). During (b), their modulation was considerably reduced or completely absent. During (c), their modulation was typically larger than during (a) but occurred with a slight phase lead re. ipsilateral head velocity. These dynamic properties of pursuit neurons are quite similar to those of gaze velocity neurons at the input and output of the flocculus.

Eye velocity neurons (located at the dorsal border of the VIth nerve nuclei) were modulated in phase with eye velocity during both paradigms (a) and (b). No modulation occurred during (c).

These findings are compatible with the hypothesis that during foveal pursuit, eye velocity neurons receive competing eye velocity signals from pursuit neurons and vestibular neurons, and feed the resultant sum into a neural integration stage in order to generate the neural control signal for the oculomotor motoneurons. Comparable neurophysiological studies on skeletomotor pursuit systems are not available at present.

Acknowledgements

This work was supported by the Deutsche Forschungsgemeinschaft, SFB 200/A1. The technical assistance of Elke Jaworski and Anneliese Thelen for various procedures of histology, animal training, and neurophysiology is gratefully acknowledged.

References

Bach, M., Bouis, D. and Fischer, B. (1983) An accurate and linear infrared oculomotor. J. Neurosci. Methods, 9: 9–14.

Behrens, F. and Grüsser, O.-J. (1978) Movement perception and eye movements elicited by stationary visual patterns illuminated by intermittent flashes. In G. Kommerell (Ed.), Disorders of Ocular Motility, Bergmann, München, pp. 273–283.

Blanks, R. H. I., Precht, W. and Torigoe, Y. (1983) Afferent projections to the cerebellar flocculus in the pigmented rat demonstrated by retrograde transport of horseradish peroxidase. Exp. Brain Res., 52: 293–306.

Braitenberg, V., and Atwood, R. P. (1958) Morphological observations on the cerebellar cortex. J. Comp. Neurol., 109: 1–27.

Chubb, M. C. and Fuchs, A. F. (1982) Contribution of y group of vestibular nuclei and dentate nucleus of cerebellum to generation of vertical smooth eye movements. J. Neurophysiol., 48: 75–99.

Dodge, R. (1903) Five types of eye movement in the horizontal meridian plane of the field of regard. Am. J. Physiol., 8: 307–329.

Eckmiller, R. (1983) Neural control of foveal pursuit versus saccadic eye movements in primates — Single unit data and models. IEEE Trans. SMC, 13: 980–989.

Eckmiller, R. and Bauswein, E. (1984) Activity of pursuit neurons and eye velocity neurons in primate brain stem during foveal pursuit versus OKN. Soc. Neurosci. Abstr., 10: 391.

Eckmiller, R. and Mackeben, M. (1978) Pursuit eye movements and their neural control in the monkey. Pflügers Arch., 377: 15–23.

Eckmiller, R. and Mackeben, M. (1980) Pre-motor single unit activity in the monkey brain stem correlated with eye velocity during pursuit. Brain Res., 184: 210–214.

Eckmiller, R. and Westheimer, G. (1983) Compensation of oculomotor deficits in monkeys with neonatal cerebellar ablations. Exp. Brain Res., 49: 315–326.

Eckmiller, R., Meisami, E. and Westheimer, G. (1984) Neuroanatomical status of monkeys showing functional compensation following neonatal cerebellar lesions. Exp. Brain Res., 56: 59–71.

Freund, H.-J. (1983) Motor unit and muscle activity in voluntary motor control. Physiol. Rev., 63: 387–436.

Kase, M., Noda, H., Suzuki, D. A. and Miller, D. C. (1979) Target velocity signals of visual tracking in vermal Purkinje cells of the monkey. Science, 205: 717–720.

Kornhuber, H. H. (1971) Motor functions of cerebellum and basal ganglia: the cerebellocortical saccadic (ballistic) clock, the cerebellonuclear hold regulator, and the basal ganglia ramp (voluntary speed smooth movement) generator. Kybernetik, 8: 157–162.

Langer, T. P. and Kaneko, C. R. S. (1984) Brainstem afferents to the abducens nucleus in the monkey. Soc. Neurosci. Abstr., 10: 987.

Le Grand, Y. (1972) Spectral luminosity. In D. Jameson and L. M. Hurvich (Eds.), Handbook of Sensory Physiology, Vol. VII, Springer, Berlin, pp. 413–433.

Lisberger, S. G. and Fuchs, A. F. (1978) Role of primate flocculus during rapid behavioral modification of vestibulo-ocular reflex. I. Purkinje cell activity during visually guided horizontal smooth-pursuit eye movements and passive head rotation. J. Neurophysiol., 41: 733–763.

Lorente de Nó, R. (1933) Vestibulo-ocular reflex arc. Arch. Neurol. Psychiat., 30: 245–291.

Miles, F. A. and Evarts, E. V. (1979) Concepts of motor organization. Annu. Rev. Psychol., 30: 327–362.

Miles, F. A., Fuller, J. H., Braitman, D. J. and Dow, B. M. (1980) Long-term adaptive changes in primate vestibuloocular reflex. III. Electrophysiological observations in flocculus of normal monkeys. J. Neurophysiol., 43: 1437–1476.

Noda, H. and Suzuki, D. A. (1979) The role of the flocculus of the monkey in fixation and smooth pursuit eye movements. J. Physiol. (Lond.), 294: 335–348.

Ranson, S. W. and Hinsey, J. C. (1930) Reflexes in the hind limbs of cats after transection of the spinal cord at various levels. Am. J. Physiol., 94: 471–495.

Robinson, D. A. (1971) Models of oculomotor neural organization. In P. Bach-y-Rita, C. C. Collins and J. E. Hyde (Eds.), The Control of Eye Movements, Academic Press, New York, pp. 519–543.

Robinson, D. A. (1973) Models of the saccadic eye movement control system. Kybernetik, 14: 71–83.

Steinbach, M. J. (1976) Pursuing the perceptual rather than the

retinal stimulus. Vision Res., 16: 1371–1376.
Suzuki, D. A., Noda, H. and Kase, M. (1981) Visual and pursuit eye movement-related activity in posterior vermis of the monkey cerebellum. J. Neurophysiol., 46: 1120–1139.
Tatton, W. G. and Bruce, I. C. (1981) Comment: A scheme for the interactions between motor programs and sensory input. Can. J. Physiol. Pharmacol., 59: 691–699.
Ter Braak, J. W. G. (1936) Untersuchungen über optokinetischen Nystagmus. Arch. Neerl. Physiol., 21: 308–376.
Tomlinson, R. D. and Robinson, D. A. (1984) Signals in vestibular nucleus mediating vertical eye movements in the monkey. J. Neurophysiol., 51: 1121–1136.

Westheimer, G. and Blair, S. M. (1974) Functional organization of primate oculomotor system revealed by cerebellectomy. Exp. Brain Res., 21: 463–472.
Wheeless, L. L., Cohen, G. H. and Boynton, R. M. (1967) Luminance as a parameter of the eye-movement control system. J. Opt. Soc. Am., 57: 394–400.
Winterson, B. J. and Steinman, R. M. (1978) The effect of luminance on human smooth pursuit of perifoveal and foveal targets. Vision Res., 18: 1165–1172.
Zee, D. S., Yamazaki, A., Butler, P. H. and Gücer, G. (1981) Effects of ablation of flocculus and paraflocculus on eye movements in primate. J. Neurophysiol., 46: 878–899.

Neuronal mechanisms underlying eye-head coordination

A. Berthoz and A. Grantyn

Laboratoire de Physiologie Neurosensorielle, CNRS, 15 rue de l'Ecole de Médecine, 75270 Paris Cedex 06, France

Introduction

The study of eye-head coordination is a complex matter for several reasons. Firstly, it is well known that throughout phylogeny the development of various oculomotor subsystems, in parallel with the appearance of the fovea and the migration of the eyes from a lateral to a frontal position, has deeply modified the functional relation between eye and head (see Dieringer et al., 1983; Graf and Simpson, 1985). Secondly, the requirements of eye-head coordination may be quite different, depending on the nature of particular motor paradigms, such as grooming, shaking, eating, etc ... Two extreme types of visuo-motor strategies are encountered in all species: one is the stabilising strategy, which tends to immobilise images of the surrounding world on the retina by maintaining gaze on a fixed point in space; the other is orienting, which tends to shift the direction of gaze from one point in space to another. There exists a third strategy aiming at stabilizing the image of a continuously moving object on the retina: this behaviour is observed in foveated species only and is called pursuit.

The stabilisation of visual images on the retina is performed, as described in other chapters of this volume, by the vestibulo-ocular reflex (VOR), optokinetic nystagmus (OKN) or pursuit. But it can also be regulated automatically by other sensory motor modules such as the vestibulocollic reflex (VCR), the cervico-ocular reflex (COR), the cervico-collic reflex (CCR), whose interplay has been studied in detail by Peterson and his colleagues in recent years (Peterson and Golberg, 1982; and reviewed in Berthoz, 1985).

A basic concept for the understanding of eye-head coordination during orienting reactions has been proposed by Bizzi et al. (1971), who gave convincing evidence for central preprogramming of gaze shift in the monkey by a parallel motor command sent to both eye and head motor centres, with a peripheral regulation and recentering of eye position by the VOR. They have also identified several strategies in which the timing of eye and neck command were different. Lestienne and al. (1984) have, in addition, proposed that in the monkey some brainstem neurons would code gaze shifts and not either eye or head movements.

The interaction of stabilising and orienting strategies in the alert animal has also been extensively studied in the cat in recent years by Roucoux et al. (1980) and Guitton et al. (1980, 1984). Studies reviewed by Berthoz (1985) have also revealed that another important manifestation of eye-head coordinating mechanisms is the sensory substitution, which occurs after lesions, or during alteration, of sensory cues: it is well known that sensory cues (visual, vestibular, tactile, proprioceptive) are used by the central nervous system to constitute an internal representation of head motion in space by combining their information. Each cue differs from the other by: (a) the parameter of head motion it can measure (position, velocity, acceleration), (b) its frequency range, and (c) its geometrical characteristics. After a peripheral lesion which precludes the use of a given sensory cue, various sensory motor modules can substitute each other. For instance, the COR can take over the VOR function, but only in a limited range, due to each subsystem's dynamic properties. Consequently, all these sensory motor modules show dynamic complementarity in normal behaviour and dynamic substitution in case of malfunction.

When trying to understand the neuronal operations which underlie eye-head coordination, all these aspects have to be kept in mind and the route is still quite long, until we can unravel these mechanisms. Fortunately, modern techniques of neurobiology allow us to investigate these questions in alert animals, in which we can observe neuronal operations and relate structure to function.

The purpose of this chapter is not to enter into details of methodology which are described in other publications, but to put forward and document some facts and hypotheses obtained in our laboratory, particularly concerning one of the modules of eye-head and, potentially, eye-ear-head coordination. This module underlies a close coupling between the ponto-medullary circuits generating horizontal eye movements and those controlling the dorsal neck muscles in the cat. The result is a combined orienting movement of eye and head towards one side, and it is subserved by at least two neuronal types which have been fully identified: a certain group of ipsilateral reticulo-spinal neurons and the contralateral tecto-reticulo-spinal neurons.

Methods

The following section gives a synopsis of the methods which were used in the experiments described below. They have been described in detail by Yoshida et al. (1982), Vidal et al. (1982, 1983a,b) and Grantyn and Grantyn (1980, 1982).

Surgical procedures

Experiments were performed on adult cats. Figs. 6 and 7 show diagrammatic representations of typical experimental paradigms. The animals underwent the following surgical procedures.

(a) Coils of teflon-coated, stainless steel wire were implanted on the eyeball to measure eye movements with the search coil method. (b) Stimulating needle electrodes were placed chronically in the superior colliculus for orthodromic activation of tecto-reticulo-spinal neurons and in the spinal cord for antidromic activation of reticulo-spinal neurons. (c) Electromyographic bipolar electrodes made of teflon-coated multistrand stainless steel wires were implanted chronically in several neck muscles: splenius, longissimus capitis, obliquus capitis cranialis and caudalis. (d) A small portion of the occipital bone was removed to allow access of recording microelectrodes to the brainstem. An opening of about 5 mm in diameter was made and a funnel-shaped chamber formed with dental cement. The dura was removed and the cerebellar surface covered with silicone film (Silastic). The chamber was closed with semi-solid bone wax in between the experiments. (e) A metal platform with three bolts was cemented stereotaxically onto the skull to restrain the animal's head during recording sessions. At the same time, the tip of a hypodermic needle was fixed on the chamber close to the opening as a reference point for a stereotaxic orientation of microelectrode tracks.

Recording conditions

Following the recovery from surgical procedures, alert animals were placed in the stereotaxic apparatus with their head fixed in a 25° nose-down position in order to orient the horizontal semicircular canals in the horizontal plane. The body of the animal was gently restrained with a cloth bag and an elastic bandage. No drugs were used to modify the state of alertness. The animal together with the stereotaxic frame, micromanipulator and solenoids for the generation of magnetic fields were firmly fixed on a turntable for vestibular and/or optokinetic stimulation.

Eye movement recording was made using Skalar magnetic search coil system with a DC band-width to 200 Hz (3 dB), providing both horizontal and vertical components of eye movements in one eye. The sensitivity is 0.1 volt per degree with a resolution of about 5" of arc. Calibration of eye movements was made by rotating the field coils around the animal by steps of 5, 10 and 20°. The overall precision is about 30' of arc. The straight-ahead position was calculated by taking the centre of the oculomotor range or by making the cat track a target moving horizontally or vertically through the centre of visual field.

EMG of neck muscles was recorded and passed through a rectifier and an integrator device (5 msecond integration time constant).

Neuronal activity was recorded by means of glass microelectrodes filled with a 10% solution of horseradish peroxidase (HRP, Worthington) in 0.5 M KCl, buffered by Tris (pH 7.6). The resistance of these electrodes is in the range of 12–20 MΩ. The microelectrodes penetrated the brainstem through the intact cerebellum and allowed intra-axonic recording and HRP injections. Only neurons which were activated monosynaptically by stimulation of the contralateral superior colliculus, and antidromically by the spinal cord were retained for the present report.

Intra-axonal injection of HRP

After proper identification of each axon, HRP was injected electrophoretically by passing a positive current (15–30 nA) through the micro-electrode for several minutes. After a period of 12–24 hours, animals were anesthetized and perfused through the ascending aorta with a normal saline solution followed by 3 litres of fixative (0.8% paraformaldehyde, 1.0% gluteraldehyde, pH 7.4). The brain was stored at 4°C in a solution of phosphate buffer (pH 7.4) and 30% sucrose and subsequently cut in 100-μm thick coronal sections on a freezing microtome. Following incubation in a solution of $CoCl_2$, the sections were reacted with diaminobenzidine and H_2O_2 in a modification of the technique described by Bishop et al. (1976). In some cases, the sections were counterstained with cresyl violet. The drawing and reconstructions shown were made with the aid of a drawing tube.

Data processing

Eye movement components, EMG of neck muscles and neuronal activity were recorded on an analog tape and then processed on an HP 5451 B and HP 1000 computer system. Horizontal and vertical eye velocity was calculated after smoothing by a non-phase-shifting mathematical filter (low pass, with cut off at 200 Hz). A detailed analysis of neuronal and motor events during and around the saccade was made possible by marking the onset and end of the saccade with the computer. The neuronal firing rate was evaluated by calculating the instantaneous firing rate.

Results

Behavioural observations on eye-head coordination in the cat

In this section we shall review experiments done previously which have revealed the presence of a powerful eye movement signal in the activity of dorsal neck muscles in the cat. We shall only summarize some results concerning the relation between horizontal gaze signals and neck muscle activity, although some recent results have begun to clarify this question for vertical gaze.

Horizontal eye movement signals in dorsal neck muscles of the alert cat during orienting

Vidal et al. (1982) have shown that the tonic component of the electromyographic activity of several dorsal neck muscles in the cat with immobilized head is clearly related to the horizontal component of eye position during spontaneous eye movements. The records are available for all compartments of mm. splenius, obliquus capitis caudalis and cranialis, and from longissimus capitis, which are all known to contribute to horizontal rotation of the head (Strauss-Durckheim, 1845). These muscles all exibited a strong tonic modulation of their activity

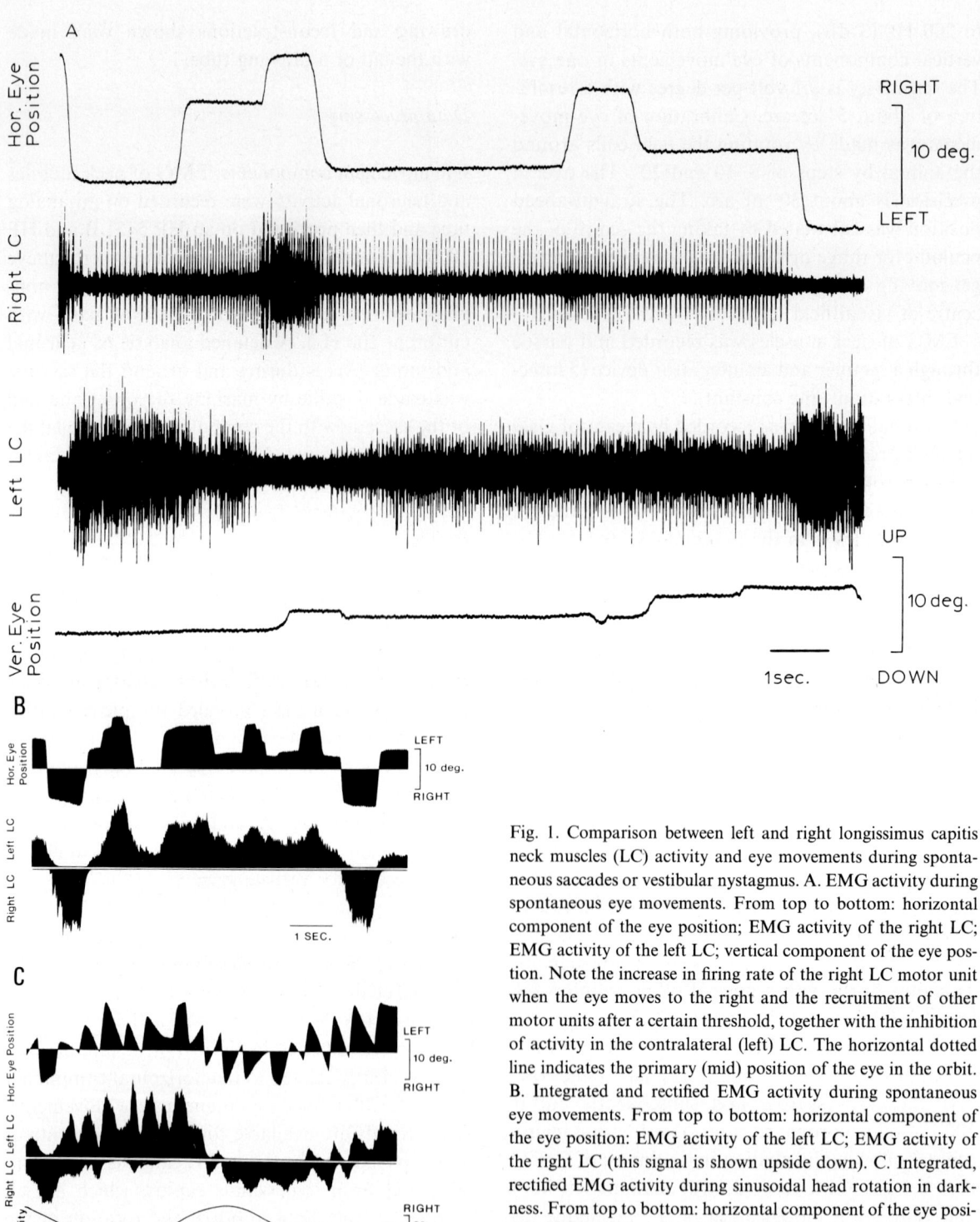

Fig. 1. Comparison between left and right longissimus capitis neck muscles (LC) activity and eye movements during spontaneous saccades or vestibular nystagmus. A. EMG activity during spontaneous eye movements. From top to bottom: horizontal component of the eye position; EMG activity of the right LC; EMG activity of the left LC; vertical component of the eye position. Note the increase in firing rate of the right LC motor unit when the eye moves to the right and the recruitment of other motor units after a certain threshold, together with the inhibition of activity in the contralateral (left) LC. The horizontal dotted line indicates the primary (mid) position of the eye in the orbit. B. Integrated and rectified EMG activity during spontaneous eye movements. From top to bottom: horizontal component of the eye position: EMG activity of the left LC; EMG activity of the right LC (this signal is shown upside down). C. Integrated, rectified EMG activity during sinusoidal head rotation in darkness. From top to bottom: horizontal component of the eye position; EMG activity of the left LC; EMG activity of the right LC (this signal is shown upside down); head velocity. From Vidal et al. (1982).

proportional to the horizontal component of the ipsilateral eye position. An example of recording from the longissimus capitis is shown in Fig. 1A and B, from Vidal et al. (1982).

Berthoz et al. (1982) have recorded simultaneously from a left abducens motoneuron and from two single motor units, respectively, in the left and right longissimus capitis muscle. The firing rate of the abducens motoneuron was related to horizontal eye position during fixation, with a slope of 4.8 spikes per second per degree with an eye position threshold of about 6° to the right. The two motor units had rate versus horizontal eye position curves with slopes of, respectively, 3.9 and 3.7 spikes per second per degree, with a threshold of a few degrees with respect to the mid-position of the eye in the orbit. Two mechanisms contribute to the global increase of muscle activity related to change in eye position: (a) an increase in motor unit discharge rate which is roughly proportional to ipsilateral eye position, and (b) a recruitment of motor units with increasing eccentricity from the mid-position of the eye. This last mechanism is responsible for the apparent exponential shape of the curves relating integrated EMG to horizontal eye position.

The remarkable fact is that a given neck muscle is never active, its motoneurons probably being powerfully inhibited, when the eye is directed to the contralateral side. A small overlap with respect to the mid-position of the eye in the orbit (primary position) does exist, and some motor units may discharge at low frequency when the animal looks up to about 3–5° contralaterally.

An extensive study of this relationship for nearly all dorsal neck muscles which is currently being made shows variations from one muscle to the other. This probably corresponds to the fact that each muscle has pulling directions which are distributed in a complex manner in the vectorial motor space of the neck or that the same muscles may have several functional roles, related, for instance, to head turning or postural control.

In conclusion, a parallel tonic activation or coupling can be observed between abducens motoneurons on one side and ipsilateral neck motoneurons of horizontal rotators of the neck. A switching of activity from the left to the right neck muscles occurs, for instance, whenever the eyes go from left to right. This "oculo-collic coupling" is present not only in the cat. Lestienne et al. (1984) have shown that in the head-fixed monkey the dorsal neck EMG is related to the horizontal component of eye position during orienting or pursuit. However, in the primate the decoupling of neck muscle activity from eye position is observed more frequently than in the cat.

In addition to this tonic component, a phasic activation of neck motoneurons occurs during saccades to the ipsilateral side (see Figs. 4–7). This transient saccade-related coupling has been found by Fuller (1980) in the rabbit, by Roucoux et al. (1982) following electrical stimulation of the superior colliculus in the cat, and by Bizzi et al. (1971) in the monkey. Consequently, one has to assume an existence of neuronal groups (populations) generating tonic and/or phasic signals which can be utilized in parallel by both ocular and neck motoneurons. We shall now review the evidence concerning the influence of these gaze-related signals on stabilizing vestibulo-collic reflexes.

Modulation of the VCR by signals related to horizontal gaze

Horizontal VCR. If a cat with head immobilized is rotated around a vertical axis in darkness, one could expect to record in neck muscles a discharge corresponding to the horizontal vestibulo-collic reflex, the properties of which have been extensively studied in the decerebrate cat (Ezure and Sasaki, 1978; Bilotto et al., 1982; Peterson and Goldberg, 1982). However, Vidal et al. (1982) have shown that, in intact unanesthetized cat, EMG activity of splenius, obliquus and longissimus capitis muscles still follows the horizontal component of eye position, even during sinusoidal rotation of the animal in darkness in the plane of the horizontal semi-circular canal.

A surprising observation shown in Fig. 1C is that during head rotation to the right, in spite of a compensatory slow phase of nystagmus directed to the left, the mean position of the eye in the orbit (beating-field) is displaced to the right, i.e., in the direction of head motion. This shift of gaze in the anticompensatory direction is due to the action of the quick phases of vestibular nystagmus (similar to the beating field of optokinetic nystagmus). It gives a tonic activation of the right neck muscle which suppresses the VCR. This behaviour may be interpreted as an orienting reaction. A similar behaviour has been reported during transient head rotations in man (Melvill-Jones, 1964) and in cat (Berthoz et al., 1975).

Vertical VCR. The VCR in the frontal plane has been described quantitatively in decerebrate cats (Berthoz and Anderson, 1971; Schor and Miller, 1981). In our laboratory, Darlot et al. (1985) have studied the neck muscle activity in alert cats during tilting in the frontal plane and have measured the modulation of the VCR in this plane by horizontal eye position signals. Fig. 2 shows that during lateral tilt the VCR evoked by sinusoidal rotation is modulated, together with the horizontal component of eye position. Although the pattern of muscle activity during tilt oscillations often showed non-linear behaviour (bursting), the authors performed, when justified, a linear frequency analysis of the relation between tilt angle and neck muscle EMG. The results show that the vestibulo-collic reflex has a higher gain for rotation in the frontal plane than in the horizontal plane. This could be due to a contribution of the otoliths. The coupling between EMG and the horizontal eye position com-

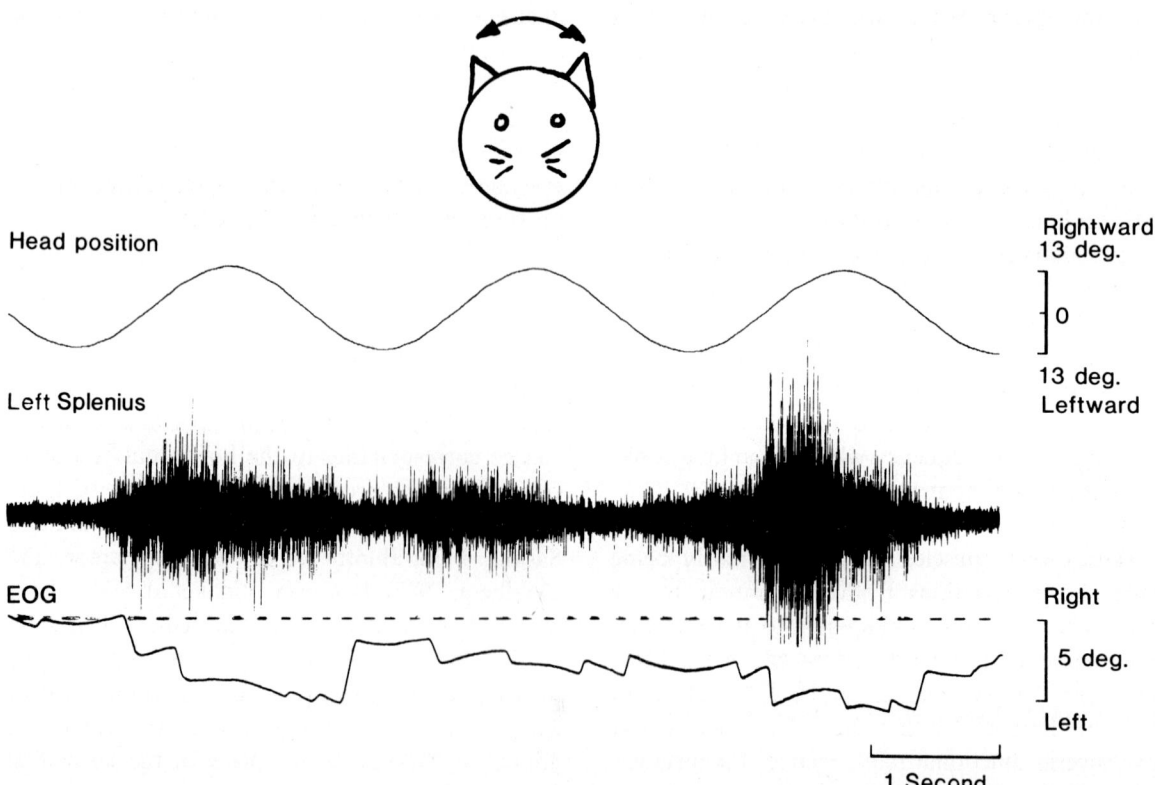

Fig. 2. Interaction between eye position signals and the VCR in the frontal plane. From top to bottom: recording of head angular position during sinusoidal rotation in the frontal plane on each side of the vertical (see diagram). EMG of left splenius neck muscles showing horizontal component of eye position. Note that the amplitude of the VCR is linked with the eccentricity of the eye position to the left. From Darlot et al. (1985).

ponent has been studied by dividing the EMG in a mean (*DC*) level and a sinusoidal modulation of amplitude (*A*) related to the sinusoidal head tilt. Both *DC* and *A* increase with ipsilateral horizontal eye displacement, but *DC* seems to increase exponentially and *A* linearly. This modulation of VCR is functionally meaningful, as described simply in the following example: if the body of the free moving animal would be tilted, say to the left, the VCR would pull the head back to the right by activating the right neck muscles; this would be very functional for stabilising the head in space. However, if the strategy is to tilt the head and body to the left, for instance, in order to look at a mouse located on the ground to the left, the VCR becomes non-adaptive. In this case the deviation of gaze to the left automatically suppresses VCR activity in the right neck muscle and increases activity on the right through the oculo-collic coupling mechanism.

Therefore, the vestibulo-collic reflex is modulated in both the horizontal and frontal planes by a gaze-related signal. Roucoux et al. (1982) proposed that, in the horizontal plane, one of the functions of this signal is to perform an automatic transition from the retinotopic coordinate system to the craniotopic coordinate system.

Modulation of neck EMG during optokinetic stimulation

Optokinetic stimulation by large moving visual scenes is known to induce postural reactions, which have been reviewed elsewhere. During optokinetic nystagmus the activity of dorsal neck muscles is also modulated in relation with eye movements (Vidal et al., 1983a, b), which holds true for all compartments of the splenius muscle (Wilson et al., 1983). A visuo-motor tonic component independent of eye movement may also be present, as suggested by studies in humans, and by Thoden et al. (1977) in the cat. However, this point requires a still more rigorous investigation.

In conclusion, behavioural studies reveal the existence of a coupling mechanism with tonic (eye position) and phasic (saccadic) components. The tonic coupling is present throughout phylogeny and, probably, also in man, as was suggested by Bennet and Savill in 1889. This is probably a specific synergy which, in higher species, can be overridden by other synergies or reflex modules, or even completely when, for instance, the animal or human fixates visually an object turning with the head.

Neuronal mechanisms underlying eye-head synergy during orienting

The first neuronal candidates to mediate this ipsiversive coupling or synergy between eye and head are the second-order type I vestibulo-spinal neurons, which have been studied in the alert cat with intracellular techniques by Yoshida et al. (1981), McCrea et al. (1980, 1981) and Berthoz et al. (1981). They have demonstrated the existence of an eye position signal modulating the firing rate of these neurons and proved that secondary type I neurons carrying horizontal eye position signal and projecting to the VIth nucleus also project to the spinal cord. Isu and Yokota (1983) have confirmed that a group of second-order type I neurons, located in a fairly restricted region of the ventrolateral part of the medial vestibular nucleus, had this dual projection to the abducens nucleus and the spinal cord.

However, it has been argued (Berthoz, 1985) that (a) the vestibulo-collic reflex is crossed and cannot subserve the ipsiversive eye-head synergy and (b) horizontal second-order neurons carry often a large head velocity signal which is not present in the neck muscle activity.

Therefore, it is necessary to search for another population of neurons. Our attention was directed towards reticulo-spinal neurons located in the pontine and ponto-medullary reticular formation in the periabducens region.

Reticulo-spinal neurons mediating the ipsiversive orienting synergy

Evidence for a role of reticulo-spinal neurons located in this area in the eye-head synergy emerges from the observations summarized by Peterson (1984): (a) anatomical or electrophysiological stud-

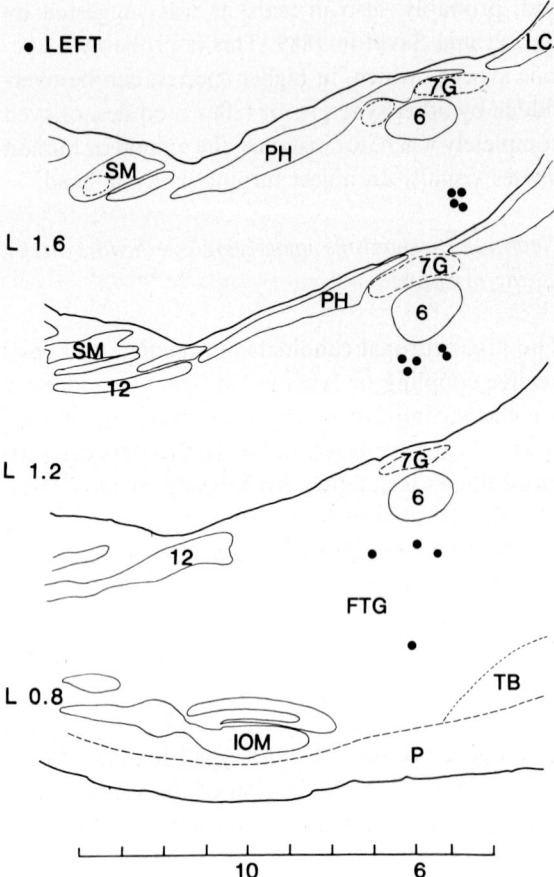

Fig. 3. Location of the recorded reticular neurons. Locations (black dots) in the brainstem are shown on three parasagittal sections at different lateralities. FTG, gigantocellular tegmental field; IOM, medial accessory inferior olive; LC, locus coeruleus: P, pyramidal tract; PH, prepositus hypoglossi; 7G, genu of the facial nerve; SM, medial nucleus of the solitary tract; TB, trapezoid body. The scale at the bottom indicates (in mm) the posterior location with respect to the frontal zero of Berman's atlas. From Vidal et al. (1983a, b).

ies concerning the branching of reticulo-spinal neurons in the brain stem (Grantyn et al., 1980) and spinal cord (Peterson et al., 1978; Kuypers and Huisman, 1982); (b) behavioural observations following localised brainstem lesions in rat (Sirkin et al., 1980; Sirkin and Teitelbaum, 1983); (c) single cell recording in the monkey (Whittington et al., 1984).

However, no direct proof was available in the alert cat, most of the studies having been performed on anesthetized or decerebrated preparations (apart from Whittington et al., 1984). Vidal et al. (1983a,b) performed recordings in the periabducens area of the ponto-medullary reticular formation, which contains medial reticulo-spinal neurons projecting to the neck (Peterson et al., 1978). They found several types of reticular neurons whose activity was related with the tonic and/or phasic components of dorsal neck muscle activity. The cells discharged together with the ipsilateral horizontal component of eye movements and, as shown in the example of Figs. 4 and 5, their firing rate was closely linked to the ipsilateral neck EMG. They were found in the area ventral to the VIth nucleus (Fig. 3). However, the areas rostral to the abducens nucleus were not explored in this work. The cells were often found in small clusters and had properties ranging from "tonic" to "burst tonic", with average horizontal eye position threshold of about 1–2° to the contralateral side ($n = 9$) for "burst-tonic" neurons, with an average slope of firing rate versus horizontal eye position of about 5 spikes per degree per second during fixations.

These data suggested that a group of ipsilateral reticular neurons was indeed mediating the eye-neck synergy. However, the data of Vidal et al. (1983a) were derived from extracellular recording from neurons which were not identified as reticulo-spinal cells. Therefore, we attempted (Grantyn et al., 1985) to obtain a more precise identification of these neurons with the technique of intra-axonic HRP injection in the alert cat coupled with antidromic identification by stimulation of the cervical spinal cord. The experimental paradigm is illustrated in Fig. 6A. The axons of reticulo-spinal neurons were penetrated at the level of the abducens nucleus in the alert cat. Stimulating electrodes were placed in the contralateral superior colliculus and spinal cord. The animal faced a screen, in front of which the experimenters moved small, attention-attracting objects in order to induce orienting behaviour. Fig. 6B shows the activity of a neuron which increased the discharge rate when the cat was

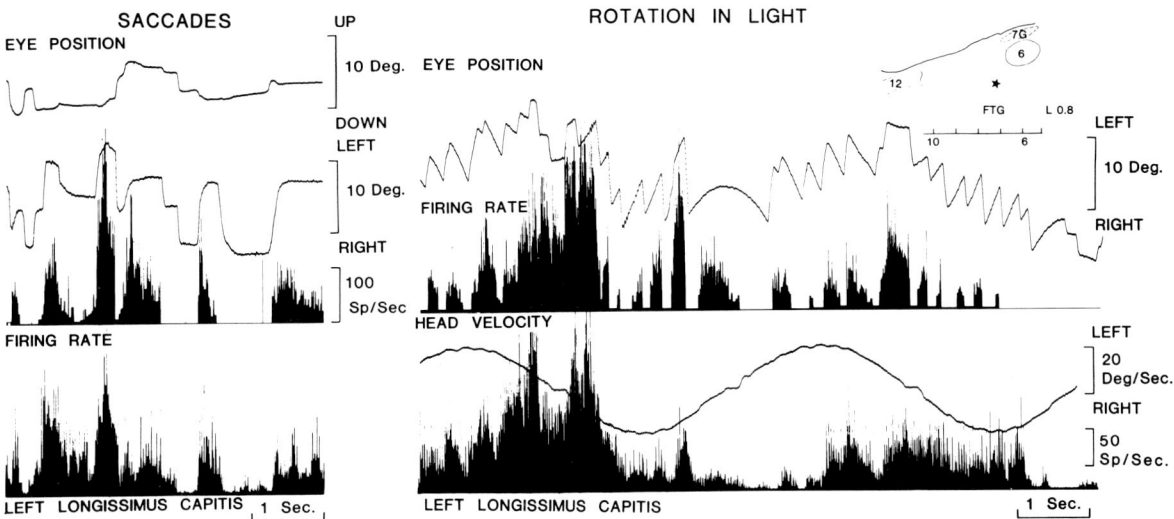

Fig. 4. Discharge characteristics of a "burst-tonic" reticular neuron. Left: firing pattern of the neuron during spontaneous saccades. From top to bottom: vertical and horizontal components of eye position, instantaneous firing rate of the neuron, integrated EMG of the left longissimus capitis muscle. Right: firing pattern of the neuron during sinusoidal horizontal rotation in the light (combined vestibular and optokinetic nystagmus). From top to bottom: horizontal component of eye position, firing rate of the neuron, head velocity, integrated EMG of longissimus capitis muscle.

orienting to the right. This record shows the vertical and horizontal components of the eye movement. The mid-position of the eye in the orbit is indicated by dashed horizontal lines, and the shaded area shows when the eye was to the right of the mid-position. The EMG of the right longissimus capitis reveals both a tonic component related to rightward eye position and a phasic burst which occurs mainly when the cat makes saccades to the right (vertical dotted lines).

The reticular neuron is completely silent when the eye is to the left side of the orbit. When the cat looks to the right the discharge rate is very closely related to electromyographic activity and, as can be seen on the record, slightly leads saccade. A measurement of latencies between the onset of neuronal firing and a saccade has a limited meaning in this case because when the eye moves from a leftward to a rightward position the neuron obviously has an eye position threshold which may considerably modify this latency. When the saccades occur during a tonic discharge the latency is also difficult to measure.

The morphological reconstruction of this neuron is shown on Fig. 6C. The soma was located in the nucleus reticularis pontis caudalis, about 1 mm rostral to the VIth nucleus. On its course towards the spinal cord the main axon of this neuron issued 13 collaterals, which terminated in the VIth nucleus, nucleus prepositus hypoglossi, medial vestibular nucleus, facial nucleus and nucleus intercalatus. The highest density of terminals (boutons terminaux et en passant) is observed in the abducens (collaterals 1, 2) and facial (collaterals 3, 4) nuclei. The third major target structure of this particular neuron was the so-called dorsal FTG (gigantocellular tegmental field), known as a source of direct excitatory and inhibitory inputs to cervical motoneurons (Peterson, 1984). Distal segments of dorsally directed collaterals (Nos. 1, 2, 4, 8–11) establish connections with restricted portions of the medial vestibular and prepositus/intercalatus nuclei, for which the participation in the control of eye movements is well established.

Therefore, the information carried by the neuron is sent not only to the spinal cord, but also to struc-

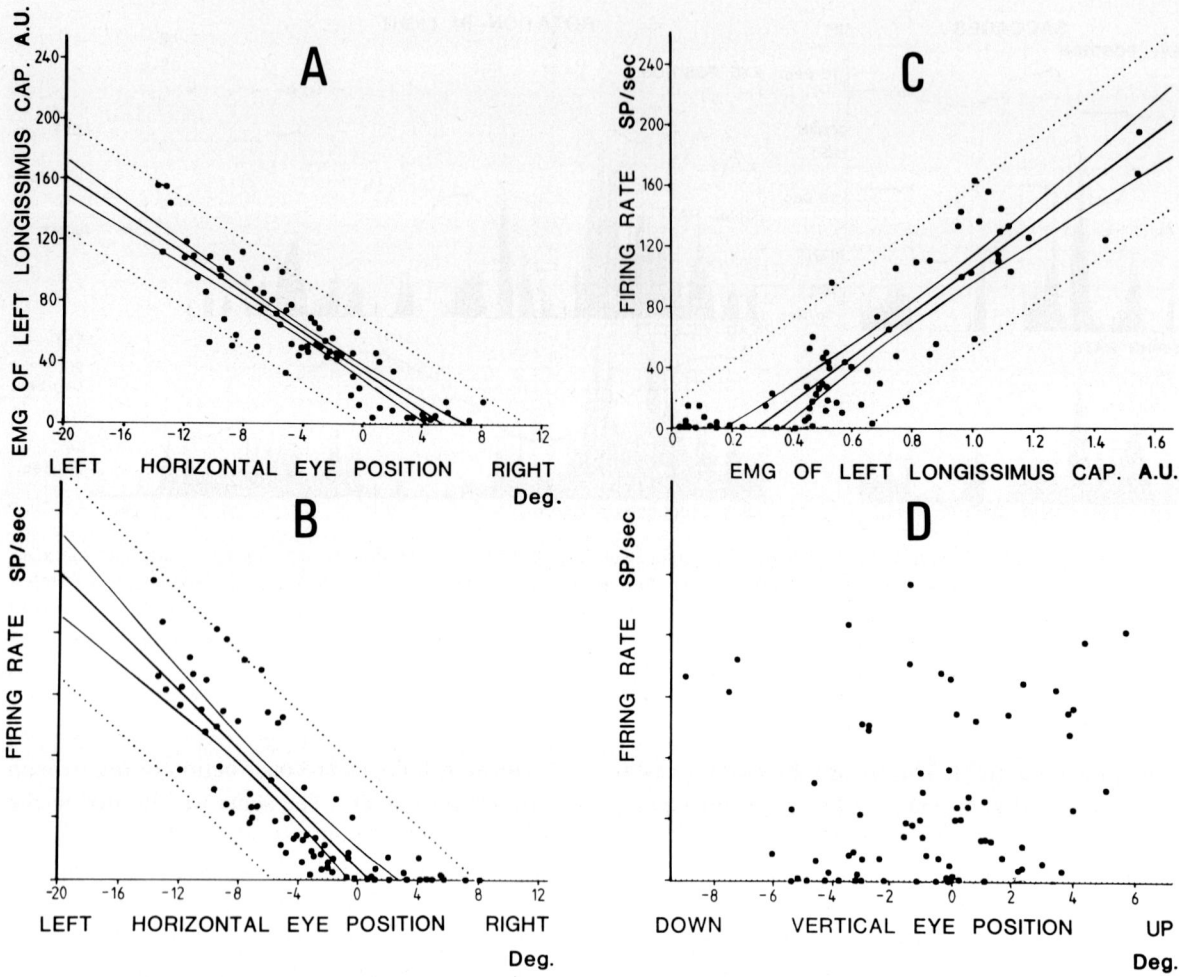

Fig. 5. Quantitative analysis of the relationship between the firing rate of a periabducens reticular neuron, eye position and neck muscle activity. A. Relationship between EMG of ipsilateral left longissimus capitis muscle (integrated EMG in arbitrary units, A.U.) and horizontal component of eye position. Data obtained as described in Methods. The straight line is the regression line, continuous lines on each side indicate the confidence interval at 95% for the regression line, and dotted lines indicate the confidence interval at the same level for the population of points. B. Relationship between the firing rate of neuron and horizontal component of eye position. Same notations as in A for the statistical analysis. C. Relationship between the firing rate of the neuron and EMG of the ipsilateral left longissimus capitis muscle. Same notation as above. D. Relationship between the firing rate of the neuron and the vertical component of eye position. No correlation was found. From Vidal et al. (1983a).

tures which are known to be closely concerned with the control of eye movements. The terminations in the medial part of the facial nucleus, which has been shown to contain motoneurons controlling ear muscles (Courville, 1966; Papez, 1927; Henkel and Edwards, 1978), suggest that this neuron actually may control not only eye-head coordination, but an even more complex synergy which involves orienting movements of the eye, the head and the ears.

In conclusion, this finding together with a detailed analysis of these neurons (Grantyn et al., 1985) demonstrates that ipsilaterally projecting excitatory reticulo-spinal neurons subserve the orienting eye-head coupling which has been found in the behavioural experiments reviewed above. All the characteristics (threshold, firing pattern, directional profile) of the neuronal activity of these neurons are close to the discharge of neck motoneurons. This suggests that, in this particular case, neck motor activity is controlled at brainstem level. This obviously does not mean that neck motoneurons cannot be activated by other routes, and we have some records which clearly show strong neck muscle activation occurring in the absence of any discharge from this neuron. What we propose is that when the cat makes an orienting movement the ipsilateral neck muscle is subjected to a dominating control of reticulo-spinal neurons just described. This dominance may depend on the gating function of other descending systems which have not yet been properly analyzed.

This is compatible with the suggestions made by Kuypers and his colleagues (for review, see Kuypers and Huisman, 1982) concerning the control of axial musculature by reticulo-spinal pathways. It is also in accord with the findings of Alstermark et al. (1983a, b), who showed that reticulo-spinal neurons in the brainstem relay the disynaptic cortical influences on neck motoneurons. It is most probable that the group of reticulo-spinal neurons which we are dealing with receives a number of inputs from the labyrinth (Peterson, 1984), the cerebellum (Eccles et al., 1975) and the superior colliculus (Grantyn et al., 1980). This last proposition is illustrated by the fact that the neuron of Fig. 6 was monosynaptically activated by stimulation of the contralateral superior colliculus (SC). Given what is known about the contribution of the SC to saccade generation (Guitton et al., 1980; Roucoux et al., 1982), the SC could provide a phasic input responsible for the bursts of EMG seen during saccades. Therefore, we have studied the discharge of tecto-reticulo-spinal neurons during visuo-motor orienting behaviour. The electrophysiological and morphological identification of this neuronal population has been elaborated by Grantyn and Grantyn (1982).

Tecto-reticulo-spinal neurons (TRSN) contributing to the phasic component of orienting synergy

It is well known that projection neurons from the SC provide, in the monkey, vectorial coding of saccades during visuo-motor behaviour (see the articles by Sparks and Jay (Section IV-B) and Wurtz and Hikosaka (Section IV-A). The physiological properties of unidentified neurons in deep and intermediate layers of the SC have been studied recently by Harris (1980), Peck et al. (1980) and Straschill and Schick (1977). However, the precise physiological properties of projection neurons which link the SC to the brainstem structures involved in eye and head movement control were not investigated. In the cat, Grantyn et al. (1976, 1979) have described the synaptic efferent connections of tectal neurons to horizontal ocular motoneurons, and Grantyn and Grantyn (1982) have studied the axonal branching patterns and sites of termination of the tecto-reticulo-spinal neurons (TRSN). Some of the collaterals of TRSN do project to the ponto-bulbar areas which contain the somata of reticulo-spinal neurons (RSNs) described above. In addition, we have seen that RSNs which have a discharge rate related to ipsilateral eye and head movements do receive mono- or disynaptic activation from the contralateral SC. Therefore, it is reasonable to assume that TRSNs are one of the important inputs to RSNs. We have recently made an extensive study of the properties of TRSNs by combining intra-axonic recording of the activity of these neurons within the predorsal bundle at abducens nucleus level, and intra-axonic injection of HRP (Grantyn and Berthoz, 1983, 1984). TRSNs were identified electrophysiologically (Fig. 7) by their short-latency (0.3–0.5 mseconds), direct orthodromic response to the SC stimulation through chronically implanted needle electrodes, and antidromic invasion by stimulation through chronically implanted electrodes located in the anterior funiculus at C1 or C2 levels of the spinal cord. Fig. 7C,

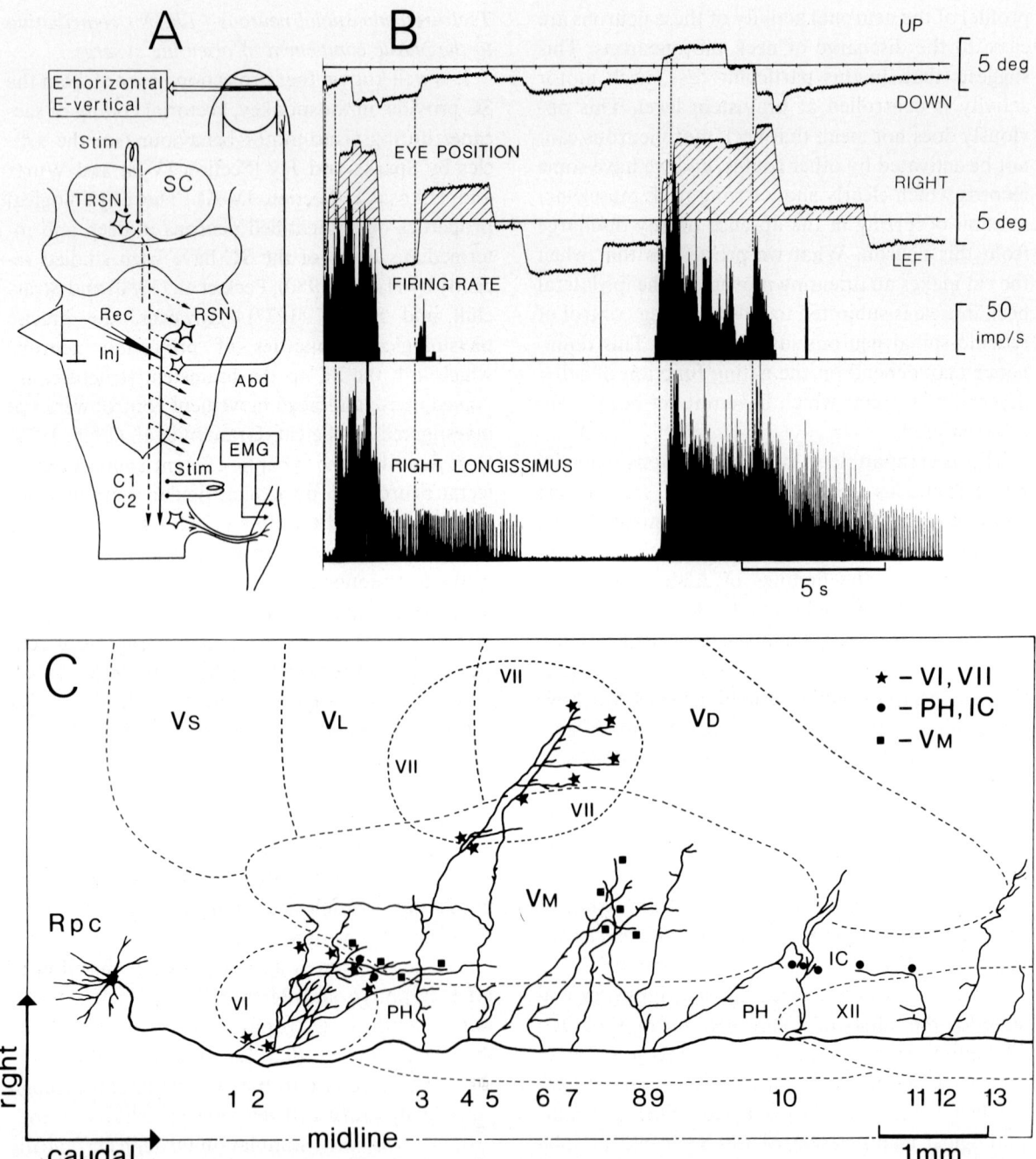

Fig. 6. Physiological and morphological properties of a reticulo-spinal neuron. A. Schematic description of experimental paradigm. TRSN, tecto-reticulo-spinal neuron; RSN, reticulo-spinal neuron; Abd, abducens nucleus; SC, superior colliculus. Two bipolar stimulation electrodes (Stim) are placed in deep layer of the SC and in spinal cord. Intracellular micro-electrode is shown in the RSN axon for intra-axonic recording (Rec) and injection (Inj) of HRP. EMG of neck muscles is recorded by chronically implanted wire electrodes. Horizontal (E-horizontal), vertical (E-vertical) components of eye movements are recorded by the search coil technique. B. Firing pattern of a right side RSN and its relation with eye movements and neck EMG. From top to bottom: vertical and horizontal

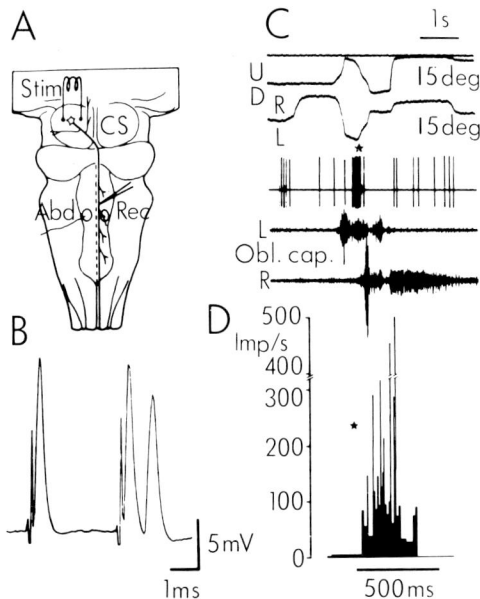

Fig. 7. Electrophysiological identification of a TRSN and its activity during orienting reaction in an alert cat. A. Dorsal view of brainstem showing locations of stimulating and recording electrodes. B. Intra-axonal recording of a direct orthodromic spike response to stimulation of contralateral superior colliculus (CS). C. Activity of same neuron during orienting towards a novel object (brush) introduced near the centre of visual field and rapidly withdrawn to right. From top to bottom: vertical and horizontal eye position (U, up; D, down; R, right; L, left), neuronal discharge, EMG of left (L) and right (R) m. obliquus capitis anterior. Note following of the moving object by double saccade to right (star) and phasic activation of right EMG. This eye-neck synergy is preceded by an intense burst discharge of the neuron located in the left CS. D. Instantaneous frequency plot of burst marked by star in C. Modified from Grantyn and Berthoz (1985).

D shows a typical example of the behaviour of a TRSN during an eye-head orienting synergy. The head-fixed cat was presented on the left side with an object which was moving to the right. The animal made the following sequence of movements: (a) firstly, an upward and leftward saccade, to foveate on the target; simultaneously, there was a strong phasic activation of the left obliquus capitis neck muscle; (b) then, secondly, a succession of two saccades to follow the object during its movement to the right, with a downward and rightward eye movement associated with a sharp burst of the right obliquus capitis when the eye crossed the mid-position in the orbit. The TRSN generated an intense burst (star), the characteristics of which are shown in detail in Fig. 7D. This burst preceded the rightward eye movement and phasic neck activation.

We found that TRSNs differ with respect to their relationship to the visuo-motor behaviour. However, a subpopulation of these neurons which can be called visuo-motor has common features. They are characterized by a poor responsiveness to stationary light flashes, directionally selective responses to moving stimuli and large receptive fields with a vaguely defined leading edge. Many give an enhanced visual response to attention-attracting three-dimentional objects. They never discharge during spontaneous saccades in darkness. Strong bursts may attain instantaneous firing rates as high as 300–700 imp/sec, but mean frequencies are generally 120–130 imp/sec. The exact nature of the signal coded by these neurons is not fully understood,

---

components of eye position, firing rate of the right side RSN and integrated EMG of right longissimus capitis muscle (arbitary units). Note that the neuron only fires when eye position is on the ipsilateral side (right) of the orbit (the horizontal straight lines on the eye movement records indicate mid-position of the eye in the orbit). Shaded areas show when the horizontal component is to the right. Note also bursts of activity which are associated with saccades to the right in both the firing rate and the EMG. C. Morphology of RSN whose discharge pattern is shown in B. HRP was injected in the axon 0.4 mm anterior to collateral 1. Reconstruction in projection on horizontal plane. Parts of collaterals bearing no symbols are distributed in the dorsal half of the reticular core, except for collaterals 3, 4 and 6, which take a ventro-lateral course. Parts of collaterals supplying other nuclei (abducens, facialis, medial vestibular, prepositus hypoglossi and intercalatus) are denoted by different key symbols (see upper right of C). Abbreviations: IC, nucleus intercalatus; PH, nucleus prepositus hypoglossi; RPC, nucleus reticularis pontis caudalis; Vd, VL, VM, VS, descending, lateral, medial and superior vestibular nuclei, respectively; VI, nucleus abducentis; VII, nucleus on facialis (Grantyn and Berthoz, unpublished observations).

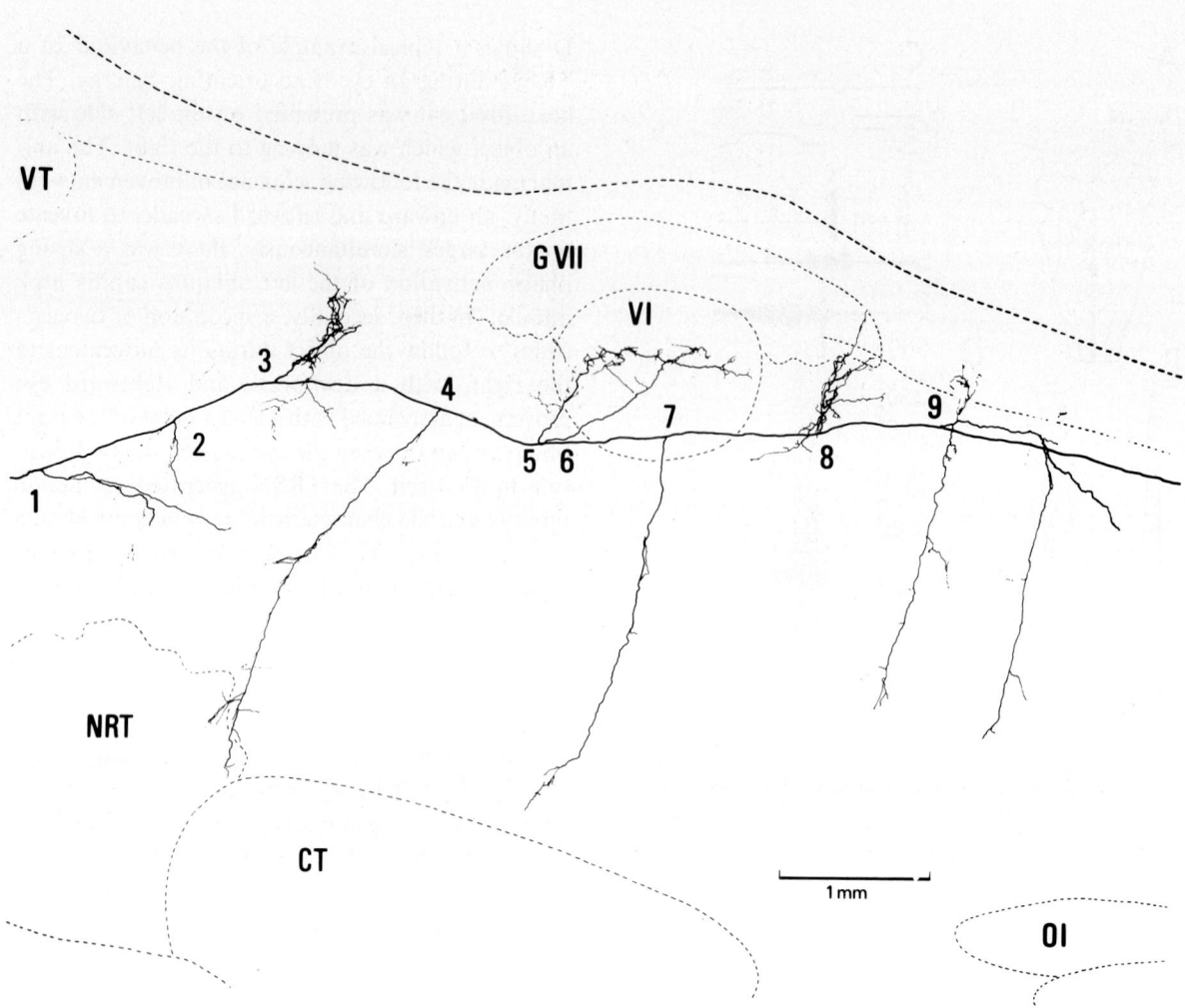

Fig. 8. Reconstruction in the sagittal plane of the axonal collaterals of the tecto-reticulo-spinal neuron shown in Fig. 7 in the pons and rostral medulla. CT, trapezoid body; GVII, genu of the facial nerve; NRT, nucleus reticularis segmenti pontis; OI, inferior olive; VT, ventral tegmental nucleus (of Gudden). The surface of the IVth ventricle is indicated by a thick dotted line. The inferior border of the propositus nucleus is indicated by a thin dotted line. From Grantyn and Berthoz (1985).

but they probably code dynamic parameters related to the saccades needed to capture visually the moving target, rather than reconstruct the target position.

As shown in Fig. 8, the pattern of collaterals in the brainstem of the neuron shown in Fig. 7 is compatible with a direct action of this neuron on several structures important for eye and head movement control. Collateral 3, in particular, projects to the dorsal aspect of the nucleus reticularis pontis caudalis. This is precisely the same area where the somata of reticulo-spinal neurons described above have been found. Collateral 4 distributes within the paramedian part of the nucleus reticularis pontis caudalis, with thin finely branched multiple plexus not seen in dorsal collaterals. Collaterals 5 and 6 distribute in the abducens nucleus. Collateral 7 traverses the nucleus reticularis gigantocellularis. Collateral 8 terminates in the area of burst inhibitory neurons (Hikosaka and Kawakami, 1977; Yoshida et al., 1982), containing also the reticulo-cervical RSNs (Peterson, 1984). Collateral 9 terminates in the ventral border of the nucleus prepositus hypoglossi and gives ventral branches to the nucleus reticularis gigantocellularis. This suggests that the apparently "diffuse" projection of TRSN is in fact an extremely specific distribution of the signals carried by these neurons to various target neurons, which, in turn, utilize them in their computing processes.

Discussion

Taken together, the observations we have described lead to several conclusions on the functional aspects of eye-head coordination and on the underlying neuronal mechanisms. It should be pointed out that our results, obtained in cats with heads fixed, do reveal some important features of gaze control which can be generalized to head-free animals (Crommelinck et al., 1982). Indeed, the eye-head coupling in freely moving animals appears to be dominated by different strategies. We have discussed already that cats, depending on the behavioural context, can adopt either a compensatory (VCR) or an orienting (anticompensatory) mode of eye-head coordination. In addition, the animal can use a "suppression strategy", in order to follow a target moving at the same angular velocity as its head. Such choices of strategies would require switching mechanisms which are still far from being understood. An important observation bearing on this subject is that the second-order vestibular neurons projecting to the spinal cord still bear the head velocity signal during orienting, when VCR is non-adaptive (Berthoz et al., 1981; Yoshida, K., Vidal, P. P. and Berthoz, A.,unpublished data). It can then be suggested that the VCR is suppressed, or "gated", at the segmental level, and that the propriospinal interneuron pools may play an important role in this operation.

We agree with Fuller et al. (1983), who underlined an extreme diversity of strategies in normal behaviour. However, we propose that extremely complex and ever-changing strategies are, in fact, based upon a finite repertoire of subsystems which are relatively simple but which can generate, by subtle interplay, an appearance of unlimited behavioural versatility. The ipsiversive orienting synergy dealt with above is an important element of the repertoire. We shall now discuss some peripheral and central components of this functional subsystem.

Behaviour of motor units in the neck muscles

The tonic component of neck-EMG related to the horizontal eye position

At the level of neck muscles a number of questions are still to be answered. First of all, a quantitative analysis of firing rate and recruitment order has not yet been performed for tonic motor units. It would be of interest to see, for example, if the recruitment order of neck motor units is related to different eye position threshold of RSNs. Likewise, the exact mechanism of inhibition of contralateral neck muscle activity during ipsiversive orienting is still unknown. According to the microstimulation studies by Peterson (1977), such neurons should be located in the dorsal FTG at the level of and posterior to the abducens nucleus.

The behavioural properties of RSNs projecting to the cervical segments should also be related to the pulling directions of neck muscles. According to recent findings by Vidal et al. (1985), the head of the cat, contrary to everyday thinking, is positioned on the cervical vertebral column oriented perpendicularly to gravity. Consequently, orienting in the horizontal plane can be accomplished only, or preferentially, by rotation of the head around the axis of the first vertebra. This finding explains well why the RSNs with monosynaptic projection to neck motoneurons do not innervate lower spinal segments (Peterson, 1977). Recent experiments by Denise, P. and Darlot, C. (unpublished data) support the idea of selective coupling between horizontal eye and neck rotators, so far as they demonstrate that motoneurons of axial muscles of the trunk do not carry a signal reflecting the horizontal eye position. Since body turning is considered as a natural component of adversive (orienting) reactions (Hess et al., 1946), the neuronal substrates which integrate the eye-head synergy with axial and limb movements may represent an important subject for future studies.

The phasic component of neck-EMG

In general, the phasic bursts of neck-EMG are synchronous with ipsilateral saccades, this being true not only for the cat but also for other species. The origin of the saccade-related phasic input to neck motoneurons has not yet been elucidated. In 1971, Anderson et al., based on stimulation experiments, stated largely that "the tecto-reticulo-spinal pathway constitutes the most important pathway for activation of neck motoneurons". At present, we can specify that tecto-reticulo-spinal neurons (TRSN) do generate phasic discharges related to contraversive saccades to phasic components of the contralateral neck-EMG (Grantyn and Berthoz, 1983, 1985, and unpublished results). Bearing in mind the monosynaptic projection of TRSNs to RSNs (Grantyn et al., 1980), it is reasonable to suppose that at least some of the latter could repeat faithfully the descending TRSN signal and provide phasic input to neck motoneurons. Clearly, the relative contributions of the direct tecto-spinal projection and of the di- (or poly-) synaptic tecto-reticulo-spinal pathways still remain to be evaluated.

Neuronal elements of the tecto-reticulo-spinal system

Our observations on the discharge patterns of TRSNs and RSNs in alert cats allow us, for the first time, to establish some structure-function relationship in a neuronal system underlying one of the basic behavioural strategies: the orienting gaze shift. Classical investigations by Hess et al. (1946) have demonstrated that tectal stimulation, depending on its intensity and duration, can induce graded orienting reactions towards contralateral visual field. Weaker stimulation may result in contraversive eye movements only, whereas stronger or prolonged stimulation provokes head and body turning, and locomotion. These observations were confirmed by more recent studies (Roucoux et al., 1980; Harris, 1980). Based on indirect evidence, it has been suggested that there exist separate populations of efferent neurons of the SC which control either eye or head movements (Straschill and Schick, 1977; Harris, 1980).

Grantyn and Grantyn (1982) have shown, however, that a certain class of tectal neurons, the TRSNs, display an axonal branching pattern compatible with the control of the eye-head synergy (see Fig. 8). Grantyn and Berthoz (1983, 1985) demonstrated that a substantial fraction of neurons belonging to this class generate their most intense bursts in association with contraversive saccades and phasic activation of contralateral neck-EMG during strongly motivated visual orienting. Some properties of TRSNs must be particularly stressed. From the point of view of behavioural correlations, these neurons should be regarded as "conditionally" presaccadic (see Hepp and Henn, 1983) or "conditionally" linked to phasic activity in the contralateral neck-EMG. TRSNs may burst in the absence of any motor correlates of orienting and, on the other hand, contraversive spontaneous saccades or activation of neck muscles do occur in the absence of TRSN discharges.

This flexibility of correlations with motor events can be partially explained on the basis of morphological observations. The average density of TRSN terminals in the abducens nucleus, in the paramedian pontine reticular formation (PPRF) and in the FTG appears to be low. This led Grantyn and Grantyn (1982) to propose that TRSNs may provide a generalized facilitatory background for contraversive gaze shifts (eye plus head) without being able to trigger motoneuronal spike activity or to control its frequency profile. However, we found that the distribution of TRSN terminals in the ponto-bulbar tegmentum can follow two patterns. The first would correspond well to the term "diffuse": occasional, evenly distributed boutons over a length of preterminal branch extending over several hundred μm. The second pattern is of a "specific", clustered type, suggesting that a relatively large number of contacts can be made with a single target neuron. Provided that a train of spikes generated by a given TRSN is of sufficiently high frequency, these selected target neurons may transmit the descending collicular signal with a rather high degree of fidelity. Furthermore, as can be seen in Fig. 6, an individual RSN projecting to the spinal cord and identified as a postsynaptic element of the tecto-reticular pathway replicates many of the ponto-bulbar projections of TRSNs in the abducens nucleus, in the dorsal part of the caudal pontine and gigantocellular reticular nuclei and in the nucleus prepositus hypoglossi. Considering now, for the sake of simplicity, abducens motoneurons as a selected target population one should assume that a measurable correlation between the discharge profile of a TRSN and the parameters of a saccade can be expected when, and only when, (1) the intensity of TRSN bursts in response to a sensory stimulus is close to maximal, this probably being dependent on the interplay of several forebrain structures converging to the SC, (2) the number of RSNs projecting collaterals to the abducens nucleus and receiving clustered ("specific") inputs from TRSN is sufficiently high to produce subthreshold modulation of motoneuronal discharge by acting in parallel with the direct tecto-abducens pathway.

These considerations emphasize the crucial role of RSNs in the transformation of the output signal generated in the SC during visuo-motor reactions. One of the operations can merely consist of an amplification of the collicular signal due to the parallel, convergent action of TRSNs and RSNs upon the same target areas in the lower brain-stem (compare Figs. 8 and 6C) and, probably, in the spinal cord. More complex forms of signal transformation by RSNs may be expected, considering the convergence on them of a number of descending systems (e.g., cortical, tectal, mesencephalic reticular) and of sensory pathways representing different modalities, including the vestibular (cf. Scheibel and Scheibel, 1958; Peterson, 1977, 1984). The role of multiple convergence to RSNs may consist of either gating or modification of the effects produced on each given neuron by its dominant synaptic input. Our observations on TRSNs and pontine RSNs in the alert cat render a good example of such a transformation. TSNs receiving direct collicular input do display a tonic component of discharge, related to the ipsilateral eye position and to the level of tonic EMG activity. Since TRSNs do not generate a tonic signal, this latter must be added by some other synaptic input(s) to RSNs, one of the candidates being the nucleus prepositus hypoglossi (Lopez Barneo et al., 1982)

Although the TRSNs and RSNs are definitely a part of the immediate premotor network related to ocular and spinal motoneurons, these two classes of neurons do not code the movement parameters with high precision. We have pointed out already the flexibility of correlations with the saccades and the dependence of such correlations on the discharge frequency in the case of TRSN bursts (Grantyn and Berthoz, 1985). Neither TRSNs nor RSNs considered here are comparable with excitatory or inhibitory burst neurons of the periabducens area, which show much tighter correlations with saccade parameters (Kaneko et al., 1981; Yoshida et al., 1982). Nevertheless, the joint action of TRSNs and their target neurons, the RSNs, does result in a pulse-step input to motoneurons, subserving the orienting eye-head and probably ear synergy. It is conceivable that these neurons represent an archaic system of urgent but low-precision orienting. Its interactions with other descending systems assuring a precise foveation remain to be investigated.

References

Alstermark, B., Pinter, M. and Sasaki, S., (1983a) Brainstem relay of disynaptic pyramidal EPSPs to neck motoneurons in the cat. Brain Res., 259: 147–150.

Alstermark, B., Pinter, M. and Sasaki, S. (1983b) Convergence on reticulospinal neurons mediating contralateral pyramidal disynaptic EPSPs to neck motoneurons. Brain Res., 259: 151–154.

Anderson, M. E., Yoshida, M. and Wilson, V. J. (1971) Influence of superior colliculus on cat neck motoneurons. J. Neurophysiol., 34: 898–907.

Bennet, A. H. and Savill, T. (1889) A case of permanent conjugate deviation of the eyes and head, the result of a lesion limited to the sixth nucleus; with remarks on associated lateral movements of the eye balls, and rotation of the head and neck. Brain, 12: 102–116.

Berthoz, A. (1985) Adaptive mechanisms in eye-head coordination. In A. Berthoz and G. Melvill Jones (Eds.), Adaptive

Mechanisms in Gaze Control, Elsevier, Amsterdam pp. 177–201.
Berthoz, A. and Anderson, J. H. (1971) Frequency analysis of vestibular influence on extensor motoneurons. II Relationship between neck and fore-limb extensors. Brain Res., 34: 346–380.
Berthoz, A., Jeannerod, M., Vital-Durand, F. and Oliveras, J. L. (1975) Development of vestibulo-ocular responses in visually deprived kittens. Exp. Brain Res., 23: 425–442.
Berthoz, A., Yoshida, K. and Vidal, P. P. (1981) Horizontal eye movement signals in second order vestibular nuclei neurons in the alert cat. Ann. NY Acad. Sci., 374: 144–156.
Berthoz, A., Vidal, P. P. and Corvisier, J. (1982) Brainstem neurons mediating horizontal eye position signals to dorsal neck muscles of the alert cat. In A. Roucoux and M. Crommelinck (Eds.), Physiological and Pathological Aspects of Eye Movements, Junk, The Hague, pp. 385–398.
Bilotto, G., Goldberg, J., Peterson, B. W. and Wilson, V. J. (1982) Dynamic properties of vestibular reflexes in the decerebrate cat. Exp. Brain Res., 47: 343–352.
Bishop, G. A., McCrea, R. A. and Kitai, S. T. (1976) Afferent projection to the nucleus interpositus and lateral nucleus of the cat cerebellum. Anat. Rec., 184: 360.
Bizzi, E., Kalil, R. E. and Tagliasco, V. (1971) Eye head coordination in monkeys: evidence for centrally patterned organization. Science, 173: 452–454.
Courville, J. (1966) The nucleus of the facial nerve. The relation between cellular groups and peripheral branches of the nerve. Brain Res., 1: 338–354.
Crommelinck, M., Roucoux, A. and Veraart, C. (1982) The relation of neck muscle activity to horizontal eye position in the cat. II. Head free. In A. Roucoux and M. Crommelinck (Eds.), Physiological and Pathological Aspects of Eye Movements, Junk, The Hague, pp. 379–384.
Darlot, C., Denise, P. and Droulez, J. (1985) Modulation by horizontal eye position of the vestibulo-collic reflex induced by tilting in the frontal plane in the alert cat. Exp. Brain Res., 58: 510–519.
Dieringer, N., Cocheran, S. L. and Precht, W. (1983) Differences in the central organization of gaze stabilizing reflexes between frog and turtle. J. Comp. Physiol., 153: 495–508.
Eccles, J. C., Nicoll, R. A., Schwarz, W. F., Taborikova, H. and Willey, T. J. (1975) Reticulospinal neurons with and without monosynaptic inputs from cerebellar nuclei, J. Neurophysiol., 381: 513–530.
Ezure, K. and Sasaki, S. (1978) Frequency-response analysis of vestibular induced neck reflex in the cat. I. Characteristics of neural transmission from horizontal semicircular canals to neck motoneurons. J. Neurophysiol., 41: 445–458.
Fuller, J. H. (1980) Linkage of eye and head movements in the alert rabbit. Brain Res., 194: 219–222.
Fuller, J. H., Maldonado, H. and Schlag, J. (1983) Vestibular-oculomotor interaction in cat eye-head movements. Brain Res., 271: 241–250.

Graf, W. and Simpson, J. I. (1985) The selection of reference frames by nature and by its investigators. In A. Berthoz and G. Melvill Jones (Eds.), Adaptive Mechanisms in Gaze Control, Elsevier, Amsterdam, pp. 1–16.
Grantyn, A. and Berthoz, A. (1983) Discharge patterns of tecto-bulbo-spinal neurons during visuo-motor reactions in the alert cat. Am. Soc. Neurosci. Abstr., 9: 751.
Grantyn, A. and Berthoz, A. (1985) Burst activity identified tecto-reticulo-spinal neurons in the alert cat. Exp. Brain Res., 57: 417–421.
Grantyn, A. and Grantyn, R. (1976) Synaptic actions of tecto-fugal pathways on abducens motoneurons in the cat. Brain Res., 105: 269–285.
Grantyn, A. and Grantyn, R. (1982) Axonal patterns and sites of termination of cat superior colliculus neurons projecting in the tecto-bulbo-spinal tract. Exp. Brain Res., 46: 243–256.
Grantyn, A., Grantyn, R., Robine, K. P. and Berthoz, A. (1979) Electroanatomy of tectal efferent connections related to eye movements in the horizontal plane. Exp. Brain Res., 37: 149–172.
Grantyn, R., Baker, R. and Grantyn, A. (1980) Morphological and physiological identification of excitatory pontine reticular neurons projecting to the cat abducens nucleus and spinal cord. Brain Res., 198: 221–228.
Grantyn, A., Berthoz, A. and Ong-Meang, V. (1985) Pontine reticulo-spinal neurons are a component of reticular circuits controlling eye-head synergies. Am. Soc. Neurosci. Abstr., 11: 1039.
Guitton, D., Crommelinck, M. and Roucoux, A. (1980) Stimulation of the superior colliculus in the alert cat. I. Eye movements and neck EMG activity evoked when the head is restrained. Exp. Brain Res., 39: 63–73.
Guitton, D., Douglas, R. M. and Volle, M. (1984) Eye head coordination in cats. J. Neurophysiol., 52: 1030–1050.
Harris, L. R. (1980) The superior colliculus and movements of the eyes and head in cats. J. Physiol. (Lond.), 300: 367–391.
Henkel, C. K. and Edwards, S. B. (1978) The superior colliculus control of pinna movements in the cat: possible anatomical connections. J. Comp. Neurol., 182: 763–776.
Hepp, K. and Henn, V. (1983) Spatio-temporal recoding of rapid eye movement signals in the monkey paramedian pontine reticular formation (PPRF). Exp. Brain Res., 52: 105–120.
Hess, W. R., Bürgi, S. and Bucher, V. (1946) Motor function of tectal and tegmental area. Mschr. Psychiat. Neurol., 112: 1–52.
Hikosaka, O. and Kawakami, T. (1977) Inhibitory reticular neurons related to the quick phase of vestibular nystagmus. Their location and projection. Exp. Brain Res., 27: 377–396.
Isu, N. and Yokota, J. (1983) Morphophysiological study on the divergent projection of axon collaterals of medial vestibular nucleus neurons in the cat. Exp. Brain Res., 53: 151–162.
Kaneko, C. R. S., Evinger, C. and Fuchs, A. F. (1981) The role of cat pontine burst neurons in the generation of saccadic eye movements. J. Neurophysiol., 46: 387–408.

Kuypers, H. J. G. M. and Huisman, A. M. (1982) The new anatomy of descending brain pathways. In B. Sjölund and A. Björklund (Eds.), Brainstem Control of Spinal Mechanisms, Elsevier, Amsterdam, pp. 29–54.

Lestienne, F., Vidal, P. P. and Berthoz, A. (1984) Gaze changing behaviour in head restrained monkey. Exp. Brain Res., 53: 349–356.

Lopez-Barneo, J., Darlot, C., Berthoz, A. and Baker, R. (1982) Neuronal activity in prepositus nucleus correlated with eye movement in the alert cat. J. Neurophysiol., 47: 329–352.

McCrea, R. A., Yoshida, K., Berthoz, A. and Baker, R. (1980) Eye movement related activity and morphology of second order vestibular neurons terminating in the cat abducens nucleus. Exp. Brain Res., 40: 468–473.

McCrea, R., Yoshida, K., Evinger, C. and Berthoz, A. (1981) The location, axonal arborizations and termination sites of eye movement related secondary vestibular neurons demonstrated by intraaxonal HRP injection in the alert cat. In A. F. Fuchs and W. Becker (Eds.), Progress in Oculomotor Research, Vol. 12, Elsevier/North-Holland, Amsterdam, pp. 379–386.

Melvill-Jones, G. (1964) Predominance of anti-compensatory oculomotor responses during rapid head rotation. Aerosp. Med., 35: 965–988.

Papez, J. W. (1927) Subdivisions of the facial nucleus. J. Comp. Neurol., 43: 159–191.

Peck, C. K., Schlag-Rey, M. and Schlag, J. (1980) Visuo-oculomotor properties of cells in the superior colliculus of the alert cat. J. Comp. Neurol., 194: 97–116.

Peterson, B. W. (1977) Identification of reticulospinal projections that may participate in gaze control. In R. Baker and A. Berthoz (Eds.), Control of Gaze by Brainstem Neurons, Elsevier, New York, pp. 143–152.

Peterson, B. W. (1984) The reticulospinal system and its role in the control of movement. In C. D. Barnes (Ed.), Brainstem Control of Spinal Cord Function, Academic Press, New York, pp. 27–86.

Peterson, B. W. and Goldberg, J. (1982) Role of vestibular and neck reflexes in controlling eye and head position. In A. Roucoux and M. Crommelinck (Eds.), Physiological and Pathological Aspects of Eye Movements, Junk, The Hague, pp. 351–364.

Peterson, B. W., Pitts, N. G., Fukushima, K. and Mackel, R. (1978) Reticulo-spinal excitation and inhibition of neck motoneurons. Exp. Brain Res., 32: 417–489.

Roucoux, A., Guitton, D. and Crommelinck, M. (1980) Stimulation of the superior colliculus in the alert cat. II. Eye and head movements evoked when the head is unrestrained. Exp. Brain Res. 39: 75–86.

Roucoux, A., Vidal, P. P., Veraart, C., Crommelinck, M. and Berthoz, A. (1982) The relation of neck muscle activity to horizontal eye position in the alert cat. I. Head fixed. In A. Roucoux and M. Crommelinck (Eds.), Physiological and Pathological Aspects of Eye Movements, Junk, The Hague, pp. 371–378.

Scheibel, M. E. and Scheibel, A. B. (1958) Structural substrates for integrative patterns in the brainstem reticular core. In H. H. Jasper, L. D. Proctor, R. S. Knighton, W. C. Noshag and R. T. Costello (Eds.), Reticular Formation of the Brain, Little, Brown Co., Boston, pp. 31–55.

Schor, R. H. and Miller, A. (1981) Vestibular reflexes in neck and forelimb muscles evoked by roll tilt. J. Neurophysiol., 46: 167–178.

Sirkin, D. W. and Teitelbaum, P. (1983) The pontine reticular formation is part of the output pathway for amphetamine — and apomorphine — induced lateral head movements: evidence from experimental lesions in the rat. Brain Res., 260: 281–296.

Sirkin, D. W., Schallert, T. and Teitelbaum, P. (1980) Involvement of the pontine reticular formation in head movements and labyrinthine righting in the rat. Exp. Neurol., 69: 435–457.

Straschill, M. and Schick, F. (1977) Discharge of superior colliculus neurons during head and eye movements of the alert cat. Exp. Brain Res., 27: 131–141.

Strauss-Durckheim, H. (1845) Anatomie Descriptive et Comparée du Chat, T. II, Paris.

Thoden, U., Dichgans, J. and Savidis, T. (1977) Direction specific optokinetic modulation of monosynaptic hind limb reflexes in cats. Exp. Brain. Res., 30: 155–160.

Vidal, P. P., Roucoux, A. and Berthoz, A. (1982) Horizontal eye position related activity in neck muscles of the alert cat. Exp. Brain Res., 46: 448–453.

Vidal, P. P., Corvisier, J. and Berthoz, A. (1983a) Eye and neck motor signals in periabducens reticular neurons of the alert cat. Exp. Brain Res., 53: 16–28.

Vidal, P. P., Roucoux, A., Berthoz, A. and Crommelinck, M. (1983b) Eye position related activity in deep neck muscles of the alert cat. In E. R. Pfaltz (Ed.), Neurophysiological and Clinical Aspects of Vestibular Disorders. Advances in Otorhino-laryngology, Vol. 30, Karger Basel, pp. 27–30.

Vidal, P. P., Graf, W. and Berthoz, A. (1985) The orientation of the cortical vertebral column in unrestrained, awake animals. I. Resting position. Exp. Brain Res., in press.

Whittington, D. A., Lestienne, F. and Bizzi, E. (1984) Behaviour of preoculomotor burst neurons during eye-head coordination. Exp. Brain Res., 55: 215–222.

Wilson, V. J., Precht, W. and Dieringer, N. (1983) Responses of cat's splenius muscle to optokinetic stimulation. Exp. Brain Res. 50: 153–156.

Yoshida, K., Berthoz, A., Vidal, P. P. and McCrea, P. (1981) Eye movement related activity of identified second order vestibular neurons in the cat. In A. F. Fuchs and W. Becker (Eds.), Progress in Oculomotor Research, Vol. 12, Elsevier/North-Holland, Amsterdam, pp. 371–378.

Yoshida, K., McCrea, R., Berthoz, A. and Vidal, P. P. (1982) Morphological and physiological characteristics of inhibitory burst neurons controlling horizontal rapid eye movements in the alert cat. J. Neurophysiol., 48: 761–784.

H.-J. Freund, U. Büttner, B. Cohen and J. Noth
Progress in Brain Research, Vol. 64.
© 1986 Elsevier Science Publishers B.V. (Biomedical Division)

Regulation of multi-joint arm posture and movement

E. Bizzi, F. A. Mussa-Ivaldi and N. Hogan

Massachusetts Institute of Technology, Department of Psychology and Whitaker College, Cambridge, MA 02139, U.S.A.

Introduction

The aim of this paper is to discuss the control strategies adopted by the central nervous system (CNS) to execute movements and maintain posture. To this end, we believe it is necessary to look first at the mechanical properties of the musculo-skeletal apparatus. Such an approach is based on the assumption that the functional properties of the motor system have been developed by the need not only to control, but also to take advantage of the mechanical properties of the musculo-skeletal apparatus. A case for this approach was made years ago by Feldman (1974a), who investigated the spring-like properties of the human arm. Muscles do indeed behave like tunable springs in the sense that the force generated by them is a function of length and level of neural activation (Rack and Westbury, 1974). In addition, muscles are arranged about the joints in an agonist-antagonist configuration. If muscles have spring-like properties, then a limb's posture is maintained when the forces exerted by the agonist and antagonist muscle groups are equal and opposite. This implies that when a force is applied, the limb is displaced by an amount proportional to both the external force, and the stiffness of the muscles. When the external force is removed, the limb should return to the original position. This prediction is nothing else than a restatement of Hooke's Law, but in a biological context. Evidence supporting the idea that muscles in vivo indeed have spring-like properties is briefly discussed in the first part of this report. In the second part, the implication of these findings for trajectory control is discussed.

Multi-joint spring-like behavior

Recently, we have investigated the way in which the CNS controls the muscle spring-like properties in the context of multi-joint arm posture and movement (Hogan, 1984, 1985; Mussa-Ivaldi et al., 1984, 1985). It should be emphasized that the muscle spring-like behavior in the multiple-joint case generates a richer and more complex situation when compared with analogous studies restricted to a single joint. For example, in the multi-joint case, the forces and displacements around neighboring joints are not independent, because of the existence of muscles which span two joints (such as biceps brachii). This interaction between all of the muscles is conveniently taken into account by considering the net stiffness at the hand. We have experimentally determined the relation between force and displacement of the end-point of the limb by displacing the end-point from an equilibrium position and measuring the steady-state force opposing the displacement.

We have shown that when the hand is displaced from a maintained posture and held at zero velocity, arm muscles generate a restoring force which, when the arm is released, returns the hand to the initial position in a manner which is entirely compatible with what would be expected of a spring

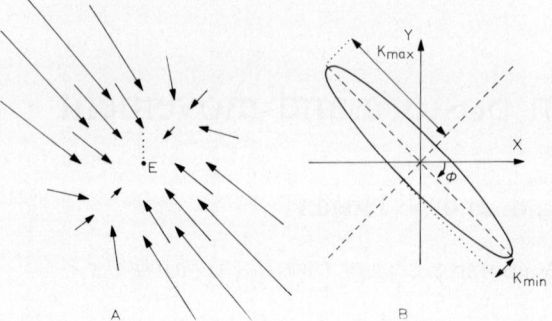

Fig. 1. Two representations of the postural force field. A. Pincushion diagram: force vectors $\underline{F}$ (arrows) are shown in correspondence to each displacement from the equilibrium point, E. B. Stiffness ellipse: the stiffness matrix which generates the force field is plotted with respect to a frame centered at the equilibrium point. The ellipse has a size (its area), an orientation (the angle ϕ) and a shape (the ratio K_{max}/K_{min}).

system. By recording the response to displacement of variable size and direction, we have succeeded in describing the field of elastic forces associated with the hand. At any given hand position, this field was characterized by a shape, a magnitude and an orientation (Fig. 1). We also found that the stiffness field

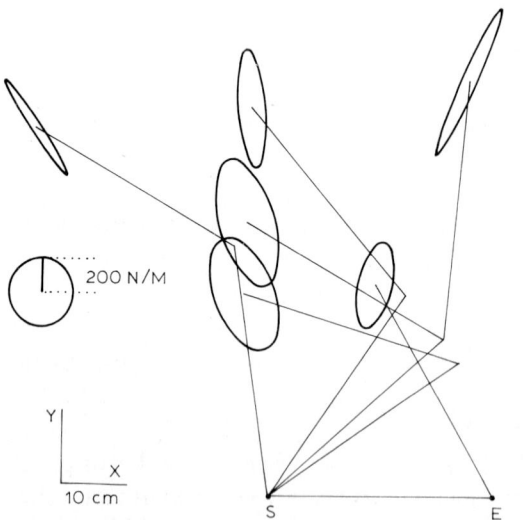

Fig. 2. Stiffness ellipses obtained from a subject during posture in six work-space locations. S, shoulder joint; E, elbow joint. The calibration for the stiffness is given by the circle, which represents an isotropic stiffness of 200 N/m.

associated with hand posture varies substantially at different positions of the hand in the work space.

Specifically, the shape and the orientation display a common pattern, which can be summarized as follows: the stiffness is more isotropic (circular) in proximal positions and more anisotropic (elongated) in distal positions; the direction of maximum stiffness is approximately oriented along a radial line joining the hand to the shoulder (Fig. 2).

Several factors may contribute to such regular variations. First, the mechanical advantage of a force applied at the hand which is a function of the elbow and shoulder joint angles. Second, the muscle insertions which are subject to variations in their moment arms as the joint angles change in the work space. Third, since the neural input to the muscles changes their spring-like properties (Rack and Westbury, 1969, 1974; Gottlieb and Agarwal, 1978), the observed variation in the stiffness may be due to the different levels of neural activation associated with different postures. In an effort to distinguish between these factors, we simulated the effect of a constant joint stiffness and found the simulated changes of end-point stiffness to be different from those recorded from our subjects. The systematic difference between these simulations and our experimental data suggests that changes in neural input contribute significantly to the determination of the hand stiffness.

When the stiffness was recorded in the same subject at intervals of days or months, there was a remarkable constancy in its shape and orientation. In contrast, it varied substantially in magnitude (up to 100%). These variations can be attributed either to a change in the level of "arousal" of the subject or to the after-effects of a prior experimental condition in which the subjects experienced postural disturbances. The variability in magnitude, coupled with the relative invariance in orientation and shape, is a strong indication that the increase in the motoneuronal activity, which is responsible for the increased magnitude of the stiffness, must be delivered in a well-controlled way. A change in stiffness magnitude at constant shape and orientation can be achieved only by a uniformly scaled change in the individual stiffnesses of all the elastic elements. It suggests that the alpha motoneuron activities are subject to coordinative constraints resulting either from coupling among different motoneuronal pools or from supraspinal signals activating these pools.

Formal test of muscle elastic behavior

We have devised a way to test the spring-like behavior of the multi-joint arm system. In general, an elastic field can be viewed as a potential energy valley. To explain what is meant by this term, consider that when a spring is stretched, potential energy is stored in it, giving rise to a force related to the amount of stretch. When the potential energy is plotted as a function of position, it assumes the shape of a valley, with the bottom (minimum potential energy) representing the equilibrium position of the spring. Vector calculus gives us a precise definition of spring-like behavior versus non-spring-like behavior. If the force/position relation is spring-like, then it defines a potential field. The potential energy is completely determined by the force/length relationship

$$\text{potential energy} = \int_{l_1}^{l_2} (\text{force}) \, d\,(\text{length}),$$

where l_1 and l_2 are initial and final positions). It may be proven that this potential energy can be defined if (and only if) the stiffness tensor is symmetric.

Experimentally, we have determined the muscle stiffness properties by imposing a displacement to the hand, and measuring the static restoring forces as a function of hand displacement. We have then computed the elements of the stiffness tensor and checked for symmetric and anti-symmetric terms. By comparing the magnitude of the symmetric and anti-symmetric components of the stiffness, we were able to quantify the extent to which the muscles are spring-like. Our results have indicated that the stiffness is essentially symmetric and this rigorously proves, for the first time, the spring-like nature of hand posture. In addition, these data allowed us to derive some important conclusions about the reflex regulation of the posture. In fact, the symmetry of the hand stiffness matrix implies that the matrix relating joint torques to joint displacements is also symmetric. The symmetry of the joint stiffness, in turn, indicates that a displacement of the elbow induces a torque at the shoulder which is equal to the elbow torque induced by a shoulder displacement. In other words, the spring-like behavior experimentally observed in hand posture results in the constraint that the mechanical coupling between the joints should be symmetric. If this is so, then heteronomous proprioceptive reflexes must have equal gain; a conclusion that could not have been reached on the basis of single-joint experiments.

From posture to movement: single joint experiments

The studies described in the previous section on multi-joint arm posture and previous experimental work on visually triggered head and arm posture in trained monkeys have shown that final position of the limb is an equilibrium point between sets of opposing forces (Bizzi et al., 1976; Polit and Bizzi, 1978). This view may be illustrated by reference to a simple mechanical analogue in which the muscles are represented by a pair of springs acting across a hinge in the agonist/antagonist configuration (Fig.

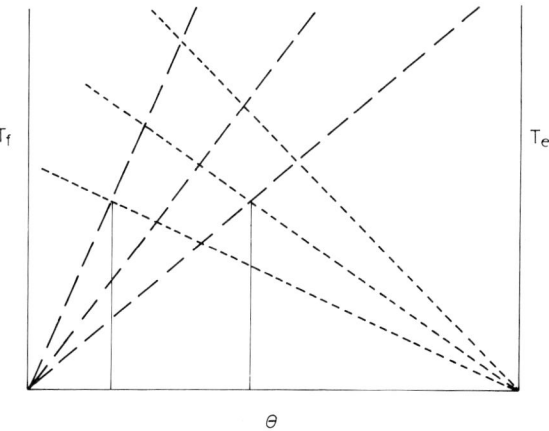

Fig. 3. Schematic representation of flexor (T_f) and extensor (T_e) length-tension curves. θ represents joint angle. From Bizzi et al. (1982).

3). If the control signal were to specify a new length-tension relationship for the springs, movement would occur until a new equilibrium point was reached. In accordance with this hypothesis, movements are, at the simplest level, transitions in posture. This hypothesis is attractive because it suggests that the CNS controls movements through a process specifying only the final position via a pattern of muscle activation. However, our results show that in the case of simple forearm movements the control signal induces a gradual shift of the equilibrium point and not a step-like shift in final equilibrium point.

The movements which we have examined involve pointing with the forearm to a visible target. Their velocity profile displays one peak and the electromyographic (EMG) activity typically appears as a burst gradually blending with the tonic activity characteristic of the holding phase.

In monkeys, three experimental paradigms were used to determine whether the motor control adopts the simple strategy of "final position control". The basic experimental set-up was the same in each case. The monkey sat in a primate chair with its forearm fastened to an apparatus permitting flexion and extension about the elbow in the horizontal plane. Several small target lights were spaced at 10° intervals along an arc centered on the axis of rotation of the elbow. The monkey had been trained to point to whichever light was on and to hold the arm for about 1 second in an electrically defined target zone 12–15° wide centered on the light in order to obtain a reward of water. A torque motor in series with the shaft of the arm apparatus was used to apply postural disturbances to the arm.

The first set of experiments was conducted in both intact and deafferented animals (Bizzi et al., 1982, 1984), in the absence of visual feedback. In randomly selected trials, a target was presented and the arm was clamped in its initial position before the onset of visually triggered movements, and then released at various times after the onset of evoked agonist EMG activity. The duration of the holding period (i.e., the time between the onset of EMG activity in the agonists and release of the arm) was varied randomly from 100 to 600 msecs. The acceleration of the arm immediately after its release was plotted as a function of the holding period (Fig. 4). In both intact and deafferented monkeys, the initial acceleration increased gradually with the duration of the holding period, for holding periods up to 400–600 msecs, and the movements were therefore progressively faster after the release of the arm.

These findings suggest that the simple forearm movements studied do not result from rapid shifts in the equilibrium point between agonist and antagonist muscle groups. According to the hypothesis of final position control, we would expect the steady-state equilibrium position to be achieved after a delay due only to the dynamics of muscle contraction. Individual motor units, recruited at low levels of force, reach their peak force 60–80 msecs after the onset of the action potential in the muscle fiber (Collatos et al., 1977). For a movement of at least 600 msecs duration, however, we found that the mechanical expression of the alpha motoneuronal activity did not reach steady-state until at least 450 msecs had elapsed after the onset of action potentials in the muscles.

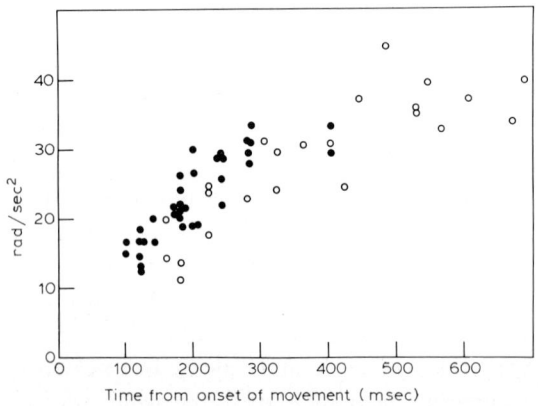

Fig. 4. The forearm of intact and deafferented animals was held in its initial position while the animal attempted to move toward a target light, and was released at various times. This figure is a plot of acceleration immediately following release versus holding time. The abscissa shows time in msecs; the ordinate shows radians per second squared. ●, intact animal; ○, deafferented animal. From Bizzi et al. (1984).

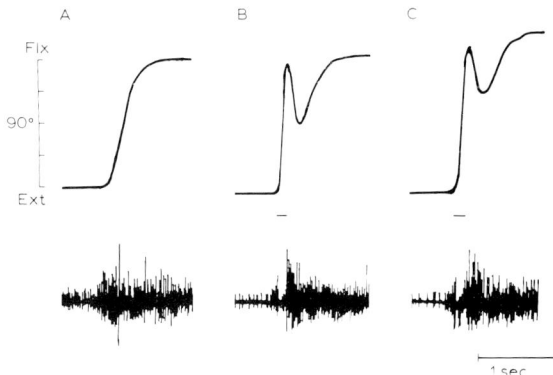

Fig. 5. Forearm movements with an assisting torque pulse in an intact animal. The upper trace shows arm position with an elbow angle of 90° at the midpoint of the scale; the lower trace shows flexor (biceps) EMG. The bar beneath the position trace indicates duration of the torque pulse. A. Control movement without a torque pulse. B, C. Two movements with torque pulses. The arm reached the target position early in the movement, transiently returned to an intermediate position, and then moved back to the target position. Note the unloading reflex in the EMG trace. Flx, flexion; Ext, extension. Position scale representing angular excursion = 60°. From Bizzi et al. (1984).

Similar conclusions were drawn from the second and third sets of experiments, which involved quickly forcing the forearm to the target position. In this set of experiments, as the intact monkey began to move toward a new target position, a brief torque pulse (150 mseconds), whose onset was triggered by the initial increase in EMG activity in the agonist muscles, drove the elbow quickly to the intended final position. However, instead of remaining in this position, the forearm returned to a point intermediate between the initial and final positions before reversing direction again and moving back towards the target position (Fig. 5). During the return movement to the intermediate position, which required extension, the flexor muscles showed EMG activity. Again, the findings suggest that these simple forearm movements cannot be ascribed to a rapid shift in the equilibrium point. According to the hypothesis of final position control, we would expect the equilibrium position to be achieved after a delay due only to the dynamics of muscle contraction (60–80 mseconds) and would

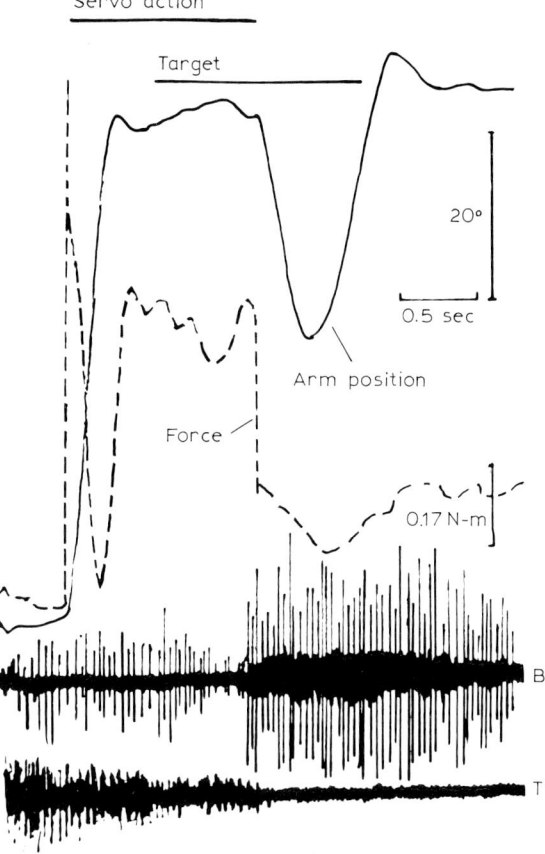

Fig. 6. Forearm movements of deafferented monkeys with a holding action in the final position. While the target remained off, the servo moved the arm to the target position, the target light was activated, and the servo was turned off. The arm returned to a position intermediate between the initial and target positions before moving back to the target position. Similar results were obtained in many trials in two monkeys. The upper bar indicates duration of servo action. The lower bar indicates onset of the target light. The broad trace shows arm position; the dashed trace shows torque. B, flexor (biceps); T, extensor (triceps). From Bizzi et al. (1984).

have no explanation for the return movement (Collatos et al., 1977).

The third set of experiments, performed in deafferented monkeys, provided further evidence against the hypothesis that the trajectory was controlled only by specifying the final position (Fig. 6). The arm was suddenly displaced to one of the target positions and maintained there by the servo action of the torque motor. The monkey could not have expected a reward, because the light at the target position had not been illuminated. In fact, because of the absence of any proprioceptive or visual information regarding arm position, the monkey was unaware of the displacement, Now, with the arm still constrained in the new position, the light at that position was illuminated. To the trained monkey, its appearance was a signal to start the neural processes involved in pointing to the target. We detected the onset of this process through the appearance of EMG activity in the proper set of muscles, after the usual reaction time. After a predetermined time (80–150 mseconds) had elapsed following the onset of the EMG activity, the torque motor was turned off, releasing the arm. Since the arm was in the correct position for receiving a reward, it is remarkable that the arm did not remain stationary after release. Instead, the arm first moved toward the position from which it had originally been displaced, and then changed direction and returned to the target position. This finding cannot be explained if muscles are regarded merely as generators of force, but is readily explained if the length-dependence of muscle force is taken into account. It should be pointed out that if the alpha motoneuronal activity evoked by the target light had rapidly achieved the level appropriate for the new final position, then no return movement should have taken place. The occurrence of the return movement indicates that the control signal is specified by a gradual shift toward the final position. This conclusion is consistent with the observation that the amplitude of the movement toward the final position decreased as the period of servo restraint of the arm was prolonged. Finally, when the servo action was maintained after the appearance of the evoked EMG activity for a period corresponding to the normal movement duration, the arm showed no significant movement after its release.

These findings suggest the existence of a gradually changing control signal during movement of the forearm from one equilibrium position to another and are not consistent with the hypothesis of a single, step-like shift to a final equilibrium point (Cooke, 1979; Kelso and Holt, 1980). Thus, in the transition from the intitial to the final position, the alpha motoneuronal activity defines a series of equilibrium positions, which constitute a trajectory whose endpoint is the desired final position. It should be emphasized that this hypothesis is based on analysis of forearm movements performed at moderate speeds and that the character of the control signal may vary with the type of movement.

From posture to movement: multi-joint experiments

The hypothesis that movements are centrally represented as gradual shifts in the equilibrium position of the limbs has also been tested for planar multi-joint arm movements (McKeon et al., 1984). Subjects were asked to perform pointing movements between two targets while gripping the handle of a two-link planar manipulandum. Unexpected activation of the clutch at J1 at the beginning of a movement (see Fig. 7) caused subsequent hand movement to be along an arc with radius equal to the length of the more proximal (J2) link of the manipulandum. The target locations and the timing of the clutch engagement were arranged such that the constrained path took the handle away from the intended path. The clutch could then be released

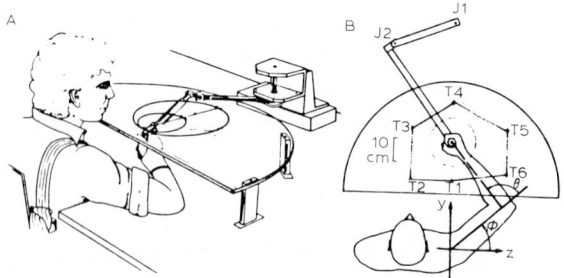

Fig. 7. Oblique (A) and plan (B) views of a seated subject grasping the handle of the hand-position transducer. The right arm was raised to shoulder level and moved in a horizontal work space. Movement of the handle was measured by way of potentiometers located at the two mechanical joints of the apparatus (J1, J2). The subject was positioned so that J1 lay on the Y axis. The two links of the apparatus were made of aluminium tubes. A clutch was mounted on the joint J1 of the apparatus. When it was activated, the handle was constrained to move in a circular path around J2. From Abend et al. (1982).

at different times, thereby removing the path constraint.

Following clutch release, a tendency for the path to return to the intended path rather than proceed directly to the final position was observed. In further experiments, handle force was measured. Movement duration was within the range 600–1200 mseconds. While the clutch was engaged, handle force was found to be always strongly oriented so as to restore the hand to the unconstrained path and not to the end-point of the path (McKeon et al., 1984). These findings allow us to extend to multi-joint arm movements the hypothesis that trajectories are executed as a sequence of equilibrium points of the hand.

Summary and conclusions

We have described the mechanical behavior subserving arm posture by providing a compact representation of the elastic field associated with the end-point of the limb. This field is described by the stiffness which relates forces to displacements and which is characterized by shape, size and orientation. The hand is at static equilibrium at the center of the field. In addition, we put forward a unique demonstration of the degree to which the neuromuscular system is spring-like. In the second part of the paper, we have presented experimental evidence supporting the hypothesis that arm movements are generated and controlled as a gradual shift of the end-point elastic field.

Acknowledgements

This research was supported by National Institute of Neurological Disease and Stroke Research Grant NS09343, National Institute of Arthritis, Metabolism, and Digestive Diseases Grant AM26710, and National Eye Institute Grant EY02621. Dr. Mussa-Ivaldi is supported by a CNR Fellowship.

References

Abend, W., Bizzi, E. and Morasso, P. (1982) Human arm trajectory formation. Brain, 105: 331–348.

Bizzi, E., Polit, A. and Morasso, P. (1976) Mechanisms underlying achievement of final head position. J. Neurophysiol., 39: 435–444.

Bizzi, E., Accornero, N., Chapple, W. and Hogan, N. (1982) Arm trajectory formation in monkeys. Exp. Brain Res., 46: 139–143.

Bizzi, E., Accornero, N., Chapple, W. and Hogan, N. (1984) Posture control and trajectory formation during arm movement. J. Neurosci., 4: 2738–2744.

Collatos, T. C., Edgerton, V. R., Smith, J. I. and Botterman, B. R. (1977) Contractile properties and fiber type compositions of flexors and extensors of elbow joint in cat: implications for motor control. J. Neurophysiol., 40: 1291–1300.

Cooke, J. D. (1979) Dependence of human arm movements on limb mechanical properties. Brain Res., 165: 366–369.

Feldman, A. G. (1974a) Change of muscle length due to shift in the equilibrium point of the muscle-load system. Biofizika, 19: 534–538.

Feldman, A. G. (1974b) Control of muscle length. Biofizika, 19: 749–751.

Gottlieb, G. L. and Agarwal, G. C. (1978) Dependence of human ankle compliance on joint angle. J. Biomech., 11: 177–181.

Hogan, N. (1984) An organizing principle for a class of voluntary movements. J. Neurosci., 4: 2745–2754.

Hogan, N. (1985) The mechanics of multi-joint posture and movement control. Biol. Cybern., 52: 315–331.

Kelso, J. A. S. and Holt, K. G. (1980) Exploring a vibratory system analysis of human movement production. J. Neurophysiol., 43: 1183–1196.

McKeon, B., Hogan, N. and Bizzi, E. (1984) Effect of temporary path constraint during planar arm movement. Abstracts, Society for Neuroscience, 14th Annual Meeting, Anaheim, CA.

Mussa-Ivaldi, F. A., Hogan, N. and Bizzi, E. (1984) Invariant features of hand postural stiffness. Abstracts, Society for Neuroscience, 14th Annual Meeting, Anaheim, CA.

Mussa-Ivaldi, F. A., Hogan, N. and Bizzi, E. (1985) Neural, mechanical and geometric factors subserving arm posture in humans. J. Neurosci., 5: 2732–2743.

Polit, A. and Bizzi, E. (1978) Processes controlling arm movements in monkeys. Science, 201: 1235–1237.

Rack, P. M. H. and Westbury, D. R. (1969) The effects of length and stimulus rate on tension in the isometric cat soleus muscle. J. Physiol. (Lond.), 204: 443–460.

Rack, P. M. H. and Westbury, D. R. (1974) The short range stiffness of active mammalian muscle and its effect on mechanical properties. J. Physiol. (Lond.), 240: 331–350.

Are corrections in accurate arm movements corrective?

Marc Jeannerod

Laboratoire de Neuropsychologie Expérimentale, INSERM, Unité 94, 16 Avenue du Doyen Lépine, Bron, France

Introduction

It has been commonly accepted, since Woodworth (1899), that accuracy of aiming movements of the arm results from interplay between "initial adjustment" and "current control". The initial adjustment reflects, in Woodworth's terms, the intention of the movement as a whole, i.e., its coordination and its extent. An error in initial adjustment will produce misdirection of the arm. Current control is responsible for final adjustment of the movement by way of the influence of vision. Woodworth had observed that movements executed at normal speed are slower at the end or even completed by little extra movements, although movements executed at high speed lack these final adjustments, because in the latter case he thought vision is not allowed enough time to exert its control on movement accuracy.

Later, Craik (1947) modelled the arm movement control system during tracking a moving target, as a system periodically generating ballistic corrections with a constant undershooting of target position. Accordingly, during tracking the system would systematically lag target position. When target would come to a stop the movement would approximate its position after a delay corresponding to one sampling period. Assuming, as Craik did, that ballistic corrections are too short by about 10% with respect to error, the final approximation after target stop would drive the moving arm within 1% of target position. In addition, such a system would be devoid of oscillations around a stationary target, due to the property of ballistic systems to be insensitive to feedback signals during the movement itself.

A refined version of the same model was proposed by Crossman and Goodeve in 1963 (see Crossman and Goodeve, 1983). These authors recorded hand trajectories during the task of pointing at targets of varying width. When the target was small and high accuracy was required, the deceleration phase of these movements approximated an exponential function. By contrast, when the target was so large that the movement was virtually aimless, the velocity profile was symmetrical, and lacked the exponential decay before the stop. The authors considered that the symmetrical velocity curve observed in aimless movements was the result of a single initial impulsion, as already hypothesized by Woodworth, and that the exponential decay observed in precise movements was in fact produced by a succession of overlapping and diminishing smaller curves of symmetrical shape. In other words, they thought that precise movements were composed of iterative single pulses approximating target position more and more closely.

At any rate, this difference between movements with and without a precise goal is interesting because it demonstrates that the longer deceleration observed when a high accuracy is required must be due to an active process for bringing the movement at the target, rather than to passive counteracting forces. A longer deceleration implies that a certain level of velocity is maintained in the later part of the trajectory in order to cover residual distance before the stop. In other words, a movement directed at a small target would unavoidably undershoot target position if it had a symmetrical velocity profile. In fact, significance of asymmetry of the velocity curve is difficult to interpret, particularly in the case of moving segments with a high load, such as the arm. In that case, the apparent smoothness of the deceleration curve could be an effect of filtering out smaller reaccelerations during the deceleration phase. Precise recordings of arm trajectories during pointing movements directed at large or small targets were made by Soechting (1984). This author observed that although the initial phase of the movement (up to the velocity peak) was highly stereotyped, the deceleration phase was much more variable. When the movement was aimed at a small target, duration of the deceleration phase was prolonged by comparison with movements aimed at larger targets. When the target was small it was approached at a low velocity, and in many instances the velocity profile showed a secondary peak before contact with the target was made.

An important aspect of the double impulse theory of Crossman and Goodeve (1983; see also Keele, 1968, 1981) is that the secondary movement is supposed to be a visually triggered correction. Accordingly, in the action of reaching, the motor system would first generate a movement independently from visual feedback and, after a delay (some 200–250 mseconds according to the classical estimate of Keele and Posner (1968)) needed for visual computation of the residual distance (error) between the limb and the target, would generate a correction. There are difficulties with this conception, however. First, the time for visual feedback to be effective can be much shorter than 200 mseconds (e.g., Carlton, 1981), and, therefore, visual feedback could improve final accuracy by acting during the movement generated by the initial impulse, and not only after completion of that movement. Second, as will be shown here, secondary movements may be present in situations where no visual feedback from the moving limb is available, which excludes visual corrective mechanisms.

Methods

One essential aspect of this study was to select a motor task requiring a high degree of precision. Movements involving prehension of small three-dimensional objects were selected. Correct grasping of an object implies simultaneous contact of the object by the thumb and the other fingers which form the hand grip. Such a simultaneity requires (1) that the amplitude of the arm movement that carries the hand exactly corresponds to the distance of the object with respect to the body, and (2) that arm movement and closure of the finger grip are rightly synchronized.

Apparatus

The apparatus consisted of a box, 68 cm high, 100 cm wide and 70 cm deep, resting on a table. It was divided horizontally by a semi-reflecting mirror into two equal compartments (Fig. 1). Subjects were seated in front of the box with their forehead resting on the front panel. They looked through a window within the upper compartment and placed their right hand in the lower compartment. Three-dimensional target objects were placed in the lower compartment along the subjects' sagittal axis. These were small (2–6 cm) solid objects such as a sphere or a cube. Distance from the body could be varied (e.g., 25, 32, 40 cm). Two experimental situations were used. In the control situation (visual feedback condition), subjects could see the lower compartment through the mirror. In this situation, they saw both the target object and their hand when they performed a prehension movement toward it. In the other situation, however (no visual feedback condition), sight of the hand was not possible. A mask was inserted below the mirror, so that the lower còmpartment was no longer visible. Target objects were displayed from the top of the upper compartment. Since the mirror was placed half-way between the target display and the table, subjects could see in the mirror a virtual image of the object projecting at the table level. Another object identical to that

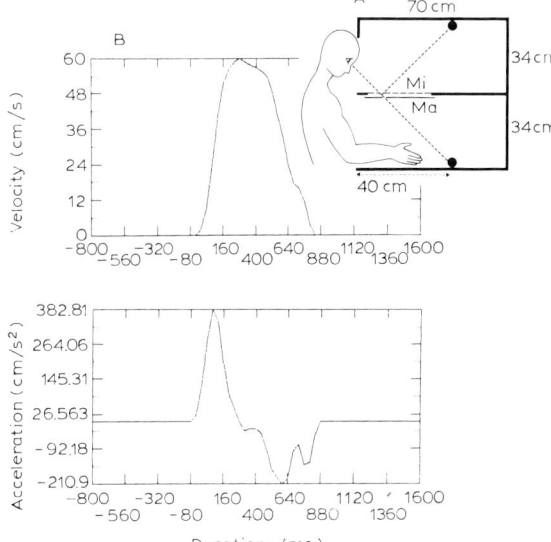

Fig. 1. A. Apparatus for manipulating visual feedback during prehension movements (from Jeannerod, 1984). When the mask (Ma) below the mirror (Mi) is withdrawn the subject sees his hand during part of his movement (visual feedback condition). When the mask is placed below the mirror (no visual feedback condition), the hand is no longer visible. B. Velocity and acceleration profiles of arm during a single prehension movement. Subject 6, target placed at 32 cm from body. No visual feedback condition. Total movement duration: 800 mseconds. Time to velocity peak: 280 mseconds. Onset of reacceleration (parameter A): 600 mseconds. Curves have been smoothed by using a least-square polynomial approximation. Frequency cut-off: 5 Hz.

seen in the mirror was placed directly on the table in exact coincidence with the virtual image. Thus, subjects reached for the virtual object below the mirror without seeing their hand, and met the second, real, object at the expected location.

Subjects and procedure

Subjects were seven young, right-handed volunteers. During the experiment, subjects had to place their right hand on a starting block near their body axis, with the forearm in the prone position and the fingers semiflexed. They were required to perform rapid and accurate movements, to grasp the target object as precisely as possible and to carry it near the starting block. No formal time constraint was given. At the beginning of each trial a new object was displayed while the subjects kept their eyes closed. At an acoustic signal they opened their eyes, and had to wait 2–10 seconds until a small light was turned on in front of them, before performing the reaching movement.

Each subject first received a few practice trials in the complete visual feedback condition. The idea was that subjects would be able to stabilize their velocity-accuracy tradeoff before the experimental trials started. Each subject then received a total of 20 experimental trials.

Data analysis

The radial aspect of the subject's hand was filmed with a cine-camera running at 50 frames per second. Data were processed by projecting frame by frame the image of the movement on a screen, with a 1×1 magnification. Duration of the movement was measured as the number of frames between the first detectable arm displacement and contact with the target object. Data from each second frame was kept for further analysis (i.e., time resolution was 40 mseconds).

The position of anatomical details on the wrist was plotted over successive frames. Distance between successive positions gave a measure of the instantaneous tangential velocity for the arm trajectory. From the same frames the relative positions of the tip of the index finger and the tip of the thumb were also plotted. This gave a measure of the size of the finger grip and its change over time. Due to the resting posture imposed on the hand and the shape of the objects, no rotation of the wrist occurred during the movement. It was assumed that the arm trajectory (and consequently the finger displacement) was rectilinear in the proximo-distal dimension, i.e., was effected in a plane parallel to the plane of the film. As far as it could be verified in the present study, this assumption appeared to be a reasonable one.

Those trials where the fingers appeared to come in contact with the table before contacting the object (an event which could be noted only during processing of the film) were discarded. Position, velocity and acceleration profiles were built for the arm trajectory and the finger grip size of each movement, with the help of a graphic programme on a MINC 11 computer.

Results

The complete set of results from this study has been previously reported (Jeannerod, 1984). In the present paper, attention will be focused mostly on the kinematic aspects of arm movements during prehension.

No visual feedback condition

Duration (T) of the movements was found to vary across subjects. For movements directed at targets at 40 cm distance, mean duration ranged from 674 mseconds in one subject up to 1013 mseconds in another one. This large variability can be explained by the fact that no time constraints were given for execution. Intrasubject variability was relatively low, since coefficients of variation for duration were around 10% in most subjects.

Trajectory of the arm

The general pattern of the transportation component was that of a U-shaped trajectory. The hand was first raised from the resting position and then lowered down to the object. The profile of tangential velocity of this trajectory was consistently marked by a sharp rise up to a peak, followed by a less steep deceleration. Mean peak velocity ranged between 56 cm/sec and 82 cm/sec. Time to the peak velocity was 308 mseconds from movement onset, on average (see Fig. 1).

In the three subjects where this was tested, i.e., subjects 5, 6 and 7, peak velocity was found to increase linearly with target distance. Correlation coefficients were 0.91, 0.93 and 0.92, respectively ($P < .001$). Fig. 2 shows this relationship in the three subjects.

The deceleration of the arm trajectory was consistently marked by a break point where the tangential velocity tended to become constant or even to reincrease before the movement was stopped at the contact with the object. The time of occurrence of this break point (parameter A) was measured for each movement on the curve of acceleration vs. time displayed graphically by the computer. The criterion for the determination of A was the value

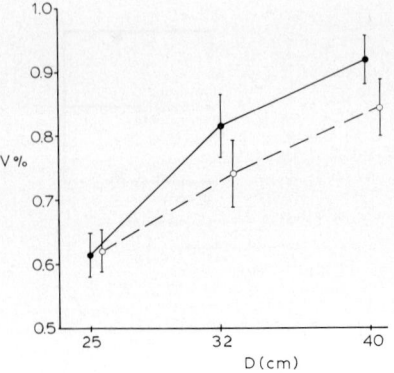

Fig. 2. Relationship of mean peak velocity of the transportation component to distance of the target. Values of peak velocity have been normalized with respect to the highest value for each subject. Solid line, no visual feedback condition (subjects 5, 6, 7). Dashed line, no vision condition (subjects 6, 7). The latter condition involved the same constraint as the no visual feedback condition, except that in addition vision of the target object was cut at the time of movement onset (Jeannerod, 1984).

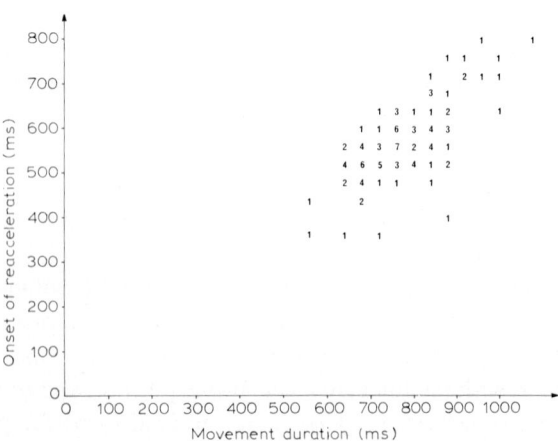

Fig. 3. Onset of reacceleration of the arm as a function of total duration of prehension movements. Digits indicate number of occurrences.

on the time axis of the lowest point on the acceleration graph (see Fig. 1). Fig. 3 shows the repartition of A values as a function of total movement duration (T) of the corresponding movements. It can be seen that the break point consistently occurred at a time which corresponded to 70–80% of total movement duration. The correlation of $A = f(T)$ was found to be significant in 6/7 subjects. In subjects 5, 6 and 7, whose averaged movements are shown in Fig. 4, correlation coefficients were 0.71 ($P < .01$), 0.86 ($P < .001$) and 0.83 ($P < .001$), respectively. As a consequence of the relatively invariant position of A on the time axis, the duration of $T - A$ (i.e., the duration of the secondary movement) tended to represent a constant ratio of total movement duration. This point is further documented by the fact that averaging movements of different durations did not alter the shape of the velocity profiles of these movements (Figs. 4 and 5). Obviously, if the break point occurred at different times from movement to movement and was not scaled to movement duration, it would be masked by the process of averaging.

The precise nature, in kinematic terms, of the break point is not easy to determine. This point corresponds on the acceleration profiles to a secondary "peak", during the deceleration phase. Although

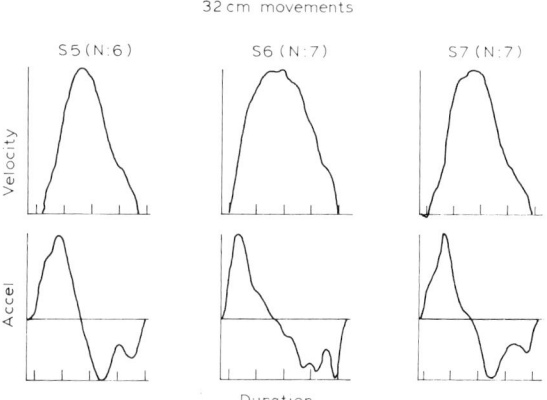

Fig. 4. Averaged arm movements during prehension. Velocity and acceleration profiles corresponding to several movements have been averaged in subjects 5, 6 and 7. Curves have been smoothed using the same technique as in Fig. 1B.

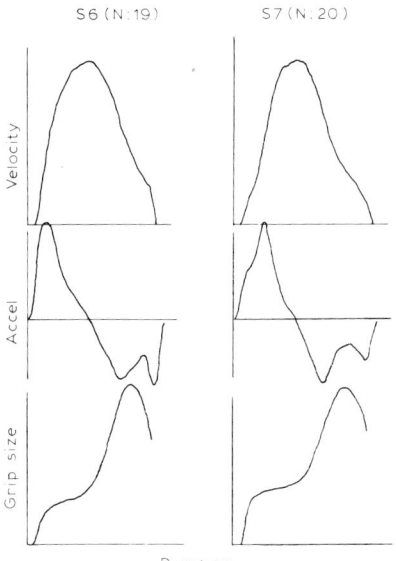

Fig. 5. Averaged prehension movements. 19 and 20 movements have been averaged in subjects 6 and 7, respectively. Upper two curves are averaged velocity and acceleration profiles as a function of time for the transportation component. Lower curve is averaged finger grip size as a function of time (manipulation component) from the corresponding movements.

this peak very rarely reached positive values of acceleration, it was nevertheless likely to represent reacceleration, partly damped by the load of the arm. Indeed, the slope of the curve before the peak was much steeper than would be required for a passive return to zero, an argument which favors the occurrence of an active process counteracting deceleration.

Finger grip

The resting position imposed on the subjects' hand before performing the movement implied semiflexion of the fingers. As the arm displacement was started, the fingers began to stretch and the grip size increased rapidly up to a maximum. At a later stage, the fingers were flexed again and the grip size was reduced in order to match the size of the target object. The size of the maximal grip aperture was a function of the anticipated size of the object, i.e., it was larger when the movements were directed at larger objects. The relationship of the grip size to

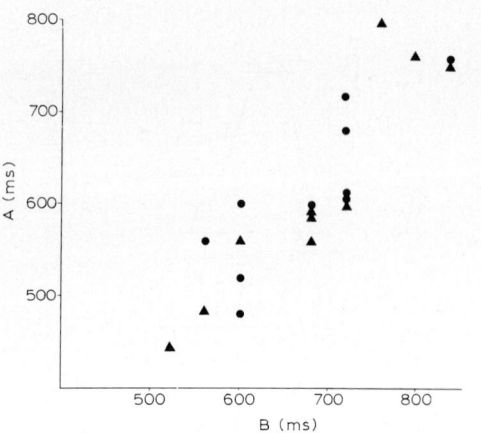

Fig. 6. Correlation between the onset of reacceleration of the transportation component (parameter A) and the time occurrence of the maximal grip aperture (parameter B) in subject 7. Note similar distribution for movements performed in the no visual feedback condition (●) and in the no vision condition (▲) (Jeannerod, 1984).

the object size has been described in more detail in a previous study (Jeannerod, 1981). In that paper, emphasis was put on the fact that the transportation component remained unaffected when the prehension movements were directed at objects of different sizes.

The position in time of the point of maximal grip aperture (parameter B) appeared to occur within 74–81% of total movement duration, except in 1/7 subjects, where it occurred earlier. In addition, the values of B for each given movement were found to be very close to those of A for the same movements. Fig. 5 demonstrates this point for subjects 6 and 7 in showing that the maximum grip aperture corresponds to the onset of reacceleration of the arm. A strong correlation was found between the values of the two parameters. As an example, A and B have been plotted against each other for the 20 reaching movements of subject 7 (Fig. 6). In this case the correlation coefficient for $A = f(B)$ was 0.89 ($P < .001$). The same degree of significance was obtained with five other subjects (r ranging between 0.76 and 0.88). Finally, in one subject, r was only 0.49 ($P < .1$).

Visual feedback condition

Prehension movements performed under visual control of the moving limb had a significantly longer duration. In addition, the value of the parameter A was less than in the no visual feedback condition. Decrease in the value of A together with increase in movement duration resulted in increase of the value $T - A$ of the secondary movement.

Discussion

Occurrence of arm reacceleration in the last 1/4 of prehension movements could fit the correction hypothesis put forward to account for the role of visual feedback in movement accuracy (see Introduction). However, the fact that secondary movements are still present when no visual feedback from the arm is available is an argument against a corrective role of vision.

The mode of control operating in arm movements is thus different from that observed in eye movements. In the case of ocular saccades secondary movements (termed correction saccades) seem to depend on visual feedback. This was demonstrated in 1975 by Prablanc and Jeannerod. In their experiment, subjects had to track by eye targets appearing in their peripheral visual field. Targets could either remain lighted for the duration of the trials (target step), or be turned off after 20–200 mseconds (target pulse). In the target-step situation main saccades were systematically followed by correction saccades (at least when target location was beyond 5° from central fixation). In the target-pulse situation, which involved the target being turned off before the main saccade was initiated, virtually no correction saccades were observed (they were present in only 1% of cases) so that undershoot of the main saccade with respect to target position remained uncorrected. The same result was obtained more recently by Mather (1985).

Prablanc and Jeannerod's (1975) results, however, were somewhat in contradiction with those obtained previously by Becker and Fuchs (1969). The latter authors had been able to show that secondary saccades were still observed when eye movements were executed in the dark. They argued that in executing eye movements toward a target the main and the secondary saccades are released as a single pre-programmed "package", whether visual feedback is available or not. Discrepancy between the results of the two groups may be explained by differences in experimental conditions. One of those differences is the size of target jumps used in each experiment (40°, Becker and Fuchs, 1969; 5–20°, Prablanc and Jeannerod, 1975. For a discussion of this point, see Prablanc et al., 1978). Another difference is the way the suppression of visual feedback was produced. Although in Prablanc and Jeannerod's experiment the target was turned off immediately prior to the movement, in the Becker and Fuchs experiment the target position was first learned by the subjects by moving their eyes between two lights; then the lights were turned off and a series of movements was executed in total darkness. It can be argued that in such a condition of prolonged absence of a visible target, the internal image used as a target for the eye movement rapidly deteriorates and loses its calibration with respect to the body position. This internal target, however, even though of a degraded spatial value, still can be used as a real target (Koerner, 1975), which would explain persistence of "correction" saccades to approximate its position. By contrast, in Prablanc and Jeannerod's experiment saccades were aimed at a real target which unexpectedly disappeared for a brief period of time at the onset of the movement.

In addition, another set of results published in the same paper (Prablanc and Jeannerod, 1975) tended to confirm that visual feedback is needed at the end of the main saccade for correcting eye movement amplitude. In that experiment, the main saccade was triggered by a short (20 msecond) target pulse, a situation where no correction saccade occurred and the undershoot remained uncorrected. However, if a second 20-msecond pulse was presented at the same location within a short delay (50 mseconds) after the end of the main saccade, a correction saccade occurred, which corrected the undershoot.

This difference in control modes between eye and arm movements can be accounted for by the respective characteristics of the two categories of movements. Arm movements such as reaching and grasping have many degrees of freedom. It is hard to believe that the complex muscular commands involved in the control of accuracy of such movements all could be handled by visual feedback alone. Visual feedback is typically a position feedback related to the endpoint of the limb, but it cannot reflect the intrinsic aspects of the movement (such as coordination between segments) that have to be controlled for achieving terminal accuracy. By contrast, saccadic eye movements are controlled by fewer muscles, they do not involve coordination between segments and are normally not subjected to changes in load of the eye. The only parameter to be controlled in this case is the difference between retinal position of the target and the fovea. In addition, contribution of proprioceptive feedback seems to be very limited in controlling eye movements. These might be the reasons why visual feedback is both necessary and sufficient for achieving saccade accuracy.

By contrast, reaccelerations observed in arm movements should probably not be looked at as corrections, but rather as an effect of the central patterning of motor output. Accordingly, they could represent "positioning" movements (Annett et al., 1958) or target "acquisition" phases (Welford, 1968), i.e., constraints appearing in movements involving several segments and requiring a high degree of precision. Relative synchrony of arm reacceleration with finger closure, as observed in the present results, is evocative of a central coordination. In this respect, it is interesting to note that segmental movements during prehension are coordinated in time, not in space. Coordination and corrections based on sensory feedback (visual or proprioceptive) would require positional cues, either from limb position with respect to the target, or to the body. These cues were not available for the visual modality in our experiment. It remains to be demonstrated whether proprioception might effectively represent at the central level a signal for intersegmental coordination. This point has been discussed in another paper (Jeannerod et al., 1984).

Acknowledgement

I thank C. Prablanc for his permission to use his computer programmes.

References

Annett, J., Golby, C. W. and Kay, H. (1958) The measurement of elements in an assembly task. The information output of the human motor system. Q. J. Exp. Psychol., 10: 1–11.
Becker, W. and Fuchs, A. F. (1969) Further properties of the human saccadic system: eye movements and correction saccades with and without visual fixation points. Vision Res., 9: 1247–1258.
Carlton, L. G. (1981) Processing visual feedback information for movement control. J. Exp. Psychol., Hum. Percept. Perf. 7: 1019–1030.
Craik, K. J. W. (1947) Theory of the human operator in control systems. I. The operator as an engineering system. Br. J. Psychol., 38: 56–61.
Crossman, E. R. F. W. and Goodeve, P. J. (1983) Feedback control of hand movements and Fitts law. Paper presented at the Mtg of Exp. Soc., Cambridge (1963). Reprinted in Q. J. Exp. Psychol., 35A: 251–278.
Jeannerod, M. (1981) Intersegmental coordination during reaching at natural visual objects. In J. Long and A. Baddeley (Eds.), Attention and Performance, Vol. IX, Erlbaum, Hillsdale, pp. 153–168.
Jeannerod, M. (1984) The timing of natural prehension movements. J. Mot. Behav., 16: 235–254.
Jeannerod, M., Michel, F., and Prablanc, C. (1984) The control of hand movements in a case of hemianaesthesia following a parietal lesion. Brain, 107: 899–920.
Keele, S. W. (1968) Movement control in skilled motor performance. Psychol. Bull., 70: 387–404.
Keele, S. W. (1981) Behavioral analysis of movement. In: V. B. Brooks (Ed.), Handbook of Physiology, Section I: The Nervous System, Vol. II: Motor Control, Part 2, Williams and Wilkins, Baltimore, pp. 1391–1414.
Keele, S. W. and Posner, M. I. (1968) Processing of visual feedback in rapid movements. J. Exp. Psychol., 77: 155–158.
Koerner, F. (1975) Untersuchungen über die nichtvisuelle Kontrolle von Augenbevegungen. Adv. Ophtal., 31: 100–158.
Mather, J. A. (1985) Some aspects of the organization of the oculomotor system. J. Mot. Behav., 17: 373–383.
Prablanc, C. and Jeannerod, M. (1975) Corrective saccades: dependence on retinal reaffernt signals. Vision Res., 15: 465–469.
Prablanc, C., Masse, D. and Echallier, F. (1978) Corrective mechanisms in visually goal-directed large saccades. Vision Res., 18: 557–560.
Soechting, J. F. (1984) Effect of target size on spatial and temporal characteristics of a pointing movement in man. Exp. Brain Res., 54: 121–132.
Welford, A. J. (1968) Fundamentals of Skills. Methuen Co. Ltd, London.
Woodworth, R. S. (1899) The accuracy of voluntary movements. Psychol. Rev., Monograph suppl., 3: 114.

Discussion

D. A. Robinson

Departments of Ophthalmology and Biomedical Engineering, The Johns Hopkins University, 601 North Broadway, Baltimore, MD 21205, U.S.A.

The seven papers in this session strike one for their diversity rather than their similarities. True, four of the papers deal with movements of the finger, hand and/or arm, but their goals as well as their techniques seem, at least at the level presented, rather different. Dr. Bizzi examines the arm as a two-joint system (shoulder and elbow) and measures its stiffness in a two-dimensional plane. The results should contribute to an understanding of the time course of the neural commands that control the musculature of each joint during rapid reaching movements as revealed by the results of suddenly perturbing the movement in midflight. Dr. Jeannerod examines coordination of the wrist and fingers in reaching to pick up a ball without visual feedback from the hand. This task differs from Dr. Bizzi's in that a physical object is to be encountered so that a single ballistic movement runs the risk of crashing into it. Understandably then, the movement is decomposed into a rapid phase that brings the hand and fingers close to the ball, and then a final phase in which the hand approaches more slowly and the thumb-finger distance is adjusted to the ball diameter. Dr. Noth measures the mechanical impedance of the finger using phase plots which display the results in a very clear and graphic way. Using an ischemic block he separates the impedance into that due to viscoelastic properties of the finger and that due to two reflex arcs. Characteristic shifts in the phase plot reveal abnormalities with, for example, cerebellar disease. Dr. Freund addresses yet another question: how fast can limbs or fingers be made to oscillate? Frequencies as high as 16 Hz can be observed and such movements are characterized by an isochrony principle in that their frequency is independent of amplitude. Note that some of these tasks are goal-directed, some plan physical contact with a goal, some are isometric, some essentially isotonic, some very fast; indeed, none of them share enough characteristics to be assigned to a common movement subsystem or a common movement strategy.

From the standpoint of the subject of this meeting — comparing oculomotor and skeletalmotor systems — one might compare these contributions to, say, four reports on the saccadic system, had they been put together in a single session (take, for example, the contributions of Drs. Goldberg, Sparks, Wurtz and Henn). The latter studies could immediately be related to each other because they all address themselves to a single, identifiable system, the purpose of which is well understood. They differ in techniques and regions of the CNS studied but they are unified as parts of a single system. Even if we were to compare the studies of limb movements to four studies within the entire oculomotor system, the latter papers would still be unified by a system that largely consists of only five subsystems. Not to belabor the obvious, the great heterogeneity in skeletalmotor studies arises from the inability to tease out individual subsystems of motor control, identify their purpose and study them in isolation. Whether this is even possible is moot. The question arises of whether, if we cannot do this, motor physiology will be forever doomed to studying bits and pieces of special, simplified situations, without ever being able to raise their sights to the larger issues. Unfortunately, the search for subsystems is fraught with more teleology, phylogeny and mathematical modelling than most investigators feel comfortable with. Perhaps the science of robotics will show the way.

A second difference, at once apparent, is that few studies appear anymore, even in oculomotor symposia, on the oculomotor periphery. Obviously, problems remain and treatment of disorders remains important, but because of an overall simplicity of the eye and its muscles, interest has passed deeper into the CNS as we try to understand where the signals come from and how they are created and shaped before coming to the motoneuron. Nor need we worry about short or long feedback loops from proprioception. The case is quite otherwise in skeletalmotor control, as this conference shows. Obviously, there is much concern with neural activity at higher levels of motor control, but the four papers in this session on limb control show how terribly dependent we still are on the biomechanics of the particular set of joints and muscles being considered at the moment and the effects of feedback loops that cause all these muscles to react seemingly at the whim of the CNS in defiance of generalized, mathematical tractability. Dr. Matthews remarked that so many of these loops are now appearing, of various latencies, that we should stop referring to them as a stretch reflex and give them different names. Dr. Noth illustrated the problem mentioned above by pointing out that it is difficult to think of a name for such a loop if you don't know its function. Clearly, these peripheral problems, fortunately absent in the oculomotor system, pose a formidable barrier to progress in skeletalmotor control.

A good portion of premotor circuitry and signal processing has been worked out in the oculomotor system. When Dr. Eckmiller describes neurons near the abducens nucleus that encode an eye-velocity signal in its discharge rate, he may reasonably be expected to suppose that, like other eye-velocity commands, it will proceed directly (if not monosynaptically) to the abducens motoneurons and indirectly through the neural integrator in the nearby prepositus and vestibular nuclei to supply the correct mix of velocity and position commands to make the eyes pursue. Of course, this needs to be demonstrated eventually, but the point is that his findings rest comfortably against a backdrop of common knowledge concerning signal processing prior to delivery to the motoneurons. Similarly, when Dr. Henn delivers excitotoxins to the pontine reticular formation, he knows that it contains burst neurons that deliver an eye-velocity command for saccades to the motoneurons and the neural integrator. The purpose was not to show what is already known but to sort out effects on vertical saccades and show that the neural integrator itself was not located there. Again, his findings rest on a crystallizing picture of premotor circuitry.

Unfortunately, such is not the case in the skeletalmotor system. The region corresponding to the pontine and medullary reticular formations in the vicinity of the abducens nuclei, the final staging area of all horizontal, conjugate eye movements, is undoubtedly the internuncial gray areas of the spinal cord. That these internuncials vastly outnumber the motoneurons assures us that they too play an important role in processing signals for the motoneurons. Our lack of knowledge in this area, due to the present difficulties in recording from it in moving animals, represents a major roadblock in building a bridge between the motoneurons and higher centers such as motor cortex and identifying any possible separation of activity into functional subsystems.

Dr. Berthoz, in this session, finds himself caught between the oculomotor and skeletalmotor camps. Head movements may offer an interesting bridge between the simplicities of the one and the difficulties of the other. Neck muscles are certainly rich in spindles, like the eye muscles, but, also like the eye, we seldom use our heads to manipulate external loads so the use of proprioceptive feedback loops may be less common or severe as for the limbs. Head movements are most frequently coupled to eye movements to serve vision so it is, perhaps, not so surprising to see, as Berthoz does, neurons in the same premotor areas of the brain stem subserving eye movements, that carry eye and head position signals to the cervical spinal cord. Serving eye movements is also, probably, a separable identifiable function for head movements. The head may also depend less on neck proprioception because it contains the vestibular apparatus; superb transducers of head position and motion. It may well be that craniomotor control may allow us to try to extend our good luck in the oculomotor system to a system that is more complex but, perhaps, not quite so complex as limb control.

The title of this section, Functional organisation of movement, causes me to come back to my original theme: the greatest advantage one has in the oculomotor system is that one knows the function of each of its subsystems and the greatest problem in skeletal motor systems is that it has not been so decomposed. Without it, progress will be slow indeed. It is, in my view, a theoretical problem. We don't know if it is solveable but, on the other hand, no one seems to be trying.

SECTION VI

Adaptive Control and Psychophysical Aspects

Chapter 5 Clinical and Psychophysical Aspects

Parametric adjustments in the oculomotor system

F. A. Miles

Laboratory of Sensorimotor Research, National Eye Institute, National Institutes of Health, Bethesda, MD 20205, U.S.A.

Introduction

Much of the current interest in the neural control of eye movements emanates from a general feeling that the oculomotor system is one of the simpler, more machine-like sensorimotor systems. The discrete, well-defined nature of the input and output, with invariant loading and modular central organization, all encourage a quantitative, systems approach to characterize its various operations. Precise descriptions of input-output relationships abound, generally the result of classical forcing functions beloved of engineers — sinusoids and steps — and studies that do not specify performance in terms of gain, phase shift, time constant, and so forth are apt to be discounted as anecdotal. The linear systems approach has proved to be an extraordinarily powerful tool, not only at the system level, but also at the level of the individual components — receptors, neuronal networks and motor apparatus. Conceptually, the field has been subsumed by the engineers, whose unromantic concern with the brain is merely to define its transfer function.

This machine-like quality, however, does not mean that the oculomotor system is totally hardwired and inflexible. Gonshor and Melvill Jones's report in 1971 showing that when subjects wore reversing prism spectacles their vestibulo-ocular reflex (VOR) underwent adaptive alteration, alerted the field to yet a further attractive feature of the oculomotor system — its adaptive versatility. The VOR functions to keep the eyes stable with respect to the stationary surroundings during head rotations and so prevents the movements of the head from disrupting the retinal image. The reflex operates open-loop since the semicircular canal receptors, which sense the input (head rotation), are in no way influenced by the eye movements which constitute the output. To be wholly successful, the output should match the input in amplitude (gain of unity) and show 180° of phase shift. Though less than perfect, the reflex is nonetheless very effective, and the adaptive mechanisms that were able to adjust the reflex to the extreme demands of reversing prisms are assumed to play a crucial role in the establishment and maintenance of normal performance. Without such an adaptive arrangement it is difficult to imagine how the system could establish an appropriate gain during development and survive the rigors of aging, minor disease, trauma, fatigue and so forth.

Over the last decade, other subdivisions of the oculomotor system that were recognized to function essentially open-loop — the saccadic system for instance — were found to be sensitive to visual disruption, and it seems that each year more and more parameters of oculomotor control are shown to be protected by some adaptive neural mechanism. Most recently, it has been realized that closed-loop systems such as those mediating visual tracking also benefit from such gain regulation. This should not have been surprising since, whatever the organizational structure of a control system, its performance will be adversely affected if its internal parameters have less than optimal values. Of course, the system's dynamics would be a crucial factor here and there is accumulating evidence that these too are subject to adaptive regulation.

One of the striking features of the oculomotor system is its modular organization: The vestibular, saccadic, vergence and visual tracking subdivisions generally fulfill distinctly different functions and have largely independent central processing. All are now known to be subject to some form of internal parametric adjustment and to utilize highly selected visual cues to detect and correct inappropriate performance (dysmetria). In order to ascertain whether a particular parameter is regulated by an adaptive mechanism, it has been usual to introduce some disturbance into the control loop to render the current value of the parameter in question inappropriate. Generally this has been done with a reversible, non-invasive optical challenge that was tailor made to stress only the parameter(s) of interest; the system's adaptive capability was then assessed from its ability to compensate.

The vestibulo-ocular reflex

Ordinarily, the retinal image of the surrounding world is kept reasonably stable during head movements by counter rotations of the eyes that are produced primarily by the VOR. Magnifying (or reducing) spectacles increase (or decrease) the magnitude of the eye movements required to compensate for any given head rotation and selectively challenge the nervous system's ability to regulate the gain of the VOR. If worn for a few days, such spectacles lead to an increase (or decrease) in the gain of the VOR (Miles and Fuller, 1974; Gauthier and Robinson, 1975; Miles and Eighmy, 1980; Gauthier et al., 1983). The magnification factors typically used here were quite large ($\times 2$ and $\times 0.5$), and during the adaptation period the subject is severely hampered because he is unable to keep his retinal image stable when he turns his head (Miles and Fuller, 1974); although there are visually driven reflexes that would help the subject to track the moving images that he sees through the spectacles, these have severely limited dynamic capabilities and so are never as effective as an appropriate VOR. Anyone who has had the prescription for his or her spectacles changed will have experienced these phenomena, if only mildly, each diopter producing a change in the magnification factor of about 3% (Rønne, 1923; Collewijn et al., 1983). While the extreme challenge of telescopic spectacles leads to rather gradual changes in VOR gain that are measured in days, the more modest stress of 5D spectacles, for example, can be fully compensated in only 30 minutes (Collewijn et al., 1981b, 1983). Spectacles, or equivalent optical arrangements, have now been used to demonstrate the existence of adaptive gain control in the VOR of a variety of species: humans (Gauthier and Robinson, 1975; Gonshor and Melvill Jones, 1976a, b; Berthoz et al., 1981; Melvill Jones and Gonshor, 1982; Collewijn et al., 1983); monkeys (Miles and Fuller, 1974; Miles and Eighmy, 1980; Paige, 1983); baboons (Gauthier et al., 1983); cats (Melvill Jones and Davies, 1976; Robinson, 1976; Keller and Precht, 1979; Godaux et al., 1983); rabbits (Collewijn and Grootendorst, 1978, 1979; Ito et al., 1979a; Nagao, 1983); birds (Wallman et al., 1982) and fish (Schairer and Bennett, 1977, 1978, 1981).

The left-right reversing prisms used by Gonshor and Melvill Jones (1976a, b) present a much more complex challenge to the VOR: in addition to reversing the visual input associated with horizontal (yaw) rotations of the head (stressing the horizontal VOR), they also reverse the visual input associated with rolling the head from side to side (stressing the torsional VOR), but do not alter the visual input associated with pitch rotations of the head (which stimulate the vertical VOR). The nervous system is able to respond appropriately to this asymmetric optical challenge, selectively attenuating the compensatory eye movements associated with rotations about the yaw and roll axes while leaving those concerned with rotations about the pitch axis unaffected (Berthoz et al., 1981). Such directional selectivity is also evident in the cat's adaptive response to cross-axis stimulation: rotating the animal vertically, while moving the visual surroundings horizontally, gradually leads to the appearance of a horizontal component in the compensatory eye movements generated during vertical test rotations in the dark (Schultheis and Robinson, 1981). Such orthogonal components are also evident in the vestibulo-ocular responses of human subjects whose visual input has been rotated 30° in the frontal, or roll plane, using a pair of rotated dove prisms (Callan and Ebenholtz, 1982).

Changes in VOR gain are elicited by the various optical devices whether the head rotations giving rise to the vestibular stimulation occur voluntarily during the normal course of events or are passively imposed by oscillating the subject on a platform. In the latter case, however, sinusoidal oscillation at a particular frequency leads to gain changes that are generally greatest at the adapting frequency (Robinson, 1976; Collewijn and Grootendorst, 1979; Schairer and Bennett, 1981; Wallman et al., 1982; Nagao, 1983; Lisberger et al., 1983; Godaux et al., 1983). In the rabbit, this frequency selectivity is very marked, and after the platform has stopped the eyes may even continue to oscillate (in the dark) at the adapting frequency (Collewijn and Grootendorst, 1979). This led the authors to suggest that the adaptive mechanism in this species stores patterns of motion which are emitted whenever the sensory-motor conditions match those that prevailed at the time of storage. In the primate, frequency selectivity is less sharply tuned and characteristic, orderly phase shifts are evident at test frequencies above and below the adapting frequency (Lisberger et al., 1983)*. This has led to the suggestion that the central pathways in the primate are organized into parallel, overlapping temporal-frequency channels that act as bandpass filters (Miles et al., 1985). This adaptive equalizer model functions conceptually like the spectrum equalizer in a high-fidelity sound reproduction system, which emphasizes or de-emphasizes portions of the audio spectrum to match the acoustics of the auditorium. The channels in the VOR are assumed to differ in their dynamic properties and to each have independently adjustable gain elements. A key point here is that the adaptive mechanism can address selected channels because of their phase differences: adjustments are assumed to depend on precise phase coherence (or temporal coincidence) between the vestibular and error inputs to the modifiable element. Simulation reveals that such an arrangement could operate as an adaptive tuning mechanism, effectively compensating for the frequency-dependent dynamics of the labyrinthine receptors and the oculomotor plant.

The site of adaptation

Cognizant of Marr's (1969) theory invoking the cerebellar cortex as an important site for motor learning, Ito (1972) suggested that the long-term changes in VOR gain were mediated by modifiable synapses in the floccular lobes of the cerebellum. Based largely on his assessment of the anatomical arrangements in the rabbit, Ito suggested that the flocculus was a side-loop of the reflex whose contribution was regulated in the long term by climbing fiber inputs. Climbing fibers had been shown to receive visual inputs (Maekawa and Simpson, 1973; Simpson and Alley, 1974), which it was assumed would allow them to sense the retinal image slip associated with head rotations and in some way regulate the efficacy of the coincidental vestibular mossy fiber inputs to the Purkinje output cells. Subsequent recordings from the Purkinje cells (P cells) in the flocculus of the albino rabbit revealed differences between the discharge modulations evoked by vestibular stimulation in normal and adapted animals (Dufossé et al., 1978a). However, these data are difficult to interpret because neither the site of the recording nor the origin of the recorded modulations are known: the adaptation procedure most probably resulted in modifications restricted to the horizontal VOR, but since the exact loci of the recordings in the adapted animals were not known it is not possible to ascertain which of the recorded cells were in the zone most likely to be concerned with the horizontal VOR; changes in the efficacy of

---

* Similar trends are evident in the phase data for cats (Godaux et al., 1983) and birds (Wallman et al., 1982).

the horizontal vestibular signals were inferred solely from a statistical comparison of the subset of P cells that modulated in phase with contralateral head movement — selected on the grounds that there was a preponderance of such cells in areas from which microstimulation is known to elicit horizontal eye movements; the signal content of the discharges was not determined and secondary effects due to non-vestibular signals — such as those related to eye movements (Miyashita, 1984) — cannot be reliably assessed. Unfortunately, there are so many assumptions here that no firm conclusions are possible from this study.

A most ingenious series of experiments by Collewijn and Grootendorst (1978, 1979) has since shown that the adaptive mechanism in the pigmented rabbit senses errors in the gain of the VOR by matching visual inputs to compensatory eye movements rather than to head movements (or vestibular inputs). In fact, in the laboratory, it was possible to contrive matters so that VOR gain could be increased by visual inputs alone, using sinusoidal optokinetic stimulation with no head movement*. These findings suggest that a re-appraisal of the original Ito model and of the role of the flocculus is in order. Lesions of the flocculus have been shown to compromise the adaptive capability of the VOR in every species so far examined (Robinson, 1976; Schairer and Bennett, 1981; Nagao, 1983; Lisberger et al., 1984) and, as a consequence, this structure continues to be the focus of studies concerned with the site of adaptation. However, the clear suggestion from some recent studies in the primate is that the flocculus in this species is not the site of the modifiable elements but rather supplies the error information that guides the induction of changes elsewhere, presumably the brain stem.

Unlike the rabbit, man and monkey do not show increases in VOR gain with persistent optokinetic stimulation in the absence of vestibular stimulation (Collewijn et al., 1981a, 1983; Miles and Lisberger, 1981a; Lisberger et al., 1984). This and other data suggest that the adaptive mechanism in the primate relates retinal slip to ongoing head movements. That semicircular canal primary afferents and the cells that they innervate in the brain stem are unaffected by adaptation is known from recordings in the vestibular nerve and nuclei (Lisberger and Miles, 1980; Miles and Braitman, 1980). The flocculus is known to play an important role in visual tracking in primates (Zee et al., 1981) and the discharges of many P cells in the primate flocculus effectively encode horizontal or vertical gaze velocity during visual tracking by summing together head velocity (vestibular) and eye velocity signals (Lisberger and Fuchs, 1978; Miles et al., 1980b). Recordings from these cells in normal and adapted monkeys have revealed that the strength of the horizontal vestibular component of discharge varies along with the gain of the horizontal VOR (Miles et al., 1980a). Based on the current model of these gaze velocity P cells and their link to the VOR, it was concluded that the recorded changes were the exact converse of those that would have been expected if these cells had been part of the modifiable gain element. On the other hand, the changes were exactly in accord with the idea that the gaze velocity P cells were encoding the error signals responsible for the induction of gain changes elsewhere in the VOR pathway. It was argued that whenever the VOR gain was inappropriate the subject had to use visual tracking to improve retinal image stability during head turns; persistent tracking during head turns would therefore be a direct index of the error in the VOR and any central correlate of the same — such as the discharges of the gaze velocity P cells — could in theory guide re-calibration of the reflex and supplement or even substitute for frank visual error signals (Miles and Lisberger, 1981b). In this scheme, the retinal slip associated with head movements is only the first in a complex chain of events that culminates in adaptation. In fact, it is known that adaptation can still proceed even when pursuit tracking is so effective that visual errors during head turns are completely eliminated or even per-

---

* The same observation has been made on fish (Schairer and Bennett, 1978), but a recent attempt to replicate the finding in rabbits was unsuccessful (Nagao, 1983), probably because responses were not tested at the appropriate (adapting) frequency.

sistently reversed by over-shoot: retinal slip per se is clearly not directly guiding adaptation here (Collewijn et al., 1983). Such data led to the suggestion that in the primate the tracking response during head turns constitutes the system's most reliable estimate of VOR gain error (Miles, 1982). It is interesting in this regard that large-field visual stimulation is not necessary for adaptation: changes in VOR gain can be induced by tracking quite small targets that either are seen through spectacles (Collewijn et al., 1983), or have been linked to head movements so that they move as if seen through spectacles (Miles and Lisberger, 1981a; Lisberger et al., 1984).

All of these data on the primate are consistent with the view that the adaptive mechanism uses the gaze velocity signals encoded in the discharges of many P cells in the flocculus to evaluate and correct long-term VOR gain errors. However, as yet positive proof for this position is lacking. It can still be argued that changes in VOR gain are mediated by synaptic modifications in the floccular cortex that affect P cells other than the so-called gaze velocity type, and a recent study claims to have recorded from such cells (Watanabe, 1984). This study recorded the P cell discharge modulations evoked by horizontal oscillations in the dark, and reported changes in both amplitude and phase in association with changes in the horizontal VOR gain. Unlike earlier studies, this one used the eye movements evoked by microstimulation at the recording sites to classify the cells and to assess their likely ability to modulate VOR gain. Unfortunately, this study did not assess the signal content of the P cell discharges, and the etiology of the observed changes during oscillation testing — so crucial for the resolution of cause/effect issues — is not known. It is also unclear whether the attempt to rule out secondary effects by lesioning the brain stem and eliminating compensatory eye movements was actually successful.

Lesions of that part of the inferior olive which supplies climbing fiber inputs to the flocculus have been shown to eliminate adaptive gain control in the VOR of the rabbit and cat (Ito and Miyashita, 1975; Haddad et al., 1980). However, it has been reported that the destruction of climbing fibers causes P cells to lose their customary inhibitory action on vestibular relay cells in the brain stem (Dufossé et al., 1978b; Ito et al., 1978, 1979b)*, so that lesions of the olive might be expected to merely mimic lesions of the flocculus. Lidocaine injections into the inferior olive in the cat have been shown to cause an immediate increase in the gain of the VOR, regardless of its initial value (Demer and Robinson, 1982). Given the ultra-low discharge rates of climbing fibers, this would infer that they exert some modulating influence on the transmission of vestibular signals through the floccular cortex, complicating the interpretation of deficits following olivary lesions yet further.

In conclusion, the site of the modifiable elements responsible for the adaptive regulation of VOR gain remains unknown, and the exact role of the flocculus — as the locus of the underlying changes and/or the source of the error information used to guide the induction of such changes elsewhere — remains unresolved. Perhaps it is time for a new approach. One promising new development is the finding in cats that depletion of brain catecholamines with intracisternal injections of 6-hydroxydopamine results in major deficits in the animal's ability to reduce the gain of its VOR (Keller and Smith, 1983).

Saccadic eye movements

Magnifying the visual image with spectacles that move with the head in no way alters the task of the saccadic system, which senses eccentric targets and programs rapid eye movements that will bring their images into the fovea. If, however, the optical magnification were to be achieved by contact lenses that moved with the eyes, then the challenge would be quite different. Contact lenses do not affect the compensatory eye movements required to maintain retinal image stability during head turns but do al-

---

* Although one attempt to replicate this result was not successful (Montarolo et al., 1981).

ter the apparent eccentricity of the images. That is to say, they affect the input to the saccadic system: contact lenses cause saccadic dysmetria. In the laboratory, this effect has been achieved by consistently shifting the target while the subject is in the act of trying to aquire it with a saccade. Depending on the nature of the shift, subjects at first consistently under- or over-shoot the target with their primary saccades and must follow up with unusually large secondary correctives. Provided that the target shifts are not too large, the subjects fail even to perceive them. Nonetheless, the subjects soon begin to compensate and in minutes are acquiring the displaced targets with their primary saccades with their customary accuracy (McLaughlin, 1967; Vossius, 1972; Henson, 1978; Miller et al., 1981; Wolf et al., 1985).

Recent studies concerning the saccadic system's ability to compensate for more profound dysmetrias, such as those that result from weakness of the extraocular muscles, have uncovered some long-term adaptive processes that require days for completion. Kommerell and colleagues (1976) recorded eye movements in patients with partial, unilateral abducens nerve palsies who, because they happened to have better vision in their paretic eye, were in the habit of using that eye in preference to the visually impaired one with normal control. In fact, saccades made by the paretic eye were more accurate than those of the non-paretic eye, which were hypermetric. After patching the paretic eye for a few days, the visually impaired eye became orthometric while the covered (paretic) eye became hypometric. That both eyes were affected in the same way was crucial to the thesis that the adaptive changes were in the brain and not the muscles: in the monocular viewing situation, corresponding muscles of the two eyes (e.g., right lateral rectus and left medial rectus) receive the same innervation (Hering's Law); thus, the fact that the reduction in saccadic amplitude was also evident in the covered eye indicated that the changes underlying the improvement in the accuracy of the non-paretic viewing eye were central and not peripheral.

Abel and coworkers (1978), using a similar approach with a patient with a unilateral IIIrd nerve palsy but normal vision in both eyes, found that patching the non-paretic eye led to increases in the saccadic innervation to that eye, which rendered it severely hypermetric. Further, this adaptation occurred without altering the peak velocity-amplitude relationship of the saccades produced by the normal eye. This suggested that saccadic amplitude was being regulated through adjustments of the duration — and not the velocity — of the programmed movement. This in turn was taken to indicate that the programmed pulse of innervation that rapidly moves the eye to a new position is subject to adaptive regulation by processes that operate on its duration rather than its amplitude.

The patients in the above studies consistently used only one of their eyes. When they were first obliged, by patching, to use their other eye, they not only had difficulty acquiring targets with their primary saccades, as already mentioned, but also had problems maintaining stable fixation afterwards, their eyes tending to drift consistently onwards or backwards with a roughly exponential waveform for 100 mseconds or longer: so-called post-saccadic drift. Once more, however, visual experience resulted in the gradual elimination of the problem in the viewing eye, while the covered eye gradually developed the reverse problem, i.e., post-saccadic drifts in the converse direction. Clearly, the improvement in the viewing eye must have been achieved through adjustments in the innervation. The maintenance of good ocular stability immediately after the execution of a saccade depends on the programming of a new level, or step, of innervation that is exactly appropriate for holding the eye at its newly acquired position against the elastic forces encountered there. If the step of innervation is too large for the antecedent pulse then the eye will drift onwards, and if it is too small the eye will drift back. The system's ability to eliminate post-saccadic drift is taken to indicate that the step component of the saccadic program also is subject to adaptive regulation.

Optican and Robinson (1980) studied these same adaptive mechanisms in monkeys by surgically weakening the medial and lateral recti muscles of one eye. Following patching of the intact eye, the eye with weakened muscles gradually recovered normal saccadic accuracy and post-saccadic stability provided that the cerebellum was intact: midline lesions of the cerebellum compromised the pulse adaptation underlying the recovery of accuracy, while lateral lesions involving the flocculus and paraflocculus compromised the step adaptation underlying the recovery of post-saccadic stability. This clearly established the existence of two separate adaptive mechanisms that were dependent on the integrity of different parts of the cerebellum and operated to regulate two separate parameters of saccadic performance. This study also showed that these adaptive processes were each capable of considerable selectivity and could moderate their influence in accordance with the varying needs of different orbital positions and directions of movement.

The animals in the above study with midline cerebellar lesions were particularly interesting because they managed to eliminate post-saccadic drift while continuing to make hypometric saccades (Optican and Robinson, 1980). This indicates that the step of innervation is not regulated in absolute terms but is merely matched to the antecedent pulse — even when, as in this case, the pulse is dysmetric and fails to acquire the target. This notion of pulse-step matching suggested that the adaptive mechanism regulating the amplitude of the step component might be concerned solely with the suppression of post-saccadic ocular drift and detect errors by merely sensing post-saccadic retinal image slip. This hypothesis was recently tested in monkeys using a visual display positioned under computer control to permit the scene to be drifted after each saccade in such a way as to simulate exactly the visual consequences of pulse-step mismatch (Optican and Miles, 1985). Over a period of days this resulted in the appearance of pronounced post-saccadic ocular drifts with roughly exponential decaying waveforms such as might be expected to follow a central adjustment of the saccadic pulse-step ratio. Drifting the visual scene, of course, results in displacement as well as movement of the images, and either parameter might be the adequate stimulus to adaptation. However, changing the post-saccadic pattern of movement so that each drift was first exactly offset by an abrupt displacement did not affect the adaptation. The fact that the adapting paradigm now involved only transient displacement of the scene meant that the system's response — post-saccadic ocular drift — was now maladaptive insofar as it resulted in a net displacement of the eye with respect to the scene: the adaptive mechanism seems to be sensitive to velocity rather than position errors, which is consistent with the idea that it uses post-saccadic slip to sense and correct pulse-step mismatch (Optican and Miles, 1985).

The above experiments involving artifically imposed post-saccadic drift generally employed an exponential pattern of movement with a time constant of 50 mseconds, which approximated the time constant of the ocular drift seen in the earlier study on monkeys with surgically weakened muscles (Optican and Robinson, 1980). It had been assumed that the time constant of the post-saccadic ocular drift induced by these paradigms would always be a function solely of orbital mechanics as the eye passively assumed the final position dictated by the step of innervation. However, halving or doubling the time constant of the artificially imposed drifts resulted in corresponding changes (albeit smaller) in the time constant of the subsequent post-saccadic ocular drifts (Optican and Miles, 1985). It seems reasonable to assume that orbital mechanics would not be affected by these paradigms, hence the clear suggestion here is that the transition from pulse to step is not so sudden that, in the event of a mismatch, the gradual settling of the eye is merely a passive mechanical one. A recent study of the extraocular motoneuron discharges responsible for saccadic eye movements in the monkey has emphasized the existence of a so-called slide component of discharge, which prolongs the transition between the pulse and step components of innervation (Goldstein, 1983). It would seem from this that there are three components to the saccadic neural program — pulse, slide, step — and all appear to be subject to adaptive regulation.

Visual tracking

While it is true that closed-loop negative feedback control systems are less sensitive to fluctuations in internal parameters, there is always an optimal range of preferred values: if the forward loop gain were very low the system would be sluggish and display a large steady-state error; if the gain were very high the system would be much more brisk but show overshoot and oscillation. The optimal, preferred gain would represent a compromise, being that which would give a reasonably brisk response rate, acceptable steady-state error and adequate stability.

Visual tracking, whereby images drifting across the retina elicit eye movements that work to eliminate that drift, is essentially a closed-loop operation. All animals with mobile eyes use a visual tracking system, often referred to as the optokinetic reflex, to help stabilize their eyes with respect to the stationary surroundings. If they so choose, primates can also track small targets that move across the stationary background using the so-called pursuit system. Unfortunately, it is often difficult to make a clear distinction between the systems mediating these two kinds of tracking. Further, while retinal image slip is a powerful input to these tracking systems, it is not the only one, and they do not function simply as velocity servo systems. Motivational factors are also known to exert a considerable influence on visual tracking, a particularly troublesome factor for anyone trying to investigate parametric regulation: paradigms that challenge the tracking system to increase or decrease its gain may also unwittingly encourage the subject to try harder (or less hard); in this event, any improvement (or deterioration) in tracking performance is unlikely to be accepted as evidence for parametric regulation. Nonetheless, recent studies have provided some evidence for the existence of long-term adaptive mechanisms operating to regulate a large number of control parameters in these tracking systems.

The first of these studies, on monkeys, was concerned with the visual tracking mechanisms that help to stabilize the eyes in space, and measured the initial ocular following responses elicited by unexpected, brief (100 mseconds) movements of the visual scene (Kawano and Miles, 1983). Animals were never trained to track these movements and were never reinforced for their responses; furthermore, the speed, direction and onset time of the test ramps were always randomized. Surprisingly, such movements of the scene invariably elicited machine-like tracking responses at latencies commonly as short as 50 mseconds. To ascertain if the forward loop gain of the system generating these ocular following responses was subject to adaptive regulation, animals were exposed to brief velocity-step movements of the scene; these were designed to initiate ocular following and then transiently induce retinal events such as might be expected if the gain was clearly too low or too high. To this end, the scene was first drifted at a particular speed for 150 mseconds, after which time the speed was either stepped up (to induce "undershoot") or, in other experiments, stepped down (to induce "overshoot") for a further 150 mseconds. Each such sequence was terminated by blanking the scene for half a second, and was repeated at irregular intervals, randomizing the direction of movement and the magnitude of the speed changes. Again, tracking performance was never reinforced. Over a 3-day period, step-up experience resulted in clear increases in the tracking responses to the standard 100-msecond test ramps, while step-down resulted in the converse. Adaptation was selective for both direction and speed, so that responses to movements in one direction could be altered independently of those in other directions, and responses to low speeds ($<40°$/sec) could be altered independently of those to high ($>40°$/sec). Modifying the velocity-step paradigm to produce sudden changes in direction rather than speed also elicited adaptation: if the velocity-step paradigm involved 90° changes in the direction of movement while keeping the speed constant, then the tracking responses acquired corresponding orthogonal components. Clearly, the internal parameters governing ocular following responses are subject to extensive visually mediated adaptive regulation.

The second of the studies examined the pursuit tracking performance of a human patient with unilateral abducens nerve palsy following patching of the normal eye (Optican et al., 1982). Ordinarily, this patient relied entirely on his normal eye, and when this was patched for a few days and subsequently tested on a pursuit tracking task it showed evidence of an adaptive increase in innervation that was orbital position dependent: when the normal eye now attempted to perform any tracking task that would have involved the paretic muscle during the period of patching, it now showed overshoot and even some oscillation (at about 3 Hz) about the moving target. Thus, the nervous system had attempted to compensate rather precisely for the shortcomings due to the paretic muscle.

Vergence and accommodation

The transfer of fixation between targets that are at different distances from the observer raises additional problems: in order to maintain correct focus — and hence clear vision — the focal power of the eye lens must be adjusted (accommodation), and in order to maintain binocular alignment — and hence single vision — appropriate vergence eye movements must be executed. Accommodation and vergence are each subject to independent, negative feedback control, the former operating through the ciliary muscles and lens to reduce blur, and the latter through the extraocular muscles and globe to eliminate retinal image disparity, i.e., bring the two retinal images into sharp correspondence so that a single, fused image is perceived. Since both systems function to track the fixation target as it moves towards or away from the observer, that is, in depth, it is perhaps not surprising that the neural control of the intrinsic and extrinsic eye muscles mediating these two responses is partly shared. During monocular viewing, when the disparity cues driving vergence are absent, changes in accommodation are associated with parallel changes in vergence: the so-called accommodative vergence response (Mueller, 1826; Maddox, 1886). Also, during pinhole viewing, when the blur cues driving accommodation are absent, changes in vergence are associated with parallel changes in accommodation: the so-called vergence accommodation response (Fincham and Walton, 1957). It is assumed that these responses are mediated by cross-links between the two negative feedback control systems, and since each gives rise to an output that does not affect its input, each operates open-loop. The vergence accommodation reflex appears to be much the more important of the two and it is the prime mechanism by which large changes in accommodation are achieved: the blur-driven accommodation reflex is quite sluggish and secondary (Semmlow and Wetzel, 1979). Fincham and Walton (1957) showed that the vergence accommodation response was capable of eliciting changes in accommodation that were close to ideal, at least in young subjects, and recent experiments suggest that the system uses visually mediated adaptive mechanisms to achieve this performance. Though of uncertain functional significance, the accommodative vergence reflex is also able to respond to an adaptive challenge.

In normal binocular viewing conditions, accommodation and vergence operate in concert, and the parameter that determines the strength of the geometric link between them is the separation of the two eyes: the greater the separation, the greater the required change in vergence per unit change in accommodation. Increasing the apparent separation of the two eyes by means of laterally-displacing periscopic spectacles has been shown to cause appropriate, adaptive changes in both the accommodative vergence and vergence accommodation responses — increases and decreases, respectively (Miles and Judge, 1982). 30 minutes were sufficient to elicit 50% changes. However, the adaptive mechanism failed to respond to the challenge of medially-displacing periscopic (cyclopean) spectacles that decreased the apparent separation of the eyes to zero. It is possible that the challenge was too extreme in this case, or required more than the 30 minutes of experience employed in this study.

Contact lenses alter the accommodation required to maintain sharp retinal images at all viewing distances by a fixed amount, while not altering the vergence angle required to maintain binocular alignment of the eyes. Positive lenses, for example, reduce the required accommodation associated with the vergence angle at any given viewing distance; this immediately leads to an increase in the convergence associated with any given level of accommodation. If the lenses are left in place for a few minutes, this over-convergence persists (as an esophoria) in the monocular viewing situation (Schor, 1979). Medially- or laterally-displacing wedge prisms have the converse effect insofar as they affect the angle between the eyes required to maintain alignment on any given object but do not affect the required accommodation. Base-out prisms, for example, increase the required vergence angle associated with fixation targets at any given distance by a fixed amount. Like positive lenses, base-out prisms lead to an increase in the convergence associated with any given level of accommodation, and again this over-convergence persists as an esophoria during monocular testing. Schor (1979, 1980) has argued convincingly that such adaptive effects can be accounted for by merely incorporating a leaky integrator with a long time constant into the forward path of the vergence control system. It is important to realize that while lenses and wedge prisms produce changes in the stimuli to accommodation and vergence, respectively, which are the same at all viewing distances, the effect of the periscopic spectacles is in inverse relation to the viewing distance. Thus, so far as the coupling between accommodation and vergence is concerned, lenses and wedge prisms stress the system's ability to regulate the bias while the periscopes challenge the system's ability to regulate the gain.

Anisometropes, whose spectacle prescription is slightly different for the two eyes, manage to contend with the differing magnification factors quite successfully. The eye confronted with the more positive lens, and hence more magnified image, must always make correspondingly larger movements than the other eye to maintain binocular alignment and single vision. This means that the two eyes experience unequal prismatic deviations during eccentric fixation, e.g., if the right spectacle lens is the more positive one then binocular alignment on objects at any given distance requires progressively increasing convergence during leftward gaze and progressively decreasing convergence during rightward gaze. Of course, vertical eccentric deviations will also be greater for the right eye, and it should be noted that vertical binocular alignment is unrelated to the viewing distance. It has been shown that during monocular viewing the alignment of the eye behind the patch in the corrected anisometrope varies with gaze position exactly in accordance with the varying prismatic demands of the spectacles (Ellerbrock and Fry, 1942; Ellerbrock, 1948, Allen, 1974). More recently, Henson and Dharamshi (1982) have shown that if gaze is confined to a particular direction during the adaptation to wedge prisms, then the changes evident in the alignment of the covered eye in the monocular test situation (phoria) are greatest at that position. Furthermore, they showed that normal subjects can successfully adapt their resting phoria to small amounts of optically induced incomittance achieved with a contact lens/spectacle lens combination in front of one eye; this induced a prismatic deviation which increased as the line of sight deviated from the optical center of the spectacle lens. The adaptive mechanisms operating here are presumably important for the establishment and maintenance of Hering's Law.

Closing remarks

It is clear that appropriate optical techniques are now available with which to challenge many of the major parameters governing oculomotor function. In many, but not all, instances it is known that the nervous system is able to respond positively to this challenge through adaptive processes that operate directly on the gain of the parameter in question. Such adaptive gain control has been demonstrated in a rich variety of species, including fish, birds and mammals. Carefully selected visual challenges generally elicit equally selective adaptation, but not always. Sometimes two subsystems appear to share a modifiable element: this is thought to be the reason for the common finding that changes in the gain of the VOR often result in parallel changes in the optokinetic reflex (Lisberger et al., 1981; Demer, 1981; Zasorin et al., 1983).

Much of the initial interest in adaptive phenomena was motivated by concern with so-called plastic mechanisms underlying long-term learning, but it is clear that not all of the responses are necessarily of this type. One indication of this is the rate of adaptation, which can vary widely from one regulatory mechanism to another, ranging from minutes (even seconds) to days. Long-term plastic adjustments occur over hours or days and show good retention of the altered state when the subject remains in darkness or is otherwise deprived of visual feedback. Presumably, slow changes of this kind are solely concerned with the maintenance of long-term stability. The changes in VOR gain associated with telescopic spectacles and the recovery of saccadic eye movements following surgically induced dysmetria appear to be of this type (Miles and Eighmy, 1980; Optican and Robinson, 1980; Paige, 1983). The assumption here is that some semi-permanent change in synaptic efficacy has occurred within the neuronal networks subserving this reflex. However, one would not invoke such mechanisms to explain rapid, transient adjustments that can occur in seconds. An example is the human subject's ability to alter his compensatory eye movements during VOR testing in the dark merely by imagining objects that move with him (Barr et al., 1976; Collewijn et al., 1981a; Baloh et al., 1984). In this instance, the subject exerts some kind of cognitive influence on his compensatory eye movements which now no longer merely reflect the influence of the semicircular canals and the usual VOR. Such changes seem to be part of a strategy to deal quickly with an evanescent though presumably recurring challenge. The subject is here exercising an option to override or modulate the usual reflex, presumably because the reflex is recognized as counter-productive. However, given the strong dependence on vestibular mechanisms for the maintenance of stability, this approach would seem prudent only where the subject himself provides the input stimulus, as in combined head and eye tracking (Robinson, 1982) or eye-hand coordination.

Such observations caution against any assumption of invariance when dealing with oculomotor reflexes in different paradigms. Indeed, recent observations on the visual tracking responses of monkeys reveal considerable versatility in this regard. One particularly intriguing observation specifically concerns the vertical optokinetic response, the magnitude of which is very sensitive to the orientation of the head: tracking responses to stimuli that move upwards with respect to the head are considerably more vigorous when the animal is placed on its side than when it is in the more usual upright position (Matsuo and Cohen, 1984). Another curious finding is that the initial visual tracking responses elicited by unexpected movements of the visual scene, which were mentioned earlier, are often transiently enhanced after saccadic eye movements (Kawano and Miles, 1984). This post-saccadic enhancement results from the visual stimulation produced by the saccade sweeping the retina across the visual scene (Kawano and Miles, unpublished observations). Thus, when no such visual stimulation is produced, as when a vertical saccade is made while viewing vertical stripes, for example, then no enhancement results: saccadic eye movements per se are not sufficient to elicit the enhancement. Furthermore, saccades are not necessary: the post-saccadic enhancement effect could be evoked by merely shifting the visual scene in a saccade-like way. Such observations suggest the need for extraordinary attention to detail when examining oculomotor responses.

References

Abel, L. A., Schmidt, D., Dell'Osso, L. F. and Daroff, R. B. (1978) Saccadic system plasticity in humans. Ann. Neurol., 4: 313–318.

Allen, D. C. (1974) Vertical prism adaptation in anisometropes. Am. J. Opt. Physiol. Optics, 51: 252–259.

Baloh, R. W., Lyerly, K., Yee, R. D. and Honrubia, V. (1984)

Voluntary control of the human vestibulo-ocular reflex. Acta Otolaryngol., 97: 1–6.

Barr, C. C., Schultheis, L. W. and Robinson, D. A. (1976) Voluntary, non-visual control of the human vestibulo-ocular reflex. Acta Otolaryngol., 81: 365–375.

Berthoz, A., Melvill Jones, G. and Bégué, A. E. (1981) Differential visual adaptation of vertical canal-dependent vestibulo-ocular reflexes. Exp. Brain Res., 44: 19–26.

Callan, J. W. and Ebenholtz, S. M. (1982) Directional changes in the vestibular ocular response as a result of adaptation to optical tilt. Vison Res., 22: 37–42.

Collewijn, H. and Grootendorst, A. F. (1978) Adaptation of the rabbit's vestibulo-ocular reflex to modified visual input: Importance of stimulus conditions. Arch. Ital. Biol., 116: 273–280.

Collewijn, H. and Grootendorst, A. F. (1979) Adaptation of optokinetic and vestibulo-ocular reflexes to modified visual input in the rabbit. In R. Granit and O. Pompeiano (Eds.), Reflex Control of Posture and Movement. Progress in Brain Research, Vol. 50, Elsevier, Amsterdam, pp. 771–781.

Collewijn, H., Martins, A. J. and Steinman, R. M. (1981a) Natural retinal image motion: origin and change. Ann. N.Y. Acad. Sci., 374: 312–329.

Collewijn, H., Martins, A. J. and Steinman, R. M. (1981b) The time course of adaptation of human compensatory eye movements. Doc. Ophth. Proc., 30: 123–133.

Collewijn, H., Martins, A. J. and Steinman, R. M. (1983) Compensatory eye movements during active and passive head movements: Fast adaptation to changes in visual magnification. J. Physiol., 340: 259–286.

Demer, J. L. (1981) The variable gain element of the vestibulo-ocular reflex is common to the optokinetic system of the cat. Brain Res., 229: 1–13.

Demer, J. L. and Robinson, D. A. (1982) Effects of reversible lesions and stimulation of olivocerebellar system on vestibuloocular reflex plasticity. J. Neurophysiol., 47: 1084–1107.

Dufossé, M., Ito, M., Jastreboff, P. J. and Miyashita, Y. (1978a) A neuronal correlate in rabbit's cerebellum to adaptive modifcation of the vestibulo-ocular reflex. Brain Res., 150: 611–616.

Dufossé, M., Ito, M. and Miyashita, Y. (1978b) Diminution and reversal of eye movements induced by local stimulation of rabbit cerebellar flocculus after partial destruction of the inferior olive. Exp. Brain Res., 33: 139–141.

Ellerbrock, V. J. (1948) Further study of effects induced by anisometropic corrections. Am. J. Optom. Arch. Am. Acad. Optom., 25: 430–437.

Ellerbrock, V. J. and Fry, G. A. (1942) Effects induced by anisometropic corrections. Am. J. Optom. Arch. Am. Acad. Optom., 19: 444–459.

Fincham, E. F. and Walton, J. (1957) The reciprocal actions of accommodation and convergence. J. Physiol., 137: 488–508.

Gauthier, G. M. and Robinson, D. A. (1975) Adaptation of the human vestibulo-ocular reflex to magnifying lenses. Brain Res., 92: 331–335.

Gauthier, G. M., Marchetti, E. and Pellet, J. (1983) Cerebellar control of vestibulo-ocular reflex (VOR) studied with injection of Harmaline in the trained baboon. Arch. Ital. Biol., 121: 19–36.

Godaux, E., Halleux, J. and Gobert, C. (1983) Adaptive change of the vestibulo-ocular reflex in the cat: The effects of a long-term frequency-selective procedure. Exp. Brain Res., 49: 28–34.

Goldstein, H. P. (1983) The Neural Encoding of Saccades in the Rhesus Monkey. Ph.D. Thesis, Johns Hopkins University.

Gonshor, A. and Melvill Jones, G. (1971) Plasticity in the adult human vestibulo-ocular reflex arc. Proc. Can. Fed. Biol. Soc., 14: 11.

Gonshor, A. and Melvill Jones, G. (1976a) Short-term adaptive changes in the human vestibulo-ocular reflex arc. J. Physiol., 256: 361–379.

Gonshor, A. and Melvill Jones, G. (1976b) Extreme vestibulo-ocular adaptation induced by prolonged optical reversal of vision. J. Physiol., 256: 381–414.

Haddad, G. M., Demer, J. L. and Robinson, D. A. (1980) The effect of lesions of the dorsal cap of the inferior olive on the vestibulo-ocular and optokinetic systems of the cat. Brain Res., 185: 265–275.

Henson, D. B. (1978) Corrective saccades: effects of altering visual feedback. Vision Res., 18: 63–67.

Henson, D. B. and Dharamshi, B. G. (1982) Oculomotor adaptation to induced heterophoria and anisometropia. Invest. Ophthalmol., 22: 234–240.

Ito, M. (1972) Neural design of the cerebellar motor control system. Brain Res., 40: 81–84.

Ito, M. and Miyashita, Y. (1975) The effects of chronic destruction of the inferior olive upon visual modification of the horizontal vestibulo-ocular reflex of rabbits. Proc. Jpn. Acad., 50: 716–720.

Ito, M., Jastreboff, P. J. and Miyashita, Y. (1979a) Adaptive modification of the rabbit's horizontal vestibulo-ocular reflex during sustained vestibular and optokinetic stimulation. Exp. Brain Res., 37: 17–30.

Ito, M., Orlov, I. and Shimoyama, I. (1978) Reduction of the cerebellar stimulus effect of rat Deiters neurons after chemical destruction of the inferior olive. Exp. Brain Res., 33: 143–145.

Ito, M., Nisimaru, N. and Shibuki, K. (1979b) Destruction of inferior olive induces rapid depression in synaptic action of cerebellar Purkinje cells. Nature, 277: 568–569.

Kawano, K. and Miles, F. A. (1983) Adaptive plasticity in short-latency ocular following responses of monkey. Soc. Neurosci. Abstr., 9: 868.

Kawano, K. and Miles, F. A. (1984) Ocular following responses of monkey: post-saccadic enhancement and dependence on spatio-temporal characteristics of the visual stimulus. Soc. Neurosci. Abstr., 10: 390.

Keller, E. L. and Precht, W. (1979) Adaptive modification of central vestibular neurons in response to visual stimulation through reversing prisms. J. Neurophysiol., 42: 896–911.

Keller, E. L. and Smith, M. J. (1983) Suppressed visual adaptation of the vestibuloocular reflex in catecholamine-depleted cats. Brain Res., 258: 323–327.

Kommerell, G., Olivier, D. and Theopold, H. (1976) Adaptive programming of phasic and tonic components in saccadic eye movements. Investigations in patients with abducens palsy. Invest. Ophthalmol., 15: 657–660

Lisberger, S. G. and Fuchs, A. F. (1978) Role of primate flocculus during rapid behavioral modification of vestibuloocular reflex. I. Purkinje cell activity during visually guided horizontal smooth-pursuit eye movements and passive head rotation. J. Neurophysiol., 41: 733–763.

Lisberger, S. G. and Miles, F. A. (1980) Role of primate medial vestibular nucleus in long-term adaptive plasticity of vestibuloocular reflex. J. Neurophysiol., 43: 1725–1745.

Lisberger, S. G., Miles, F. A., Optican, L. M. and Eighmy, B. B. (1981) Optokinetic response in monkey: underlying mechanisms and their sensitivity to long-term adaptive changes in vestibuloocular reflex. J. Neurophysiol., 45: 869–890.

Lisberger, S. G., Miles, F. A. and Optican, L. M. (1983) Frequency-selective adaptation: evidence for channels in the vestibulo-ocular reflex? J. Neurosci., 3: 1234–1244.

Lisberger, S. G., Miles, F. A. and Zee, D. S. (1984) Signals used to compute errors in the monkey vestibulo-ocular reflex: possible role of the flocculus. J. Neurophysiol., 52: 1140–1153.

Maddox, E. E. (1886) Investigations on the relationship between convergence and accommodation of the eyes. J. Anat., 20: 475–508, 565–584.

Maekawa, K. and Simpson, J. I. (1973) Climbing fiber responses evoked in vestibulo-cerebellum of rabbit from visual system. J. Neurophysiol., 36: 649–666.

Marr, D. (1969) A theory of cerebellar cortex. J. Physiol. London, 202: 437–470.

Matsuo, V. and Cohen, B. (1984) Vertical optokinetic nystagmus and vestibular nystagmus in the monkey: up-down asymmetry and effects of gravity. Exp. Brain Res., 53: 197–216.

McLaughlin, S. C. (1967) Parametric adjustment in saccadic eye movements. Percept. Psychophys., 2: 359–362.

Melvill Jones, G. and Davies, P. (1976) Adaptation of cat vestibuloocular reflex to 200 days of optically reversed vision. Brain Res., 103: 551–554.

Melvill Jones, G. and Gonshor, A. (1982) Oculomotor response to rapid head oscillation (0.5–5.0 Hz) after prolonged adaptation to vision-reversal. Exp. Brain Res., 45: 45–58.

Miles, F. A. (1982) Adaptive gain control in the vestibulo-ocular reflex. In G. Lennerstrand, D. S. Zee and E. L. Keller (Eds.), Functional Basis of Ocular Motility Disorders, Pergamon, Oxford, pp. 325–336.

Miles, F. A. and Braitman, D. J. (1980) Long-term adaptive changes in primate vestibuloocular reflex. II. Electrophysiological observations on semicircular canal primary afferents. J. Neurophysiol., 43: 1426–1436.

Miles, F. A. and Eighmy, B. B. (1980) Long-term adaptive changes in primate vestibulo-ocular reflex. I. Behavioral observations. J. Neurophysiol., 43: 1406–1425.

Miles, F. A. and Fuller, J. H. (1974) Adaptive plasticity in the vestibulo-ocular responses of the rhesus monkey. Brain Res., 30: 512–516.

Miles, F. A. and Judge, S. J. (1982) Optically-induced changes in the neural coupling between vergence eye movements and accommodation in human subjects. In G. Lennerstrand, D. S. Zee and E. L. Keller (Eds.), Functional Basis of Ocular Motility Disorders, Pergamon, Oxford, pp. 93–96.

Miles, F. A. and Lisberger, S. G. (1981a) The "error" signals subserving adaptive gain control in the primate vestibuloocular reflex. Ann. NY Acad. Sci., 374: 513–525.

Miles, F. A. and Lisberger, S. G. (1981b) Plasticity in the vestibuloocular reflex: a new hypothesis. Annu. Rev. Neurosci., 4: 273–299.

Miles, F. A., Braitman, D. J. and Dow, B. M. (1980a) Long-term adaptive changes in primate vestibuloocular reflex. IV. Electrophysiological observations in flocculus of adapted monkeys. J. Neurophysiol., 43: 1477–1493.

Miles, F. A., Fuller, J. H., Braitman, D. J. and Dow, B. M. (1980b) Long-term adaptive changes in primate vestibuloocular reflex. III. Electrophysiological observations in flocculus of normal monkeys. J. Neurophysiol., 43: 1437–1476.

Miles, F. A., Optican, L. M. and Lisberger, S. G. (1985) An adaptive equalizer model of the primate vestibulo-ocular reflex. Rev. Oculomotor Res., 1: 313–326.

Miller, J. M., Anstis, T. and Templeton, W. B. (1981) Saccadic plasticity: parametric adaptive control by retinal feedback. J. Exp. Psych., 7: 356–366.

Miyashita, Y. (1984) Eye velocity responsiveness and its proprioceptive component in the floccular Purkinje cells of the alert pigmented rabbit. Exp. Brain Res., 55: 81–90.

Montarolo, P. G., Raschi, F. and Strata, P. (1981) Are the climbing fibres essential for the Purkinje cell inhibitory action? Exp. Brain Res., 42: 215–218.

Mueller, J. (1826) In W. Baly (Ed.), Elements of Physiology, Vol. 2, (Translated from German, 1843), Taylor and Walton, London, pp. 1147–1148.

Nagao, S. (1983) Effects of vestibulocerebellar lesions upon dynamic characteristics and adaptation of vestibulo-ocular and optokinetic responses in pigmented rabbits. Exp. Brain Res., 53: 36–46.

Optican, L. M. and Miles, F. A. (1985) Visually induced adaptive changes in primate oculomotor control signals. J. Neurophysiol., 54: 940–958.

Optican, L. M. and Robinson, D. A. (1980) Cerebellar-dependent adaptive control of primate saccadic system. J. Neurophysiol., 44: 1058–1076.

Optican, L. M., Chu, F. C., Hays, A. V., Reingold, D. B. and Zee, D. S. (1982) Adaptive changes in oculomotor performance in abducens nerve palsy. Soc. Neurosci. Abstr., 8: 418.

Paige, G. D. (1983) Vestibuloocular reflex and its interactions with visual following mechanisms in the squirrel monkey. II.

Response characteristics and plasticity following unilateral inactivation of horizontal canal. J. Neurophysiol., 49: 152–168.

Robinson, D. A. (1976) Adaptive gain control of vestibuloocular reflex by the cerebellum. J. Neurophysiol., 39: 954–969.

Robinson, D. A. (1982) A model of cancellation of the vestibulo-ocular reflex. In G. Lennerstrand, D. S. Zee and E. L. Keller (Eds.), Functional Basis of Ocular Motility Disorders, Pergamon, Oxford, pp. 5–13.

Rønne, H. (1923) False movements appearing during vision through spectacle glasses; their significance with respect to experience in wearing spectacles and their connection with the vestibular apparatus. Acta Ophthalmol., 1: 55–62.

Schairer, J. O. and Bennett, M. V. L. (1977) Adaptive gain control in vestibulo-ocular reflex in goldfish. Soc. Neurosci. Abstr., 3: 157.

Schairer, J. O. and Bennett, M. V. L. (1978) VOR gain changes produced by target rotation without head movement in goldfish. Soc. Neurosci. Abstr., 4: 167.

Schairer, J. O. and Bennett, M. V. L. (1981) Cerebellectomy in goldfish prevents adaptive gain control of the VOR without affecting the optokinetic system. In T. Gualtierotti (Ed.), The Vestibular System: Functions and Morphology, Springer-Verlag, New York, pp. 463–477.

Schor, C. M. (1979) The relationship between fusional vergence eye movements and fixation disparity. Vision Res., 19: 1359–1367.

Schor, C. M. (1980) Fixation disparity: a steady-state error. Am. J. Optom., 57: 618–631.

Schultheis, L. X. and Robinson, D. A. (1981) Directional plasticity of the vestibulo-ocular reflex in the cat. Ann. NY Acad. Sci., 374: 504–512.

Semmlow, J. L. and Wetzel, P. (1979) Dynamic contributions of binocular vergence components. J. Opt. Soc. Am., 69: 639–645.

Simpson, J. I. and Alley, K. E. (1974) Visual climbing fiber input to rabbit vestibulo-cerebellum: A source of direction-specific information. Brain Res., 82: 302–308.

Vossius, G. (1972) Adaptive control of saccadic eye movement. Bibl. Ophthal., 82: 244–250.

Wallman, J., Velez, J., Weinstein, B. and Green, A. E. (1982) Avian vestibuloocular reflex: adaptive plasticity and developmental changes. J. Neurophysiol., 48: 952–967.

Watanabe, E. (1984) Neuronal events correlated with long-term adaptation of the horizontal vestibulo-ocular reflex in the primate flocculus. Brain Res., 297: 169–174.

Wolf, W., Deubel, H. and Hauske, G. (1985) Properties of parametric adjustment in the saccadic system. In A. G. Gale and F. Johnson (Eds.), Theoretical and Applied Aspects of Eye Movement Research, Elsevier/North-Holland, Amsterdam, in press.

Zasorin, N. L., Baloh, R. W., Yee, R. D. and Honrubia, V. (1983) Influence of vestibulo-ocular reflex gain on human optokinetic responses. Exp. Brain Res., 51: 271–274.

Zee, D. S., Yamazaki, A., Butler, P. H. and Gucer, G. (1981) Effects of ablation of flocculus and paraflocculus on eye movements in primates. J. Neurophysiol., 46: 878–899.

Recovery of some vestibuloocular and vestibulospinal functions following unilateral labyrinthectomy

Wolfgang Precht[†]

Institut für Hirnforschung der Universität Zürich, August-Forelstrasse 1, 8029 Zürich, Switzerland

Introduction

Following the pioneering work of Von Bechterew (1883), numerous studies on the mechanisms of functional recovery from unilateral peripheral vestibular lesions have been performed, making the vestibular lesion model one of the best-studied neural recovery models. Undoubtedly, the long-lasting interest in this model was initiated by the observation that the severe symptoms which are seen immediately after removal of one vestibular labyrinth abate rather quickly with time. The recovery from some of the deficits is, in fact, so complete that a naive observer cannot tell a damaged from an intact animal, both at rest as well as during locomotion. Besides the presence of an easily demonstrable recovery of function, the vestibular lesion model offers several other features which make it an attractive model for the study of neural plasticity or, more specifically, of sensorimotor functions: (1) The extent of the lesion of the labyrinth and/or the vestibular nerve can be precisely controlled, and reproducible lesions can be made easily. Since the vestibular receptors do not regenerate after the lesion, all the compensatory processes leading to recovery of function must be generated by the central nervous system. (2) The normal sensorimotor function of the vestibular system as well as its interactions with other sensory systems have been well studied in recent years, at both the behavioral and single unit level, thus allowing precise definitions of control values. (3) The lesion-evoked functional deficits and their recovery are precisely measurable and (4) deficits following a unilateral labyrinthine lesion are similar in a large variety of species, offering the possibility of studying similarities as well as differences in the strategies and mechanisms of their recovery.

Following unilateral labyrinthectomy the central nervous system has to cope with two major groups of motor deficits. Firstly, the symmetrical tonic influence exerted by the vestibular receptors via vestibular afferents on posture of the head, body and eyes in the resting condition is altered by unilateral withdrawal of resting activity in vestibular nerve fibers. This unilateral loss of resting activity, in turn, results in an imbalance of the output of the vestibular nuclei to the oculo- and spinal motor systems, causing the well known "vestibular lesion syndrome". It consists of severe postural asymmetries of head, body and eyes as well as eye and head nystagmus (cf. Schaefer and Meyer, 1974). It is the task of the central nervous system to establish, as quickly as possible, a new balance in the innervation of the motor systems.

The second and equally important task of the nervous system consists in the adjustment of the lesion-induced gain deficits of vestibular reflexes during head and body movements; unilateral lesion has interrupted the delicate central interactions between the two labyrinths, so that what used to be done by the joint action of two end organs now has to be achieved by only one labyrinth.

In the following a brief account of the recent progress in this field will be given. The review will concentrate on behavioral and single unit work performed in mammals, mainly the rat and cat (for review of work in other species, see Schaefer and Meyer, 1974; Precht and Dieringer, 1985). Furthermore, emphasis will be on the results obtained with the vestibuloocular system since it has been studied in much greater detail, particularly as far as its dynamic performance is concerned. However, the vestibulospinal system will be dealt with in conjunction with the recovery of head posture after lesion.

Recovery of balance of head and eye position

Head position

After unilateral labyrinthectomy, a large head tilt angle about the longitudinal (roll) axis, damaged side down, is observed in both rat (Llinás and Walton, 1979; Sirkin et al., 1984) and cat (Putkonen et al., 1977). No consistent head nystagmus was observed. Occasionally one observes slow lateral head drifts towards the lesion side, interrupted irregularly by quick movements to the intact side. Tonic lateral head deviations were likewise not observed. However, such deviations may be seen in other species (see Schaefer and Meyer, 1974).

From the above it appears that the most consistent, and therefore quantifiable, lesion parameter is the tilt angle of the head. While recovery from abnormal head tilt takes several days in the cat (Putkonen et al., 1977), it occurs within hours in the rat (Llinás and Walton, 1979; Sirkin et al., 1984). As shown in Fig. 1A, almost normal head positions are reached within 4–6 hours after labyrinthectomy. Since the lesion was performed under chloral hydrate anesthesia, and time zero denotes the moment of labyrinthine lesion, the time course of recovery shown in Fig. 1A includes the time necessary to recover from anesthesia and, therefore, cannot be taken as the real recovery time. In fact, the latter may have been much shorter, had the lesion been performed without anesthesia.

It is interesting to note that albino and pigmented strains of rats appear to recover normal head position with similar time courses, indicating that the visual system, known to be severely defective in albino strains (see Precht and Cazin, 1979), plays no major role in this fast recovery process. This conclusion is supported by the finding that recovery time of head posture in blinded pigmented rats is similar to that seen in albinos and in visually intact pigmented conspecifics (Fig. 1).

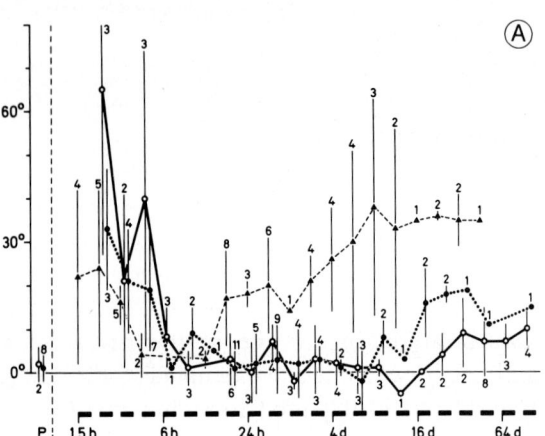

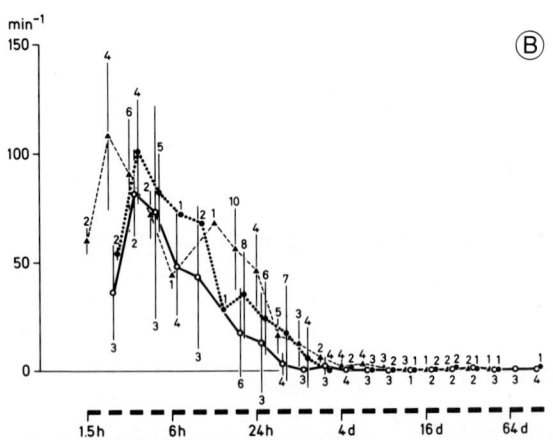

Fig. 1. Recovery of head position and ocular stability following unilateral labyrinthectomy in the rat. A. Lateral head tilt (means and standard deviations) as a function of time after labyrinthectomy (time zero) in albino rats (▲), pigmented DA rats (○) and blinded pigmented DA rats (●). The number of measurements assumed by each mean and standard deviation is indicated by the number above or below the standard deviation bar. B. Nystagmic beat frequency as a function of time after unilateral labyrinthectomy. Symbols are the same as in A (from Sirkin et al., 1984).

Following the initial rapid recovery of head posture, the albino strain showed a marked secondary increase in head tilt angle (Fig. 1A). Since this "decompensation" was not observed in blinded pigmented rats it appears to be a strain-specific phenomenon. Similar secondary increases were noted in the cat (Putkonen et al., 1977). At present no explanation can be given for this delayed decompensation occurring in some species.

Eye position

Two major abnormalities in eye position were observed after unilateral labyrinthectomy: (1) a tonic eye deviation, and (2) ocular nystagmus. The tonic eye deviation in the rat consisted of a downward deviation of the eye ipsilateral to the lesion while the contralateral eye deviated upwards. This deviation was correlated roughly with tonic head tilt described above: it disappeared with head tilt and it also reappeared when the head tilt showed a secondary increase. Ocular nystagmus, however, was mainly beating in the horizontal plane, with the quick phase directed to the intact side. In the cat the lesion-induced nystagmus disappears gradually within 3–5 days after the lesion (Precht et al., 1966; Haddad et al., 1977; Maioli et al., 1983), the recovery being somewhat faster when measured in the light. Very similar findings were obtained in the rat (Llinás and Walton, 1979; Sirkin et al., 1984). As shown in Fig. 1B, nystagmus beat frequency measured in the light reached a maximum within a few hours after the lesion was made, and declined to zero by 4 days. Again, there were no major differences between the different strains studied. No decompensation occurred at the later stages.

Comparison between recovery from head tilt and ocular nystagmus

The time courses of head tilt (eye deviation) and ocular nystagmus beat frequency after unilateral labyrinthectomy in the rat were very different from each other, the former symptom showing a rapid initial decrease followed — in the albino strain — by a secondary increase, and the latter showed a more gradual decrease. Such a clear difference has not been observed in the cat. Here, nystagmus appears to recover faster than head tilt, although measurements of head tilt have only been studied in a few animals. On the other hand, ocular balance recovery time was similar in rats and cats. That the recovery process for different lesion-evoked symptoms are to some degree independent has been noted by several investigators in several species (cf. Schaefer and Meyer, 1974). It has also been noted that additional lesions, placed in animals that had already compensated, affected certain systems quite differently. Thus, compensation of ocular nystagmus is generally more resistant to additional lesions (cerebellar, spinal, proprioceptive) than is head or body posture (Azzena, 1969; Lacour et al., 1976; Jensen, 1979). We may actually expect such differences, for the symptoms of labyrinthectomy not only involve several motor subsystems, but also they are caused by the loss of input from two different classes of sensory organs: semicircular canals and otolith organs. The differences in central processing of these two kinds of sensory signals may account for the observed differences in time of recovery of head tilt and tonic eye deviation (both probably due to loss of otolith function) and ocular nystagmus (loss of canal function).

This brief account of the recovery from head and ocular postural imbalance shows that there exists a strong pressure to restore normal head and eye position following a unilateral vestibular lesion. The speed with which this is achieved and the final degree of balance may show species-specific differences and, within a given species, different symptoms or systems may recover to a different degree or with varying time courses.

Neuronal correlates of balance control

In the intact animal the mean resting activity in the bilateral vestibular nerves and nuclei is very similar. There are species-specific differences in mean resting activity, ranging from very low values in amphibia to extremely high values in primates (cf.

Precht, 1978). Sudden removal of one vestibular input strongly reduces the resting rate in central vestibular canal and otolith neurons on the deafferented side (Shimazu and Precht, 1966; Hoshino and Pompeiano, 1977). On the intact side, resting activity of canal neurons increases approximately 2-fold, due to removal of crossed vestibular inhibition (Shimazu and Precht, 1966; Markham et al., 1977). This strong asymmetry in mean resting rate readily explains the initial imbalance of head and eyes. Several weeks after the lesion the mean resting activities of vestibular neurons on the two sides are again similar (Precht et al., 1966; McCabe et al., 1972; Azzena et al., 1977; Jensen, 1979; Ried et al., 1984). This finding could explain the observed behavioral balance (see above). However, on the basis of recent findings by Ried et al. (1984), this conclusion requires an important specification. It was noted that the overall population of vestibular neurons (type I) responding to horizontal rotation was significantly lower on the deafferented side when compared to that on the intact side. It is, of course, possible that many of the units showing a resting rate but no response to rotation are, in fact, former canal neurons contributing to balance but no longer to response dynamics. If, however, many former canal neurons became silent in chronic animals, a strong imbalance would exist between the two vestibular nuclei, and the ocular balance observed in this stage would be brought about by other structures as well. That other brain regions are involved in balance control has long been known, and recently has been suggested in the rat, based on lesion and ^{14}C-labeled 2-deoxy-D-glucose studies (Llinás and Walton, 1979).

In spite of the above complications, it still remains to be explained how some vestibular neurons regain a new resting rate during the recovery period. Recent experiments have shown that the cells in the ganglion Scarpae which survive structurally and functionally after a peripheral vestibular lesion cannot account for any appreciable amount of resting rate in central neurons (Sirkin et al., 1984). Likewise, the intact labyrinth cannot be a crucial source since, after its removal, Von Bechterew's phenomenon occurs, indicating that neurons on the first operated site are now dominating. At present, the most likely possibility is that central vestibular neurons are driven by the joint action of remaining inputs (e.g., spinal, cerebellar, vestibular), although the contribution of some gradual build-up of intrinsic activity cannot be excluded. Since recovery of balance is severely impaired when animals are kept in sensory deprived conditions after the lesion (cf. Schaefer and Meyer, 1974; Putkonen et al., 1977), it appears that the remaining sensory systems play — directly or indirectly — an important role in the drive for recovery of balance.

Recovery of the VOR as it occurs spontaneously

In the preceding paragraph it was demonstrated that the balance of the innervation of head and eyes at rest occurred within a relatively short period after unilateral labyrinthectomy. Now we shall ask the question of how dynamic vestibular reflexes recover from a vestibular lesion. At present, quantitative data are available only for the horizontal vestibuloocular reflex (VOR) of the cat. Other reflexes, such as the vertical VOR and vestibulocollic reflexes, await investigation.

Before describing the VOR after lesion, a few comments are required concerning its normal performance. Within a certain range the VOR is a linear system (Robinson, 1976; Donaghy, 1980; Maioli et al., 1983) which serves the stabilization of the retinal image during active or passive head and body movements. A pair of semicircular canals — here, the horizontal canals — work in a push-pull fashion, i.e., the VOR generated by head displacements depends on the reciprocal interaction of the two canals. Whenever one canal is excited, the coplanar partner is disfacilitated. Since the magnitude of disfacilitation depends on the level of resting rate in vestibular neurons, strong stimuli eventually cause saturation. As shown in Fig. 2, eye velocity can match stimulus velocity with a gain of close to 1 up to approximately 50°/sec. At higher velocities partial saturation occurs, i.e., the input-output relationship has a lower slope. This fact is impor-

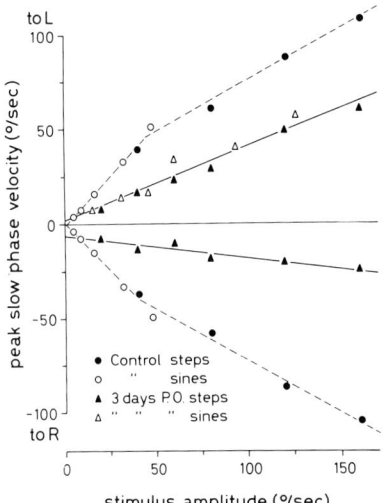

Fig. 2. Horizontal VOR measurements in the cat taken in the dark, before and 3 days after unilateral labyrinthectomy. Note, in controls, the occurrence of partial saturation at approximately 50°/sec stimulus velocity. A gain drop for responses in either direction and a marked asymmetry are the most prominent effects noted after the lesion. For further details see text (from Maioli et al., 1983).

tant in the present context since it dictates the use of low stimulus amplitudes (below partial saturation) for the evaluation of the maximal interaction between the two canals and the assessment of the effects of removing one of them.

Immediately after unilateral labyrinthectomy a strong ocular nystagmus occurs, resulting from an imbalance in the resting rates of central vestibular neurons (see above). Rotation of the head in this acute stage generates a symmetrical modulation of the velocity of the prevailing nystagmus. Nystagmus is not reversed since the resting rate of the neurons on the deafferented side is close to zero. Already by 1–2 days postoperatively a reversal of nystagmus is noted with stronger stimuli but the gain of the reversed response is lower than that in the direction of spontaneous nystagmus. Fig. 2 gives a representative example of the VOR responses measured in a cat, before and 3 days after right-side labyrinthectomy. The following major effects deserve mention: (1) the VOR gain drops in both directions but the decrease is larger on rotation to the lesion side; (2) the decrease of the gain following rotation to the intact side is approximately 50% compared to the gain of the non-saturating part of the controls; (3) no more partial saturation is noted; (4) a complete saturation of responses occurs on strong stimulations towards the deafferented side.

Clearly then, several days after unilateral labyrinthectomy, the VOR gain and its symmetry are still greatly impaired and no improvement is noted. It should be realized that approximately at the same time the ocular balance at rest has almost reached normality. Apparently the balance and gain control systems adapt to the lesion disturbance in a very different way. This fact is further stressed by observing the VOR gain and symmetry at later stages. Fig. 3 shows the time course of recovery of the VOR measured in ten adult cats that had undergone labyrinthectomy on the right-hand side. Between days 5–10 postoperatively two groups of animals were noted; one group increased the gain to approximately 0.75 while it remained low in the other. No clear improvement of right-left symmetry was observed in any group. At later periods of time slow improvements of gain and particularly symmetry occurred (Fig. 3). It should be emphasized, however, that VOR measurements were taken in the dark to test the true vestibular improvement.

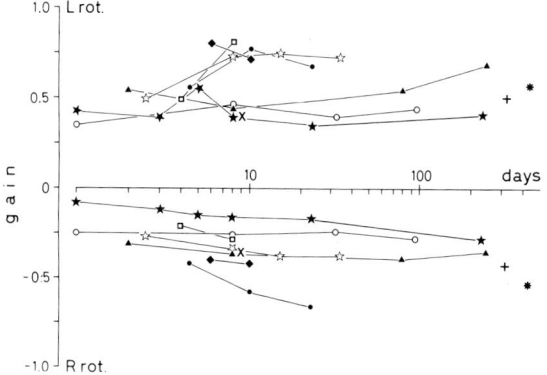

Fig. 3. Time course of VOR gain changes following unilateral labyrinthectomy. Responses obtained from ten cats are illustrated. Gain was computed after subtracting from the responses the slow phase velocity of the spontaneous nystagmus (when present) (from Maioli et al., 1983). L rot., R rot., left and right rotation, respectively.

When the animals were tested in the combined vestibular-visual situation the gain and symmetry of the combined responses were much improved compared to the pure VOR. Furthermore, it may be assumed that the performance of the VOR might have been even better if the head had been free to move since neck-ocular reflexes have been shown, in the primate, to adapt plastically and substitute partially for the VOR deficiencies (Dichgans et al., 1973), as does the optokinetic system (Precht et al., 1981). Observation of the freely moving animals in large cages where they were kept together with other cats, in fact, indicated that their locomotor abilities were rather normal and often could not be distinguished from those of intact conspecifics. This indicates that the above mentioned sensory systems effectively contributed to gaze stabilization. The question then is why the VOR, known to have remarkable plastic abilities, did not improve very much in one group of animals while it did in others? This point will be taken up again in the next section.

As already pointed out, there exists a striking difference between the time it takes to recover balance and gain. If balance had occurred as a result of approximately symmetrical resting rates between the vestibular nuclei on the two sides, the situation should be very similar to that in which one canal has been rendered non-functional by plugging its lumen. In this case no nystagmus occurs, since the resting rate remains symmetrical. Also, the VOR is symmetrical in this preparation (Money and Scott, 1962; Zuckermann, 1967). However, as shown above, in labyrinthectomized animals the VOR remains asymmetric long after balance has been achieved. A possible explanation for the persisting asymmetry comes from the finding that the number of vestibular neurons responding to rotation is very much reduced on the deafferented side when compared to the intact vestibular nucleus (Ried et al., 1984). The reason for this dearth of canal responses on the deafferented side is not known, but it must be related to the lesion of the input since it does not occur after canal plugging.

Recovery of the VOR as it occurs with "vestibular training"

Numerous studies have shown that the VOR uses visual information to modify plastically its gain whenever functional demands require it (Gonshor and Melvill Jones, 1976a,b; Robinson, 1976; Ito et al., 1979; Keller and Precht, 1979; Miles and Lisberger, 1981). Surprisingly, this powerful adaptive gain control mechanism does not seem to work reliably in unilaterally labyrinthectomized cats (Wolfe and Kos, 1977; Maioli et al., 1983) and rabbits (Baarsma and Collewijn, 1975), in which a gain increase would be highly desirable to compensate for the 50% decrease (see above). It was shown (Fig. 3) that when a gain increase occurs in some animals this happens within 5–10 days after the lesion. The animals that miss this period have a low gain for many months after the lesion. The question arising then is whether in these latter cases VOR plasticity mechanisms are severely impaired because of the lesion per se or whether the strongly reduced motor activity, and hence vestibular, optokinetic and proprioceptive stimulations, typical of the early postoperative period, prevents the gain control system from receiving a sufficient amount of visual error signal to operate. Clinical observations speak in favor of the second possibility: early post-lesion movement exercises, particularly of the head, induce a higher degree of compensation (Cawthrone, 1944; Cooksey, 1946). On the other hand, when animals were visually deprived after the labyrinthine lesion, recovery was much reduced or even prevented (Lacour and Xerri, 1981). To assess if the VOR gain control system is still operative after unilateral labyrinthectomy, we oscillated adult vestibularly lesioned cats in front of a patterned visual surround so as to force the animals to experience a situation of vestibular-visual conflict (Maioli and Precht, 1984). This type of stimulation is known to speed up adaptive VOR gain changes in intact animals made to wear magnifying/reducing lenses or left-right reversing prisms. Gain changes occur within 2–3 hours of oscillation (Robinson, 1976; Keller and Precht, 1979).

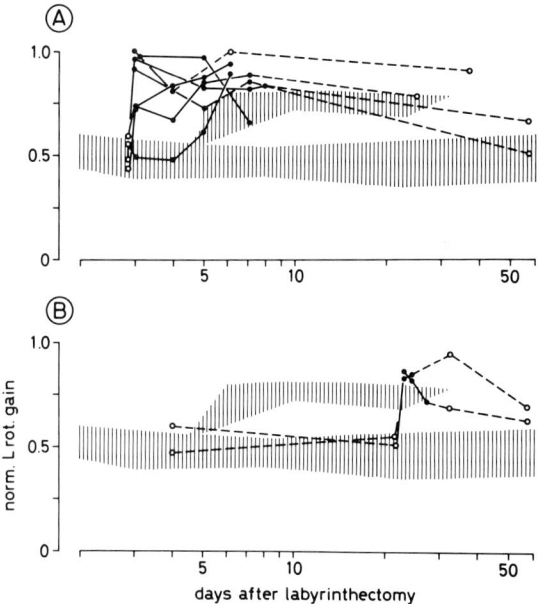

Fig. 4. Time course of VOR gain in unilaterally labyrinthectomized cats before, during and after the training period. Measurements taken during the training period are interconnected by continuous lines; periods of observations without training are indicated by dashed lines. Open circles correspond to measurements taken before forced oscillations or when no training was done on that day; filled circles refer to values measured after training sessions. Shaded areas represent the range of VOR gain time course in spontaneously recovering cats derived from Fig. 3. VOR gains were normalized relative to control values measured before the lesion. A. Time course of VOR gain in seven cats of the early-trained group. B. Same in two cats of the late-trained group (from Maioli and Precht, 1984). L rot., left rotation.

In our experiments cats were divided in two groups. The cats of the first group received forced rotation starting on the third postoperative day, when, in most cases, spontaneous nystagmus had dissipated. In the second group, cats were allowed to recover without training for 23 days in the light, whereupon training was started. No spontaneous recovery of VOR gain was observed in these animals up to that time. Fig. 4 summarizes the results obtained in both groups of cats: (1) A prompt gain increase resulting from a few hours of training was seen in nearly all cats of both groups. (2) In the early trained group (Fig. 4A), training was initiated significantly before the time at which spontaneous gain increase occurred in some cats of the non-trained animals (Fig. 3). Nevertheless, training turned out to be very effective. (3) Adaptive gain control functions in chronic animals which showed no spontaneous improvement (Fig. 4B). (4) The induced gain changes were often larger than those observed in some of the spontaneously recovering animals. (5) After training was discontinued, a clear tendency towards a gain decrease over time was observed. (6) Although training induced considerable improvements in VOR gain, it had no effect on response symmetry.

Optokinetic responses were measured before and after the training and a clear improvement by the training was noted. However, the recovery was not significantly better than that observed in spontaneously recovering animals (Precht et al., 1981).

Combining the results described in the previous and present section, it is clear that VOR gain control, although unaffected by the vestibular lesion, is often unable to take part in the compensation process. It is crucial to realize that in the chronic post-lesion stage a considerable compensation of overall behavioral motor deficits is observed in all cats. This indicates that a sustained amount of functional recovery can be accomplished without VOR recalibration. Apparently VOR deficits are compensated by sensory substitution, e.g., through the optokinetic (Precht et al., 1981) and/or neck proprioceptive inputs (Dichgans et al., 1973; Kasai and Zee, 1978) or by adapting suitable locomotor strategies. It may be argued that a particular compensation strategy is established early after the lesion, when the VOR gain control, even though potentially available, is strongly ineffective because of the reduced motor activity. During this early period adequate vestibular stimulation — evoked by active or passive head movements — can enhance the role of VOR recovery in the compensation of the gaze stabilization deficits. In our early trained cats, long-lasting improvements of VOR gain occurred in 50% of the animals. In a later period, when a satisfactory behavioral compensation is observed, it is still possible to increase the VOR by training, but the effects do not last. Apparently, recalibration is no longer needed because substitution processes can handle effectively the loss of one labyrinth. In this context, it should be realized that some species have an inherently low VOR gain (Benson, 1970; Baarsma and Collewijn, 1974) and yet under certain experimental conditions can quickly adapt that gain to higher values. In both the inherently low gain, intact individuals as well as in the chronic low VOR gain, lesioned cats, recalibration is not needed because this is the way the organisms have adusted their behavior and central sensorimotor integration processes to the functional demands.

References

Azzena, G. B. (1969) Role of the spinal cord in compensating the effects of hemilabyrinthectomy. Arch. Ital. Biol., 107: 43–53.

Azzena, G. B., Mameli, O. and Tolu, E. (1977) Vestibular units during decompensation. Experientia, 33: 234–236.

Baarsma, E. A. and Collewijn, H. (1974) Vestibulo-ocular and optokinetic reactions to rotation and their interaction in the rabbit. J. Physiol., 238: 603–625.

Baarsma, E. A. and Collewijn, H. (1975) Changes in compensatory eye movements after unilateral labyrinthectomy in the rabbit. Arch. Otorhinolaryngol., 211: 219–230.

Benson, A. J. (1970) Interactions between semicircular canals and gravireceptors. In E. B. Douglas (Ed.), Recent Advances in Aerospace Medicine, Reidel Publishing Company, Amsterdam, pp. 249–261.

Cawthrone, T. (1944) The physiological basis for head exercises. J. Chart. Soc. Physiother., 29: 106–107.

Cooksey, F. S. (1946) Rehabilitation in vestibular injuries. Proc. Roy. Soc. Med., 39: 273–275.

Dichgans, J., Bizzi, E., Morasso, P. and Tagliasco, V. (1973) Mechanisms underlying recovery of eye-head coordination following bilateral labyrinthectomy in monkeys. Exp. Brain Res., 18: 548–562.

Donaghy, M. (1980) The cat's vestibulo-ocular reflex. J. Physiol. (Lond.), 300: 337–351.

Gonshor, A. and Melvill Jones, G. (1976a) Short-term adaptive changes in the human vestibulo-ocular reflex arc. J. Physiol., 256: 361–379.

Gonshor, A. and Melvill Jones, G. (1976b) Extreme vestibulo-ocular adaptation induced by prolonged optical reversal of vision. J. Physiol., 256: 381–414.

Haddad, G. M., Friendlich, A. R. and Robinson, D. A. (1977) Compensation of nystagmus after VIIth nerve lesions in vestibulo-cerebellectomized cats. Brain Res., 135: 192–196.

Hoshino, K. and Pompeiano, O. (1977) Crossed responses of lateral vestibular neurons to macular labyrinthine stimulation. Brain Res., 131: 152–157.

Ito, M., Jastreboff, P. J. and Miyashita, Y. (1979) Adaptive modification of the rabbit's horizontal vestibulo-ocular reflex during sustained vestibular and optokinetic stimulation. Exp. Brain Res., 37: 17–30.

Jensen, D. W. (1979) Reflex control of acute postural asymmetry and compensatory symmetry after a unilateral vestibular lesion. Neuroscience, 4: 1059–1073.

Kasai, T. and Zee, D. S. (1978) Eye-head coordination in labyrinthine-defective human beings. Brain Res., 144: 123–141.

Keller, E. L. and Precht, W. (1979) Adaptive modification of central vestibular neurons in response to visual stimulation through reversing prisms. J. Neurophysiol., 42: 896–911.

Lacour, M. and Xerri, C. (1981) Vestibular compensation: new perspectives. In H. Flohr and W. Precht (Eds.), Lesion-induced Neuronal Plasticity in Sensorimotor Systems, Springer, Berlin, pp. 240–253.

Lacour, M., Roll, J. P. and Appaix, M. (1976) Modifications and development of spinal reflexes in the alert baboon (Papio papio) following a unilateral vestibular neurotomy. Brain Res., 113: 255–269.

Llinás, R. and Walton, K. (1979) Vestibular compensation: a distributed property of the central nervous system. In H. Asanuma and V. J. Wilson (Eds.), Integration in the Nervous System, A Symposium in Honor of David P. C. Lloyd and Rafael Lorente de Nó, Igaku-Shoin Ltd., Tokyo, pp. 145–166.

Maioli, C. and Precht, W. (1984) On the role of vestibulo-ocular reflex plasticity in recovery after unilateral peripheral vestibular lesions. Exp. Brain Res., 59: 267–272.

Maioli, C., Precht, W. and Ried, S. (1983) Short- and long-term modifications of vestibulo-ocular response dynamics following unilateral vestibular nerve lesions in the cat. Exp. Brain Res., 50: 259–274.

Markham, Ch. H., Yagi, T. and Curthoys, I. S. (1977) The contribution of the contralateral labyrinth to second-order vestibular neuronal activity in the cat. Brain Res., 138: 99–109.

McCabe, B. F., Ryu, J. H. and Sekitani, T. (1972) Further experiments on vestibular compensation. Laryngoscope, 82: 381–396.

Miles, F. A. and Lisberger, S. G. (1981) Plasticity in the vestibulo-ocular reflex: A new hypothesis. Annu. Rev. Neurosci., 4: 273–299.

Money, K. E. and Scott, J. W. (1962) Functions of separate sensory receptors of nonauditory labyrinth of the cat. Am. J. Physiol., 202: 1211–1220.

Precht, W. (1978) Neuronal operations in the vestibular system. In V. Braitenberg (Ed.), Studies of Brain Function, Vol. 2, Springer, Berlin, p. 225.

Precht, W. and Cazin, L. (1979) Functional deficits in the optokinetic system of albino rats. Exp. Brain Res., 37: 183–186.

Precht, W. and Dieringer, N. (1985) Neuronal events paralleling functional recovery following peripheral vestibular lesions. In

G. Melvill Jones and A. Berthoz (Eds.), Adaptive Mechanisms in Gaze Control, Elsevier, Amsterdam, pp. 251–268.

Precht, W., Shimazu, H. and Markham, C. H. (1966) A mechanism of central compensation of vestibular function following hemilabyrinthectomy. J. Neurophysiol., 29: 996–1010.

Precht, W., Maioli, C., Dieringer, N. and Cochran, S. (1981) Mechanisms of compensation of the vestibulo-ocular reflex after vestibular neurotomy. In H. Flohr and W. Precht (Eds.), Lesion-induced Neuronal Plasticity in Sensorimotor Systems, Springer, Berlin, pp. 221–230.

Putkonen, P. T. S., Courjon, J. H. and Jeannerod, M. (1977) Compensation of postural effects of hemilabyrinthectomy in the cat. A sensory substitution process? Exp. Brain Res., 28: 249–257.

Ried, S., Maioli, C. and Precht, W. (1984) Vestibular nuclear neuron activity in chronically hemilabyrinthectomized cats. Acta Oto-Laryng. (Stockholm), 98: 1–13.

Robinson, D. A. (1976) Adaptive gain control of vestibuloocular reflex by the cerebellum. J. Neurophysiol., 39: 954–969.

Schaefer, K. P. and Meyer, D. L. (1974) Compensation of vestibular lesions. In H. H. Kornhuber (Ed.), Handbook of Sensory Physiology, Vestibular System, Part 2: Psychophysics, Applied Aspects and General Interpretations, Vol. 6/2, Springer, Berlin, pp. 463–490.

Shimazu, H. and Precht, W. (1966) Inhibition of central vestibular neurons from the contralateral labyrinth and its mediating pathway. J. Neurophysiol., 29: 467–492.

Sirkin, D. W., Precht, W. and Courjon, J.-H. (1984) Initial, rapid phase of recovery from unilateral vestibular lesion in rat not dependent on survival of central portion of vestibular nerve. Brain Res., 302: 245–256.

Von Bechterew, W. (1883) Ergebnisse der Durchschneidung des N. acusticus, nebst Erörterung der Bedeutung der semicirculären Kanäle für das Körpergleichgewicht. Pflügers Arch., 30: 312–347.

Wolfe, J. W. and Kos, C. M. (1977) Nystagmic responses of the rhesus monkey to rotational stimulation following unilateral labyrinthectomy: Final report. Trans. Am. Acad. Ophthalmol. Orolaryngol., 84: 38–45.

Zuckerman, H. (1967) The physiological adaptation to unilateral semicircular canal inactivation. McGill Med. J., 36: 8–13.

The effect of gaze motor signals and spatially directed attention on eye movements and visual perception

O.-J. Grüsser

Department of Physiology, Freie Universität, Arnimallee 22, 1000 Berlin 33, Germany

Introduction

Since the first discussions about sensory perception by the pre-Socratic Greek philosophers (Diels and Kranz, 1974), perception has been interpreted essentially in two different ways: as a passive phenomenon (e.g., Aristotle and his pupils) or as the result of an interaction of active efferent signals originating in the sense organs or the brain and the afferent signal flow. Empedocles (about 492–430 B.C.) believed visual perception to be caused predominantly by a reflection of "internal" light emitted from the eye to the objects (cf. Diels and Kranz, 1974). Democrites of Abdera (about 460–370 B.C.) and Plato (427–347 B.C.) elaborated on Empedocles' interaction theory. In "Timaios", Plato proposed the following model: visual rays, emitted from the eye, form together with the external light a signal-transmitting structure, the "body of light", which touches the objects and thus receives movement which is transmitted back to the eye, reaching the soul via the sense organ (Fig. 1a). This extraocular interaction theory, later accepted by the majority of the Stoic philosophers and the church fathers, was not modified until more than 1300 years later. One of the most outstanding Arabian physicians and philosophers, Ibn-al-Haitam (in Latin, Alhazen, 965–1038 A.D.; Wiedemann, 1910; Bauer, 1911), believed that an interaction between the efferent spiritus visibilis and the light from the outer world occurs in the crystalline lens (Fig. 1b). Nikolaus Cusanus (1401–1446 A.D.) in his books "Liber de Mente" and "Compendium" also discussed Plato's interaction theory and argued that the efferent signals are generated by motor acts and attention directed towards the objects one wishes to see (for details, see Grüsser, 1986). Only after Alcmaeon of Croton's (late 6th, early 5th century B.C.) age-old idea about light generated in the eye (pressure phosphenes) was experimentally refuted by Morgagni (1741) and G. A. Languth (1742) did the intraocular interaction theory disappear from physiological discussions, and the Aristotelian view of perception as a passive process seemed to have won. Paradoxically, Aristotle himself published the first experimental observation which eventually led to a revival of the interaction theory in a new form. In his book "On Dreams" he described an experiment with an afterimage: "And if, after looking at the sun or some other bright object, we close our eyelids, then we can see, if we observe carefully, an image of the same colour wherever the line of sight moves. It changes to red and then to purple until it fades to black and disappears finally".

In modern sensory physiology, afterimage movement was first described by Erasmus Darwin (1794/1796) and his son Robert W. Darwin (1789), by Charles Bell (1823) and Jan Purkinje (1825a,b): An afterimage is seen remaining stationary in the extrapersonal space when the eyes are moved passively in the dark. When the center of gaze moves actively, the afterimage is seen moving. Stationary

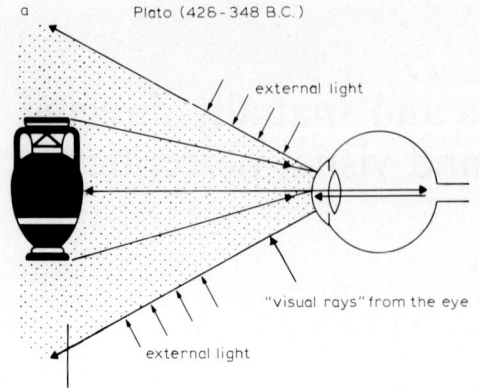

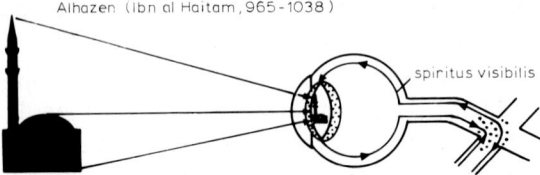

Bell's and Purkyně's observations (1823, 1825)

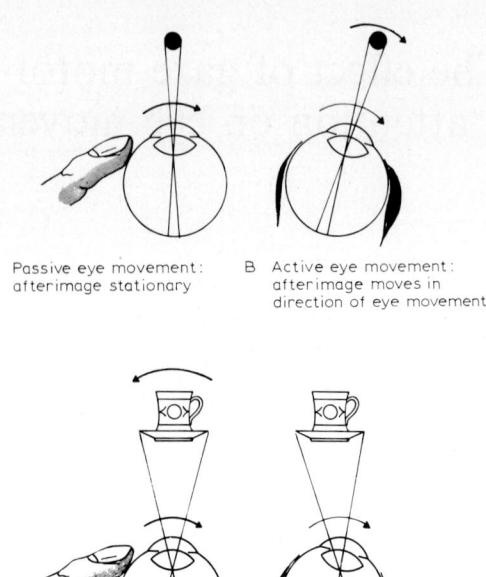

A Passive eye movement: afterimage stationary

B Active eye movement: afterimage moves in direction of eye movement

C Passive eye movement visual object stationary: apparent movement in direction opposite to eye movement

D Active eye movement visual object stationary: object is seen stationary

Fig. 1. Schemes of the interaction theory of visual perception. (a) Model proposed by Plato ("Timaios"): during the course of visual perception, visual rays generated in the organism leave the eye and interact with the external light, forming the "cone of vision", which has its top in the eye and its base on the object perceived. The cone of vision touches the objects, and therefore is mechanically vibrating. This vibration is sent back to the eye. This signal leads to visual perception when it is sent to the cognitive components of the soul, which are believed to be located in the brain. (b) Interaction theory of Alhazen. Efferent visual signals (spiritus visibilis) generated in the brain (optic chiasm) enter the eyes and interact at the site of the crystalline lense with the external light reflected from the objects. The result of this interaction is fed back to the optic nerve and transmitted by the optic nerve to the chiasm, where it is combined with the corresponding information from the other eye and generates object perception.

Fig. 2. Afterimage experiment of Bell (1823) and Purkinje (1825a,b). When a foveal afterimage is seen in the dark and the eyes are moved actively, afterimage movement or change in position is perceived. However, when the eye is moved passively, the afterimage remains stationary in the visual space. Thus, the afterimage movement and stability is opposed to that observed when an object of the extrapersonal space is perceived with active and passive eye movements: the object seemed stationary in the case of active eye movement, while it is seen moving in the case of passive eye movements.

real objects are seen in apparent motion when the eyes are moved passively; they were seen stationary when the eyes moved actively (Fig. 2). As a meticulous observer, Purkinje was aware of the experimental limitations of the latter statement: When the center of gaze pursues an object moving in front of a patterned visual background, an apparent shift in the background in the opposite direction to the gaze movement appears, but the speed of the background shift is considerably lower than the angular velocity of the center of gaze and is restricted to the foveal and parafoveal region of the visual field (cf. also Filehne, 1922).

Purkinje emphasized the importance of motor acts in visual movement perception and compared these observations with the sensations when a tactile stimulus is moved across the skin: when the hand is stationary, the stimulus moving across the palm is perceived moving; when the hand itself moves across the stationary object, the latter is perceived as stationary. When the tactile stimulus is stationary on the palm but the hand moves with the object, the latter is perceived in motion. Purkinje's conclusions were further elaborated by Von Helmholtz (1896), who thought that the apparent motion of an afterimage during active eye movements was caused by internal feedback signals ("effort of will") and reinforced his view with Von Graefe's observation (1854) that a patient with an acute palsy of the rectus externus muscle perceives the stationary objects moving in the direction of the intended outward eye movement (monocular observation). Ewald Hering (1861, 1879) and Ernst Mach (1886) also recognized the importance of motor commands interacting with the afferent visual signal flow for the perception of visual movement and the perceived constancy of the extrapersonal visual space coordinates. Mach and Hering, following Purkinje, postulated that the neuronal signals controlling voluntary eye movements are fed back within the central nervous system ("outflow" hypothesis) and not only modify movement perception, but also recalibrate the spatial values of the retinal signals ("Ortswert der Netzhaut", cf. pp. 128–129 in Mach, 1886). This matching of retinal coordinates with that of extrapersonal space (coordinate transformation) is not only necessary for the correct perception of the directions in the extrapersonal space, but also for adequate goal-directed movements.

An alternative explanation is provided by the assumption that kinesthetic feedback signals, originating in the mechanoreceptors of the eye muscles or other orbital structures, are used to cancel the afferent visual movement signals within the central nervous system (inflow hypothesis). The outflow hypothesis was further elaborated by Von Uexküll (1928). His block diagram contains essentially all components (Fig. 3) which were later used by Von Holst and Mittelstaedt (1950). Efference copy signals (corollary discharge, described also by Sperry, 1950; Teuber 1960), representing the goal-directed commands controlling the movement of that part of the body which contains the respective sense organ, interact within the central nervous system with the "reafferent" signal flow from that sense organ.

In the following I will deal with data on gaze movement, visual movement and space perception, which support the outflow hypothesis, but also emphasize the importance of spatially directed visual attention. In particular, I will describe: (a) visual movement perception induced by saccades or eye pursuit movements evoked by the intention to gaze at an extrafoveal visual target "stabilized" on the retina; (b) visual movement perception evoked by eye pursuit movements or optokinetic nystagmus, when stationary spatially periodic stimulus patterns are illuminated stroboscopically (Sigma-movement); (c) visual movement perception when an immobilized eye is stimulated and the subject intentionally pursues the moving stimulus; (d) the recalibration time course of spatial values of retinal coordinates during and after saccades.

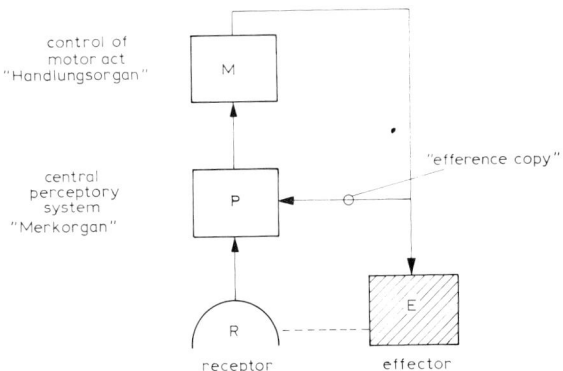

Fig. 3. Block diagram (redrawn) of J. Von Uexküll's "Merkwelt-Wirkwelt-Koppelung" (1928): Whenever active movement leads to movement of a receptor organ at the body surface, somewhere in the central nervous system a signal of that movement command is branched off and interacts with the afferent sensory signal flow.

Pursuing Aristotle's afterimage

A small, long-lasting afterimage placed in a region ±2° around the fovea centralis evoked smooth pursuit eye movements (head fixed) when the subject intended to fixate the afterimage. The angular ve-

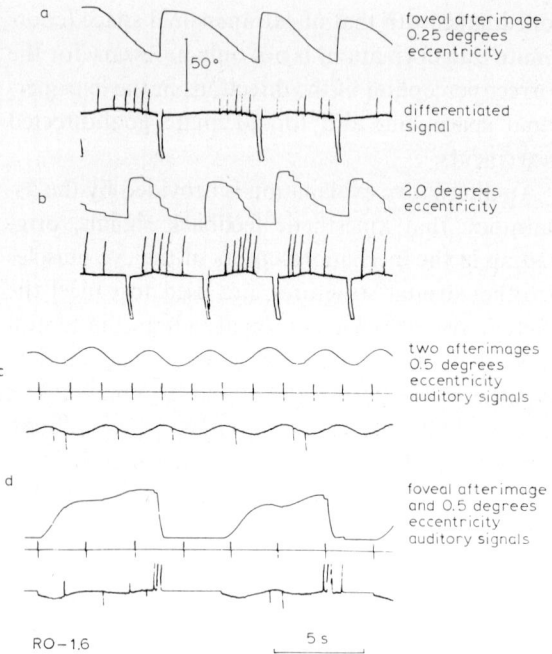

Fig. 4. Eye position recordings by means of electromagnetic search coil technique. (a) Pursuit eye movements are evoked when a small foveal afterimage of about 0.2° diameter is placed 0.25° extrafoveally and the subject gazes intentionally at this stabilized retinal image. Note acceleration of the pursuit speed with time. (b) Depending on afterimage eccentricity, attention of the subject, and an individual factor, these pursuit eye movements generated by a retinal position error signal are combined with saccades. (c) Two afterimages are placed 0.5° left and right of the fovea center. The subject's gaze commands are triggered by periodic auditory signals. With each auditory stimulus the subject shifts his attention from one afterimage to the other. The intention to fixate the extrafoveal signals led to nearly sinusoidal horizontal eye movements. When the distance of the two afterimages from the fovea center was larger than 1°, smooth pursuit eye movements appeared in combination with saccades. (d) One afterimage was placed in the fovea center, the other shifted horizontally by 1° towards the right. The subject fixated alternately the foveal and the extrafoveal afterimage. This evoked smooth pursuit eye movements and fixation periods. The latter were sometimes accompanied by a fast "saccade towards the fovea".

locity of the smooth pursuit eye movements depended on eccentricity of the afterimage and on the degree of attention with which the subject tried to fixate the afterimage (Kommerell and Klein, 1971; Collewijn and Grüsser, unpublished data). The afterimage is seen moving in the direction of the eye pursuit movements (Fig. 4a); its perceived speed was linearly related to the angular velocity of the pursuit eye movements, which usually increased with the duration of pursuit. In some observers small saccades in the direction of the pursuit movements appeared. They led to the percept of a jerky afterimage movement, but only when their amplitude exceeded about 1°.

When the afterimage was placed at a distance greater than 2° from the fovea center, attentive fixation evoked saccades predominantly, which were interrupted by smooth pursuit movements when the subject maintained his intention to fixate. The saccade amplitude was loosely correlated to the eccentricity of the afterimage (Fig. 4b); the frequency of the saccades depended on attention.

When two or more afterimages were placed at different retinal eccentricities, the apparent movement during eye pursuit movements of saccades was always the same for all afterimages and depended upon which afterimage the subject intended to fixate. Two afterimages, one on the left, the other on the right side of the fovea at $\leq 2°$ distance, aroused more or less sinusoidal pursuit eye movements and corresponding movement percepts when the subject shifted his attention at regular intervals from one afterimage to the other (Fig. 4c). Shifting attention between one afterimage placed in the fovea center, the other about 0.5° eccentrically, led to smooth pursuit eye movements, whereby the shift in attention towards the foveal afterimage either stopped smooth pursuit movement (and movement perception) abruptly or was accompanied by a small "saccade towards the fovea". Such "paradoxical" saccades were also observed when one afterimage was placed in the center of the fovea, the other 2° or more eccentrically, and the attention was shifted rapidly back and forth between the peripheral and the central afterimage.

This observation clearly indicates the existence of two components of neuronal control of smooth pursuit eye movements which to my knowledge have so far not been included in the models explaining smooth pursuit eye movement: within a range of $\pm 3°$ of the fovea center a position signal and not

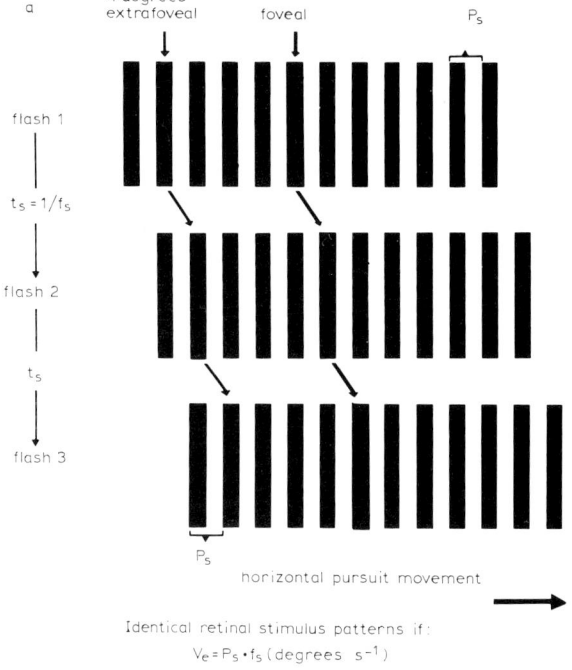

just a retinal velocity error signal also guides smooth gaze pursuit movement. In addition, in the case of different stimuli present in the visual field simultaneously, spatially directed attention determines which position signal is selected to perform this task (cf. also Collewijn et al., 1982).

Sigma-movement and Sigma-optokinetic nystagmus

The following section will deal with another experimental paradigm by which the possible impact of efference copy signals on movement perception during eye pursuit movements and OKN can be demonstrated. The Sigma paradigm (Stoper, 1967; Lamontagne, 1973) provides quasi-stabilized retinal stimuli: an "infinitely" long row of equidistant dots or stripes (P_s, Fig. 5a) was illuminated stroboscopically at a flash frequency f_s and slow pursuit gaze movements were induced at an angular velocity at which the center of gaze moved during one flash interval from one dot (stripe) to the next or the next but one, etc. Then identical retinal stimuli were

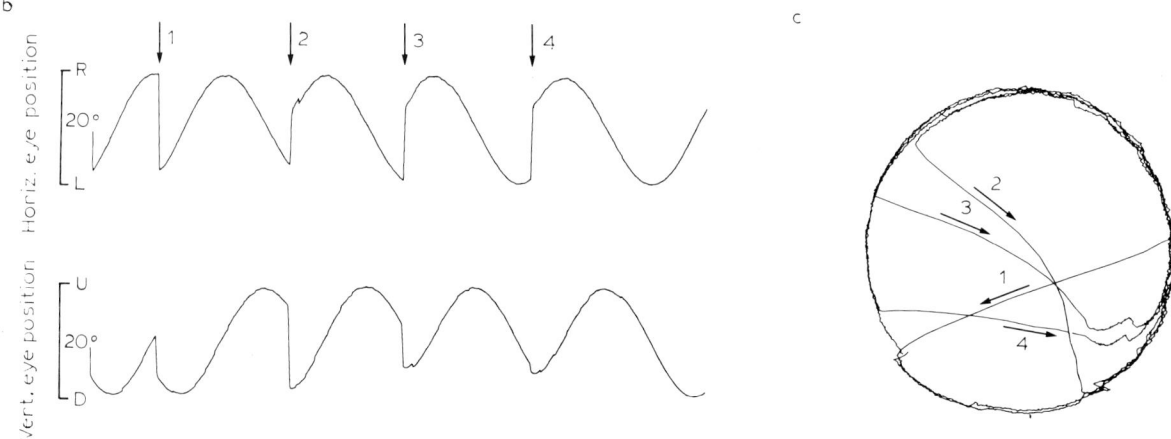

Fig. 5. Sigma-paradigm. (a) A long row of equidistant bars is illuminated stroboscopically at a flash frequency, f_s. The center of gaze moves during one flash interval from one dot to the next or the next but one, thus generating identical retinal stimulus patterns. The apparent movement perceived leads to an optokinetic nystagmus (Sigma-OKN). (b) Sigma-pursuit eye movements are evoked when a closed figure (dot circle) composed of equidistant dots is stroboscopically illuminated, and smooth pursuit eye movements are initiated which lead to an apparent movement of the circle in the direction of the eye pursuit movements, which in turn maintains the pursuit eye movements. Horizontal component of eye movement (electromagnetic search coil recordings). (c) Reconstruction of eye position from vertical and horizontal components. (b), (c) Large voluntary saccades across the circle interrupt the pursuit eye movements temporarily, but do not interrupt the apparent rotation of the dot circle. Thus, smooth pursuit movements go on at precisely the same speed (Behrens et al., 1985).

evoked from flash to flash, whereby the angular speed of eye or gaze movements V_g was

$$V_g = k \cdot P_s \cdot f_s \; [\mathrm{deg/sec}] \qquad (1)$$

k is an integer ≥ 1. A human observer who has initiated eye pursuit movements according to Eqn. 1 perceived the stroboscopically illuminated row of dots or stripes as moving continuously in the direction of the eye pursuit movements. This apparent Sigma movement guided in turn further pursuit eye movements and led to an optokinetic nystagmus (Sigma-OKN, Behrens and Grüsser, 1979, 1982), which in turn maintained the movement illusion ad libitum in an attentive subject. Sigma-movement perception — as movement perception in the afterimage experiments — is aroused by efference copy signals, since the retinal displacement signals are on the average null — at least for Sigma-pursuit movements in an attentive subject. Sigma-phenomena could be elicited not only by one-dimensional periodic stimuli, but also when a circle, ellipse or any other closed figure composed of equidistant dots had been stroboscopically illuminated (Fig. 5b,

Behrens and Grüsser, 1979, 1982; Adler et al. 1981; Van der Steen et al., 1983). Under such stimulus conditions only the fovea received identical stimuli from flash to flash; nevertheless, the subjects perceived a large part of the circle or ellipse rotating in the direction of the eye pursuit movements.

The level of attention could change the gain of Sigma-OKN slightly but did not alter the apparent speed. This observation is easily explained when one assumes that retinal displacement signals are added to the internal efference copy signals, as proposed by the scheme in Fig. 3. When stroboscopically illuminated stationary stripe patterns were projected to extrafoveal regions of the visual field, Sigma-OKN could also be aroused when attention was shifted towards the extrafoveal pattern without shifting the center of gaze to it. Thus, when two or more stripe patterns of different spatial periods, P_s, were present within the visual field, attention determined which retinal signal was used to guide the smooth pursuit component of Sigma-OKN (Fig. 6, Behrens and Grüsser, 1982; Collewijn et al., 1982).

Sigma-phenomena were also elicitable with periodic stimulus patterns which were generated on

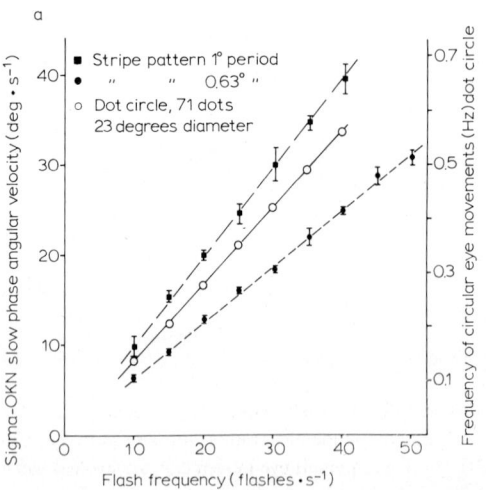
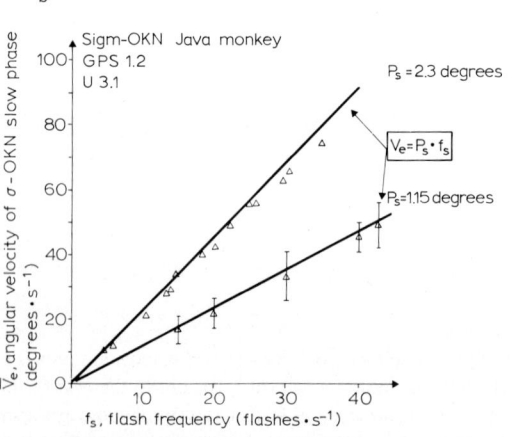

Fig. 6. Sigma-OKN. (a) Relationship between flash frequency (abscissa) and angular velocity of horizontal Sigma-OKN slow phase (left side ordinate) obtained with two different vertical stripe patterns ($P_s = 1.0$ or $0.63°$). The line with the open circles represents the relationship between flash frequency and the frequency of circular eye movements (right side ordinate) obtained with a dot circle of 71 dots and 23° in diameter (from Behrens and Grüsser, 1979). (b) Horizontal Sigma-OKN in Java monkey. Same relationship as in (a). Vertical stripe pattern of two different spatial periods ($P_s = 1.15$ and $2.3°$; from Grüsser et al., 1979).

the cyclopean retina. For example, a 16 or 24 vertical stripe Julesz stereogram (Julesz and Payne, 1968) was seen by all subjects with normal stereovision as a stereostripe pattern when both eyes were illuminated at flash frequencies $f_s \geq 2$ flashes/sec. When the subjects induced smooth pursuit eye movements across the stationary stereopattern by fixating a small spot of light moving at a speed corresponding to Eqn. 1, the whole stereopattern was seen moving in the direction of the eye movements. During this movement illusion the surface structure of the individual stripes changed (because the distribution of the black and white random dots varied between respective stripes of the stereogram), but all subjects could elicit Sigma-OKN and maintain a continuous movement illusion. Again, Eqn. 1 was applicable (Adler and Grüsser, 1982). In addition, Sigma-movement and Sigma-OKN were also elicitable when a time delay, Δt, between the left and right eye stimuli was introduced instead of synchronous dichoptic flashes. With alternating dichoptic stimuli ($\Delta t = 1/2 f_s$) the stereocomponents of the stripe pattern disappeared but the stripes were still seen moving in the direction of the eye pursuit movements and a corresponding Sigma-OKN was aroused.

From these findings we concluded that the interaction of efference copy signals and afferent visual information flow leading to Sigma phenomena used for the control of gaze movements takes place beyond the visual cortices (V1–V4). This view is confirmed by more recent clinical findings (Buettner et al., 1982; Buettner and Fettner, personal communication): Sigma-OKN disappeared when an extensive lesion of the parietal lobe was present. In addition, the cerebellar flocculus seems to play a role in the generation of Sigma-movements.

Sigma-movement and corresponding gaze pursuit movements could also be aroused by stroboscopically illuminated three-dimensional objects composed of spatially periodic components. The eyes then performed smooth pursuit movements at a speed determined by the center of gaze moving from flash to flash from one of the periodical objects (rods or balls) to the next, independent of the change in angle, distance, shape and relative orientation with respect to the subject's eye. Moreover, Sigma phenomena were not restricted to gaze movement solely by means of eye or head movements but were also elicitable when the subjects walked by or around the object at an appropriate speed. An example of data obtained in such experiments is shown in Fig. 7 (for further details, see Adler and Grüsser, 1982; Adler et al., 1981; Grüsser, 1986).

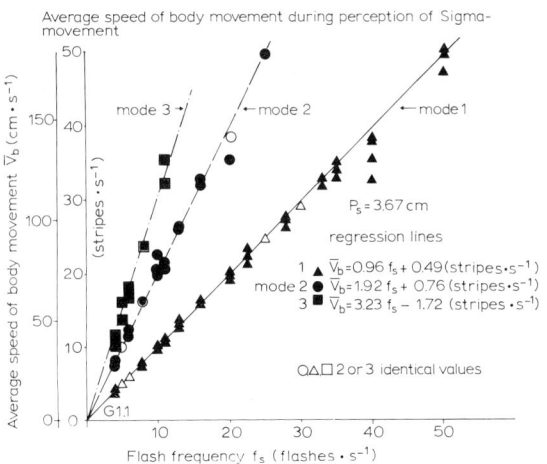

Fig. 7. Sigma-movement is also evoked when a stationary periodic stripe pattern is illuminated stroboscopically and the subject can walk along the stripe pattern after having initiated eye pursuit movements. Apparent rotation of the stripe cylinder in the direction of the eye pursuit movement is maintained independent of whether the center of gaze is moved by eye, head or whole body movements. Data presented in this figure were obtained when the subject walked along the vertical stripe pattern fixed on the inner wall of a cylinder, 280 cm in diameter. Period of vertical stripes, 3.67 cm; data obtained in modes 1, 2 and 3.

Animal models to study Sigma-movement and Sigma-OKN

To study efference copy mechanisms by means of microelectrode recordings one has to apply a reliable animal model. Since it appeared very difficult to train monkeys to pursue an extrafoveal afterimage, we tested whether Sigma-OKN could be aroused in animals. This is indeed the case (mon-

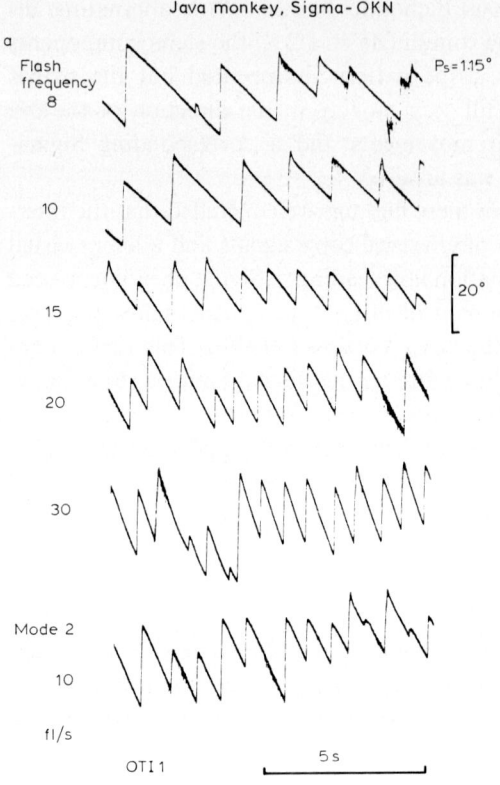

keys: Grüsser et al., 1979; rabbits: Nikolay et al., 1979; Busch et al., 1979). Essentially all findings obtained in humans with Sigma-OKN and the laws expressed by Eqn. 1 were also found to be valid for Java monkeys, while for rabbits the gain, as expressed by k of Eqn. 1, was about 0.7 (Fig. 8a).

Sigma-OKN was maintained in both rabbits and monkeys when flash sequences with a considerable random variation in successive intervals were applied instead of exactly periodic flashes. Like humans, monkeys also seem to perceive with Sigma-stimulus conditions fairly smooth visual movement, and within a considerable range of temporal flash "jitter" the speed of the OKN slow phase was not affected (Fig. 8b). This finding was at first surprising, but could be explained by the assumption that the mechanisms generating the smooth pursuit eye movement (or smooth phase of Sigma-OKN) operate with a fairly large time constant of several hundred mseconds, thus tolerating deviations between the predicted and the perceived position of the apparent moving stimulus.

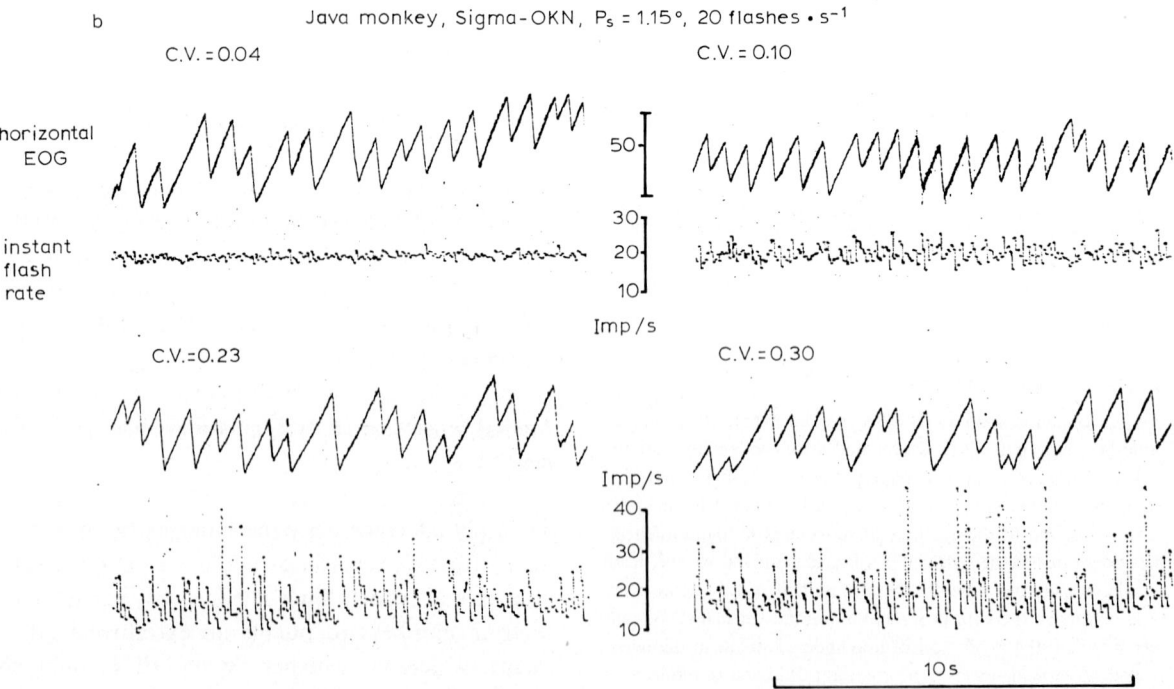

Fig. 8. (a) Horizontal Sigma-OKN recorded in Java monkey (*Macaca fascicularis*). Recording of electrooculogram by implanted electrodes. Note that the speed of the slow-phase OKN increases with flash frequency as indicated. (b) Recording of Sigma-OKN in Java monkey. Vertical stripe pattern of 1.15° period. Average flash rate, 20 flashes/sec. Flash sequence of increasing irregularity. The different amounts of temporal noise in the flash sequence are characterized by the coefficient of variation (C.V.) of the flash interval distribution, which approximates a Gaussian distribution (from Adler et al., 1981).

Eye movements and movement perception aroused by movement stimulation of the retina of an immobilized eye

Injecting 3–5 cc of a local anaesthetic around the eyeball behind the orbita completely immobilizes the eye for 30–60 minutes but does not impair signal transfer by the optic nerve when the injections are administered properly (Kornmüller, 1931; Grüsser et al., 1981). When the immobilized eye was stimulated by a moving pattern which the subject tried to pursue, the perceived speed of the pattern increased with the duration of pursuit. Recording the movements of the other normal eye, kept in darkness, we found that the speed of the pursuit eye movements or of the optokinetic nystagmus slow phase clearly exhibited an accelerating property (Fig. 9a). This non-linearity became all the more evident the longer the pursuit was maintained, i.e., with optokinetic stripe patterns it depended upon instructing the subject to pursue one selected stripe of the vertical stripe pattern as long as possible or to see as many stripes as possible, i.e., to perform a high frequency, small amplitude OKN. Data shown in Fig. 9a indicate that it seems to be rather meaningless to define a general open loop gain for such conditions, since OKN gain depended essentially on the duration of the smooth pursuit component of OKN. A similar statement was found to be true when an oscillating small spot of light instead of the moving stripe pattern was pursued (Fig. 9b). The quasi-sinusoidal eye movements aroused in the non-seeing eye by constant-amplitude, horizontal, sinewave stimulation of the immobilized retina led to sinusoidal eye movements of increasing amplitude and a corresponding increase in the perceived amplitude.

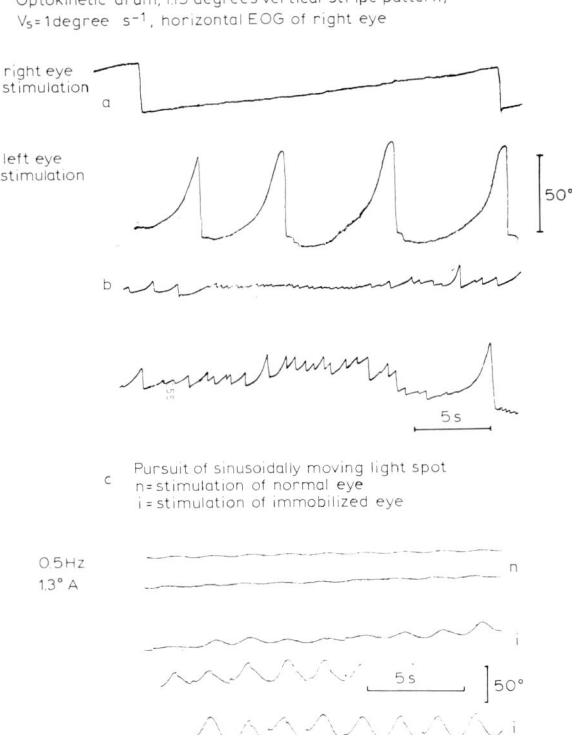

Fig. 9. Eye movements evoked by stimulation of an immobilized eye. (a) Optokinetic nystagmus (DC-EOG recordings) of the right eye evoked by optokinetic stimulation of the right eye or the immobilized left eye. According to the instructions the subject pursued a selected stripe of the 1.15° period vertical stripe pattern as long as possible (attentive optokinetic pursuit nystagmus). Note the non-linear time course of eye position. (b) As in (a), but the subject was instructed to gaze at successive stripes. A regular small amplitude OKN was evoked. (c) Horizontal pursuit eye movements evoked by the intention to pursue sinusoidally moving stimulus (horizontal direction) applied to the immobilized eye (0.5 Hz, 4° amplitude). Note the non-linear response property and the increase in amplitude with duration of stimulation.

Time constant of per- and post-saccadic recalibration of retinal spatial values as measured by a new after-image technique

While in the preceding sections the relationship between gaze movement and visual movement perception was discussed, I will describe in the following some observations on how the perception of spatial directions depends on gaze movements.

During horizontal back and forth saccades performed at a maximum alternation frequency (3–4.5 saccades/sec) across a structured background the stationary objects seem to move back and forth, especially those located within an "inner" region of 20° of the field of gaze. This observation of oscillopsia indicates that recalibration of spatial values

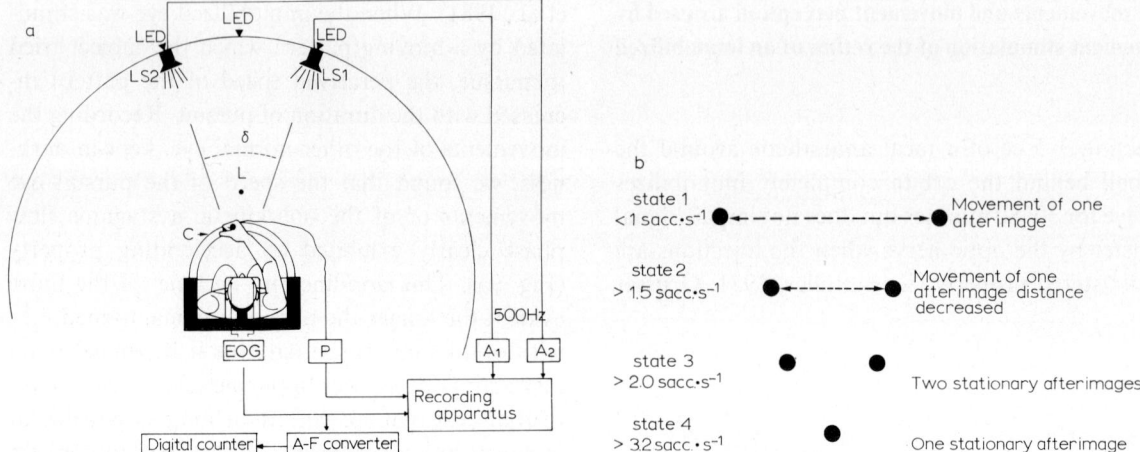

Fig. 10. (a) Scheme of the experimental set-up to measure the time course of "recalibration" of spatial retinal values during and after saccades. The subject sat with the head tightly fixed in the center of a vertical cylinder, 280 cm in diameter. Two loudspeakers (LS) were placed on the wall of the cylinder at eye height and an angular distance of 39°. Three light-emitting diodes (LED) served for calibration of DC-electrooculogram. Before the measurements the subjects had to fixate a strong light source, L, or a photoflash monocularly to imprint a small long-lasting foveal afterimage. When looking at the sounding loudspeakers in total darkness, the subject perceived a shift in the afterimage position and "pointed" with the movable handle on a semicircular rail (C) towards the respective end position of the afterimage. (b) Illustration of the four states of afterimage perception during horizontal auditory saccades performed at different rates as indicated. For further explanation see text.

of retinal coordinates takes some time (Purkinje, 1825a, b). We measured the time constant of this recalibration process by means of "auditory" saccades performed in total darkness: as targets two alternately sounding loudspeakers were placed at eye level (Fig. 10a). The subjects were instructed to shift their attention and gaze as quickly as possible to the respective audible sound source. The head of the subject was firmly fixed. The alternation frequency determined the voluntary saccade frequency up to 4.5 saccades/sec. At a saccade frequency < 0.8 saccades/sec the subjects observed saccadic movement (or change in position) of a small foveal afterimage (<0.2° diameter), but the afterimage seemed to attain its final position more slowly than the eyes (state 1, Fig. 10b). When the saccade frequency was above 1.5 saccades/sec, the perceived amplitude of afterimage movement decreased with increasing saccade frequency (state 2). When saccade frequency was above 2–2.2 saccades/sec, the subject perceived two afterimages simultaneously, which then appeared to be stationary at the saccadic end position (state 3, Fig. 10b). At a saccade frequency above 3.2–3.6 saccades/sec only one stationary afterimage was seen in a midposition between the two auditory targets (state 4). However, DC-EOG recordings of the eye movements revealed that the saccade amplitude remained constant up to 4.2–4.5 saccades/sec.

From the amplitude of the perceived afterimage movement (or the distance of the two afterimages observed in state 3), the time constant of the coordinate transformation of retinal spatial values could be measured (for details, see Grüsser and Krizić, 1984; Grüsser et al., 1985). A simple mathematical model (Fig. 11) could be used to explain the findings. It provided a new step in the discussion about efference copy signals since it states a distinct time course for their interaction with the afferent visual signal flow and for the recalibration of the spatial values of retinal coordinates.

In four observations with migraine phosphenes (two subjects) these afterimage experiments could be extended. Under these conditions migraine phos-

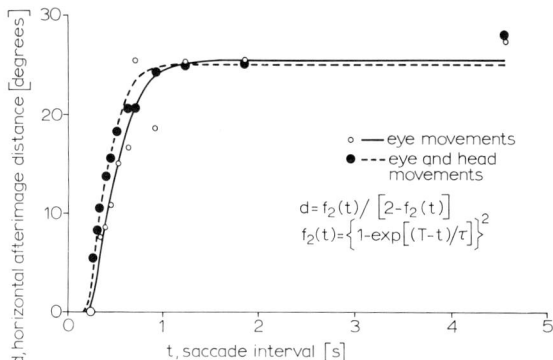

Fig. 11. Change in amplitude of afterimage movement (d, ordinate) is plotted as a function of horizontal saccade temporal intervals (abscissa). The continuous line represents the coordinate transformation function for d in measurements with the head fixed, the dashed line with eye and head movements. Data from one subject. In the equation describing d as a function of the duration t of the saccade interval, T is the dead time, τ the time constant of the coordinate transformation, b is a constant and A the amplitude of the gaze movement (48° in this experiment).

phenes and afterimages behaved identically. We combined a foveal afterimage with a migraine phosphene located about 2° outside the fovea. During fast horizontal back and forth saccades, no change in the relative position of migraine phosphene and afterimage was observed. Thus, the interaction between afferent visual signal flow and the recalibrating efference copy signals occurs at a cortical level beyond the primary visual cortex, where the migraine phosphene is believed to originate (cf. Jung, 1979; Baumgartner, 1982).

In more recent experiments we extended the experimental paradigm shown in Fig. 10a: the subject's head was free and the subject was asked to look at the sounding target by means of fast head movements. This instruction, of course, led to combined eye-head "saccades" (Bizzi, 1974). Surprisingly, it was found that the speed of recalibration of spatial values of retinal coordinates increased in most subjects, i.e., the time constant τ and/or the dead time T of the model of Fig. 11 decreased (Grüsser et al., 1985, 1986). It is still not clear which neuronal mechanisms are responsible for this change in the time constants of retinal coordinate transformations: efference copy signals from the head movement commands, afferent vestibular signals or neck receptor signals are candidates.

Five conclusions

(1) When we observe a single object moving across a structured visual background, attentive selection of the object from the manifold objects visible is a prerequisite for gaze pursuit movements. Hereby, gaze might change its position in space by means of saccades and/or smooth pursuit eye, head or body movements. Error signals controlling this movement are evidently not only retinal slip velocity signals (target velocity minus gaze velocity) but also retinal position errors, namely the distance between target and fovea center. Retinal position errors change smooth pursuit velocity and might lead to goal-directed saccades. Both mechanisms are intended to bring the target near the fovea center. From the data described in the section entitled "Pursuing Aristotle's afterimage" it is evident that also for this task the central nervous system processes efference copy signals representing the movement commands of the gaze control system. These efference copy signals are added to retinal signals in the central nervous system and generate a representation of target velocity in the extrapersonal space. Evidently, it is the perceived movement which guides the gaze pursuit (for details, see the discussion in Henn et al., 1980). The accelerating speed of gaze when an extrafoveal afterimage is pursued can be used to estimate the time course of the efference copy signals feedback. With some algebraic computation one finds for the change in position of gaze (relative to the coordinate of the extrapersonal space $P_g(t)$):

$$P_g(t) = gP_aT \sum_{i=0}^{i=n} (n-i)\,\beta^i \text{ [degrees]} \quad (2)$$

Hereby, P_a is the distance of the afterimage from the fovea, g a weighting factor for this distance, T the delay of the feedback cycle between efference copy signal and movement perception, n and i are integers and β the gain of the movement control signals. When this gain is 1, an approximation which is valid for highly attentive pursuit, Eqn. 2 is simplified to

$$P_g(t) = gP_a\left(\frac{t^2}{T} + t\right) \text{ [degrees]} \qquad (3)$$

Hereby, $t (= i \cdot T)$ is the time since the onset of eye pursuit movements. From the data as shown in Fig. 4, the time T could be estimated, and also the weighting factor g.

(2) The argument that β of Eqn. 2 is near 1 can be deduced from the findings on Sigma-pursuit eye movements. With closed figures composed of equidistant dots the average gain of smooth pursuit is 1; the same is true for highly attentive pursuit of an "infinite" horizontal row of dots or equidistant vertical stripes. Also, for Sigma-movement a variation in gain is observed, certainly depending on the level of attention on the part of the subject. Whenever this variation leads to considerable retinal position errors (difference between foveal center and pursued target), either correcting saccades appear or pursuit speed is changed.

(3) In the experiments with movement stimulation of an immobilized eye the retinal angular velocity led to an OKN gain near 1 when the pursuit mode was interrupted by saccades within 0.2 seconds. In this case these backward saccades evidently led to a set-back in the gain. However, when attentive pursuit was applied for as long as possible, accelerating pursuit eye movements were found which are predicted by Eqn. 2. Nevertheless, the maintained retinal error signal in this case was the retinal angular velocity and not a position signal, although it acted in the same way in principle as the position error.

(4) In all the conditions described in the preceding paragraphs attention played an essential role. Hereby, not only did the pursuit gain depend on the general level of attention, but attention in this context meant attentive selection of a certain visual object in the extrapersonal space as the goal of gaze tracking movements.

(5) Finally, a second type of efference copy signal has to be discussed. When we pursue a target moving across the extrapersonal space, movement of this target is always related to the coordinates of space which are perceived as stable since their directions do not change essentially when the center of gaze changes its position. This observation means that a continuous "updating" of foveal coordinate values relative to those of the extrapersonal space is necessary. This updating can work with some fuzzy border conditions, since the framework of extrapersonal space coordinates is probably also maintained by vestibular and proprioceptive signals. Nevertheless, it is necessary that the spatial values of the fovea are matched to those of the extrapersonal space. The data described in the section on per- and postsaccadic recalibration of retinal spatial values indicate that considerable time is necessary to achieve this goal (further discussion in Grüsser et al., 1985, 1986).

Summary

Gaze movement signals are controlled by retinal "error" signals, namely target distance from fovea and retinal slip velocity. In addition, the perceived movement of the pursued target relative to extrapersonal space coordinates plays an essential role in gaze control. The latter value is elaborated by the sum of retinal error signals and efference copy signals of motor commands controlling gaze. Three examples are described which measure quantitatively the impact of these efference copy signals: perceived movement and eye movements evoked by an extrafoveal afterimage, Sigma-movement, and Sigma-OKN, and movement perception aroused by stimulation of an immobilized eye.

Efference copy signals are not only necessary for movement perception and gaze motor control but also to recalibrate the retinal spatial values relative to the coordinates of the extrapersonal space when the eyes move. The time constant of this coordinate transformation associated with eye saccades could be measured by a new afterimage technique. It was found that this process outlasts the saccades considerably.

Acknowledgements

The investigations were supported by a grant from the Deutsche Forschungsgemeinschaft (Gr 161), and in part by a Twinning Grant from the European Science Foundation, ETP, Strasbourg. Experiments described in the section entitled "Pursuing Aristotle's afterimage" were performed in collaboration with Professor H. Collewijn at the Department of Physiology, Erasmus Universiteit, Rotterdam. I thank Mrs. J. Dames for her help in the English translation of the manuscript and Mr. M. Winzer for drawing the figures.

References

Adler, B. and Grüsser, O.-J. (1982) Sigma-movement and optokinetic nystagmus elicited by stroboscopically illuminated stereopatterns, Exp. Brain Res., 47: 353–364.

Adler, B., Collewijn, H., Curio, G., Grüsser, O.-J., Pause, M., Schreiter, U. and Weiss, L. (1981) Sigma-movement and Sigma-nystagmus: a new tool to investigate the gaze pursuit system and visual movement perception in man and monkey. Ann. N.Y. Acad. Sci., 374: 284–302.

Aristotle, Volume 8 (1975) Parva naturalia, translation by W. S. Hett, Heinemann, London, pp. 348–373.

Bauer, H. (1911) Die Psychologie Alhazens auf Grund von Alhazens Optik, Aschendorf, Münster i.W.

Baumgartner, G. (1982) Visuelle Wahrnehmungsstörungen und Halluzinationen bei Epilepsie und andere Hirnerkrankungen. In I. Karbowski (Ed.), Halluzinationen bei Epilepsien und ihre Differentialdiagnose, Verlag Hans Huber, Bern, pp. 9–24.

Behrens, F. and Grüsser, O.-J. (1979) Smooth pursuit eye movements and optokinetic nystagmus elicited by intermittently illuminated stationary patterns. Exp. Brain Res., 37: 317–336.

Behrens, F. and Grüsser, O.-J. (1982) On the additivity of Sigma- and Phi-movement in visual perception and oculomotor control. Human Neurobiol., 1: 121–127.

Bell, C. (1823) On the motions of the eye, and illustrations of the uses of the muscles and nerves of the orbit. Phil. Trans. Roy. Soc. London, 113: 166–186.

Bizzi, E. (1974) The coordination of eye-head movement. Sci. Am., 231: 100–106.

Buettner, U. W., Dichgans, J. and Grüsser, O.-J. (1982) Efferent motion perception (Sigma-movements) and Sigma-pursuit in neurological patients. In G. Lennerstrand, D. S. Zee and E. L. Keller (Eds.), Functional Basis of Ocular Motility Disorders, Pergamon Press, Oxford, pp. 359–361.

Busch, F., Grüsser, O.-J. and Nikolay, H. (1979) Additivity of Sigma and Phi-optokinetic nystagmus in rabbits. Pflügers Arch., 382: R45.

Collewijn, H., Curio, G. and Grüsser, O.-J. (1982) Spatially selective visual attention and generation of eye pursuit movements. Human Neurobiol., 1: 129–139.

Cusanus, N. (1963) Liber de Mente. Quoted in E. Cassirer, Individuum und Kosmos in der Philosophie der Renaissance, Wiss. Buchgesellschaft, Darmstadt.

Cusanus, N. (1982) Compendium, 1488, Meiner, Hamburg.

Darwin, E. (1794/1796) Zoonomia; or the laws of organic life, Volume I, II. J. Johnson, London, reprint: (1974) AMS Press, New York, pp. 568, 722.

Darwin, R. W. (1789) On the ocular spectra of light and colours. Phil. Trans., 76: 313. Reprint in Darwin, E. (1794).

Diels, H. and Kranz, W. (1974) Die Fragmente der Vorsokratiker, Vol. I, 6th edn, Weidmann.

Filehne, W. (1922) Über das optische Wahrnehmen von Bewegungen. Z. Sinnesphysiol., 53: 134–145.

Grüsser, O.-J. (1986) Efference copy and visual perception. A review. Rev. Sensory Physiol., in preparation.

Grüsser, O.-J. and Krizić, A. (1984) Time constant of per- and postsaccadic recalibration of retinal spatial values as measured by a new afterimage method. Invest. Ophthalmol. Vis. Sci., 25: ARVO Suppl. 263.

Grüsser, O.-J., Pause, M. and Schreiter, U. (1979) Three methods to elicit Sigma-OKN in Java monkeys. Exp. Brain Res., 35: 519–526.

Grüsser, O.-J., Kulikowski, J., Pause, M. and Wollensak, J. (1981) Optokinetic nystagmus, Sigma-optokinetic nystagmus and eye pursuit movements elicited by stimulation of an immobilized eye. J. Physiol., 320: 21.

Grüsser, O.-J., Kirsten, M., Krizić, A. and Weiss, L. (1985) The time course of retinal coordinate transformation during and after saccades evoked by auditory stimuli in the dark. Pflügers Arch., 403: R67.

Grüsser, O.-J., Krizić, A. and Weiss, L. (1986) Afterimage movement during saccades in the dark. Vision Res., in press.

Henn, V., Cohen, B. and Young, L. R. (Eds.) (1980) Visual vestibular interaction in motion perception and the generation of nystagmus. Neurosci. Res. Prog. Bull., 18: 459–651.

Hering, E. (1861) Vom Ortssinne der Netzhaut, Beiträge zur Physiologie, Heft 1, Leipzig.

Hering, E. (1879) Der Raumsinn und die Bewegungen des Auges. In L. Hermann (Ed.), Handbuch der Physiologie, Vol. 3, Vogel, Leipzig, pp. 343–601.

Jeannerod, M., Kennedy, H. and Magnin, M. (1979) Corollary discharge: Its possible implications in visual and oculomotor interactions. Neuropsychologia, 17: 241–258.

Julesz, B. and Payne, R. A. (1968) Differences between monocular and binocular stroboscopic movement perception. Vision Res., 8: 433–444.

Jung, R. (1979) Translokation corticaler Migränephosphene bei Augenbewegungen und vestibulären Reizen. Neuropsychologia, 17: 173–185.

Kommerell, G. and Klein, U. (1971) Über die visuelle Regelung der Okulomotorik: die optomotorische Wirkung exzentrischer Nachbilder. Vision Res., 11: 905–920.

Kornmüller, A. E. (1931) Eine experimentelle Anästhesie der äußeren Augenmuskeln am Menschen und ihre Auswirkungen. J. Psychol. Neurol. Lpz., 41: 354–366.

Lamontagne, C. (1973) A new experimental paradigm for the investigation of the secondary system of human visual motion perception. Perception, 2: 167–180.

Languth, D. G. (1742) De luce ex pressione oculi, Medical dissertation, Wittenberg.

Mach, E. (1886) Die Analyse der Empfindungen und das Verhältnis des Physischen zum Psychischen, English translation: The Analysis of Sensations and the Relation of the Physical to the Psychical, (1959) Dover, New York.

Morgagni, G. B. (1741) Adversaria Anatomica Omnia, Lugdanŭm, Batavia.

Nikolay, H., Pause, M. and Schreiter, U. (1979) Optokinetic responses of rabbits to stroboscopically illuminated stationary patterns. Neurosci. Lett., Suppl. 3: S107.

Plato "Timaios" in: Sämtliche Werke, Vol. 3 (1969), Hegner, Köln, pp. 93–191.

Purkinje, J. (1825a) Beobachtungen und Versuche zur Physiologie der Sinne II.: Neue Beiträge zur Kenntniss des Sehens in subjectiver Hinsicht, G. Reimer, Berlin.

Purkinje, J. (1825b) Über die Scheinbewegungen, welche im subjectiven Umfange des Gesichtssinnes vorkommen, Bull. der naturwissenschaftlichen Sektion der Schlesischen Gesellschaft IV, pp. 9, 10.

Sperry, R. W. (1950) Neural basis of the spontaneous optokinetic response produced by visual inversion. J. Comp. Physiol. Psychol., 43: 482–489.

Stoper, A. E. (1967) Vision during pursuit movement: the role of oculomotor information, Ph.D. Thesis, Brandeis University.

Teuber, H. L. (1960) Perception. In J. Field and H. W. Magoun (Eds.), Handbook of Physiology. Neurophysiology, Vol. III. American Physiological Society, Washington DC, pp. 1595–1668.

Von Graefe, A, (1854) Beiträge zur Physiologie und Pathologie der schiefen Augenmuskeln. Arch. f. Ophthalm., I(1): 1–81.

Von Helmholtz, H. (1896) Handbuch der Physiologischen Optik, 2nd edn., Voss, Hamburg (1st edn., Leipzig, 1866).

Von Holst, E. and Mittelstaedt, H. (1950) Das Reafferenzprinzip. Wechselwirkung zwischen Zentralnervensystem und Peripherie. Naturwissenschaften, 37: 464–476.

Van der Steen, J., Taminga, E. R. and Collewijn, H. (1983) A comparison of oculomotor pursuit of a target in circular, real, Beta or Sigma-motion. Vision Res., 23: 1655–1661.

Von Uexküll, J. (1928) Theoretische Biologie, 2nd edn., Springer, Berlin, Reprint (1973) Suhrkamp, Frankfurt a.M.

Wiedemann, E. (1910) Zu Ibn al Heitams Optik. Arch. Ges. Naturwiss. u. Technik, 3: 1–53.

Discussion

A. Berthoz

Laboratoire de Physiologie Neurosensielle, CNRS, 15 Rue de l'Ecole de Médicine, 75270 Paris Cedex 06, France

Possible role of non feedback mechanisms in adaptive behavior (discussion of the paper by Miles)

Nashner was interested by the fact that Miles, in his experiments, observed a process, also seen in postural control, in which two mechanisms seem to interact: One is feedback control which works through gain adjustment, the other is the use of different "behavioral forms" (a term used here by Nashner in the place of "strategy"). In this case one observes a gain change which is not a true feedback gain change but an early index of the fact that the subject is actually changing his "behavioral form". He suggested that some of the saccadic amplitude changes observed by Miles are in fact shifts in "behavioral forms". Miles concurred with this suggestion and took the adaptive change in the VOR as an example. He recalled that the VOR gain change can be obtained rapidly simply by instructing the subject to imagine the target moving with him or on the wall, demonstrating that the compensatory eye movements are obviously not only determined by the semi-circular canals. However, he pointed out that a better instruction may be to use eye-hand coordination rather than imagining a target on the wall, in order to allow the subject to predict the task.

There is support for the idea of a dual mechanism in adaptive control. I have suggested in a recent review (Berthoz, 1985) that indeed the first steps in adaptation, when either a sensory cue is distorted or missing, or when a central or peripheral lesion dictates a need for adaptation, are the following:

First, there are gain or phase changes by feedback or feedforward control if in the range of the normal function. Secondly, the repertoire of available subsystems ("behavioral forms" described by Nashner) is searched for a combination which may substitute or complement the defective function. Finally, if the previous steps are not sufficient or if some changes have to be stabilized, then synaptic plasticity occurs. In particular, I have proposed that the saccadic system may play an adaptive role in correcting saccadic dysmetria, but also in substituting for defective subsystems, even the VOR. Extremely rapid changes, and even apparent reversal of VOR, can be accomplished in man by this type of mechanism during adaptive experiments with prism reversal (see reviews in Melvill-Jones and Berthoz, 1985).

Miles emphasized that we have often concentrated on long-term adaptive changes even though it has been known for a long time that rapid changes can occur in a number of oculomotor parameters. He reminded the audience that McLaughlin (1967) had observed very rapid changes in the amplitudes of saccadic eye movements when the targets for these eye movements were displaced at the time the subject tried to acquire them. These changes occurred in spite of the fact that the subjects did not perceive the target shifts. Other studies on this topic were done by Miller et al. (1981) and Wolf et al. (1984). Grüsser proposed another paradigm based upon his own observations in man. He predicted that if a monkey made a saccade across an empty field and the experimeter then moved a patterned field that appeared suddenly, there would be an effect within 200 mseconds.

Mechanisms of vestibular compensation (questions concerning the paper by Precht)

Jeannerod asked Precht about the cerebellum in the compensation process. Precht stated that it has been shown in several species that the cerebellum plays a modifying but not an essential role in balance compensation. Less is known about the recovery of the gain, although Jeannerod and his colleagues have shown that the cerebellum is probably necessary. It is probable that the plastic capacity of the normal VOR to adapt would have been impaired if the flocculus had been lesioned.

Cohen commented that Precht's results would have interesting implications for the recovery of patients after hemilabyrinthectomy. He wondered if the head movements of these two groups of animals had been measured. For example, Oman (unpublished data) has measured the head movements of astronauts over a certain period of time, using the integration of accelometers. He wondered if there was any change in the OKN gain or in OKAN of these two groups of animals.

Precht responded that he had not yet measured head movements. The OKN gain did not differ in the non-trained and the trained group. Thus, the training in itself was not facilitating OKN recovery. OKAN was measured but data have not yet been analysed.

Origin of accelerating smooth eye movements during after-image tracking (discussion of the paper by Grüsser)

Eckmiller commented that in the two experiments of Grüsser, the "pursuit-like" eye movements that he had recorded were accelerating movements resulting from a small position error with respect to the fovea, without any retinal slip velocity signal. Grüsser responded that the perceived movement is always added to the position error. Because they add successively, one can predict a hyperbolic increase in image velocity. Eckmiller proposed that the acceleration could be explained by an internally generated motor velocity signal, which is updated by the position error on the retina by means of a simple integration process. He pointed to the fact that Grüsser has introduced an additional concept which gives functional importance to an efferent copy signal in the simple scheme, based on a motor program generator. Eckmiller wondered how the two mechanisms interacted.

Grüsser described how he viewed the integration process (see Fig. 1): for example, a 0.5° position error between the fovea and an afterimage induces a gaze movement. This movement induces a perception of movement because the internal movement generator has a branch which leads to a percept. The efferent copy adds to the position error, which increases the movement velocity further, and therefore leads to an acceleration. The interaction occurs in the brain and is not due to an external physical interaction. To support this view, Grüsser mentioned that stationary, stroboscopically illuminated stereo-stripes can induce Sigma-OKN and apparent motion. The results of Büttner (section

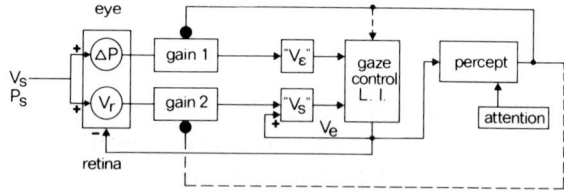

Fig. 1. Block diagram of the two mechanisms controlling pursuit eye movements. The retinal error signal, ΔP, i.e., the distance between target and fovea, leads to a gaze velocity signal V_e after an attention-dependent gain. This is added to the second retinal error signal, the retinal slip velocity V_r, which leads to a gaze motor signal V_s after attention-dependent gain control. To that signal the actual smooth pursuit eye of gaze velocity V_e is added. The percept corresponds to this efference copy signal V_e. Perceived position or velocity changes in turn the gain of the two retinal error signals. Hereby attention selects the target. The pursuit controlled by ΔP only works for a distance range of about ±0.3° around fovea centralis. When ΔP is larger, the saccadic system is activated. This system is not included in the block diagram (from Grüsser, unpublished data).

IV-B) suggest that the interaction between efference copy signals and afferent signals about visual motion is a parietal lobe function. Grüsser had previously shown that Sigma-pursuit can be used to localize a defect of smooth pursuit eye movements. The study of 127 patients showed that after lesions of the cerebellum and the parietal cortex there were no Sigma-pursuit movements. This means that the hypothesised smooth pursuit command and efference copy mechanism is no longer functioning, although in patients with other lesions that produce defective smooth pursuit movements, there is good Sigma-pursuit.

Loeb asked whether the generation of saccade would interrupt the smooth rate of the acceleration. Grüsser answered that if the saccade goes in the opposite direction, the acceleration is slowed, but it can be facilitated by saccades in the same direction. In the case of OKN, every backward saccade interrupts the acceleration.

Efferent motor copy does play a role in saccadic eye movements

Sparks summarized experiments which were aimed at demonstrating that an efferent motor command, and not proprioception, was used to guide a saccade to its target when the eye was disturbed during the saccade. He first verified that, in the monkey, as in other species, extra-ocular proprioceptive signals reach the central nervous system through the ophthalmic branch of the trigeminal nerve. HRP was injected in the extraocular muscles, and the only labelled cells were found in the trigeminal ganglion. When the ophthalmic branch of the trigeminal nerve was sectioned and HRP injected at the periphery, no labelled cells were found in the trigeminal ganglion or in the brainstem. In two animals the ophthalmic branch was sectioned bilaterally. The animals then had to fixate a dot in total darkness. The target then was flashed briefly at some eccentricity for 50 mseconds; it disappeared before the animal could move its eyes. The monkey was required to look to the remembered position of the target in order to obtain a liquid reward. Randomly, in 30% of the trials, after the target had disappeared, but before the animal had initiated a saccade to the target, the superior colliculus was stimulated to drive the eyes to another position in the orbit. Normal animals and animals with bilateral nerve sections are able to compensate for this perturbation and to generate a new saccade to the position of the target in space.

There were no background cues as to the location of this target, and after the stimulation-induced perturbation no stimulus was present. Therefore, no retinal update was possible. Since the trajectory of the compensatory saccade was not based upon visual cues, it must have been based upon precise knowledge of the stimulation-induced change in eye position. Although the bilateral nerve section eliminated extraocular muscle proprioception cues, it did not affect performance of this task. The most probable explanation is that the motor command can be used to generate and guide subsequent movements of the eyes (Guthrie et al., 1983).

In support of the view that the parameters of the saccade are indeed available at premotor level, Berthoz and co-workers (Yoshida et al., 1982) have demonstrated in the cat and Van Gisbergen et al. (1981) have demonstrated in the monkey that premotor burst neurons code saccadic eye displacement by the number of spikes in the burst, saccadic eye velocity by the instantaneous firing rate and the duration of saccades by the duration of the burst. The branching of these neurons to structures other than the motor nuclei (Yoshida et al., 1982) establishes the morphological basis for an efferent copy of the motor command.

References

Berthoz, A. (1985) Adaptive mechanisms in eye-head coordination. In A. Berthoz and G. Melvill Jones (Eds.), Adaptive Mechanisms in Gaze Control, Elsevier, Amsterdam, pp. 177–202.

Guthrie, B. L., Porter, J. P. and Sparks, D. L. (1983) Corollary discharge provides accurate eye position information to the oculomotor system. Science, 221: 1193–1195.

Melville-Jones, G. and Berthoz, A. (Eds.) (1985) Adaptive Mechanisms in Gaze Control, Reviews in Oculomotor Research, Vol. 1, Elsevier, Amsterdam.

McLaughlin, S. (1967) Parametric adjustments in saccadic eye movements. Percept. Psychophys., 2: 359–362.

Miller, J. M., Anstis, T. and Templeton, W. B. (1981) Saccadic plasticity, parametric adaptive control by retinal feedback. J. Exp. Psychol. Human Percept. Perf., 7: 356–366.

Van Gisbergen, J. A., Robinson, D. A. and Gielen, S. A. (1981) A quantitative analysis of generation of saccadic eye movements by burst neurons. J. Neurophysiol., 45: 417–442.

Wolf, W., Deubel, H. and Hauske, G. (1984) Properties of parametric adjustment in the saccadic system. In A. Gale and F. Johnson (Eds.), Theoretical and Applied Aspects of Eye Movement Research, Elsevier, Amsterdam, pp. 79–86.

Yoshida, K., McCrea, R., Berthoz, A. and Vidal, P.-P. (1982) Morphological and physiological characteristics of inhibitory burst neurons controlling horizontal rapid eye movements in the alert cat. J. Neurophysiol., 48: 761–784.

# SECTION VII

General Concepts

Is the oculomotor system a cartoon of motor control?

David A. Robinson

Departments of Ophthalmology and Biomedical Engineering, The Johns Hopkins University, Baltimore, MD 21205, U.S.A.

Introduction

One advantage in studying the oculomotor system is that it is contained entirely within the cranial vault so that one can, theoretically, record from all of its neurons. This has allowed one to start at the motoneuron, characterize its discharge rate, and then step centrally, synapse by synapse, trying to relate the discharge rate of successively premotor neurons to that of the motoneuron, building bridges of causality as one goes. The case is quite otherwise for spinal motor control. Very few recordings have been made of spinal motoneurons and premotor neurons in the spinal cords of behaving animals. As in oculomotor physiology as well, recordings have been made in cerebral cortex and cerebellum, but with no understanding of signal processing in the cord there is no way to relate these high-level signals to the movements they presumably are causing. While a top-down approach is useful in some cases, beginning at the top in spinal motor control, where signal coding is in its most complex form, it has not been very instructive in understanding movement control. The bottom-up approach, possible in the oculomotor system, has paid off in providing us glimpses, however dim, of how premotor circuits generate eye movements.

As a result, oculomotor physiologists have a good deal more data about premotor signals than do spinal cord physiologists. The key, however, to advancements in the oculomotor system is that the many simplifying features of eye movements make these data more interpretable. As described below, these features allow the discharge rates of premotor neurons to be related to external variables such as eye and head movement, permitting easy interpretation of the role played in signal processing. Yet it is these simplifying features themselves that are worrisome. Do they make the oculomotor system so different from other motor systems that what is learned about the one has no bearing on the others? I shall argue that this is the case if one wishes to study all the load and disturbance compensation systems attendant on limb control since the eye does not need such systems, but at a higher level in the planning and strategies of movement control there is no reason to suppose that the oculomotor system is qualitatively different. It is just simpler. The oculomotor system is a cartoon of motor control in the sense that a cartoon extracts the essence of a picture in just a few lines, avoiding unessential detail. In this regard, oculomotor studies may be expected to contribute to the understanding of motor control in general.

Features special to the oculomotor system

Points well accepted in oculomotor physiology will not be belabored by references. Such references may be found in reviews such as Robinson (1981).

Dimensionality

For all practical purposes the eyeball rotates

around its center, so there is only one joint. This is an obvious and enormous simplification compared to multi-articulated limbs and helps considerably in simplifying the relation between eye position and motoneuron activity. One should, however, not fail to appreciate that the eye moves in three dimensions, and while recent findings suggest that the coordinates of the semicircular canals are important in the vestibulo-ocular reflex (Simpson et al., 1981), the situation is far more complex for saccades, and, like motor physiologists in general, we have essentially no understanding of how sensory and motor maps are translated into movement specifications and what coordinate systems are used.

Geometry

The muscles wrap around the eyeball so that the moment arm for the muscle's force remains constant (the globe radius) as the eye moves, thus eliminating one of the greatest sources of nonlinearity in limb muscles. The muscles are straight and parallel-fibered. The contribution of each motor unit adds directly to the torque on the eye.

Motoneurons and stretch reflexes

Reciprocal innervation is always obeyed. Co-contraction is never observed. There is no stretch reflex, although there are lots of spindles and tendon organs. Lack of these reflexes is no surprise since the mechanics of the load does not change and external forces are not anticipated. Consequently, it is even possible to relate the discharge rate, R_m, of a motoneuron to eye position, E (in, say, the horizontal plane), in the monkey, by a mathematical equation,

$$R_m = R_0 + kE + r\dot{E} = 100 + 4E + \dot{E} \quad (1)$$

where k and r reflect elastic and viscous mechanical properties of the muscles and orbital tissues and R_0 is the background rate, in spikes/sec, for fixation straight ahead. The numerical values describe the typical motoneuron. There are cases, such as saccades, where this equation is only approximated, but the main point is that such an equation can be written at all. It clearly cannot in the spinal cord, where load changes, external forces and co-contractions are the rule, not the exception.

It is here one worries about the cartoon label. The control of skeletal muscle carries with it an array of reflexes designed to compensate for these external changes and to see the movement through to completion, or quickly substitute an alternate way to achieve the goal. The oculomotor system has none of this; one must go elsewhere to study such things. On the other hand, one can turn this problem into a virtue and study signal command generation in a system uncluttered by all these compensatory reflexes. Further, many rapid limb movements are made with a fixed load, often zero, in an open-loop fashion — errors are corrected after, not during, the movement — and therefore are similar in strategy to eye movements. Thus, we can utilize the cartoon feature to penetrate into command generation in systems with strategies common to all motor control.

Separability and simplicity of function

If one tries to determine what some cell is doing in controlling a movement it is an enormous advantage to know that it belongs to a subsystem with a simple, known function. The oculomotor system can be broken down into five major subsystems: saccadic, pursuit, vergence, optokinetic, and the vestibulo-ocular reflex (VOR). The functions of these systems are well recognized (see, e.g., Robinson, 1981) and are very easy to understand and describe mathematically. The ability to understand the discharge rates of neurons in this context is, oddly, appreciated by few oculomotor neurophysiologists. Without it, the behavior of central oculomotor neurons would be as incomprehensible as is the behavior of other intracranial neurons in spinal motor control.

Let one example suffice. The VOR is formed around a skeletal three-neuron arc: the first is the primary vestibular afferent that supplies the signal from the semicircular canals,

$$R_{vl} = 90 - 0.4\dot{H} \qquad (2)$$

where $\dot{H}$ is head angular velocity and the resting discharge rate is 90 spikes/sec. This signal, carried by the typical afferent, obviously reports head velocity to the brain stem. The last neuron in the three-neuron arc is the motoneuron obeying Eqn. 1. The task of understanding the VOR is that of understanding how neurons convert the signal in Eqn. 2 to that of Eqn. 1. The signal, R_2, carried by the middle neuron is obviously informative. In a trained monkey, one can hold some variables constant while varying others, and consequently find

$$R_2 = 115 + 2.4E + 0.4\dot{E}_p - 1.1\dot{H} - |\dot{E}_r|. \qquad (3)$$

When the monkey fixates straight ahead, the neuron fires at 115 spikes/sec but changes by $2.4E$ when it fixates in one direction or the other by the angle E. In addition, it modulates by $0.4\dot{E}_p$ spikes/sec during pursuit movements at velocity $\dot{E}_p$ °/sec. The signal $-1.1\dot{H}$ is relayed from the canals (Eqn. 2) to the motoneurons (Eqn. 1), where it becomes the term $\dot{E}$, since the purpose of the VOR is to make $\dot{E}$ equal to $-\dot{H}$. The term $-|\dot{E}_r|$ indicates that during rapid eye movements, when eye velocity, $\dot{E}_r$, is large, in any direction (absolute value sign), the neuron is completely inhibited (minus sign) and stops firing.

It is not our purpose here to speculate on how and why the signal transformation from Eqns. 2 to 3 to 1 occurs in this curious fashion. For such speculation see Pola and Robinson (1978). What is important is that one can write such an equation as Eqn. 3 at all. It is made possible because there are only a few types of eye movements, they can be isolated from each other, each performs a simple function in a stereotyped way, so the signals on premotor neurons can easily be related to physical sensory and motor variables. Nothing comparable comes to mind in spinal cord neurophysiology, although one should add parenthetically that no one has looked.

The activity of many other oculomotor cell types in the brain stem has been analyzed in the fashion of Eqn. 3 (see e.g., Tomlinson and Robinson, 1984) and it is not unreasonable to think that with more data, especially anatomical, we will soon "finish" the VOR; that is, understand, at least in broad outlines, how its task is accomplished by neural networks — an idea heretical to most of motor control. Again, the spectre of the cartoon appears, even in the area of the generation of movement commands, and for the VOR there may be little defense because the sensory drive from the canals is remarkable among all sensory systems for the simplicity of its signal (Eqn. 2). This is not the case, however, for visuomotor systems, where problems arise of sensory maps, motor maps, spatial-temporal transformations, coordinate transformations; problems common to all of motor control. In these areas the oculomotor system is a cartoon only in the sense that we may be able to take advantage of the simplifying features to penetrate deeper than others into fundamental problems of motor control.

Areas common to eye and limb control

Plasticity

Intense research into parametric adaptive control, also called plasticity or motor learning, began when Gonshor and Melvill Jones (1971, 1976) first demonstrated plasticity in the VOR. Since then, it has been demonstrated in the saccadic system, vergence-accommodation system, in several other forms in the VOR (reviewed by Robinson and Optican, 1981) and, more recently, in the pursuit system (Optican et al., 1982). It is thus ubiquitous in the oculomotor system and, since its function is to maintain calibration of movement parameters and thereby eliminate dysmetria, no one supposes that such control is not common to all motor systems.

While it has been shown that the olivary — climbing fiber — Purkinje cell pathway is essential in most forms of plasticity (Ito, 1982) there is still debate on whether the modifiable synapses that presumably mediate it reside in the cerebellum. This issue is so well known that it is unnecessary to review it here. It is, however, important to point out that what we learn about it in the oculomotor system will very probably be directly applicable to spinal motor control. Again, the oculomotor system is a cartoon in the best sense. The VOR, for example, is so simple that it will be very odd if, in the near future, we do not locate the modifiable synapses, and thus lead the way in motor plasticity in general.

Position vs. change of position

A curious story is emerging in oculomotor physiology: the signals that emerge from central systems to premotor circuits are coded as eye velocity commands. In the VOR, for example, the signal $-\dot{H}$ (Eqns. 2, 3) is an eye velocity command, $\dot{E}$. Eqns. 1 and 3 show that an eye position signal, E, is required so it is necessary to propose some circuit that can produce E, given $\dot{E}$. Mathematically, this is called integration so this circuit is called a neural integrator (Robinson, 1968). Models of how this is done have been proposed (Cannon et al., 1983) but the point here is that however it is done, it is done.

For the saccadic system, the command emerges from central processing on so-called medium-lead burst neurons. Their discharge rate is roughly proportional to saccadic eye velocity. This signal too must be integrated and a combination of a position and velocity command sent to the motoneurons (Eqn. 1). Practical and theoretical reasons demand that the same integrator integrate both vestibular and saccadic velocity signals (Robinson, 1975). A class of Purkinje cells, called gaze-velocity Purkinje cells, in the flocculus code the pursuit velocity commands. These signals are believed to be relayed to the motoneurons via the y group of the vestibular nuclei. Thus, we have three major oculomotor systems sharing a common premotor circuit driven entirely by velocity commands. This is shown in Fig. 1.

What about the spinal cord? We know that in many tasks the motoneuron must carry a limb-position signal. It must, then, also appear on premotor neurons, but there have been too few recordings to be able to say much about this. At higher levels, in the cranial vault where one can record, one seldom finds signals that tonically report limb position, muscle length or joint angle. Most signals reflect only a change in these variables. Are the signals for a change (phasic) transformed into the signal to be changed (tonic) somewhere in the cord near the motoneurons? In the oculomotor system we see the same thing. The eye-position signal is seen profusely in the vestibular and prepositus hypoglossal nuclei, both within dendritic reach of the motoneurons, but seldom further away. It is not usually seen on Purkinje cells, it is seen weakly in the thalamus, it is not seen in the basal ganglia, superior colliculi or any region of cerebral cortex. Signals representing changes in eye position abound in these areas. Unfortunately, we will not know if Fig. 1 is an arrangement unique to eye movements until we have recordings from premotor circuits in the spinal cord.

Strategies in rapid visuomotor systems

The smooth pursuit system offers a good cartoon of one type of motor control. An instructive car-

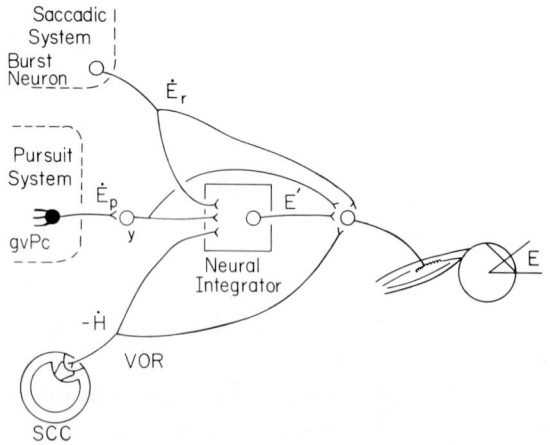

Fig. 1. Final motor signal processing begins with an eye velocity command $-\dot{H}$, $\dot{E}_p$, and $\dot{E}_r$ on afferents from the semicircular canals (SCC), gaze-velocity Purkinje cells (gvPc) and burst neurons, respectively, for the VOR, pursuit and saccadic systems, respectively. All are integrated to produce a common eye position command, E'. This is a schematic to show the flow of signals, not necessarily the actual connections of neurons.

A

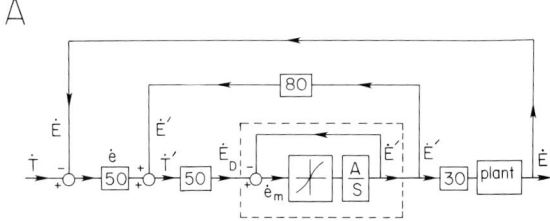

B

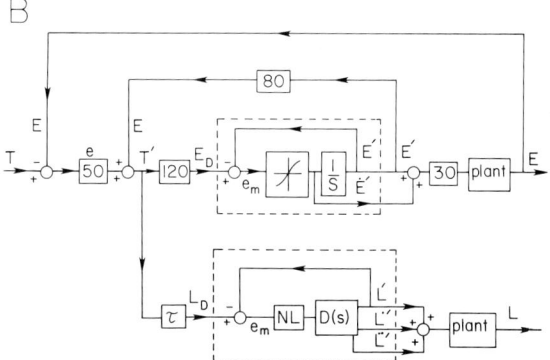

Fig. 2. Current hypotheses for central control of smooth pursuit (A), saccades (B, upper part), and rapid limb movements (B, lower). The first major strategy is to cancel the unavoidable negative feedback (of E, $\dot{E}$) by a positive feedback (of E', $\dot{E}'$). The second is to then construct an inner negative feedback loop (within dashed lines) to drive the plant variable to its desired position or velocity. T, target position; E, eye position; e, retinal error; T', central representation of T; E_D, desired eye position; e_m, motor error; E', eye position command. In A all variables are velocities rather than positions. Delays, in mseconds, are shown in boxes. L_D, desired limb position; L, physical limb position; L', $\dot{L}'$, $\ddot{L}'$, internal commands of L and its derivatives; NL, nonlinearities; $1/s$, an integrator; A, a gain; $D(s)$, a network to produce motor commands appropriate to the plant and load.

toon, because its simplicities allow one to think about central strategies and even model them. This system tries to match eye velocity to target velocity. The retina measures the difference, retinal image velocity, and sends a signal for the eye to go fast enough to reduce this error to an acceptably small value. It is thus a velocity tracking system with unity negative feedback. If A is the forward amplification factor from retina to muscles, the closed-loop, steady-state gain will be $A/(1 + A)$. Since subjects track at about 90% of target velocity, A must be 9. Dynamic behavior suggests the presence of a lag with a time constant of 400 mseconds and a pure delay, or latency, of 130 mseconds. We can now indulge in a pleasure usually denied those working in limb control: because this seems to be a pretty simple, linear system, we can simulate our model on a computer. It will surprise few to learn that this model is unstable and oscillates. Feedback loops with high gains and fast response times cannot tolerate large delays. The simulation allows us to reject this simple model.

L. R. Young, in 1968, offered a bold solution to this dilemma: get rid of the negative feedback (Young et al., 1968; Young, 1971). You cannot do this literally, because the feedback is built-in (the retina moves with the eye) but you can cancel it by internal positive feedback, as shown in Fig. 2A. This pathway is an efference copy of the eye-velocity command ($\dot{E}'$, Fig. 2A) that, added to retinal slip velocity $\dot{e}$, creates a central copy of target velocity, $\dot{T}'$. This is very effective. The system is now stable and accurate regardless of the delay. Unfortunately, the positive loop cannot encompass all of the troublesome delays, specifically 50 mseconds in the retina and 30 mseconds in the motor periphery. For stability, it is important that the delays around the negative and positive loops be equal and an 80-msecond delay in the latter accomplishes this. Put another way, it is important that reafference ($\dot{e}$) and efference copy ($\dot{E}'$) be added in the same time frame. With this addition, the system behaves as if there were no feedback at all. It is completely stable.

The use of this strategy seems compelling in the case of pursuit simply because it is very difficult to think of another way out of the dilemma of stability. Sampling is not a solution since it has been shown that the pursuit system is continuous, not sampled. Any alternate scheme is bound to get more complicated and awkward. Moreover, efference copy is a well-accepted concept supported by a variety of circumstantial evidence. The problem created by delays is not unique to pursuit. The problem may be put another way: the pursuit response only takes about 130 mseconds; the system certainly cannot rely for guidance on visual feedback that itself takes 130 mseconds. Many rapid limb movements are similar; their response time is comparable to the visual reaction time and they too are made largely in an open-loop mode. They too do not have time to wait for visual feedback, and if they tried to, they also would become unstable. Since the problem is a general one, perhaps the solution is too.

Models of the saccadic system have been proposed that also utilize internal positive feedback (Van Gisbergen et al., 1981). A simplified version is shown in the upper part of Fig. 2B. It is remarkably similar to Fig. 2A, except that it deals with eye postion rather than eye velocity. An internal copy of eye position, $\dot{E}'$, is added to retinal error, e, to create a central copy of target position T'. One must hasten to point out fundamental differences. Vision is continuous during pursuit but is interrupted during every saccade. Because of this, vision begins more or less anew after each saccade and it apparently requires about 200 mseconds before visual analysis is sufficiently complete to warrant another saccade. Consequently, the saccadic system appears refractory for about 200 mseconds and this causes it to behave like a sampled-data system. That alone would prevent the saccadic system from oscillating because of delays and negative feedback, so one cannot argue, as in pursuit, that the saccadic system must use positive feedback to achieve stability. Nevertheless, a growing body of evidence indicates that the saccadic system cannot be driven by retinal error alone but rather by some internal representation of target position in space (Mays and Sparks, 1980a, b). Consequently, there are strong reasons to assume that two visuo-motor tracking systems have shed their negative feedback and in doing so create central representations of the positions and velocities of external objects.

There is another similarity in the models of Figs. 2A and B. After the creation of $\dot{T}'$ or T', the central nervous system decides on which target to follow, and to reconstruct T' from auditory clues or memory when appropriate. After this it declares a desired eye position, E_D, or velocity, $\dot{E}_D$. Then a system, enclosed in dashed lines, drives the actual eye variable to equal the desired eye variable. This can easily be done by a feedforward system, but both models employ a negative feedback scheme instead. In both cases, this is required by the major system nonlinearity. For pursuit this is an acceleration saturation (Lisberger et al., 1981). To get an acceleration signal one must subtract $\dot{E}'$ from $\dot{E}_D$ since this velocity difference is an acceleration command. It is called the motor error, $\dot{e}_m$. This accounts for the innermost negative feedback loop and a saturation element within this loop accounts nicely for observed behavior (unpublished observations by the author). Similarly, the major nonlinearity in saccades is a velocity saturation. To get a velocity signal one can subtract E' from E_D, since a desired change in position constitutes a velocity command. The difference is the motor error e_m and a saturation element operating on it accounts for the well-known, velocity-amplitude nonlinearity of saccades.

Thus, in two visuo-oculomotor systems, attempts to deal with system non-linearities suggest the idea that after the built-in, outer negative feedback has been removed by positive feedback, the main business of executing the movement is done by negative feedback. Instability need no longer be an issue here since delays within the innermost loop are probably small compared to its response times. Perhaps other motor systems, in a similar way, can utilize the benefits of negative feedback without fear of oscillations.

An example for a limb movement is shown in the lower part of Fig. 2B. The visuo-oculomotor system, in the upper part, has already determined target position T'. If a limb movement is to be made to this target, T' becomes desired limb position, L_D, after a decision-making delay, τ, specific to each system. Note that T' and L_D are independent of subsequent eye movements, since any change in E is cancelled by the negative and positive feedback paths. A premotor circuit now quickly tries to make an internal copy, L', of limb position, L, match L_D. In accordance with the example set by the two oculomotor systems, it is suggested that this might be done by negative feedback.

This idea is hardly novel. It is of the genre of

hypotheses that movements are driven to a specified end goal. It does not state, however, that only final-position information is sent to the muscles. Obviously this circuit will attempt to compensate for the mechanical impedance of the load and will deliver to the motoneurons a signal that is a mixture of desired position, velocity, acceleration, etc., to deal with load elasticities, viscosities, inertia, etc. Fig. 1 shows that only the first two of these is required for the eye; the situation will usually be more complex in the spinal cord. The use of negative feedback allows initial position to be taken into account; the signals, forces, durations, velocities, etc., will be quite different for the same final position, depending on initial limb position. Note that none of these systems makes ballistic or preprogrammed movements. It is now known that even saccades can be altered in mid-flight. The smooth pursuit system has no refractory period, the saccadic system usually exhibits refractoriness. For limb control this will depend on the particular system and its task.

These considerations suggest that eye and limb movements share many problems in common. These problems concern the coding of sensory information, its transformation into motor objectives and the transformation into the final motor commands. If the oculomotor system is a cartoon, it is so in a good sense. Because of its simplifying features it may allow us to penetrate deeper and more quickly into the problems of central planning and execution of movement in general.

References

Cannon, S. C., Robinson, D. A. and Shamma, S. (1983) A proposed neural network for the integrator of the oculomotor system. Biol. Cybern., 49: 127–136.

Gonshor, A. and Melvill Jones, G. (1971) Plasticity in the adult human vestibulo-ocular reflex arc. Proc. Can. Fed. Biol. Soc., 14: 11.

Gonshor, A. and Melvill Jones, G. (1976) Extreme vestibulo-ocular adaptation induced by prolonged optical reversal of vision. J. Physiol., 256: 381–414.

Ito, M. (1982) Cerebellar control of the vestibulo-ocular reflex — around the flocculus hypothesis. Annu. Rev. Neurosci., 5: 275–296.

Lisberger, S. G., Evinger, C., Johanson, G. W. and Fuchs, A. F. (1981) Relationship between eye acceleration and retinal image velocity during foveal smooth pursuit in man and monkey. J. Neurophysiol., 46: 229–249.

Mays, L. E. and Sparks, D. L. (1980a) Dissociation of visual and saccade-related responses in superior colliculus neurons. J. Neurophysiol., 43: 207–232.

Mays, L. E. and Sparks, D. L. (1980b) Saccades are spatially, not retinocentrically coded. Science, 208: 1163–1165.

Optican, L. M., Chu, F. C., Hays, A. V., Reingold, D. B. and Zee, D. S. (1982) Adaptive changes of oculomotor performance in abducens nerve palsy. Soc. Neurosci. Abstr., 8: 418.

Pola, J. and Robinson, D. A. (1978) Oculomotor signals in the medial longitudinal fasciculus of the monkey. J. Neurophysiol., 41: 245–259.

Robinson, D. A. (1968) Eye movement control in primates. Science, 161: 1219–1224.

Robinson, D. A. (1975) Oculomotor control signals. In P. Bach-y-Rita and G. Lennerstrand (Eds.), Basic Mechanisms of Ocular Motility and Their Clinical Implications, Vol. 24, Pergamon Press, Oxford, pp. 337–374.

Robinson, D. A. (1981) Control of eye movements, In V. B. Brooks (Ed.), Handbook of Physiology, Vol. II, Part 2, The Nervous System, Williams & Wilkins, Baltimore, pp. 1275–1320.

Robinson, D. A. and Optican, L. M. (1981) Adaptive plasticity in the oculomotor system. In H. Flohr and W. Precht (Eds.), Lesion-induced Neuronal Plasticity in Sensorimotor Systems, Springer, Berlin, pp. 295–304.

Simpson, J. I., Graf, W. and Leonard, C. S. (1981) The coordinate system of visual climbing fibers to the flocculus. In A. F. Fuchs and W. Becker (Eds.), Progress in Oculomotor Research, Elsevier, New York, pp. 475–484.

Tomlinson, R. D. and Robinson, D. A. (1984) Signals in vestibular nucleus mediating vertical eye movements in the monkey. J. Neurophysiol., 51: 1121–1136.

Van Gisbergen, J. A. M., Robinson, D. A. and Gielen, S. (1981) A quantitative analysis of the generation of saccadic eye movements by burst neurons. J. Neurophysiol., 45: 417–442.

Young, L. R. (1971) Pursuit eye tracking movements. In P. Bach-y-Rita, C. C. Collins and J. E. Hyde (Eds.), Control of Eye Movements, Academic Press, New York, pp. 429–443.

Young, L. R., Forster, J. D. and Van Houtte, N. (1968) A revised stochastic sampled data model for eye tracking movements. Fourth Annual NASA-University Conference on Manual Control, University of Michigan, Ann Arbor, MI.

Some concluding remarks about general concepts in studies of the skeletomotor system

Mario Wiesendanger

Institut de Physiologie, Université de Fribourg, Pérolles, CH-1700 Fribourg, Switzerland

A "bottom-up" or a "top-down" approach?

The main idea of this meeting was to solicit interaction between those engaged in oculomotor research and those studying the skeletomotor system. It would be easy to point at principal differences between the two systems, but we were reminded by the organizers rather to look for common principles of organization. It is in this vein that Robinson* (cf. preceding paper) pleaded for the use of strategies which were so successful in oculomotor research and which should also be followed by those interested in the skeletomotor system, provided of course that the object of the study is not the mechanics of load. Robinson ventures the prediction that in a few years' time, a formal description of the neuronal machinery at the premotor level will be available. Although it is conceded that progress in understanding the operation of the brainstem structures has been remarkable, doubts may be raised as to the contribution this work is supposed to bring in solving some of the fundamental problems of purposive motor control. The issue which was discussed by Robinson is an old problem of research strategy: it is the question about the "bottom-up" or the "top-down" approach. It may be appropriate to echo the remarks of Teuber (1974) at a motor control conference which were in response to a similar plea made at that time by Robinson: "The issue raised by David Robinson is surely fascinating; we would probably divide the audience into those who prefer working from the ground up... and those who would rather work from the top down; and some of us, perhaps most of us, really believe one has to do both. I, for one, have always felt that we must keep the highest achievements of motor organization before us — such as speech — if we want to come to terms, properly, with more elementary ones. Besides, complexity and simplicity are relative affairs". To that I may add a further relevant citation from a recent book by Evarts et al. (1984): "Some neurophysiologists assert the importance of a detailed, if not complete, understanding of the neuromuscular synapse and the mechanics of muscle fibers before setting out on a more general study of behavior control. Others argue that before any understanding of supraspinal control of behavior is possible, the spinal and muscular systems must be thoroughly understood at a level far in advance of that currently available. And still others maintain that study of the cortex is unlikely to yield significant results until subcortical mechanisms are known with mathematical precision. We propose to attack the question in a different way. We would like to step back from the actual mechanisms involved in executing motor commands and from the various servomechanisms or obligatory reflexive mechanisms which operate the motor apparatus. We intend largely to ignore the mechanisms of movement execution and hope to gain a better understanding of higher brain function. Our approach is to "work backwards", to start from the

---
* Asterisks indicate authors contributing to this volume.

behavior, specifically its motor aspects, and to look for the influences that act to select one of the several potential behavioral patterns that could occur under any given circumstance. In order to pursue such an objective, we feel that it is unnecessary to have a complete understanding of precisely how the motor apparatus interacts with neural commands to produce a movement. Rather, an empirical recognition, not understanding, of these distinct signals may be all that is required. It is our contention, then, that the study of brain circuits which lie at the basis of higher brain function is possible without a complete analysis of the "lower" functions". What the meeting brought out so clearly is that there are many different levels of endeavor and understanding. My point is that each level has its own justification, provided that we do not lose sight of what I consider as the major issue of motricity: to seek the purposefulness in motor behavior with its concomitant stabilization of the body and of perception. In other words, even with a "bottom-up" approach, the elemental functions must be evaluated on the background of purpose (cf. also Granit, 1977).

Levels of inquiry

The necessity to have a better understanding of the mechanics of the motor apparatus, if one is dealing with control problems, was repeatedly advocated at the meeting (e.g. Noth*, Loeb*). As pointed out by Matthews*, the central nervous system has to deal with a highly unlinear machinery. Some of the complex motor unit properties were highlighted by Kernell* at the beginning of the meeting. The non-linearities are also seen in the extraocular muscles and may even be used by the central structures to code gaze (Hepp*).

The main emphasis of the meeting, however, was clearly on the central motor structures. A new dimension at structural-functional level which has become apparent in recent years, and which was discussed by Kuypers*, is the very rich "innervation" of the spinal cord by noradrenergic and serotoninergic descending pathways whose role is still a matter of speculation. It is possible that they play a role in the autonomic control; however, there is also evidence that activation of these fiber systems may drastically change spinal reflexes. Hultborn* and colleagues discovered that the serotoninergic system may be capable of "switching on" a plateau potential of motoneurones which in turn is responsible for a long-lasting stretch response. This is a rather remarkable example of a specific modulatory action of such a seemingly "diffuse" descending system.

Impressive is the degree of spatial segregation of functionally distinct subsets of neurones in the brainstem oculomotor centers, a situation which presumably is unparalleled in the somatic-motor system. I will only mention, as an example, the observations that microstimulation of successively deeper bands of the superior colliculus elicited horizontal saccades of progressively larger amplitudes, as reported by Cohen*.

Another level of inquiry which was much in the foreground of this meeting dealt with the recording from single units in the awake performing animal. Does the cell discharge reflect some sort of parameter control (such as force) or a more "holistic" aspect (such as movement trajectory)? Interpretations for the skeletomotor system are fraught with uncertainties about all possible transformations of the signals which are likely to occur in the spinal circuitry. Furthermore, co-variation does not imply causality. The method of spike-triggered averaging was put to excellent use by Fetz* and Cheney by recording the activity of single units in the motor cortex and of various limb muscles. The case of causality is much stronger when facilitatory and inhibitory effects are correlated with the occurrence of spike discharges. It is surprising that this method has hardly been exploited in the oculomotor system.

One point which has been made clear in recent years (mainly by the work of Evarts et al. (1984)) in that neuronal activity of the motor cortex does not only reflect a central command; instead, the neurones can be seen as summing points of central and peripheral signals. Once more, the problem was discussed whether the motor cortex generates reflex-like responses to load perturbations. The results of Matthews* indicate that much of what has been interpreted as "transcortical reflexes" can equally likely be interpreted in terms of spinal mechanisms. His favored and new interpretation is that late muscle responses evoked by stretch may be generated by group II afferents. However, there are still strong arguments in favor of the transcortical hypothesis which therefore, in my opinion, should not be rejected. An alternative role for proprioceptive feedback signals might be their use by higher structures for adaptive changes of the central command (this may be particularly important in a predictive situation).

Another question addressed by many investigators is whether the timing of cell discharges can provide clues as to the hierarchic position of a given structure: a "ranking" of lead time in a reaction time situation may, so it is hoped, indicate for example whether the dentate nucleus is "up-stream" or "down-stream" to the motor cortex. This sort of reasoning is borne out by today's prevailing concept of a hierarchic organization (a concept which, however, has encountered some well-founded criticism, see, e.g., Kelso and Tuller, 1981). With respect to the structures which have been most intensively studied, namely, the motor cortex (Fetz*), the premotor areas (Wise*, Strick*), the basal ganglia (DeLong*) and the cerebellum (Thach*), one should not gloss over the anatomical fact that all these structures are reciprocally connected with the motor cortex. Thus, the premotor areas not only project to the motor cortex, but the latter also projects back to the premotor areas (and one could therefore equally well say that the premotor cortex is "down-stream" to the motor cortex!). With respect to the basal ganglia, DeLong's* investigations have focused mainly on the "motor loop" which takes its origin in the sensorimotor areas and projects, via the thalamus, to premotor areas and thence to the motor cortex. It is interesting that his data plead for a role of this subsystem in motor execution rather than in movement initiation and preparation (covariation of neurones with movement parameters, sensory responses to perturbations, microstimulation effects). According to the anatomical tracing studies by Schell and Strick*, which were also reported at the meeting, the output of the basal ganglia is mainly directed to the supplementary motor area (SMA). Whether the "association loop" of DeLong* feeds back to the prefrontal cortex remains to be investigated in detail. It can generally be said that not much is known as yet about the "association loop", and therefore any generalization about basal ganglia function is premature.

New aspects on the function of the premotor cortex were presented by Wise*. Many cells appear to be "set-related", which became evident when the preparatory period before movement execution was manipulated. Such neurones are not unique in the premotor cortex, but were previously found in abundance also in prefrontal areas, in the SMA and, to a much smaller extent, even in the pre- and postcentral cortices. These single unit studies in monkeys and the electromyographic investigations in human subjects led Evarts et al. (1984) to formulate a general hypothesis about the central role of the cerebral cortex in motor behavior, namely to add flexibility in motor behavior. In contrast to "lower" organisms without cerebral cortex for which motor behavior is strongly coupled with sensory stimuli, the motor behavior in mammals becomes less stimulus-bound, in a machine-like fashion, to sensory events; an external stimulus may or may not generate motor output, and if it occurs it may be expressed in different ways which depend on the purposive context. In an experimental situation, this means that motor output is linked more to the instruction signal than to the trigger signal.

Are there common features among neurones of the cerebral cortex devoted to limb movements and to ocular movements, respectively? The reader may find that some properties of neurones in the frontal eye field (studied by Goldberg*) are strikingly similar to some of the premotor cortex and of the supplementary motor area. A clear behavioral contingency of cell discharges was also found in neurones of pars reticulata of substantia nigra (Wurtz*).

What are the cellular correlates of motor learning? This is an interesting new field which, for obvious reasons, however, is difficult to study at the single unit level. In his introductory talk, Eccles reviewed the current ideas about "cerebellar" and "cerebral cortical" learning. He mentioned especially the series of studies by Sasaki et al. (1981). The results were obtained with indwelling macroelectrodes which allow one to follow the development of slow pre-movement potentials over weeks while the animals learn a motor task. Striking increases of potential amplitudes are seen in some but not all cortical areas, changes which parallel the proficiency with which the motor task is effected.

Circumscribed lesions in neurological patients and in experimental animals may still provide useful insights about the possible function of a given structure, and this was again demonstrated at this conference. Most importantly, it is now possible to assess the extent of a lesion in patients during life with a precision never achieved previously. Also, the technical means to test motor performance have much improved, and there can be no doubt that the neurological assessment of motor functions can be placed at a high level of precision and quantification. In experimental animals, reversible lesions are of particular value, as exemplified by the series of investigations by Hore and Vilis*. A fascinating new approach discussed by Wurtz* is to manipulate reversibly a particular transmitter system by local injections of an agonist (e.g. Muscimol) or its antagonist (e.g. Bicucullin).

The quantitative assessment of motor deficits is also an important prerequisite for studies of recovery of function after acute lesions. Precht* discussed the vestibular lesion as a useful paradigm for the study of brain plasticity, a field of research so important for clinical neurology, but also a field which is still full of unsolved questions.

Motor psychophysics and the integration of synergies

The understanding of motor performance ultimately depends on our understanding of the integrative processes involved in the coupling of elemental movements and of posture into a unitary, purposeful motor act. Sherrington, W. R. Hess, Bernstein and others, by virtue of their intuition, imagination, observations and of their theoretical acumen, prepared the ground for a most productive new area of research. The reader may find it useful to consult re-editions of selected works of Bernstein (editor: Whiting, 1984) and of W. R. Hess (editor: Akert, 1981). The conceptual tradition of Bernstein was followed in more recent years by Gurfinkel and his colleagues at the Institute for Information Transmission Problems in Moscow and in several laboratories in the United States and in Europe.

One major issue in the field of what one might call "motor psychophysics" is to find out the rules which govern movement trajectories as they are performed in our daily habits. Of particular interest is the temporal sequence of activation of the various muscles and of the kinematic variables. It turns out that many movements have invariant properties. Thus, hand-writing is executed with an invariant temporal structure, i.e., independent of whether writing is done on a small piece of paper or in large letters on the blackboard. The existence of an "isochrony principle" is also evident in the bell-shaped isometric contractions which are performed in the same amount of time irrespective of the peak tension (Freund*). Two further invariant properties were discussed by Bizzi* which are not trivial and remarkable from the viewpoint of coordination: trajectories of the hand from any point to any other point are always straight lines and the velocity profiles are always bell-shaped, as also demonstrated in the grasping movements described by Jeannerod*.

If we consider again the main general principle of motor behavior — the purposeful orientation of body parts in space and the stabilization of the body and of perception — we realize that coordination of many muscle groups, i.e., the integration of synergies, becomes the key issue in understanding "higher" motor control. Consider the "orientation reaction" of a cat in response to a sudden noise, or the visually guided reaching movement of a human subject: trunk, head and eye movements are finely tuned (the "kinetic melody") and matched with postural stabilization; in the case of reaching, the hand is smoothly shaped in advance and in perfect accord with the object which will be grasped (Jeannerod*). Where are the coordinating structures? Are there neuronal ensembles which encode "higher-order" commands? Berthoz* and Schlag* indeed presented evidence for the existence of "gaze units". The synchronous activation of eye and neck muscles even suggests the existence of coupling neurones for oculomotor and somatic activity. Fascinating was the electrophysiological and anatomical demonstration of brainstem ("reticular") neurones impinging on many oculomotor as well as somatic-motor centers (Berthoz*). Perhaps the most intriguing aspect of this coordination is the evidence that the coupling is not obligatory (via "hard-wired" circuits), but on the contrary subject to profound modulation. In other words, the degree of coupling adapts to the needs, and in this respect, the situation is reminiscent of the plasticity of the vestibulo-oculor reflex (Miles*). Nashner* and his colleagues have focused their elegant studies on the plasticity of postural synergies, once more a nice demonstration of the adaptive properties of coupling acccording to the intention of the motor task. It is evident that the study of neuronal mechanisms involved in the coupling of synergies is a challenge to those engaged in oculomotor as well as in somatic-motor research.

In closing, we may ask ourselves whether or not we succeeded in fostering, in the framework of such an interdisciplinary conference on motor control, the identification of common fundamental problems and concepts which may be attacked with similar research strategies. An answer, at this point, is perhaps premature. However, the published accounts of the conference may hopefully help the reader to think further about the ambition which guided the organization of the conference. There can be no doubt that the conference was a unique opportunity for us to be exposed to so many different strategies and technical approaches. The future will show which avenues will lead to success!

References

Akert, K. (Ed.) (1981) Biological Order and Brain Organization. Selected Works of W. R. Hess, Springer, Berlin.

Evarts, E. V., Shinoda, Y. and Wise, S. P. (1984) Neurophysiological Approaches to Higher Brain Functions, John Wiley, New York.

Granit, R. (1977) The Purposive Brain, MIT Press, Cambridge.

Kelso, J. A. S. and Tuller, B. (1981) Towards a theory of apractic syndromes. Brain Lang., 12: 224–245.

Sasaki, K., Gemba, H. and Hashimoto, S. (1981) Premovement slow cortical potentials on self paced eye movements and thalamocortical and corticocortical responses in the monkey. Exp. Neurol., 72: 41–50.

Teuber, H. L. (1974) Concluding session: panel discussion on key problems in the programming of movements. Brain Res., 71: 541.

Whiting, W. T. A. (Ed.) (1984) Human Motor Actions. Bernstein Reassessed, North-Holland, Amsterdam.

Final discussion

B. Cohen

Mount Sinai School of Medicine of the City University of New York, New York, NY 10029, U.S.A.

Kuypers noted that only visual and vestibular influences had been described for eye movements. He asked if, by comparison with the skeletalmotor system, oculomotor control was really so simple. Limb movements under visual control, for example, are influenced by the vestibular system, and show, at the final level, multisensory convergence from low- and high-pressure muscle afferents, muscle spindles, joint and tendon organs and cutaneous afferents. Is it possible, he asked, that spindle afferents from extrocular muscles have a coordinating function for all extraocular muscles in sensing eye positions? He also suggested that spindles in the short neck muscles used in turning the head to shift gaze might have functions similar to those of to spindles in extraocular muscles.

Freund noted there was evidence for at least two systems for skeletal motor control, one for controlling the hand and another for controlling proximal musculature and posture, and that one could be extended to include oculomotor function. The oculomotor system, getting its cortical innervation from the premotor frontal cortex which sends projections to saccadic generators in the pons, appears to be closely related to the system that controls the proximal musculature. This could be important with respect to guiding both the hands and eyes to a common target. Such activity would be more important for the proximal muscles than the hand. The hand is a sense organ and, once being brought into contact with an object, can manipulate it and get feedback to operate independently. Vilis commented that saccades appeared to be spatially coded in central structures, whereas coding for limb movements has largely been described in terms of frequency. He asked whether this was real or apparent. A question was raised as to what the coding mechanism might be for various subsystems of the skeletalmotor system; specifically, is the activity for muscles coded in direction of movement?

The discussion then turned to comparative aspects of oculomotor and skeletalmotor control and to the relative understanding of each system. Matthews noted what he described as a tendency for oculomotor physiologists to turn away from the main stream of motor physiology and become too specialized, a theme echoed by Eccles. In attempting to attack the problem of oculomotor plasticity, for example, he felt that although many examples of plasticity had been described, no one seemed near to understanding how it is mediated. Robinson, who had originally challenged the skeletalmotor physiologists for not adopting a more theoretical approach to direct their research, countered that the bioengineering had forced oculomotor physiologists to view the system from a theoretical point of view, and that had been productive, since there is a strong possibility that in the next 10 years there will be a good outline of how the VOR works. He decried the tendency to assume that problems can never be solved, only studied. Loeb answered that the direction in which oculomotor physiology had gone, i.e., a compartmentalization of the oculomotor system into subsystems, and the responses of the system as an additive product of these subsystems, had been explored and proved unsucccessful in explaining or predicting skeletalmotor behavior. He found confirmation of this in Bizzi's experiments (section III) on robotics, artificial motion generation and control systems, which have not yielded to simple analysis. This may be because motor control is a distributed function that is not easily explainable by simple models. On the other hand, he noted that although analysis techniques are not now available for study of the skeletalmotor system, they are needed, because simplistic systems do not account for what has to be controlled.

Berthoz noted that there were a number of oculomotor problems that had not yielded to analysis, including the problem of the function of the vestibular efferents, the diversity among oculomotoneurons, how predictive control is established and how mental set influences control of the eyes. He cited the oculomotor-skeletal integration of champion skiers who do not actually look at the slope they are skiing, but rather appear to monitor a mental image of themselves going down such a slope. He noted that the problem of dynamic representation has been studied in motor control of the limbs, but has not been investigated for the eyes. He raised the possibility that efference copy may be a reflection of this process.

Fetz noted that although modelling of the oculomotor system seems quite advanced, a neural explanation of motor systems will involve more than block diagrams of lumped functions. The neural mechanisms generating motor behavior must eventually be understood in terms of interactions between identified cells. This requires quantitative analysis of the correlational linkages between functionally identified cell types, starting with the different types of premotor cells which directly affect motoneurons.

Cohen closed by noting that a close skeletalmotor analog of the oculomotor system might be found in the control of head and neck musculature during gaze shifts. It would be interesting to know if there were similar "saccadic" control for head movements during gaze shifts as for eye movements in the cerebral cortex. He also noted that many skeletalmotor systems had not been considered that had relatively constant loads and did not function across joints, such as facial, tongue and laryngeal muscles.

Subject Index

Abducens nucleus, 91, 232, 263, 314, 338
   abducens motoneurone, 329
   abducens nerve palsy, 375
   accessory abducens nucleus, 263
   internuclear neurones of the abducens nucleus, 263
   periabducens region, 331
Accommodation, 375
Accuracy, 353
Adaptation
   adaptive control, 70, 368, 386, 405, 413
   adaptive equalizer model, 369
   adaptive regulation, 374
   adaptive response, 4
   adaptive versatility, 367
Afterimage, 391
Alpha-gamma coactivation, 214
2-Amino-4-phosphonobutyric acid, 82
Anisometrope, 376
Area 6, 117
Association areas, 14, 164
Attention, 393
   spatially directed attention, 395
   visual attention, 393
Autonomic motor system, 94
Axon collaterals, 262

Balance control, 383
Ball-joint system, 31
Basal ganglia, 99, 161, 175, 188
   caudate nucleus, 161, 192
   cooling, 188
   globus pallidus, 104, 163, 188
   putamen, 161, 188
   somatotopic grouping, 164
   striatum, 161, 198
Bicuculline, 181
Biomechanics, 275
Body turning, 340

Calcium, 9, 45
Cartesian system, 37, 304

Central gray matter, 244
Central pattern generator, 277
Cerebellum, 99, 207, 225, 314, 369
   cerebellar disorder, 213, 281
   cerebellar nuclei, 209, 218
      dentate nucleus, 13, 104
      fastigial nucleus, 104
      interpositus, 104
   cerebellar-spindle axis, 222
   control of stability, 221
   cooling, 210
   flocculus, 226, 314, 369
   nodulus, 227
   paraflocculus, 227
   Purkinje cells, 220, 226
   uvula, 227
   vermis, 209, 227
Conjunction, 6, 15, 17
Contractile properties, 21
   adaptive range, 27
   usage, 27
Control theory, 221
Coordinates, 240
   Cartesian, 37, 304
   craniotopic, 309
   fovea-centered, 309
   head, 238, 321, 309
   motor, 240
   retinotopic, 331
   transformation, 413, 309
Coordination between segments, 359
Corollary discharge, 393
Corticofugal influence, 82
Corticothalamic projections, 198

Damping, 219
   elastic damping, 217
   viscous damping, 217
Deafferentation, 348
Direction selectivity, 79
Discharge properties, 22

burst-tonic discharge pattern, 134
  iso-frequency-curves, 35
  phasic-tonic discharge patterns, 133
  postspike facilitation, 135
Displacement, 345
Distributed function, 426
Dorsal root ganglia, 218
Dynamic complementarity, 326
Dynamic representation, 426
Dynamic substitution, 326
Dysmetria, 209, 210, 413
  dysmetria of the limbs, 210
  saccadic dysmetria, 209

Efference copy, 212, 246, 393, 402, 415
Energy, 341
  energetic efficiency, 275
Equilibrium position, 349
Esophoria, 376
Evolution, 111, 260
Eye, 184
  deviation, 184
  muscles, 260
  position, 134, 212, 237, 238, 248, 383
  retraction, 267
Eye-hand interaction, 291
Eye-head coordination, 325
Eye movements, 81, 89, 175
  amplitude, 248
  conjugate eye movements, 36, 91, 225, 248
  cyclotorsion, 32
  dump mechanism, 228
  horizontal eye movements, 304, 322
  immobilization, 399
  rapid eye movements, 243, 303
  saccadic eye movements, see Saccades
  smooth pursuit, 81, 89, 193, 282, 313, 394
  spontaneous eye movements, 179, 184
  velocity, 80, 228, 316
  velocity storage mechanism, 227
  vergence, 225
  vertical eye movements, 304

Finger grip, 357
Fixation, 155, 191, 193, 313
Force, 21, 136, 169, 209, 345
  length-dependence of muscle force, 350
  rate-gradation, 136
  recruitment gradation, 136
Frequency selectivity, 369
Frontal eye fields, 143, 175, 191, 198, 243, 283, 306
  anticipatory activity, 144, 148
  movement cells, 151
  movement fields, 151
  presaccadic neurons, 145
  retinotopic organization, 150
  visual cells, 145
Fusimotor system, 278

Gain control system, 386
Gaze, 184, 191
  gaze control, 198, 401
  gaze position, 195
  gaze shift, 34, 191
Golgi tendon organs, 69
Grasping, 359
Grip aperture, 357

Head, 195, 243, 246
  movements, 195, 243, 246
  posture, 382
  tilt, 382
Hierarchial organization, 269
Hippocampus, 16
  amygdala, 96
Homology, 262
Homoplasy, 262
Horseradish peroxidase (HRP), 251, 332

Ibotanic acid, 192
Inertia, 210
Inferior olive, 6, 254, 371
Internal parametric adjustment, 368
Ischemic conduction block, 297
Isochrony principle, 289

Joint, 345
  multi-joint movements, 345, 350
  single-joint movements, 345

Kainic acid, 251
Kinematics, 278, 356
Kinesthetic information, 278

Labyrinthectomy, 381
Limb, 219
  hindlimb, 274
  limb mechanics, 221
  oscillation, 208, 217
  stability of the limb, 219
Limbic structures, 96
  amygdala, 96
Load, 209
  torque load, 218
Localization of function, 113
Locomotion, 274
Loops, 46, 86, 163
  closed-loop, 71

cortico-subcortical loops, 163
feedback loop, 46, 71, 138, 213, 297
feedforward loop, 213
fusimotor-loop, 40
long-loop, 56, 86
loop gain, 374
open loop, 71
position feedback, 359
positive feedback, 415

Manipulation, 191
Microstimulation, 117, 165, 235, 247
  cerebellar, 212
  intracortical, 117, 137
Migraine phosphenes, 400
Modular organization, 368
Monoaminergic innervation, 46
Motility, 288
Motoneurone, 22
  alpha motoneurones, 214, 277
  bistable properties, 43, 45
  chronic stimulation, 27
  cortical access, 111
  gain-setting, 46
  gamma motoneurones, 214, 218
    dynamic, 278
    static, 278
  hysteresis, 32
  intraspinal site, 25
  membrane resistance, 26
  motor units, 133
  negative resistance, 45
  parasympathetic, 95
  plateau potentials, 42
  prolonged excitability increase, 40
  recruitment, 26, 257, 329
  self-sustained firing, 45
  size principle, 24, 257, 284
  sympathetic, 95
  task groups of motoneurones, 277
  types of motoneurones, 25
Motor control, 220, 279, 412
  adaptive motor control, 220
Motor cortex, 67, 105, 107, 218
  colony, 137
  columns, 166
  corticomotoneuronal (CM) cells, 112, 208
  intracortical microstimulation, 137
  primary motor cortex, 99, 117, 126
  synaptic connections, 138
Motor error, 235, 306
Motor learning, 3, 10, 153, 292, 369, 413
  adaptive, 9
Motor program, 153, 171, 319

Motor psychophysics, 422
Movement, 3, 166, 208
  acceleration, 208
  alternating, 218, 288
  amplitude, 161
  automatic, 3
  ballistic, 136, 222, 287, 353
  braking of, 208
  deceleration, 169, 208
  direction, 168
  field, 175, 235, 306
  fractionation, 111
  illusion, 397
  initiation, 159, 166, 176, 207
  involuntary, 169
  operantly conditioned, 10, 120
  parameters, 168
  preparation, 171
  ramp, 287
  serial, 288
  skilled, 292
  speed, 167
  symmetry, 208
  termination, 209
  timing, 167
  visually guided, 117
  voluntary, 170
Muscimol, 170, 181
Muscle, 21
  agonist, 208, 213
  antagonist, 134, 208, 213
  elastic behaviour, 341
  endurance, 21
  extraocular muscles, 55
  force, 21
  FR units, 22
  length, 218, 278
  lengthening, 277
  mechanical properties, 345
  multiarticular, 278
  pattern, 167
  recruitment-match, 22
  shortening, 277
  speed, 21
  speed-match, 22
  spring-like properties, 345
  S-units, 22
  visco-elastic properties, 297
Muscle spindles, 55, 56, 214, 217, 278, 297
  spindle afferent sensitivity, 219
Musculature
  axial musculature, 335
  distal musculature, 166
  postural musculature, 94
  proximal musculature, 166

Neck muscles, 94, 326
Neural integrator, 46, 414
Neurones, 134, 137
  corticomotoneuronal, 112, 135, 203
  eye-velocity, 316
  frontal eye field, 307, 309
  long-lead burst, 36
  medium-lead burst neurones, 36
  motoneurones, see Motoneurones
  neck motoneurones, 329
  oculomotor neurones, 203, 317
  omnipause, 306
  pause, 306
  phasic, 170
  premotor pursuit, 315
  pyramidal tract, 137
  rubromotoneuronal, 135
  tecto-reticulo-spinal, 326, 335
  thalamic eye position units, 195
  vestibular, 317
  vestibulo-spinal, 331
Nictitating membrane, 267
Nucleus
  interstitial nucleus of Cajal, 244
  nuclei of the accessory optic tract, 75
  nucleus cuneiformis, 244
  nucleus Kölliker-Fuxe, 95
  nucleus medialis dorsalis, 191
  nucleus of the optic tract, 75, 83
  nucleus prepositus hypoglossi, 339
  nucleus raphe magnus, 94
  nucleus raphe pallidus, 94
  nucleus reticularis gigantocellularis, 338
  nucleus reticularis pontis caudalis, 253, 333
  nucleus reticularis pontis oralis, 253
  nucleus subcoeruleus, 95
  nucleus subcuneiformis, 243
  nucleus ventralis lateralis pars medialis, 101
  nucleus ventralis lateralis pars oralis, 100
  nucleus ventralis posterior lateralis pars oralis, 102
  oculomotor nucleus, 91
  red nucleus, 244
  subthalamic nucleus, 167
Nystagmus, 212, 246, 248, 385
  gaze paretic nystagmus, 212
  optokinetic after-nystagmus, 229
  optokinetic nystagmus, 75, 89, 228, 331, 374
  Schau-Nystagmus, 313
  sigma-optokinetic nystagmus, 395
  spontaneous nystagmus, 385
  vestibular nystagmus, 228

Ocular flutter, 211
Oculo-collic coupling, 329

Orienting reactions, 325
  ipsiversive orienting synergy, 331
  visuo-motor orienting behavior, 335
Otoliths, 331

Pacinian receptors, 68
Parietal cortex, 127
  posterior parietal cortex, 198
Parkinson's disease, 169
Perception, 391
  visuo-movement perception, 393
Perturbations, 69, 139, 213
Phylogeny of the extraocular motor system, 260
Plasticity, 381, 413
Position, 218
  control, 348
  drift, 212
  error, 313
  eye position, 134, 212, 237, 238, 248, 383
  sense, 210
  wrist position, 218
Posture, 341
  hand posture, 341
  postural support, 208
Precision grip, 136
Prefrontal cortex, 11
Prehension, 358
Premotor cortex, 99, 106, 117, 126, 421
  anticipatory, 120
  directional specificity, 123
  movement-related cells, 117, 120
  set-related activity, 118, 120
  signal-related, 120
  visuospatial cues, 117
Pretectum, 75
Prisms, 376
Purposive motor behaviour, 420
Pyramidal tract, 111

Reaching, 158, 359
Reaction time, 123, 156, 159, 207
Readiness potential, 16
Reafference, 415
Reciprocal innervation, 412
Recovery, 381
Red nucleus, 244
Reflex, 3
  H-reflex, 69
  long-latency, 57, 295
  long-loop, 56
  middle-latency (M2) response, 67
  neck-ocular reflexes, 386
  short-latency, 59
  spinal autogenetic excitatory action, 65

spino-cerebello-spinal, 86
transcortical, 62, 67
Reticular formation, 89
  central tegmental tract, 253
  medial longitudinal fasciculus, 94, 304
  medial reticular formation, 91, 187, 253/254
  mesencephalic reticular formation, 243, 283
  nucleus cuneiformis, 244
  nucleus Kölliker-Fuse, 95
  nucleus raphe magnus, 94
  nucleus raphe pallidus, 94
  nucleus reticularis gigantocellularis, 338
  nucleus reticularis pontis caudalis, 253, 333
  nucleus reticularis pontis oralis, 253
  nucleus subcoeruleus, 95
  nucleus subcuneiformis, 243
  paramedian pontine reticular formation, 91, 187, 192, 304
  pontine reticular formation, 243
  reticulo-spinal neurones, 326, 331
  reticulospinal tract, 94, 112
  rubrospinal tract, 112
  ventral reticular formation, 95
Retina, 75
  retinal error, 158
  retinal slip, 77, 81, 228, 415
  retinal spatial values, 402
  retinotopic, 248
  W-cells, 78
  X-cells, 78
  Y-cells, 78
Reverberating activity, 39, 321
Robotics, 426

Saccades, 81, 89, 136, 143, 170, 175, 181, 208, 238, 303, 371
  accuracy, 182
  amplitude, 182
  contingent upon behavioral conditions, 186
  correction saccades, 158, 182, 358
  express saccades, 155
  irrepressible, 184
  latencies, 182
  learned saccades, 144
  peak velocity, 182
  post-saccadic recalibration, 399
  presaccadic activity, 143
  purposive, 143
  regular saccades, 156
  remembered targets, 176, 177
  saccade direction, 192
  saccadic system, 416
  self-initiated saccades, 199
  spontaneous, 143, 145, 246
  trajectory, 182
  visually guided, 143

visual targets, 182
Semicircular canals, 3
Sensory guidance, 292
Sensory motor integration, 71
Sensory motor interface, 235
Sensory motor modules, 326
Sensory substitution, 325
Servomechanism, 70, 213
Sigma movement, 395
Size principle, 24, 257, 284
Smooth pursuit system, 228, 414
Somatosensory responses, 166
  cutaneous receptive fields, 166
Space, 240
  auditory, 240
  visual, 151, 240
Spatio-temporal recording, 306
Spatio-temporal translation, 319, 413
Spectacles, 368, 375
Spike-triggered averaging, 138
Spinal cord in vitro preparation, 44
Spring system, 219
Stability, 221, 325, 415
  control of stability, 221
Stereovision, 397
Stiffness, 219, 298, 345
  stiffness tensor, 347
Stretch reflex, 40, 55, 64, 67, 85, 208, 219, 295
  group Ia afferents, 56
  group II afferents, 56
Substantia nigra, 104, 161, 176, 192
  multiple response relationship, 177
  pars reticulata, 163, 175
  tonic inhibition, 181
Subthalamic nucleus, 167
Superior colliculus, 75, 151, 192, 235, 243, 283, 306, 335
  antidromic stimulation, 180
  auditory signals, 238
  intermediate layer of SC, 251
  retinotopic spatial map, 187
  tectal stimulation, 340
  tecto-bulbo-spinal fibres, 247
  tecto-reticulo-spinal neurones, 326, 335
Supplementary motor area, 14, 16, 99, 117, 192

Target acquisition, 359
Tegmentum, 254
Temporal code, 31, 306
Thalamus, 99, 191
  area X, 101
  central thalamus, 191
  cerebello-thalamic projections, 104
  eye-position units, 194
  fixation units, 197

intralaminar nuclei, 161, 191
nigro-thalamic projections, 104
nucleus medialis dorsalis, 191
nucleus ventralis lateralis pars medialis, 100
nucleus ventralis lateralis pars oralis, 100
nucleus ventralis posterior lateralis pars oralis, 102
pallido-nigral termination, 102
pallido-thalamic projections, 104
thalamic internal medullary lamina, 191
ventrolateral thalamus, 102, 170
visual responses, 192
Time control, 287
Topographical map, 238
Torque, 133
ramp-and-hold torque, 133
Tracking, 217, 353
hand tracking, 217
oculomotor tracking, 291
ramp tracking, 218
visual tracking, 374
Trajectory, 31, 209, 214, 217, 238, 290, 303, 319, 349, 356
Transfer functions, 297
Transmitter, 8
aspartate, 8
GABA, 170, 176, 181, 185
glutamate, 8, 138
leucine, 94
Leu-enkephalin, 95
serotonin, 95
substance P, 95
transmitter-controlled bistability, 45
Tremor, 208, 217, 289, 300
intention tremor, 211

Velocity-to-position integrator, 304
Vergence, 375
accomodative vergence, 375
Vestibular, 3
lesion syndrome, 381
neurones, 317
nucleus, 3, 225, 386
primary vestibular afferents, 413
vestibular training, 386
vestibular-visual conflict, 386
vestibulo-collic reflex, 329
vestibulo-ocular reflex, 227, 313, 367, 412
vestibulo-spinal neurones, 331
Visual control, 358
Visual cortex, 75, 157
Visual field, 175
Visual neglect, 191
Visual receptive fields, 76, 143, 239
Visual scene, 374
Visual search, 153
Visuomotor systems, 413
Visuomotor tracking, 168

Wheatgerm agglutinin (WGA), 251